Lecture Notes in Business Information Processing

533

Series Editors

Wil van der Aalst ⓘ, *RWTH Aachen University, Aachen, Germany*
Sudha Ram ⓘ, *University of Arizona, Tucson, USA*
Michael Rosemann ⓘ, *Queensland University of Technology, Brisbane, Australia*
Clemens Szyperski, *Microsoft Research, Redmond, USA*
Giancarlo Guizzardi ⓘ, *University of Twente, Enschede, The Netherlands*

LNBIP reports state-of-the-art results in areas related to business information systems and industrial application software development – timely, at a high level, and in both printed and electronic form.

The type of material published includes

- Proceedings (published in time for the respective event)
- Postproceedings (consisting of thoroughly revised and/or extended final papers)
- Other edited monographs (such as, for example, project reports or invited volumes)
- Tutorials (coherently integrated collections of lectures given at advanced courses, seminars, schools, etc.)
- Award-winning or exceptional theses

LNBIP is abstracted/indexed in DBLP, EI and Scopus. LNBIP volumes are also submitted for the inclusion in ISI Proceedings.

Andrea Delgado · Tijs Slaats
Editors

Process Mining Workshops

ICPM 2024 International Workshops
Lyngby, Denmark, October 14–18, 2024
Revised Selected Papers

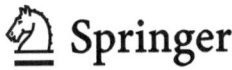 Springer

Editors
Andrea Delgado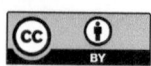
Universidad de la República
Montevideo, Uruguay

Tijs Slaats
University of Copenhagen
Copenhagen, Denmark

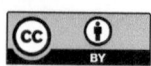

ISSN 1865-1348   ISSN 1865-1356 (electronic)
Lecture Notes in Business Information Processing
ISBN 978-3-031-82224-7   ISBN 978-3-031-82225-4 (eBook)
https://doi.org/10.1007/978-3-031-82225-4

This Springer imprint is published by the registered company Springer Nature Switzerland AG
The registered company address is: Gewerbestrasse 11, 6330 Cham, Switzerland

If disposing of this product, please recycle the paper.

Preface

The International Conference on Process Mining (ICPM), established five years ago, has consolidated as the main event for people from academia and industry to meet and exchange new ideas, discuss the latest developments and deepen collaborations and networking. This includes process mining theory, techniques and algorithms, practical applications and challenges, and supporting tools. The ICPM conference series continues to attract top quality and innovative research contributions from leading scholars and industrial researchers.

This year the conference took place in Copenhagen, Denmark, and included co-located workshops that were held on October 14, 2024. The workshops covered a wide range of current topics and featured outstanding research contributions and paper presentations. Workshops were also expanded with contributions from keynote speakers, panels, tutorials and hands-on sessions, short papers, extended abstracts and posters presentations, providing an extended and diverse space for discussion of each addressed topic.

ICPM 2024 presented thirteen workshops from which ten were traditional workshops consisting primarily of the plenary presentation of submitted and peer-reviewed papers:

- 3rd International Workshop on Collaboration Mining for Distributed Systems (COMINDS)
- 5th International Workshop on Event Data and Behavioral Analytics (EDBA)
- 3rd International Workshop on Education Meets Process Mining (EduPM)
- 1st International Workshop on Empirical Research in Process Mining (ERPM)
- 1st International Workshop on Generative Artificial Intelligence for Process Mining (GenAI4PM)
- 5th International Workshop on Leveraging Machine Learning in Process Mining (ML4PM)
- 1st International Workshop on Process Mining for Sustainability (PM4S)
- 7th International Workshop on Process-Oriented Data Science for Healthcare (PODS4H)
- 9th International Workshop on Process Querying, Manipulation, and Intelligence (PQMI)
- 4th International Workshop on Stream Management & Analytics for Process Mining (SMA4PM)

Three workshops were fully interactive, focusing on sessions that actively engaged the audience and short submissions with a more relaxed review process:

- What's the buzz with objects? Workshop (BuzzOs)
- Process Discovery Contest Workshop (PDWC)
- Processes, Laws, and Compliance Workshop (PLC)

The proceedings present and summarize the work that was discussed during the traditional workshops sessions. In total, the traditional workshops received 126 full-paper submissions of which 56 papers were accepted for publication after a single-blind review process in which submissions on average each received three reviews, leading to a total acceptance rate of about 44%. In addition 21 submissions were accepted for presentation only, including also short papers, extended abstracts and posters. Finally, 28 submissions were presented at the interactive workshops. Most traditional workshops granted a best workshop paper award and selected best papers will be invited to submit an extended version to the Process Science Journal.

We would like to thank all the members of the ICPM community who helped to make the ICPM 2024 workshops a resounding success. We particularly thank the entire organization committee for delivering such an outstanding conference. We are also grateful to the workshop organizers, the numerous reviewers and, of course, the authors for their contributions to the ICPM 2024 workshops.

November 2024

Andrea Delgado
Tijs Slaats

Organization

IEEE Task Force Steering Committee

Boudewijn van Dongen (Chair)	Eindhoven University of Technology, The Netherlands
Artem Polyvyanyy (Vice-chair)	University of Melbourne, Australia
Pnina Soffer (Vice-chair)	University of Haifa, Israel
Rafael Accorsi	Accenture, Switzerland
Peter Blank	PwC, Switzerland
Andrea Burattin	Technical University of Denmark, Denmark
Jochen De Weerdt	KU Leuven, Belgium
Claudio Di Ciccio	University of Utrecht, The Netherlands
Chiara Di Francescomarino	University of Trento, Italy
Philipp Herrmann	Horn & Company, Germany
Mieke Jans	Hasselt University, Belgium
Julian Lebherz	Standard Chartered Bank, Singapore
Sander Leemans	RWTH Aachen University, Germany
Jorge Munoz-Gama	Pontificia Universidad Catolica de Chile, Chile
Arik Senderovich	York University, Canada
Minseok Song	POSTECH, South Korea

Workshop Chairs

Andrea Delgado	Universidad de la República, Uruguay
Tijs Slaats	University of Copenhagen, Denmark

General Chair

Andrea Burattin	Technical University of Denmark, Denmark

Digital Infrastructure Chairs

Giovanni Meroni	Technical University of Denmark, Denmark
Francesca Zerbato	Eindhoven University of Technology, The Netherlands

Publicity Chairs

Amine Abbad-Andaloussi   University of St. Gallen, Switzerland
Iris Beerepoot   University of Utrecht, The Netherlands

Workshop Organizers

3rd International Workshop on Collaboration Mining for Distributed Systems (COMINDS)

Lorenzo Rossi   University of Camerino, Italy
Mahsa Pourbafrani   RWTH Aachen University, Germany
Laura González   Universidad de la República, Uruguay

5th International Workshop on Event Data and Behavioral Analytics (EDBA)

Benoît Depaire   Hasselt University, Belgium
Dirk Fahland   Eindhoven University of Technology,
            The Netherlands
Francesco Leotta   Sapienza University of Rome, Italy
Arik Senderovich   York University, Canada

3rd International Workshop on Education Meets Process Mining (EduPM)

Jorge Munoz-Gama   Pontificia Universidad Catòlica de Chile
Francesca Zerbato   Eindhoven University of Technology,
            The Netherlands
Gert Janssenswillen   Hasselt University, Belgium
Wil van der Aalst   RWTH Aachen University, Germany

1st International Workshop on Empirical Research in Process Mining (ERPM)

Djordje Djurica   Vienna University of Economics and Business,
            Austria
Kateryna Kubrak   University of Tartu, Estonia
Francesca Zerbato   Eindhoven University of Technology,
            The Netherlands
Amine Abbad-Andaloussi   University of St. Gallen, Switzerland

1st International Workshop on Generative Artificial Intelligence for Process Mining (GenAI4PM)

Maxim Vidgof	Vienna University of Economics and Business, Austria
Alessandro Berti	RWTH Aachen University, Germany
Mohammadreza Fani Sani	Microsoft

5th International Workshop on Leveraging Machine Learning in Process Mining (ML4PM)

Paolo Ceravolo	Università degli Studi di Milano, Italy
Sylvio Barbon Junior	Università degli Studi di Trieste, Italy
Vincenzo Pasquadibisceglie	Università degli Studi di Bari, Italy

1st International Workshop on Process Mining for Sustainability (PM4S)

István Koren	RWTH Aachen University, Germany
Janina Bauer	Celonis, Germany
Nina Graves	RWTH Aachen University, Germany
Birgit Penzenstadler	Chalmers University, Sweden

7th International Workshop on Process-Oriented Data Science for Healthcare (PODS4H)

Niels Martin	Hasselt University, Belgium
Carlos Fernandez-Llatas	Universitat Politècnica de València, Spain
Owen Johnson	University of Leeds, UK
Marcos Sepúlveda	Pontificia Universidad Católica de Chile, Chile
Jorge Munoz-Gama	Pontificia Universidad Católica de Chile, Chile

9th International Workshop on Process Querying, Manipulation, and Intelligence (PQMI)

Artem Polyvyanyy	University of Melbourne, Australia
Claudio Di Ciccio	Utrecht University, The Netherlands
Antonella Guzzo	University of Calabria, Italy
Arthur H. M. ter Hofstede	Queensland University of Technology, Australia

4th International Workshop on Stream Management and Analytics for Process Mining (SMA4PM)

Marwan Hassani   Eindhoven University of Technology,
                              The Netherlands
Thomas Seidl   Ludwig-Maximilians-Universität München,
                              Germany
Ahmed Awad   British University in Dubai, United Arab Emirates

Contents

3rd International Workshop on Collaboration Mining for Distributed Systems (CoMinDS 2024)

5th International Workshop on Leveraging Machine Learning in Process Mining (ML4PM 2024)

**5th International Workshop on Event Data and Behavioral Analytics
(EdbA 2024)**

**1st International Workshop on Generative Artificial Intelligence for
Process Mining (GenAI4PM 2024)**

9th International Workshop on Process Querying, Manipulation, and Intelligence (PQMI 2024)

Preface

9th International Workshop on Process Querying, Manipulation, and Intelligence (PQMI 2024)

The aim of the Ninth International Workshop on Process Querying, Manipulation, and Intelligence (PQMI 2024) was to provide a high-quality forum for researchers and practitioners to exchange research findings and ideas on methods and practices in the corresponding areas. *Process Querying* combines concepts from Big Data and Process Modeling & Analysis with Business Process Intelligence and Process Analytics to study techniques for retrieving and manipulating models of processes, both observed in the real world as per the recordings of IT systems, and envisioned as per their design in the form of conceptual representations. The ultimate aim is to systematically organize and extract process-related information for subsequent systematic use. *Process Manipulation* studies inferences from real world observations for augmenting, enhancing, and redesigning models of processes with the ultimate goal of improving real-world business processes. *Process Intelligence* looks for the symbiosis effects between artificial intelligence and process mining, encompassing such domains as knowledge representation, automated planning, reasoning, natural language processing, explainable AI, and multi-agent systems.

Techniques, methods, and tools for process querying, manipulation, and intelligence have wide-ranging applications. Examples of practical problems tackled by the themes of the workshop include business process compliance management, business process vulnerabilities detection, process variance management, process performance analysis, predictive process monitoring, process model translation, syntactical correctness checking, process model comparison, infrequent behavior detection, process instance migration, process reuse, and process standardization.

PQMI 2024 attracted thirteen high-quality submissions. Each paper was reviewed by at least three members of the Program Committee. The review process led to seven accepted papers.

The keynote by Irit Hadar entitled "Mining the Process of Process Mining: Navigating Cognition of Process Miners in Action" opened the workshop. It focuses on theories that extend the traditional cognitive paradigm, with a specific focus on hypotheses generation and testing, and demonstrated their contributions to the process mining field, using recent empirical evidence of cognitive processes underlying the process of process mining, e.g., during process querying. Understanding the cognitive challenges faced by process miners and the reasons why they arise can ensure the development of process mining methods and tools that better navigate and support the cognitive tasks of process miners.

The paper by Benedikt Knopp, Mahsa Pourbafrani, and Wil van der Aalst presents a method for Root Cause Analysis that operates on object-centric event logs (OCELs) and returns a set of association rules on the activity level. These rules associate descriptive patterns over the various object types occurring at events with patterns indicating the process outcome. The paper by Tian Li, Sander J.J. Leemans, and Artem Polyvyanyy studies the applicability of Jensen-Shannon Distance for stochastic conformance checking. Feasibility on real-life event data is also presented. The paper by Frederik Fonger, Niclas Nebelung, Arvid Lepsien, Milda Aleknonyte-Resch, and Agnes Koschmider proposes two novel event log sampling algorithms, RemainderPlus and AllBehavior, and evaluates them experimentally. Wil van der Aalst, Wied Pakusa, and Christopher T. Schwanen propose a novel algorithm that efficiently constructs optimal alignments for process trees with unique labels, i.e., in polynomial time. The paper by Luciana Barbieri, Kleber Stroeh, Edmundo Madeira, and Wil van der Aalst proposes a new strategy to combine Large Language Model capabilities with a framework for a natural language question-and-answer interface to process mining. The paper by Peter Filipp, Rene Dorsch, and Andreas Harth presents EVErPREP, a novel workflow model that leverages Event Knowledge Graphs and Semantic Web technologies to enhance event data preparation for event logs. Finally, the paper by Jakob Brand, Timotheus Kampik, Cem Okulmus, and Matthias Weidlich explores the use of standard SQL for process querying and mining tasks.

We hope the reader will enjoy reading the PQMI papers in these proceedings to learn more about the latest advances in research in process querying, manipulation, and intelligence.

We would like to thank all the authors who submitted papers for publication in this book. We are also grateful to the members of the Program Committee and the external reviewers for their excellent work in reviewing the submitted and revised papers with expertise and patience.

The PQMI Workshop Organizers

October 2024

Organization

Workshop Organizers

Antonella Guzzo   University of Calabria, Italy
Artem Polyvyanyy   University of Melbourne, Australia
Arthur ter Hofstede   Queensland University of Technology, Australia
Claudio Di Ciccio   Utrecht University, The Netherlands

Technical Support

Anandi Karunaratne   University of Melbourne, Australia
Andrei Tour   University of Melbourne, Australia

Program Committee

Abel Armas Cervantes   University of Melbourne, Australia
Agnes Koschmider   University of Bayreuth, Germany
Ahmed Awad   British University in Dubai, UAE
Anna Kalenkova   University of Adelaide, Australia
Chiara Di Francescomarino   Fondazione Bruno Kessler-IRST, Italy
Chun Ouyang   Queensland University of Technology, Australia
Eugenio Vocaturo   University of Calabria, Italy
Fabrizio M. Maggi   Free University of Bozen-Bolzano, Italy
Hyerim Bae   Pusan National University, South Korea
Jochen De Weerdt   Katholieke Universiteit Leuven, Belgium
Kanika Goel   Deloitte, India
Luciano García-Bañuelos   Tecnológico de Monterrey, Mexico
Minseok Song   Pohang University of Science and Technology, South Korea
Pnina Soffer   University of Haifa, Israel
Seppe Vanden Broucke   Katholieke Universiteit Leuven, Belgium
Stefan Schönig   University of Regensburg, Germany
Timotheus Kampik   Umeå University, Sweden

An LLM-Based Q&A Natural Language Interface to Process Mining

Luciana Barbieri[1]([✉])(iD), Kleber Stroeh[2], Edmundo R. M. Madeira[1](iD),
and Wil M. P. van der Aalst[3](iD)

[1] Institute of Computing, University of Campinas, Campinas, Brazil
{luciana.barbieri,edmundo}@ic.unicamp.br
[2] Pegasystems, São Paulo, Brazil
kleber.stroeh@pega.com
[3] RWTH Aachen University, Aachen, Germany
wvdaalst@pads.rwth-aachen.de

Abstract. Process Mining has come a long way to meet the needs of organizations that must optimize their operations. However, its use is still driven by technical users who can interpret process maps, models, graphs and other types of analyses. Business users, on the other hand, frequently report being intimidated by Process Mining tools' interfaces and not knowing "what to do next". An alternative to address this issue is providing more fluid and friendly interfaces for non-technical users based on natural language querying. Recent advances in Large Language Models (LLMs) have expanded the horizon for such interfaces. In this work we propose a new strategy to combine LLM capabilities with a framework for a natural language question-and-answer interface to Process Mining, which combines the flexibility of the former with the scalability and precision of the latter. We expand upon previous works in the area to research the dimensions of flexibility, generalization, scalability and precision. Finally, we implement such an LLM-enhanced framework and test it against a real-life compilation of questions to compare the performance of LLM-based, non LLM-based and hybrid implementations and point to directions in this field of research.

Keywords: Process Mining · Process Querying · Natural Language Interface · Large Language Models

1 Introduction

Process Mining has evolved into a mature discipline with deep impact in organizations worldwide. According to Markets and Markets, it is expected to reach a value of USD 12.1 billion by 2028 at a compound annual growth rate (CAGR) of 45.6% [13]. This growth could be further accelerated if business users joined the forces of technical users in leveraging Process Mining technologies in their daily operations. However, they often report difficulties in using the technology, citing challenges in making sense of process maps, dashboards and other representations used by tools.

© The Author(s) 2025
A. Delgado and T. Slaats (Eds.): ICPM 2024 Workshops, LNBIP 533, pp. 5–17, 2025.
https://doi.org/10.1007/978-3-031-82225-4_1

To address these difficulties, we have previously proposed a framework for a natural language interface to Process Mining tools, such that non-technical users could seize its value through questions and answers [2,3]. While other related work generally mapped Process Mining natural language questions to queries over event log data, our previous method translated these questions to logical queries that ran against existing Process Mining tools, so as to leverage the mature algorithms and techniques they provide. The method, however, applied deterministic approaches for question understanding and mapping, such as rule-based parsing, and failed short in dealing with completely new, unpredicted questions.

The recent advances in Large Language Models (LLMs), such as GPT-4 [14], have uncovered new possibilities to dealing with more open questions and expanded, therefore, the horizons of natural language-based interfaces. Commercial Process Mining tools (e.g., Celonis, SAP Signavio, Microsoft Power Automate, Mindzie, Software AG, Pegasystems, etc.) started to offer co-pilots based on such models, which shows the relevance of the topic.

In this work, we explore the integration of LLMs (GPT-4 in particular) into our previously proposed framework to overcome these generalization limitations by creating an alternative to the rule-based parser in a Process Mining question-and-answer interface.

Our approach seeks to combine the flexibility of LLMs with the power and scalability of existing Process Mining tools. Therefore, we refrain from relying entirely on LLM technologies to answer questions, since such an approach does not take advantage of valuable, dedicated Process Mining algorithms and techniques implemented in existing academic and commercial tools [1]. Furthermore, the use of LLM technologies alone brings severe limitations associated with token limits that would render them useless in bigger data scenarios, commonly found in real life.

More specifically, we (1) build upon our previous work to propose a reviewed architecture to a question-and-answer interface that leverages LLM technology for semantic parsing, (2) use the Process Mining question taxonomy proposed in [2] as the underlying basis to compose a thorough prompt to interact with the LLM, (3) implement and test the proposed architecture against a real-life database of Process Mining-related questions and (4) explore the potential of hybrid approaches that combine rule-based and LLM-based parsers in such an architecture.

The remainder of this paper is organized as follows. Section 2 reviews related work. Section 3 introduces the proposed reviewed architecture. Section 4 presents the conducted experiments and results. Section 5 concludes this paper and points out future work and directions.

2   Related Work

This section reviews related work.

2.1   Early Natural Language Interfaces for Process Mining

Earlier works in the use of natural language question answering as an interface for Process Mining have mainly relied on rule-based or machine learning approaches.

Han and other researchers at IBM identified the need for a more friendly interface to query event data about process automation execution [8]. Their work introduces the generation of an ontology on the domain of the problem that is fed into a rule-based Natural Language Interface to Databases (NLIDB) system called ATHENA, so that natural language questions could trigger queries on the process automation data.

Kobeissi et al. also propose a natural language interface for querying event data [12]. They approach it through label property graphs, that explores a graph database. The interpretation of natural language is done through a mix of machine learning and rule based approaches. The method was extended in [11] to support process behavioral queries (e.g. questions related to the sequence of executed activities).

We also approached this problem through deterministic methods previously. We started by introducing a reference architecture for a query interface to Process Mining, as well as an abstract logical representation for Process Mining queries [3]. This combination helped convert natural language questions into executing steps against a generic interface to Process Mining APIs. Later, we extended this work by introducing a taxonomy on Process Mining questions to extend the reach of the queries supported by the interface [2]. In both works, the conversion from natural language to the abstract logical representation was mainly supported by a rule based approach. Real life questions were collected from Process Mining practitioners and tested against the implementation.

All these works share, in some degree, a common limitation, which is the ability to support more generic – almost colloquial – questions, commonly used in real life.

2.2   LLM-Based Natural Language Interfaces for Process Mining

Recent developments in Generative Artificial Intelligence (GenAI) and LLMs have sparked new discussions around natural language processing in general, and, more specifically, Process Mining interfaces. Works that explore the use of LLMs to answer Process Mining questions can be categorized under the following general approaches [4].

Direct Answering. Works analyzed under this category summarize event data or process mining artifacts into text and feed it to the LLM to answer questions directly.

Pioneering works under this category include Berti et al.'s [5] exploration of GenAI capabilities of prompting direct questions or hypothesis against Process Mining inputs such as discovered Petri Nets, Direct-follows Graph (DFG) abstractions and variant information. In this work, Process Mining data is given as input to the LLM, where the processing/reasoning takes place.

Under a similar approach, Kermani et al. [10] propose an architecture for the integration of Process Mining analyses and LLM technologies, where results from the first (dashboards, process discovery, conformance checking, performance mining, organizational mining) are fed into the second through proper prompt engineering to derive interpretations and recommendations. Special attention is given to providing an optimized prompt structure to accompany the data that is processed by the LLM. Similarly to [5], working on the outcomes of previous Process Mining algorithms (discovery, conformance checking, etc.) keeps the number of tokens under control when interacting with the LLM, but limits, however, some of its application in real life scenarios, as the analyses need to take place before the use of LLMs.

Logical Representation Generation. Approaches under this category provide metadata (event log metadata, process ontologies, etc.) to an LLM to generate a logical representation, such as a structured query or executable program, corresponding to a question.

This is the case of the method proposed by Jessen et al. [9], which presents an architecture that combines metadata, ontology and LLM capabilities to translate questions into Structured Query Language (SQL) queries on an event log database. They also explore orchestrating calls through Chain-of-Thought, using zero- and few-shot learning and benchmarking results against previous works. It is unclear, however, how the handling of more specific Process Mining functionality such as process discovery or conformance checking is done without further integration into Process Mining tools.

Similarly, our proposed method uses event log metadata fed to an LLM to generate a logical representation for Process Mining questions. Distinctively, however, we propose the use of a multi-shot prompt founded on the Process Mining question taxonomy proposed in [2]. Furthermore, to the best of our knowledge, this is the first method to integrate such an LLM-based natural language interface to existing process mining tools, so that the advanced analyses and algorithms they implement can be leveraged to answer the questions.

3   Proposed Method

Our proposed method extends the architecture presented in [2] and is depicted in Fig. 1. Colored blocks correspond to the components of this extended architecture. New and revised components are depicted respectively in green and blue, while external components are shown in gray.

The user inputs a question in natural language (English) through the *Text Interface* component, such as "How many cases have been concluded today?". The question goes through an LLM-based semantic parser (components highlighted in green), which is introduced as an alternative to its rule-based counter part proposed in [2].

The role of the semantic parser is to understand the meaning of the input text (question) and convert it to a logical representation that is machine readable. This is done by taking the question in natural language, building a prompt

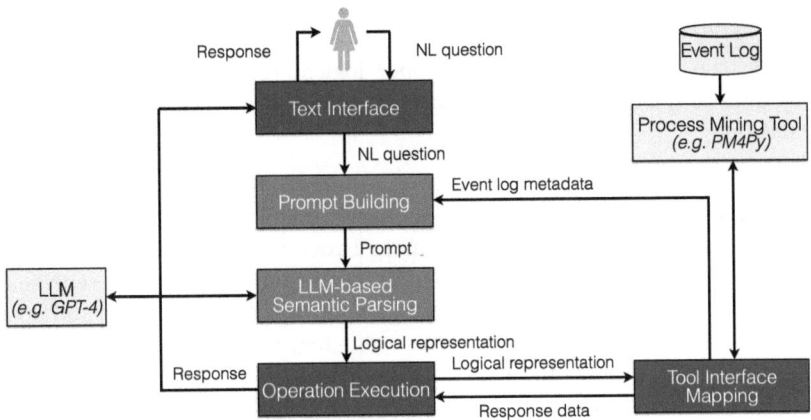

Fig. 1. LLM-based Architecture Overview

to instruct the LLM on how to create this logical representation (which is done by the *Prompt Building* component) and handing it to the model (*LLM-based Semantic Parsing* component). The resulting representation is then mapped into an API call of the underlying Process Mining tool and executed (*Operation Execution* and *Tool Interface Mapping* components). These architecture components are further detailed in the following subsections.

3.1 Logical Representation

The logical representation used to describe questions in [2] is also utilized in this work. It is an extension of the Question Decomposition Meaning Representation (QDMR) proposed in [15]. A QDMR representation comprises a sequence of operations, where each operation is applied to the results of a previous step in the sequence. Operations are inspired by SQL and include `select`, `project`, `aggregate`, `filter` and `group`, among others. The following sequence, for example, represents a question such as "What is the average duration of cases?".

```
select case
project duration #1
aggregate average #2
```

Hash tags refer to the results of a previous operation in the sequence, which may be a set of events, cases or attribute values. In the example above, for instance, `#1` refers to the results of the `select case` operation. For a detailed description of this logical representation, please refer to [2].

3.2   Prompt Building

To enable the LLM to create the proper logical representation for a Process Mining question, a multi-shot prompt [7] was engineered containing the following information:

- A textual description of the logical representation to be used, including each supported operation, its parameters and references
- A small general description of the main Process Mining terms and concepts (event log, event, activity, case, variant, etc.) and how they are represented
- Event log metadata (encoded in JSON), comprising names, types and possible values of attributes contained in the event log, which are obtained from the underlying Process Mining tool
- Metadata for the analyses supported by the underlying Process Mining tool (e.g. conformance checking and rework analysis), also encoded in JSON, including names and returned data types
- Examples of questions and their corresponding logical representations (encoded in JSON)
- Instructions on the expected response contents and format

Listings 1 to 6 depict the actual contents of the prompt. Extensive contents (e.g. metadata and example questions) are abbreviated with "..." for conciseness.

Listing 1. Logical representation description in LLM prompt

```
I'm using a logical representation for natural language questions which is
   similar to SQL. It uses a sequence of operations from the set given below,
   where ``reference" is an integer n that refers to the results of the nth
   operation in the sequence:
select concept,
project [distinct] relation of reference,
filter reference where field is [negate] value, ...
```

Listing 2. Event log metadata in LLM prompt

```
Data is organized into 2 tables: case and event, as described in JSON:
{'case': {'case': {'name': 'work_order_id', 'type': 'number'}, 'duration':
   {'name': 'duration', 'type': 'interval'}, ...}, 'event': {'timestamp':
   {'name': 'start_ts', 'type': 'timestamp'}, 'activity': {'name': 'status',
   'type': 'categorical', 'categories': ['open', 'assigned', ...]}, ...}}
```

Listing 3. Process mining terms and concepts in LLM prompt

```
The event table corresponds to the event log of a process execution. Each
   event corresponds to the execution of a single process activity or step
   and is related to a single case or process instance. A case is a temporal
   sequence of events corresponding to a ``run'' of the process. A trace or
   variant is the sequence of activities executed by a case.
```

Listing 4. Analyses metadata in LLM prompt

```
Predicates apply to specific concepts and may return different data
   depending on the concept they are applied to, as described in JSON:
{'nonconformance': {'trace': {'trace': {'type': 'text'}, 'case_count':
   {'type': 'number', 'sorting': True}}}, 'rework': {'activity': {'activity':
   {'type': 'categorical'}, 'case_count': {'type': 'number', 'sorting':
   True}}, ...}, ...}
```

Listing 5. Example questions in LLM prompt

```
These are examples of questions with their corresponding logical
   representations written in JSON:
How many cases are there in the log?,[{''operator'': ''select'',
   ''concept'': ''case'', ''ref'': []}, {''operator'': ''aggregate'',
   ''aggregate'': [''count''], ''ref'': [0]}]
List the non-conformances.,[{''operator'': ''select'', ''concept'':
   ''case'', ''ref'': []}, {''operator'': ''predicate'', ''predicate'':
   ''nonconformance'', ''ref'': [0]}] ...
```

Listing 6. Response instructions in LLM prompt

```
Respond with a single logical representation in JSON for the given question.
   The JSON representation should not contain c-style comments. If an
   operation uses multiple references, make sure they are given in the
   correct order...
```

The examples of question given in the prompt (Listing 5) are part of a hand-built set of 221 pairs of questions and logical representations. The creation of this set was done as part of this work and guided by the Process Mining question taxonomy proposed in [2]. This taxonomy provides a classification framework for questions, which is organized in seven dimensions:

- *Perspective*: the type of Process Mining (process execution data, process discovery, conformance checking, etc.) the question relates
- *Relativity*: whether the question is absolute or relative to some other data or analysis results
- *Normativity*: indicates if the question requires some normative information/-model to be answered
- *Composition*: whether the given question contains multiple questions inside itself that need separate answers
- *Filtering*: specifies if the question requires a filter to be applied to data before or after computation
- *Ambiguity*: indicates if the question can have multiple interpretations
- *Context*: denotes if the question requires additional information outside its own text to be interpreted (e.g. previous questions and answers made to the natural language interface)

Each dimension is organized hierarchically in a tree structure, so that the classification of a question is done by assigning it a leaf of each tree (dimension). For a detailed description of these dimensions, including their hierarchical breakdown, please refer to [2].

The goal when building this set of example questions was to cover as many taxonomic tree branches as possible along all of these dimensions. Table 1 presents the coverage for each dimension calculated in terms of taxonomic tree leaves represented in the question set for each dimension.

Taxonomic tree branches that are not covered by the example set are related to types of questions that are not handled by this work.

Listing 7 presents a fragment of the 221 pairs of questions and logical representations (encoded in JSON) used to build the prompt. The complete set is available at https://ic.unicamp.br/~luciana.barbieri/promptquestions.csv.

Table 1. Taxonomic coverage of the example question set

Taxonomic Dimension	Coverage
Perspective	52%
Relativity	75%
Normativity	67%
Composition	100%
Filtering	69%
Ambiguity	100%
Context	50%

Listing 7. Samples of questions and logical representations. For the complete set, see https://ic.unicamp.br/~luciana.barbieri/promptquestions.csv.

```
''How many cases are there in the log?'',[{''operator'': ''select'',
  ''concept'': ''case'', ''ref'': []}, {''operator'': ''aggregate'',
  ''aggregate'': [''count''], ''ref'': [0]}]
''List the non-conformances.'',[{''operator'': ''select'', ''concept'':
  ''case'', ''ref'': []}, {''operator'': ''predicate'', ''predicate'':
  ''nonconformance'', ''ref'': [0]}]
''What are the start activities in the process?'',[{''operator'':
  ''select'', ''concept'': ''case'', ''ref'': []}, {''operator'':
  ''predicate'', ''predicate'': ''start'', ''ref'': [0]}]
''How long does my process take, in average?'',[{''operator'': ''select'',
  ''concept'': ''case'', ''ref'': []}, {''operator'': ''project'',
  ''relation'': ''duration'', ''ref'': [0]}, {''operator'': ''aggregate'',
  ''aggregate'': [''average''], ''ref'': [1]}] ...
```

3.3   LLM-Based Parsing

The *LLM-based Parsing* component is responsible for interfacing with the external LLM by feeding it with the prompt built in the previous step (by the *Prompt Building component*) in order to obtain a logical representation for the question. In our experimental implementation, GPT-4 is the LLM of choice, so the *LLM-based Parsing* component plays its role by invoking GPT's Chat Completion API and extracting the logical representation from its response. If a valid logical representation is not present in the response text, a single retry is attempted by re-instructing GPT (in the prompt) that it should answer the question with a valid logical representation.

Other LLMs can alternatively be used for semantic parsing in the future by re-instantiating the *LLM-based Parsing* component alone.

3.4   Hybrid Parsing

As an alternative to the rule-based and pure LLM-based parsers we also propose a hybrid approach, as depicted in Fig. 2.

The idea is to initially feed the question to the original rule-based parser proposed in [2] (flow 1 represented with red dashed lines in Fig. 2).

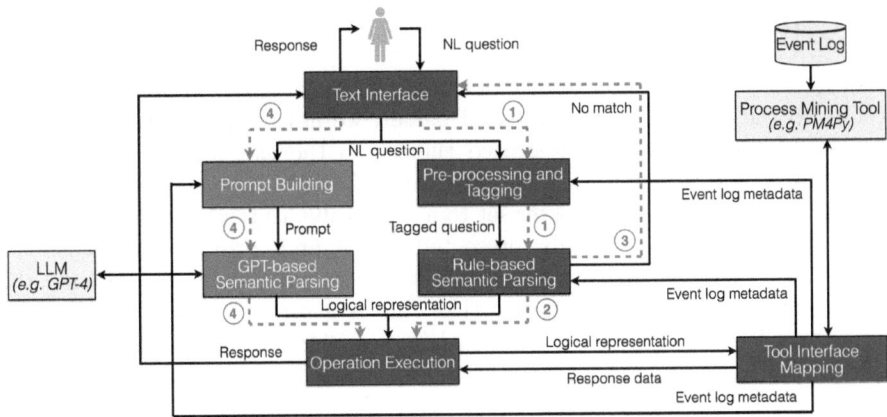

Fig. 2. Hybrid Architecture Overview

The question goes initially through the *Pre-processing and Tagging* component, which is responsible for splitting it into tokens and tagging it with part-of-speech information, (linguistic) dependency relations and recognized entities. It is then semantically parsed by the *Rule-based Semantic Parsing* component using a rule-matching approach (for more information on the *Pre-processing and Tagging* and *Rule-based Semantic Parsing* components, please refer to [2]). If a rule is triggered, the resulting logical representation is used (flow 2). Otherwise, a "no match" indication is returned (flow 3) and the question is then fed to the LLM-based parser (flow 4). The logical representation obtained from the model (Chat Completion API, in the current implementation) is used in this case.

The reasons for choosing to have the question initially parsed by the rule-based parser (and only go through the LLM-based parser when the first is not able to translate it to a logical representation) are its lower cost and response time, alongside its higher predictability.

3.5 Operation Execution and Tool Interface Mapping

After a logical representation is created for the input question, the *Operation Execution* component manages its execution. Each operation contained in the logical representation is carried out by invoking the *Tool Interface Mapping* component, with final results being returned to answer the question.

The *Tool Interface Mapping* component, on its turn, maps the logical operations to real API calls of a Process Mining tool. In our experimental implementation, PM4Py [6] is used as this underlying tool. It is an open-source library written in Python that implements a variety of process mining algorithms.

Using PM4Py's ability to handle event logs as pandas objects allows a straightforward mapping of operations such as `select`, `project`, `filter` and `aggregate` over case and event data. Predicates such as `nonconformance` and `rework`, on their turn, are directly mapped into calls to API methods that implement these analyses.

4   Experimental Results

In order to verify the applicability of the presented methods and compare their results to the existing pure rule-based parser, we have implemented the newly proposed components and integrated them into the existing architecture [2]. The gpt-4-1106-preview model was used for LLM-based parsing, with the Chat Completion API's *seed* parameter set to a fixed value to reinforce predictability.

The question set originally presented in [3] and available at https://ic. unicamp.br/~luciana.barbieri/promptquestions.csv was used to evaluate the implementation. One should notice that this is a set completely independent of the smaller, hand-built set described in Sect. 3.2 and used to build GPT's prompt. The test set is composed of 794 questions in English. Before this evaluation, each question of this set was manually analyzed to determine if it is possible to create a logical representation that could be mapped to a call and executed by the underlying Process Mining tool. The analysis concluded that, from the original 794 questions, 524 can be fully represented, mapped and executed, while this can be partially done for 96 of them. A question can be partially handled, for example, if it is a composite question for which at least one sub-question can be answered, while others cannot, such as "What are the deviations from the expected model? Why did they happen?". The remaining 174 questions cannot be handled either due to language-related problems (e.g. incomprehensible sentences), Process Mining misconceptions, or because the required functionality is not supported by the underlying Process Mining tool.

The 620 (fully or partially) answerable questions were executed against a real-life Work Force Management-based event log processed by PM4Py. However, any Process Mining event log could be used, as the testing questions are not specifically bound to any particular event log. Questions pass or partially pass a test if the obtained logical representation fully or partially answers them, respectively. If no valid logical representation is obtained or if it does not answer the question correctly, the test fails. Table 2 presents our experimental results.

Table 2. Experimental Results.

Parsing Approach	Passed	Partially Passed	Failed
Rule-based	302 (48.71%)	125 (20.16%)	193 (31.13%)
GPT-based	376 (60.65%)	108 (17.42%)	136 (21.94%)
Hybrid	350 (56.45%)	153 (24.68%)	117 (18.87%)
Ground truth	524 (84.52%)	96 (15.48%)	0 (00.00%)

When analyzing these results, one can initially observe that the GPT-based parser is able to answer more questions with a fully accurate response when compared to rule-based and hybrid approaches. Another important advantage of this parser is that it generalizes well and is able to respond abstract questions such as "What is the most complex case?" with plausible answers (it responded this particular question with the case that executed the most distinct activities). Disadvantages, on the other hand, are the higher cost and response time when compared to the rule-based parser, which can run solely on the user device. It is also worth noticing that, similarly to other AI-based models, the GPT-based parser lacks predictability (even with the use of the *seed* parameter), implying that the same question may be answered differently on separate attempts.

The hybrid approach, on its turn, was able to answer more questions correctly if we consider both full and partial responses, reducing the share of incorrect behavior (failed responses). This can be explained by the fair accuracy of the (deterministic) rule-based parser when dealing with predictable, well-behaved questions [3] being combined with the ability of the GPT-based parser to handle the more open, abstract ones. Additionally, as GPT-based parsing is only used when rule-based parsing does not find a matching rule for the question, cost and response time issues are minimized, as well as unpredictability. The drawback of the approach, however, is that it is not able to detect when the rule-based parser triggered a rule that caused a question to be partially or incorrectly answered (when the GPT-based parser might have been able to provide a fully correct answer).

5   Conclusions and Future Work

In this work, we propose a new architecture for a Q&A natural language interface for Process Mining that combines LLM technologies and Process Mining concepts organized in a taxonomy. This architecture is envisioned to balance the natural language processing capabilities of LLMs with the power of Process Mining tools, such that the first can drive interactions with the latter.

We also experiment around hybrid approaches, where LLM based implementation complements a rule-based one, in search of a better balance between generalization and precision. Finally, we test these architecture variants against real-life questions and event log, to assess their performances. In a nutshell, LLM based methods seem to help reduce failures in answering questions by increasing the number of questions that are fully or partially answered.

Based on our findings, we would like to explore the following directions of future work:

-   *Multi-agents*: interface with LLM through a multi-agent framework, such that interactions can be broken down into smaller tasks that LLMs can handle better
-   *Fine tuning*: experiment the impact of fine tuning LLMs to better understand Process Mining taxonomy
-   *Other LLMs*: compare the performance of alternative LLMs such as Gemini and Claude, among others
-   *Conversational*: evolve the question-and-answer interface to a conversational one, where context about previous interactions is used to more naturally speak to human users

Acknowledgments. We would like to thank Coordenação de Aperfeiçoamento de Pessoal de Nível Superior Brasil (CAPES) Finance Code 001, for providing the financial support for this work.

Disclosure of Interests. The authors have no competing interests to declare that are relevant to the content of this article.

References

1. van der Aalst, W.M.P.: Process management after ChatGPT: How generative and predictive AI relate to process mining (2023). http://www.linkedin.com/pulse/process-management-after-chatgpt-how-generative-ai-wil-van-der-aalst-lyyzc/
2. Barbieri, L., Madeira, E., Stroeh, K., van der Aalst, W.M.P.: A natural language querying interface for process mining. J. Intell. Inf. Syst. **61**(1), 113–142 (2023)
3. Barbieri, L., Madeira, E.R.M., Stroeh, K., van der Aalst, W.M.P.: Towards a natural language conversational interface for process mining. In: Process Mining Workshops, ICPM 2021. Springer International Publishing, Cham (2021)
4. Berti, A., Kourani, H., Hafke, H., Li, C.Y., Schuster, D.: Evaluating large language models in process mining: capabilities, benchmarks, evaluation strategies, and future challenges. arXiv preprint arXiv:2403.06749 (2024)
5. Berti, A., Schuster, D., van der Aalst, W.M.P.: Abstractions, scenarios, and prompt definitions for process mining with LLMs: a case study. In: International Conference on Business Process Management, pp. 427–439. Springer, Heidelberg (2023). https://doi.org/10.1007/978-3-031-50974-2_32
6. Berti, A., van Zelst, S., Schuster, D.: PM4Py: a process mining library for python. Softw. Impacts **17**, 100556 (2023)
7. Brown, T., et al.: Language models are few-shot learners. Adv. Neural. Inf. Process. Syst. **33**, 1877–1901 (2020)
8. Han, X., et al.: Bootstrapping natural language querying on process automation data. In: 2020 IEEE International Conference on Services Computing (SCC), pp. 170–177 (2020)
9. Jessen, U., Sroka, M., Fahland, D.: Chit-chat or deep talk: prompt engineering for process mining. arXiv preprint arXiv:2307.09909 (2023)
10. Kermani, M.A.M.A., Seddighi, H.R., Maghsoudi, M.: Revolutionizing process mining: a novel architecture for ChatGPT integration and enhanced user experience through optimized prompt engineering. arXiv preprint arXiv:2405.10689 (2024)
11. Kobeissi, M., Assy, N., Gaaloul, W., Defude, B., Benatallah, B., Haidar, B.: Natural language querying of process execution data. Inf. Syst. **116**, 102227 (2023)
12. Kobeissi, M., Assy, N., Gaaloul, W., Defude, B., Haidar, B.: An intent-based natural language interface for querying process execution data. In: 3rd International Conference on Process Mining (ICPM), pp. 152–159. IEEE (2021)
13. Markets and Markets: Process Mining Market by Offering - Global Forecast to 2028 (2023). https://www.marketsandmarkets.com/Market-Reports/process-mining-market-176608355.html
14. OpenAI: GPT-4 technical report. arXiv preprint arXiv:2303.08774 (2023)
15. Wolfson, T., et al.: Break it down: a question understanding benchmark. Trans. Assoc. Comput. Linguist. **8**, 183–198 (2020)

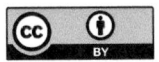

One Language to Rule Them All: Behavioural Querying of Process Data Using SQL

Jakob Brand[1], Timotheus Kampik[2,3], Cem Okulmus[3], and Matthias Weidlich[1,2(✉)]

[1] Humboldt-Universität zu Berlin, Berlin, Germany
{brandjak,matthias.weidlich}@hu-berlin.de
[2] SAP Signavio, Berlin, Germany
{timotheus.kampik,matthias.weidlich}@sap.com
[3] Umeå University, Umeå, Sweden
{tkampik,okulmus}@cs.umu.se

Abstract. State-of-the-art solutions for process mining rely on proprietary, domain-specific languages to query data recorded during business process execution. To support common analysis tasks, these languages focus on the definition of queries for behavioural patterns. Yet, the use of domain-specific languages for process mining has drawbacks: they require specific user training, lead to a decoupling of the query models for (i) data extraction and transformation, and (ii) the actual analysis, and induce engineering overhead through the development of a dedicated query engine. In this work, we therefore explore the use of standard SQL for process mining tasks. In particular, we demonstrate that the SQL concepts for row pattern recognition as realised by the `MATCH_RECOGNIZE` clause are sufficient to capture queries for behavioural patterns as specified in the SIGNAL language by SAP Signavio as well as the Process Querying Language (PQL) by Celonis. Based on a discussion of the respective language features, we outline a translation of SIGNAL and PQL queries into standard SQL. This way, we provide the basis for the adoption of widely used, general purpose query engines for process mining tasks.

Keywords: Process Querying · Process Mining · Pattern Recognition

1 Introduction

Process mining supports business process management through the analysis of event log data that has been recorded during process execution. Over the past decade, process mining has evolved from an academic field of inquiry into a widely adopted practice in large-scale organisations that is supported by special-purpose software products provided by major vendors such as Microsoft and SAP. To support a wide range of analysis tasks, *process querying* has become a

© The Author(s) 2025
A. Delgado and T. Slaats (Eds.): ICPM 2024 Workshops, LNBIP 533, pp. 18–30, 2025.
https://doi.org/10.1007/978-3-031-82225-4_2

cornerstone of existing process mining solutions and a vibrant direction of research within the community [11]. Yet, the assumption so far has mostly been that process querying is executed by special-purpose technologies, i.e., domain-specific languages that facilitate the definition of queries for behavioural patterns [5,15] (Sect. 2).

While domain-specific languages for process querying can be tailored to specific analysis needs, their usage also induces certain drawbacks. They require specific training, which narrows the user group. They also lead to a decoupling of the query models for data preparation and analysis. Since process-related data is often stored in mainstream relational database systems, the extraction, transformation and loading (ETL) of the data is typically realized in standard SQL. Finally, the use of domain-specific languages for process querying incurs engineering overhead, through the development of dedicated query engines.

In this paper, we question the need for dedicated languages for process querying. We practically demonstrate that the behavioural querying capabilities of two industry-scale process query languages can be mapped to standard SQL, most notably using the MATCH_RECOGNIZE clause as introduced with the 2016 SQL standard revision (Sect. 3). This means that process behaviour can be analysed using "mainstream" database systems. As such, our work strengthens the bridge between process query languages and database theory and applications (Sect. 4), while simultaneously raising questions about *i)* the complexity and scalability of MATCH_RECOGNIZE for behavioural querying and *ii)* the potential of ubiquitous process querying with mainstream database technologies, e.g., directly on top of enterprise system databases and in the data lake-houses that serve as the data backbone for a wide range of business applications (Sect. 5).

2   Background

Below, we give an intuitive overview of two state-of-the-art languages for process querying, i.e., SIGNAL by SAP Signavio (Sect. 2.1) and PQL by Celonis (Sect. 2.2). Then, we review the SQL MATCH_RECOGNIZE clause (Sect. 2.3).

2.1   SIGNAL by SAP Signavio

SIGNAL [5] is a language for process querying provided by SAP Signavio as part of their process mining offering. The central data model in SIGNAL is a nested table, as illustrated in Table 1. It contains information on process executions on two levels. The outer level includes attributes for a case identifier (**case_id** in Table 1) and additional case properties, if available (**customer_name** and **order_value**). For each tuple of the outer level, the inner level contains tuples that describe the individual events recorded for a case, with attributes capturing an event type (**event_name**) and timestamp (**end_time**), and potentially further properties of events (**department**).

SIGNAL supports read-only queries that are specified in an SQL-like syntax, see Listing 1. The queries refer to a single nested table (FROM clause), which

Table 1. Example of the SIGNAL columnar data format for event logs.

case_ID	customer_name	order_value	events		
			event_name	end_time	department
01	C1	599	Order received	2024-03-01 11:15	D1
			Invoice sent	2024-03-01 12:33	D2
			Payment received	2024-03-02 09:01	D2
			Order shipped	2024-03-05 14:39	D4
02	C3	149	Order received	2024-03-02 15:25	D1
			Invoice sent	2024-03-02 17:43	D2
			Timer expired	2024-03-09 17:44	D3
			Order cancelled	2024-03-09 18:02	D4

```
1  SELECT case_id
2  FROM THIS_PROCESS
3  WHERE BEHAVIOUR (event_name = 'Order received' AND 'order_value' > 300)
4      AS order_300
5  MATCHES (^order_300 ~> 'Payment received' -> 'Order shipped'$)
```

Listing 1. Example of a SIGNAL query.

is typically derived from the query context (THIS_PROCESS in Listing 1). A SIGNAL query may be *flat* and refer only to the information at the case level in the nested table, through standard SQL operators for projection, selection, and aggregation (in SELECT and WHERE clauses). A query may also be *nested*, such that the outer subquery refers to cases, while the inner subquery refers to events within cases. Such a nested query may leverage the order of events within a case as it is inferred from the events' timestamps (which is assumed to be total) in order to detect patterns based on temporal constraints (MATCHES clause). The events to consider for the evaluation of the constraints are either characterized implicitly (e.g., by referring directly to a value of the **event_name** column; 'Payment received' in Listing 1) or defined as so-called behaviours (BEHAVIOUR clause), i.e., subqueries that select the events of a case that satisfy the specified constraints.

2.2   PQL by Celonis

PQL [15] has been developed by Celonis as a query language for process mining tasks. Is adopts a so-called snowflake schema [15], as illustrated in Fig. 1. Here, the central relations are an **Activities** table and a **Cases** table. Additional information is stored in further tables with a normalized schema (a **Customers** table and an **Orders** table in our example), which is linked to the **Activities** table and **Cases** table, respectively, by foreign key relationships. These relationships have to be defined when loading data into the respective model.

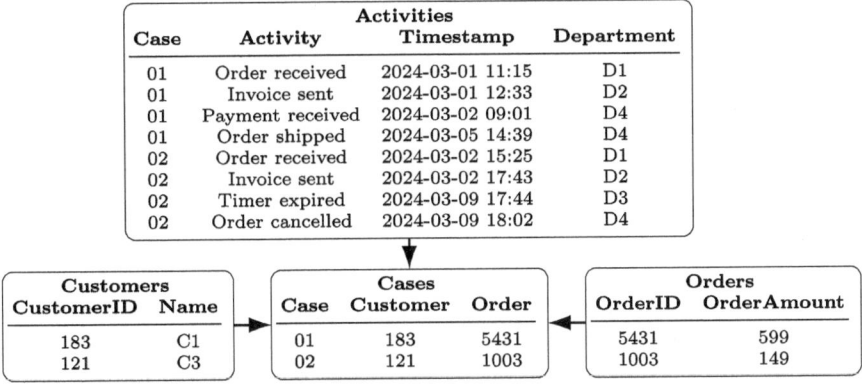

Fig. 1. Example of the PQL snowflake data model with four tables.

PQL queries are read-only and also adopt an SQL-like syntax. PQL supports a wide range of operators, from SQL-like aggregation and string modification functions through ML operators (e.g., k-means clustering) to operators for process mining tasks (e.g., a dedicated operator for conformance checking [2]).

In PQL queries, two important operations are performed implicitly based on the interpretation of the aforementioned tables in a process mining context. That is, queries over the **Activities** and **Cases** tables may refer to attributes of the additional tables, which are then joined implicitly according to the foreign keys. In addition, groupings are performed implicitly using all selected non-aggregated columns in a query.

PQL's support for the identification of behavioural patterns primarily relies on three so-called process functions that match cases showing a specific pattern of activity executions: PROCESS EQUALS enables matching based on a reduced set of regular expressions. Patterns in MATCH_PROCESS are defined in graph structure, in which vertices are activities, or sets thereof, and edges describe behavioural relations between them. The most expressive clause, MATCH_PROCESS_REGEX, defines a pattern as a regular expression. The latter resembles the behavioural matching in SIGNAL, so that we will focus on this clause in the remainder.

A MATCH_PROCESS_REGEX query is shown in Listing 2. At first, a single string column of the **Activities** table on which the matching is performed is specified. Then, a pattern is defined for behaviours via equality or wildcard matching, and transitions between them. In the example, matching is performed on a **behaviour** column that is constructed by the CASE. It has three sub-clauses, one for the each of the behaviours, which define the condition (WHEN) of the behaviour as well as its name (THEN). The latter represents the values for the **behaviour** column, which are then matched via string equality. The matching clause adds a temporary integer column to the **Cases** table with 0/1 values, indicating whether a case matches the pattern. Wrapping the clause with a FILTER = 1 condition will return all rows of all matched cases, as seen in the example.

```
1  CASE WHEN "Activities"."Activity"='Order Received'
2          AND "Activities"."OrderAmount" > 300 THEN 'order_300'
3      WHEN "Activities"."Activity"='Payment Received' THEN 'payment_received'
4      WHEN "Activities"."Activity"='Order shipped' THEN 'order_shipped'
5      ELSE '' END
6  FILTER MATCH_PROCESS_REGEX("Activities"."behaviour", ^'order_300' >>
7          ANY* >> 'payment_received' >> 'order_shipped'$) = 1;
```

Listing 2. Example of a PQL query.

As pattern detection is limited to a single string column, complex patterns on multiple/non-string columns are not directly supported. However, the CASE WHEN clause supports the evaluation of arbitrary columns and can be used beforehand to create a new string column in the **Activities** table, which indicates the satisfied constraints for each row. In our example in Listing 2, this is realized through the string values 'order_300', 'payment_received', and 'order_shipped'.

2.3 SQL Match Recognize

With the 2016 revision of the SQL standard [7], the MATCH_RECOGNIZE clause has been introduced for row pattern recognition. While a concise description can be found in [10], we summarise the main concepts of MATCH_RECOGNIZE below. Listing 3 illustrates the syntax for the MATCH_RECOGNIZE clause. It operates on an input table, as constructed by the FROM clause, which may involve joins, and produces an output table, which is then processed by SELECT and other clauses (e.g., a GROUP BY clause). The MATCH_RECOGNIZE clause involves several operators:

DEFINE: This operator is mandatory and is used to define *pattern symbols*, which are—seen semantically—matched to a set of rows that satisfy some condition. These symbols may even refer to other symbols in their definition.

PATTERN. This operator is mandatory and comprises a regular expression, which may use symbols defined in DEFINE. Notably, it is allowed to include undefined symbols, which are given a dummy predicate that is satisfied by all rows. The regular expressions may include Kleene closure ($*$ and $+$), upper and lower cardinality bounds ($\{n, m\}$), alternatives ($+$), and references to the first and last row of a table ($\hat{}$ and $\$$).

hskip-13pt ONE ROW PER MATCH / ALL ROWS PER MATCH. Upon a "match", understood as the sequence of rows which satisfies the pattern, the content of the output table is derived as follows: ONE ROW PER MATCH produces one output row for every match, i.e., provides a certain aggregation. ALL ROWS PER MATCH performs no such aggregation, and outputs each row in the sequence making up a match.

AFTER MATCH. This optional operator controls, upon a "match", where to continue pattern matching, e.g., after the first or last row (in general, or representing a specific symbol).

```
1  SELECT   <select list>
2  FROM     <source table>
3  MATCH_RECOGNIZE (
4           [ PARTITION BY <partition list> ]
5           [ ORDER BY <order by list> ]
6           [ MEASURES <measure list> ]
7           [ ONE ROW PER MATCH | ALL ROWS PER MATCH ]
8           [ AFTER MATCH <skip to option> ]
9           PATTERN ( <row pattern> )
10          [ SUBSET <subset list> ]
11          DEFINE <definition list> ) AS <table alias>;
```

Listing 3. The syntax of the MATCH_RECOGNIZE clause, as given in [10].

PARTITION BY. This optional operator groups the rows of the table given a list of columns. The MATCH_RECOGNIZE clause is then evaluated per such group.

ORDER BY. While the ordering operator is optional, it carries the same meaning as when used outside a MATCH_RECOGNIZE clause.

MEASURES. This optional operator enables access to pre-defined internal functions to populate the output with additional columns, accessible *outside* the MATCH_RECOGNIZE clause, such as match_number() and first().

hskip-13pt SUBSET. This optional operator, given a list of pattern symbols, groups them to refer to them collectively (e.g., to compute aggregates).

The MATCH_RECOGNIZE clause is available in various database management systems, such as Oracle, Snowflake, and Trino, as well as data stream processing frameworks, such as Azure Stream Analytics, Flink, and Esper.

3 Language Comparison and Translation

In this section, we compare the above languages, and outline how SIGNAL and PQL queries can be translated to SQL using the MATCH_RECOGNIZE clause.

3.1 Query Input

The input data for process querying is saved either as a nested table (in SIGNAL) or in a pre-defined schema comprising an **Activities** table, a **Cases** table and optional additional dimensions (in PQL). In SIGNAL, specifying a process identifier as input in the FROM subclause is sufficient. In PQL, the **Activities** table is specified to identify the input data. When referencing data from the dimension tables in PQL, the necessary joins are performed implicitly.

In SQL, the FROM subclause specifies the tables or views based on which the table for the evaluation of the MATCH_RECOGNIZE clause is derived. The construction of this table follows common SQL semantics. That is, a listing of multiple tables leads to the (implicit) construction of a Cartesian product, which may be avoided by specifying explicit joins or subqueries.

When translating SIGNAL and PQL queries to SQL, therefore, all tables that capture relevant process data need to be included in the FROM clause, potentially joining them over the attributes for the activity or case identifiers.

3.2 Behaviour Definition

Process querying concerns the identification of patterns over some behavioural abstraction. Using the terminology of SIGNAL, we call these abstractions *behaviours*. A behaviour is defined by a Boolean condition that is evaluated against each event of the process data, i.e., against each row of a respective table.

Patterns are then constructed by specifying relations over behaviours, incorporating the ordering of rows as established by timestamp attributes. As detailed later, a pattern resembles a regular expression (regex), i.e., the behaviours can be seen as the alphabet over which to define the regex.

To differentiate the expressiveness of behaviours, we adopt the classification of conditions as presented for MATCH_RECOGNIZE in [16]: if a condition can be evaluated on a single row, it is called an *independent condition*. For behaviours that need to be evaluated across multiple rows, the condition is called a *dependent condition*. If all rows that need to be evaluated in a dependent condition are located in the same pattern match, the condition is classified as *self-contained*.

SIGNAL. Behaviours can be defined implicitly with a string that is matched with a specified column (by default the **event_name** column). For an explicit definition, a WHERE BEHAVIOUR clause is part of the language. It supports a wide range of operators, such as comparison, logical, LIKE/ILIKE, IS NULL, and durations on event-level columns from the table. In the SIGNAL query in Listing 1, the first behaviour **order_300** is defined explicitly and matches all rows with the **event_name** 'Order received' and an **order_value** larger than 300. The second and third behaviours are implicitly defined in the MATCHES subclause.

Queries that include BEHAVIOUR and MATCHES clauses are restricted to nested tables. Therefore, the BEHAVIOUR clause operates at the inner (i.e., event) level, and comparisons to case-level aggregations like SUM or AVG are not possible. While the SIGNAL language includes LAG/LEAD operators to navigate to previous and subsequent rows in a match, they are defined as window functions that work on flattened tables and, therefore, are not applicable for row navigation in nested tables. Hence, behaviours in SIGNAL contain only independent conditions.

PQL. To define behaviours, a user may specify a single string column (by default the **activity** column) for matching it against a set of given strings. In addition, string matching may incorporate LIKE with wildcards and grouped matching.

While such behaviour definition based on string matching offers only limited expressiveness, more complex behaviours may be derived using some limited data manipulation capabilities in PQL. That is, the CASE_WHEN operator enables the creation of a temporary table based on the **Activities** table that features an additional string column **behaviour**. The latter indicates the satisfied behaviour for each row and can be incorporated in the matching operator, as discussed already for the example given in Listing 2.

In a CASE clause, multiple conditions on columns and corresponding output values (i.e., behaviour names) can be specified. The conditions are evaluated on each row individually and may include comparisons, logical operators, LIKE/ILIKE, IS NULL and BETWEEN for time intervals; they may refer to neighbouring rows using LAG/LEAD; and they can include aggregations. Note that aggregates are by default applied to groups of all non-aggregated columns and, hence, computed at least on case groups. Row navigation with LAG/LEAD, in turn, operates on the whole table by default, so that a condition for a row can refer to rows from other cases. In pattern matching, this means that a behaviour can include dependent, not self-contained conditions. By using row navigation with a PARTITION BY clause on the **case-id** (or, equivalently for case partitioning, ACTIVITY_LAG/ACTIVITY_LEAD), one can ensure self-contained, dependent conditions. If neither aggregates nor row navigation is used, the behaviour conditions are always independent.

However, when using a CASE clause for behaviour definition, each row is assigned exactly *one* behaviour. To work around this limitation, one would need to leverage the string processing capabilities of PQL. That is, for each row, each behaviour is evaluated with a separate CASE clause and the resulting string values are concatenated (CONCAT or short | |) in the **behaviour** column. In the pattern matching, the presence of a behaviour in this string is assessed using the LIKE operator, which we illustrate with the query in Listing 5 that is discussed later.

MATCH_RECOGNIZE. In the MATCH_RECOGNIZE clause, behaviours are constructed in the DEFINE clause that includes a name followed by (AS) by the respective conditions. An example is given in Listing 4, where the behaviours **order_300**, **payment_received**, and **order_shipped** are defined. The conditions may include comparisons, logical operators, LIKE/ILIKE, IS NULL; they may refer to aggregates, and neighbouring rows PREVIOUS/NEXT. Therefore, depending on the partitioning of aggregates and row navigation functions, such a query can contain either not self-contained or self-contained conditions. Only if aggregates and row navigation are not used, the behaviour conditions are independent.

By default, undefined behaviours assign the value TRUE to any row. However, a placeholder behaviour that matches any row can also be modelled more explicitly using ANY, which we use in our examples.

Turning to the translation of SIGNAL queries to SQL, the behaviours defined in a WHERE BEHAVIOUR clause and in a MATCHES clause, need to be specified in the DEFINE clause of MATCH_RECOGNIZE (as illustrated for the exemplary queries in Listing 1 and Listing 4). The same translation needs to be applied for the behaviours defined in PQL queries as part of one or more CASE clauses

```
1  SELECT case_id
2  FROM events
3  MATCH_RECOGNIZE (
4    PARTITION BY case_id
5    ORDER BY end_time
6    ONE ROW PER MATCH
7    PATTERN (^order_300 ANY* payment_received order_shipped$)
8    DEFINE order_300 AS event_name = 'Order received' AND order_value > 300,
9          payment_received AS event_name = 'Payment received',
10         order_shipped AS event_name = 'Order shipped')
```

Listing 4. Example of an SQL query with `MATCH_RECOGNIZE`.

(see Listing 2 and Listing 4). If `MATCH_PROCESS_REGEX` is used without `CASE` clauses, each behaviour in the PQL pattern is translated into an SQL behaviour using string equality or `LIKE`/`ILIKE` operators on the respective column.

We conclude that the definition of behaviours as realised in SIGNAL and PQL can be mapped to `MATCH_RECOGNIZE`.

3.3 Pattern Definition

In SIGNAL and PQL (with `MATCH_PROCESS_REGEX`), patterns are matched per case, considering the timestamp order of events. These notions of events and cases are translated to SQL using the `PARTITION BY` clause, to group the rows by the case identifier, and the `ORDER BY` clause, to order events by timestamps.

To define a pattern, all languages offer operators that are similar to regular expressions, as summarized in Table 2. Here, we first illustrate the operator semantics, using E to denote a set of events (rows) of a single case and $\succ \subseteq E \times E$ as the temporal order over E, before giving the pattern definitions in SIGNAL, PQL, and `MATCH_RECOGNIZE` in SQL. Table 2 highlights many similarities among the languages. As such, a translation of SIGNAL and PQL patterns into the `PATTERN` clause of `MATCH_RECOGNIZE` is straight-forward, except for two aspects.

First, to ensure that only a single match of a pattern per case is returned, partition-wise maximal matching needs to be enforced in SQL. That is, if a SIGNAL/PQL query does not include the *starts/ends with* operators, they need to be added in the `MATCH_RECOGNIZE` pattern as `^ANY*` and `ANY*$`.

Second, SQL lacks a pattern operator for *does not contain*. To achieve the respective semantics, an auxiliary behaviour needs to be defined with the logical NOT operator, which is then used in the pattern definition.

We illustrate these aspects of the translation with the PQL query in Listing 5. It exemplifies the aforementioned approach to represent multiple behaviours per row through string concatenation. That is, the two `CASE` clauses yield a **behaviour** column that contains a concatenated string 'beh_invoice_d2,beh_d2,' as value if a row satisfies both conditions. In addition, the PQL example includes a *does not contain* operator, which is realized by

Table 2. Operators for the definition of a pattern.

Operator	Semantics $(a, b \in E, a \neq b)$	SIGNAL	PQL	SQL
Directly follows	$a \succ b, \nexists\, c \in E \setminus \{a,b\}[a \succ c \wedge c \succ b]$	a -> b	a $\gg$ b	a b
Follows	$a \succ b$	a ~> b	a $\gg$ (ANY)* $\gg$ b	a (ANY)* b
Starts with	$\forall\, c \in E \setminus \{a\} : a \succ c$	^a	^a	^a
Ends with	$\forall\, c \in E \setminus \{a\} : c \succ a$	a$	a$	a$
Contains any	$\exists\, c \in E : a \succ c, c \succ b$	a ANY b	a $\gg$ ANY $\gg$ b	a ANY b
Does not contain	$\nexists\, c \in E$	NOT c	[!c]	/
Alternation	$a \vee b$	a | b	a | b	a | b
Permutation	$(a \succ b) \vee (b \succ a)$	(a -> b)|(b -> a)	(a $\gg$ b)|(b $\gg$ a)	PERMUTE(a, b)
Repetition (≥ 0)	$\bigcup_{i=0}^{\infty} a^i$	a*	a*	a*
Repetition (≥ 1)	$\bigcup_{i=1}^{\infty} a^i$	a+	a+	a+
0 - 1 occurrences	$a \vee \epsilon$	a?	a?	a?
x - y occurrences	$\bigcup_{i=x}^{y} a^i$	a{x, y}	a{x, y}	a{x, y}
One from set	$a \vee b \vee c$ with $c \in E \setminus \{a,b\}$	(a | (b | c))	[a,b,c]	(a | (b | c))

† The operators are available in SIGNAL, but not yet described in the public documentation.

```
1  CASE WHEN "Activities"."Activity" = 'Invoice sent'
2      AND "Activities"."Department" = 'D2' THEN 'beh_invoice_d2,',
3  ELSE ''
4  END ||
5  CASE WHEN "Activities"."Department" = 'D2' THEN 'beh_d2,',
6  ELSE ''
7  END
8  FILTER MATCH_PROCESS_REGEX("Activities"."behaviour",
9  LIKE '%beh_invoice_d2%' >> [! %'beh_d2,'%]) = 1;
```

Listing 5. PQL query with NOT operator and concatenated CASE clauses.

a check for the negated behaviour **not_d2** in the corresponding SQL query in Listing 6. Finally, the example highlights that the absence of *starts/ends with* operators in the PQL query requires the insertion of ^ANY* and ANY*$ in the SQL query to achieve an equivalent expression.

3.4 Query Output

Turning to the capabilities of the languages to define the structure of the generated output, we first note that SIGNAL and PQL operate on cases as output instances. That is, if a pattern is matched at least once, the entire corresponding case is included in the construction of the result, as detailed below.

SIGNAL. The SELECT clause may contain attributes on the case or event level, as well as aggregates over them. The output is a nested table with all specified attributes and aggregates for all matched cases. Matching in SIGNAL is existential, i.e., one satisfied match of behaviours per case is sufficient [5].

```
1  SELECT case_id
2  FROM events
3  MATCH_RECOGNIZE (
4     PARTITION BY case_id
5     ORDER BY end_time
6     ONE ROW PER MATCH
7     PATTERN (^ANY* invoice_d2 not_d2 ANY*$)
8     DEFINE invoice_d2 AS event_name = 'Invoice sent' AND department = 'D2'
9        not_d2 AS NOT(department = 'D2'))
```

Listing 6. SQL query with NOT operator.

PQL. A temporary column is added to the **Case** table, which contains 1 if a pattern is found in a case; and 0 otherwise. Using a FILTER=1 statement, all rows of all matched cases may be selected.

MATCH_RECOGNIZE. The result structure is defined in the SELECT clause, while the MEASURES clause of MATCH_RECOGNIZE further facilitates the computation of aggregates and the use of match-specific functions. When translating a SIGNAL query to SQL, columns at either case or event level as well as aggregates over them need to be included in SQL's SELECT statement. If the chosen columns are only on the case level, MATCH_RECOGNIZE is used with ONE ROW PER MATCH; otherwise ALL ROWS PER MATCH has to be selected. In PQL, when selecting matching cases by FILTER=1, all attributes from all rows of the matched cases are returned. In SQL, SELECT * with ALL ROWS PER MATCH mirrors this behaviour.

4   Related Work

Academic process query languages typically have their roots in process modelling and mining, and may thus query either process models [1,4,11] or process event data [8,9], in the latter case typically in the form of event logs. Industry-scale process query languages tend to focus on the querying of event data, presumably because process models are queried using mainstream relational and document-based approaches, where aspects specific to the domain of BPM may be lifted to the business logic level. For (process) event data, the two languages described above are *the* two key examples of domain-specific process query languages that have already been described in the literature.

However, process querying is rarely integrated into the wealth of database management research. Notable examples include approaches for the discovery of declarative process specifications, which employ standard SQL to query for behavioural patterns [12–14]. Here, the conditions that need to be verified to instantiate constraint templates are particularly suitable to be expressed as declarative queries. For imperative models, the efficient extraction of control-flow dependencies is less straight-forward, which led to efforts to implement dedicated operators directly in the database management system [3].

Turning to generic languages for process querying, little work focused on a comparison of these languages with mainstream database languages such as

SQL, or with languages that are theoretically well understood, such as Datalog. In [6], the analysis of expressive power and data complexity of SIGNAL is based on a characterisation of the core of SIGNAL using semi-positive Datalog; i.e., here the mapping from process query language to a (theoretically well understood) database query language aids formal analysis.

In contrast, our focus has been the use of standard SQL for process querying, showing that the MATCH_RECOGNIZE clause is sufficient to query for behavioural patterns as supported by SIGNAL and PQL. We believe that our results make a compelling case for the value of inquiry also in this direction, with the objective of making process querying more straightforwardly applicable, using the technologies that tend to be readily available in large-scale (enterprise) information systems.

5   Conclusions

In this paper, we demonstrated that behavioural queries in two industry-scale process query languages can be mapped to standard SQL. Our intuitive analysis raises some technical questions, most notably regarding *i)* the performance of MATCH_RECOGNIZE implementations when querying large event logs (e.g., with billions of entries) and *ii)* the theoretical data complexity and expressive power of MATCH_RECOGNIZE. Answering these questions may be particularly interesting relative to the characteristics of real-world process querying languages, whose scalability, complexity, and expressive power are (also) understudied. Beyond these technical aspects, our results can serve as a starting point enabling process querying and mining directly in the ecosystem of mainstream database systems. For example, it may enable process mining with the standard query languages of enterprise systems' relational databases, as well as in data lakehouses that collect process data of multiple organisations for the purpose of benchmarking.

References

1. Awad, A., Sakr, S.: On efficient processing of bpmn-q queries. Comput. Ind. **63**(9), 867–881 (2012)
2. Carmona, J., van Dongen, B.F., Solti, A., Weidlich, M.: Conformance Checking - Relating Processes and Models. Springer, Heidelberg (2018)
3. Dijkman, R.M., Gao, J., Syamsiyah, A., van Dongen, B.F., Grefen, P., ter Hofstede, A.H.M.: Enabling efficient process mining on large data sets: realizing an in-database process mining operator. Distrib. Parallel Datab. **38**(1), 227–253 (2020)
4. Francescomarino, C.D., Tonella, P.: The BPMN visual query language and process querying framework. In: Polyvyanyy, A. (ed.) Process Querying Methods, pp. 181–218. Springer, Heidelberg (2022). https://doi.org/10.1007/978-3-030-92875-9_7
5. Kampik, T., Lücke, A., Horstmann, J., Wheeler, M., Eickhoff, D.: Signal – the sap signavio analytics query language (2023)
6. Kampik, T., Okulmus, C.: Expressive power and complexity results for signal, an industry-scale process query language. In: BPM Forum 2024. LNBIP. Springer, Heidelberg (2024). https://doi.org/10.1007/978-3-031-70418-5_1

7. Michels, J., et al.: The new and improved sql: 2016 standard. SIGMOD Rec. **47**(2), 51–60 (2018)
8. de Murillas, E.G.L., Reijers, H.A., van der Aalst, W.M.P.: Data-aware process oriented query language. In: Polyvyanyy, A. (ed.) Process Querying Methods, pp. 49–83. Springer, Heidelberg (2022). https://doi.org/10.1007/978-3-030-92875-9_3
9. Pérez-Álvarez, J.M., Díaz, A.C., Parody, L., Quintero, A.M.R., Gómez-López, M.T.: Process instance query language and the process querying framework. In: Polyvyanyy, A. (ed.) Process Querying Methods, pp. 85–111. Springer, Heidelberg (2022). DOI: https://doi.org/10.1007/978-3-030-92875-9_4
10. Petkovic, D.: Specification of row pattern recognition in the SQL standard and its implementations. Datenbank-Spektrum **22**(2), 163–174 (2022)
11. Polyvyanyy, A.: Process query language. In: Process Querying Methods, pp. 313–341. Springer, Heidelberg (2022). https://doi.org/10.1007/978-3-030-92875-9_11
12. Riva, F., Benvenuti, D., Maggi, F.M., Marrella, A., Montali, M.: An sql-based declarative process mining framework for analyzing process data stored in relational databases. In: BPM Forum 2023. LNBIP, vol. 490, pp. 214–231. Springer, Heidelberg (2023). https://doi.org/10.1007/978-3-031-41623-1_13
13. Schönig, S., Ciccio, C.D., Mendling, J.: Configuring sql-based process mining for performance and storage optimisation. In: ACM/SIGAPP SAC 2019, pp. 94–97. ACM (2019)
14. Schönig, S., Rogge-Solti, A., Cabanillas, C., Jablonski, S., Mendling, J.: Efficient and customisable declarative process mining with SQL. In: Nurcan, S., Soffer, P., Bajec, M., Eder, J. (eds.) CAiSE 2016. LNCS, vol. 9694, pp. 290–305. Springer, Cham (2016). https://doi.org/10.1007/978-3-319-39696-5_18
15. Vogelgesang, T., Ambrosy, J., Becher, D., Seilbeck, R., Geyer-Klingeberg, J., Klenk, M.: Celonis PQL: a query language for process mining. In: Process Querying Methods, pp. 377–408. Springer, Heidelberg (2022). https://doi.org/10.1007/978-3-030-92875-9_13
16. Zhu, E., Huang, S., Chaudhuri, S.: High-performance row pattern recognition using joins. Proc. VLDB Endow. **16**(5), 1181–1194 (2023)

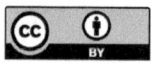

EVErPREP: Towards an Event Knowledge Graph Enhanced Workflow Model for Event Log Preparation

Peter Filipp[1]([✉])[ID], Rene Dorsch[1][ID], and Andreas Harth[1,2][ID]

[1] Fraunhofer Institute for Integrated Circuits, Nuremberg, Germany
{peter.filipp,rene.dorsch}@iis.fraunhofer.de, andreas.harth@fau.de
[2] Friedrich-Alexander University Erlangen-Nuremberg, Erlangen, Germany

Abstract. Event data preparation is a critical yet time-consuming phase in process mining projects, often slowed down by complex relational data models and a lack of domain knowledge. This paper presents EVErPREP, a novel workflow model that leverages Event Knowledge Graphs to enhance event data preparation for event logs. EVErPREP uses Semantic Web technologies to improve the exploration, extraction, and processing of event data, ultimately improving the quality and interpretability of event data and event logs. The approach is evaluated through a case study at Munich Airport's Baggage Handling System, demonstrating its effectiveness in reducing complexity and improving explainability in event data preparation. By providing a more structured and semantically enriched foundation for process mining, EVErPREP showcases increased efficiency and effectiveness of process mining projects through a semantically enriched foundation.

Keywords: Process Mining · Event Log Preparation · Knowledge Graph

1 Introduction

Process Mining (PM) has emerged as a research area that provides powerful, data-driven algorithms for improving and understanding processes. Process mining algorithms provide valuable insights into process behavior through automated discovery of process models, detection of deviations from designed processes, and analysis of key performance indicators [21]. As a result, PM has found applications in various domains, from business process workflows [22] to healthcare processes [14] and production [2].

PM algorithms are often based on event logs [20], structured records containing information about process instances, their activities, timestamps, and attributes. While event logs are crucial for PM, preparing them for analysis is a critical and often underestimated phase in PM projects, consuming up to 80% of the total project time [24]. Process Mining methodologies facilitating event log preparation have been proposed, to streamline activities that transition event data and process related domain knowledge to event logs. The Process Diagnostic Method (PDM) [1] was an early PM methodology designed to analyze processes from a single information system. However it did not address complex system environments and the planning phase of PM. The L* Life

ⓒ The Author(s) 2025
A. Delgado and T. Slaats (Eds.): ICPM 2024 Workshops, LNBIP 533, pp. 31–43, 2025.
https://doi.org/10.1007/978-3-031-82225-4_3

Cycle Model [20] has been proposed to extend the scope to include a planning and justification phase at the beginning of a PM project. The Process Mining Project Methodology (PM²) [22] further extends the preparation phase by separating it into three phases - planning, selection, and processing - and providing more detailed guidelines. Despite these methodological advances, activities related to explainability (e.g., poor documentation, unavailability of process experts), complexity (e.g., complex data structures), and data handling (e.g., identification of relevant data attributes) are still common and not sufficiently addressed by the methodologies [24], thus limiting their efficiency and effectiveness. As a result, many tasks in the preparation phase remain manual, unstructured, and knowledge-intensive [19].

To address knowledge-intensive tasks, researchers explored various processing approaches, data representations formats, and data integration methods. Event Knowledge Graphs (EKG) have demonstrated the ability to provide multiple views of event data, addressing data variety and complexity [12, 15]. RDF-based Knowledge Graphs (KG) have been widely used to facilitate data integration from multiple sources [7, 17, 18]. In addition, the application of ontologies within PM has shown promise in increasing the interpretability of event data by adding a semantic layer to the analysis [3].

Building on these advances, we propose EVErPREP, an EKG-enhanced workflow model for event log preparation. Our workflow model aims to support all event log preparation activities through the use of KGs. EVErPREP enables dynamic aggregation of data to handle different granularities, thereby reducing complexity; it supports the generation of dynamic views of event data, thereby reducing information overload in the preparation phase; and EVErPREP facilitates integrated knowledge acquisition through URIs used as identifiers for attributes and case IDs, thereby improving context availability where necessary.

Through EVErPREP, we aim to demonstrate how KG can facilitate persistent challenges in event log preparation, ultimately improving the efficiency and effectiveness of PM projects. Our contributions include:

- A workflow model for event log preparation using EKG.
- A case study from the workflow model at the Munich Airport.
- An evaluation of the workflow model's impact on event data preparation challenges in knowledge intensive tasks.

2   Background

In recent years, researchers have explored EKGs and Semantic Process Mining (SPM) to address issues related to knowledge-intensive tasks.

EKGs are studied within PM to represent and analyze event data. A KG is a system that captures and integrates information and applies a reasoner and ontologies to derive new knowledge [4]. EKGs extend this definition by including relationships between events, between events and entities, and between entities [8].

The Resource Description Framework (RDF) is widely used to represent KGs, facilitating data integration from disparate sources and multi-stakeholder environments [18]. RDF [13] provides a standardized framework for describing the instance and schema levels of a KG. SPARQL [9] is used as a powerful query language for pattern matching within graph structures. Adopting these open standards has been shown to improve the discoverability, accessibility, interoperability, and reusability of data [7, 17].

EKGs have two levels to capture information: the instance level and the schema level. The instance level of EKGs focuses on data graphs consisting of events and entities, and relationships as edges. The instance level has been studied and documented in several works [6, 11, 12, 15]. Fahland et al. [6] demonstrated that this approach enables complex analysis and facilitates the discovery of complex dynamics within processes, such as subprocesses with dynamic bottlenecks or high workloads. Khayatbashi et al. [11] compared the graph representation with object-centric event logs. They reported that data graphs can better handle relationships of complex, multifaceted processes. In addition, data graphs can overcome memory limitations by storing data on disk for processing and analysis, and can increase the efficiency of analysis by supporting different views. The schema layer specifies domain-specific meta models and the event model within ontologies. Ontologies define and formalize the knowledge of process experts through shared concepts, improving analysis through relationships and properties between and of concepts. SPM applies ontologies within PM to enable data analysis of complex data structures, and increase understandability and interpretability of process models [5, 10, 16]. Eichele et al. [5] presented a method for reasoning about and justifying of process activities, thereby improving process explainability. Nykänen et al. [16] proposed an approach that links ontology structures with event logs to achieve different levels of abstraction.

In summary, by incorporating rich metadata, EKGs and SPM provide a comprehensive framework for understanding, integrating, and analyzing complex event data, addressing many of the persistent challenges of event log preparation and analysis in PM projects.

3 EVErPREP Workflow Model

We present in this section EVErPREP. Our approach to PM preparation relies on EKGs to facilitate the discovery, accessibility, and usability of event data. Furthermore, EVErPREP assumes that data from systems and the knowledge of process experts are already integrated in the EKG. EVErPREP consists of three consecutive phases (see Fig. 1):

1. Event Knowledge Graph Exploration: Explores the graph to discover entities, events, and attributes relevant to the specific process mining research questions (PMRQs).
2. Event Log Extraction: Extracts a referenceable minimal semantic event log based on the relevant entities, events, and attributes from the EKG.
3. Event Log Processing: Consolidates and aggregates the event log using the EKG to generate different views and levels of abstraction.

3.1 Phase 1) Event Knowledge Graph Exploration

The goal of the exploration phase is to discover the data sources and domain knowledge integrated into the EKG. The exploration supports the identification of relevant entities for analysis based on the PMRQ and its scope. The input to the exploration phase is the

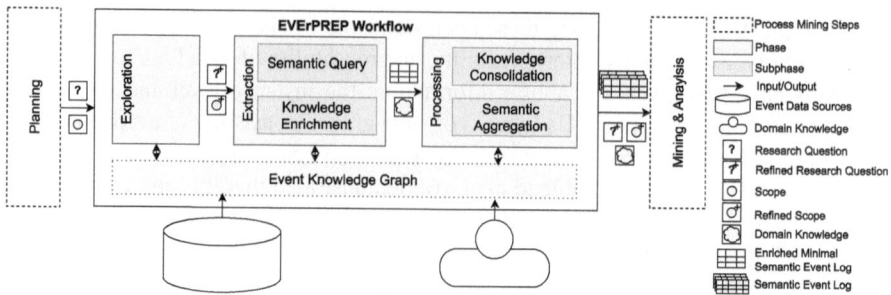

Fig. 1. EVErPREP Workflow

specific PMRQ, the scope of the PM projects, and the EKG. At the end of this phase, analysts have gained valuable knowledge about relevant entities and their context within a domain.

The exploration phase includes three main interconnected activities: graph structure analysis, knowledge retrieval, and creation of initial views. The activities are interrelated and iterative, each informing and refining the others. During graph structure analysis, analysts examine the instance and schema levels of the EKG to gather general information about the domain. Knowledge retrieval involves extracting process-related information relevant to the PMRQ and its scope from the EKG. As the analyst accumulates insights from both the graph structure analysis and the knowledge retrieval, they create and refine the initial views to guide the next steps in the process mining project.

3.2 Phase 2) Event Log Extraction

The extraction phase aims to generate an initial semantically annotated event log. The phase builds upon the results of the exploration phase and consists of two sub phases: semantic querying and knowledge enrichment.

Phase 2.1) Semantic Querying: This phase aims to specify views through semantic queries with semantic filters, simplifying the handling of complex event data early in the preparation process. This activity takes as input the domain knowledge, graph structure, retrieved entities, and PMRQ, resulting in a semantically annotated minimal event log. The event log consists only of columns for the relevant entities and the timestamps. The referencing enables knowledge acquisition through the EKG in subsequent steps.

During semantic querying, analysts formulate specific queries for the EKG, considering key objects identified in the exploration phase. SPARQL queries are applied for semantic querying and filtering of the minimal event log to reduce the amount of extracted data. The query scope is defined using the retrieved entities and the PMRQ. Cases and events of the event log are linked to their respective entities in the EKG using URIs.

Phase 2.2) Knowledge Enrichment: Following semantic querying, the knowledge enrichment phase focuses on obtaining precise descriptions of activities in the process context. This activity has as input the EKG and the minimal semantically annotated event log. The result is an enriched minimal event log extended with additional information for relevant attributes and event descriptions.

Precise descriptions can be obtained from a EKG within the instance level through attributes and entities, or within the schema level through classes. On the instance level, descriptive annotations (e.g., labels and comments) relating to the individual activities are obtained. Additional objects and attributes can be added as resources in PM or for further filtering. On the schema level, class specific information (e.g., class type, class comments and labels) can be obtained. This information aids in understanding the background of specific events or event constellations. The information at class level is particularly relevant for the semantics-based aggregation of events, which is discussed below.

3.3   Phase 3) Event Log Processing
The processing phase takes the enriched data from the extraction phase and refines it further through two sub phases: knowledge consolidation and semantic aggregation.

Phase 3.1) Knowledge Consolidation: The phase aims to integrate enriched information at the desired granularity level within the process context. This phase utilizes references from the semantic event log and the EKG as inputs. The output is a semantic event log incorporated with consolidated knowledge from the EKG, resulting in a more coherent, harmonized representation of key information. The primary challenge addressed in this step is the misalignment between EKG structure and process descriptions. EKGs typically contain varied granular knowledge, manifested as multiple labels and comments, due to inheritance hierarchies and varying detail levels in entity descriptions. This diversity, while rich in information, can complicate process analysis.

The consolidation process involves three key steps: identifying relevant knowledge, integrating diverse perspectives, and consolidation. Analysts identify relevant knowledge by determining which labels and comments from the EKG are most relevant to the PMRQ. They then integrate diverse perspectives by identifying different viewpoints on cases and events within the context of the analysis problem. Finally, the consolidation step involves choosing and combining labels and comments based on their availability and information content, ensuring activities are accurately described.

Phase 3.2) Semantic Aggregation: It aims to create an aggregated semantic event log that provides a higher-level view of the process, facilitating analysis more specific to the PMRQ while maintaining the semantic richness of the original event data. The semantic aggregation has as input the PMRQ and the enriched and consolidated information from the previous steps. The result of the semantic aggregation is an event log (e.g. in XES format) suitable for standard process mining algorithms.

The semantic aggregation process involves two main tasks: defining aggregation rules and performing contextual semantic aggregation. Aggregation rules establish semantic equivalence between event data, even when their syntactic descriptions differ. This allows for meaningful grouping of semantically similar events. Contextual semantic aggregation then applies these rules to the consolidated semantic event log data from the previous subphase, facilitating the creation of higher-level abstract activities that align with the analysis goal.

4   Case Study: Airport Munich

EVErPREP is a workflow model to facilitate the preparation phase of process mining projects in knowledge intensive processes where EKGs are already used. Our evaluation focused on answering the following research questions:

1. (RQ1) How can an Event Knowledge Graph be used to make an event log and its processing more explainable?
2. (RQ2) How can EVErPREP help to reduce complexity in event log handling?
3. (RQ3) How can EVErPREP support the accessibility of data and knowledge in PM projects?

To answer the RQs, we evaluated our approach within a case study of the Baggage Handling System (BHS) at the Airport Munich.

Characteristic of the Process: The BHS is a critical and highly complex system of the airport. It is critical because delays have a direct effect on other processes (e.g. boarding of passengers, departure flights). Complexity is created by thousands of sensors scanning the baggage at different locations within the BHS, multiple involved actors (airlines, baggage handlers), multiple modules transporting the baggage to their destination location, different business variants (handling inbound-, outbound-, and transferbaggage), and different resolution grades (baggage, passenger, container). Through the large amount of messages generated about a specific baggage, a syntactic analysis of the BHS without further domain knowledge is not suitable.

Process Mining Scope and Research Question: The Airline AirL (pseudonymized) offers a number of scheduled flights to a variety of destinations, with passengers checking in at different terminals and boarding gates. Once checked in, the baggage items are sorted transported within the different modules of the BHS until they reach the correct destination. To identify bottlenecks and understand the process of AirL better, the following PMRQ needs to be addressed: *"What is the actual baggage transfer process regarding automated baggage handling within Terminal 1 for Airline AirL?"*

Event Knowledge Graph: The EKG of the BHS uses for the schema level a domain-specific ontology, and the Simple Event Model Ontology (SEM) [23]. The domain-specific ontology describes the domain of the BHS with static concepts, such as sensor type, baggage types, airlines, and passengers. The SEM is used as a process metamodel to model events with their actors, activities, locations, and time. Actors are specific baggages, passengers, containers, and airplanes. Locations are described through the position of the sensors within the BHS. Activities are feedback from sensors that scanned baggages at specific positions within the BHS. RDF is used to instantiate the ontologies and the data from the BHS. Reasoning with OWL is used to derive hierarchies from the domain model and link differently named data points from the data sources with each other under a standardized description. Domain knowledge was derived from documentations, location specific information, and domain experts. The domain knowledge is attached to the instance and schema level concepts and relations of the EKG.

An excerpt of the EKG can be seen in Fig. 2. We used prefixes to shorten the URIs within the figure and the SPARQL query to improve readability. Common prefixes such as *rdfs:* can also be found on https://prefix.cc.

4.1 Execution of the Workflow

In this section we present the execution of EVErPREP on Munich Airport case study to answer their PMRQ. We describe the execution and the results of each step in the EVErPREP workflow.

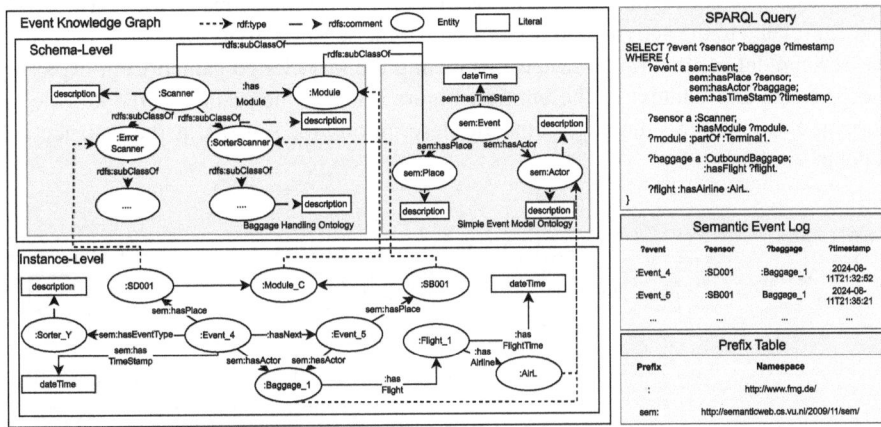

Fig. 2. Snippet of the EKG (left) with reduced relationships and basic SPARQL query and results for semantic querying (right)

Phase 1) Exploration: The goal of this phase was to discover and understand the relevant entities, relationships, and context within the EKG that were relevant to answering the PMRQ. Therefore, the EKG was explored with SPARQL queries. The initial queries were primarily designed to discover and describe concepts to answer the PMRQ. The initial queries focused on schema-level descriptions from the domain ontology to support a high-level understanding of the EKG. Based on the schema-level concepts, instances such as terminals, modules, flights, airlines, sensors, and baggage types were discovered. In addition, annotations within the BHS, such as descriptions and provenance information, were retrieved to provide additional context to the concepts. Based on the metadata and the PMRQ, a selection of relevant entities was discovered. To describe the process, relationships between entities were retrieved based on the SEM ontology and the domain ontology. The result of the exploration step with the EKG of the airport contained four core concepts, the baggage, the sensors, the locations associated with the sensors, and the events associating the baggage with the sensors.

Phase 2.1) Semantic Querying: This phase focused on creating a minimal semantic event log through semantic queries with filters, based on the insights gained from the exploration phase. The scope of the semantic query was limited to the four main concepts identified in the exploration phase and the constraints from the PMRQ. The constraints included the location to Terminal 1 and the baggage handled by the airline AirL. The events modeled with SEM were retrieved with a SPARQL query to create the semantic event log. Figure 2 shows the query and a slice of its results, which include the timestamp and URIs for the sensors, baggage, and events.

Phase 2.2) Knowledge Enrichment: The enrichment phase aimed at enriching the minimal semantic event log with detailed descriptions and contextual information for activities and events using the data within the EKG. This was limited to information that contributed to a self-explanatory process model. Due to the scope of the PMRQ, only content related to the activity and background of the sensor activity was used. To do this, the enrichment scripts traversed the EKG using the knowledge gained from exploring the structure and context of the entities. Figure 3 shows the results of the knowledge enrichment, including multiple semantic descriptions for sensors at the instance and schema levels.

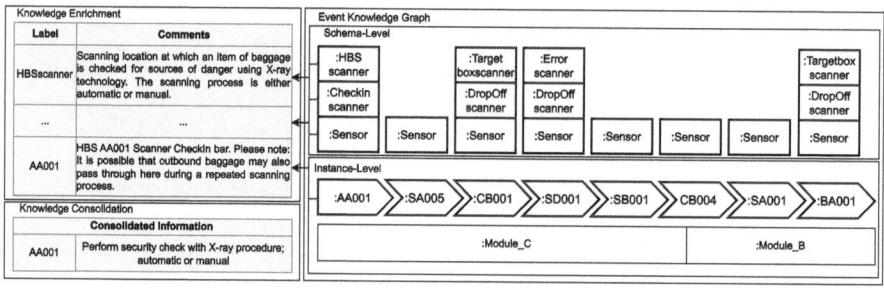

Fig. 3. Knowledge enrichment and consolidation for the sensor AA001 to combine different descriptions from the instance and schema level based on the scope and the PMRQ

Phase 3.1) Knowledge Consolidation: This phase involved integrating and harmonizing the enriched information at the desired granularity within the process context, PMRQ, and analyst understanding. Based on the results of Phase 2.2, the process model derived from the semantic event log would have contained several semantically similar variants. Consolidation was necessary because the EKG was not specifically designed to answer the specific PMRQ and therefore contains differently structured descriptions at different levels. Through consolidation, semantically similar descriptions were aligned using the OpenRefine[1] tool. An example of such an alignment is shown in Fig. 3 for the sensor with the URI *:AA001*. The alignment for all activities has been recorded in the semantic event log in a new column containing the consolidated activity description.

Phase 3.2) Semantic Aggregation: Semantic aggregation aimed to provide a higher-level view of the process by aggregating events based on semantic similarities, facilitating PMRQ-specific analysis. Thus, the aggregation is based on the enriched and

---

[1] https://openrefine.org/.

consolidated information from the semantic event log. Based on the PMRQ, hierarchies were created within the domain model for sensor types and baggage types. For each of the hierarchies, domain knowledge based on comments and labels was retrieved with SPARQL queries to create aggregations of events (see Fig. 4). The final semantic event log was based on the PMRQ associated with different levels of abstraction of the BHS to facilitate dynamic views of the process. From the semantically enriched and aggregated event log, different views were extracted in XES format for the following process mining analysis.

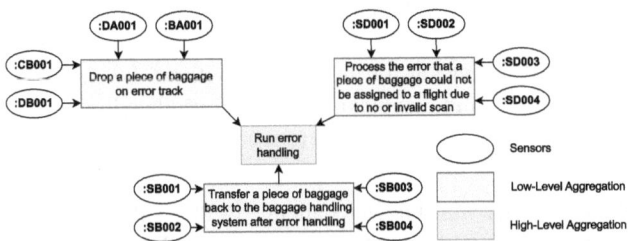

Fig. 4. Semantic aggregation to achieve a higher-level view of the process

4.2 Observations

This section presents key observations from its application to the case study regarding explainability, complexity, and data handling when EVErPREP is used for event log preparation.

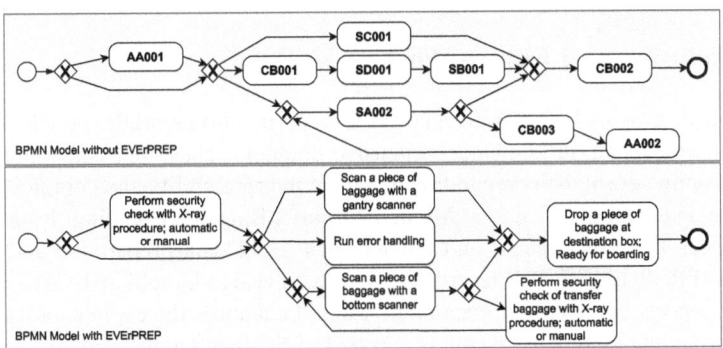

Fig. 5. Excerpt of the process model of a flight without and with EVErPREP

Explainability: A persistent challenge in PM is interpreting event logs with insufficient context, leading to misunderstandings of process behaviors [24]. Enrichment with knowledge from the EKG has significantly improved the clarity of activity descriptions within their overall context, making individual events and their sequences more comprehensible. Furthermore, the flexibility of this enrichment allows for adjusting the level of detail in process descriptions. For instance, Fig. 5 shows for the activity *AA002* the more explainable semantic description of the activities aligned with the scope of the PMRQ. This adaptability enables tailoring the information to match the analysts' knowledge level, based on the content available in the EKG.

Complexity: Managing the inherent complexity of event logs, particularly those with numerous variants, often hinders effective process analysis and interpretation [24]. Semantic aggregation, built upon semantic enrichment, has effectively reduced complexity in the extracted event logs. This approach has streamlined activity descriptions to essential, concise components. Figure 5 shows the impact of EVErPREP, its associated knowledge consolidation, and the final semantic aggregation on the process model extracted from the AirL event log for the three activities *CB001*, *SD001*, and *SB001*. The results show a reduction in complexity and improved handling of the event log for subsequent analyses, particularly in relation to more concise case variants.

Event Data Handling: A well-known challenge in PM is the handling of large event logs that are merged from a wide variety of systems [20]. The pre-existing data integration of airport systems within the EKG provides valuable information, allowing early identification of attributes relevant to specific PMRQ. This integration enables semantic querying of only essential data for core event log requirements at an early stage. Consequently, attributes irrelevant to PMRQ can be excluded from queries and further data pre-processing, contributing to a more efficient workflow.

In summary, the use of EVErPREP in the case study demonstrates that the explainability of objects, resources, and activities; the reduction in complexity; and the simplified accessibility and usability of event data contribute to a notable enhancement in the effectiveness and efficiency of the data processing step.

5   Conclusion and Future Work

This paper introduces EVErPREP, an event data preparation workflow model designed to address challenges in knowledge-intensive domains. These domains often require time-consuming event data preparation to handle interpretability and complexity issues within the data. Our case study at Munich Airport's Baggage Handling System (BHS) demonstrates the effectiveness and efficiency of event data preparation and analysis with EVErPREP. EVErPREP leverages Event Knowledge Graphs (EKGs) to improve three key aspects of event log preparation. First, it enhances the explainability of event data by providing contextual meaning. Second, it facilitates improved comprehension of complex event data through the consolidation and semantic aggregation of information, based on the structure and semantics of the underlying EKG. Third, EVErPREP improves the handling of complex event data bases by dynamically integrating attributes into the event log through dereferenceable URIs. Our case study results show that EVErPREP improves the explainability for non-domain experts of event data within the BHS. It also reduces complexity by providing more concise and meaningful activity descriptions. Furthermore, the approach simplifies data accessibility and usability, contributing to enhanced effectiveness and efficiency in the data processing step.

Future research directions include investigating the influence of EVErPREP on the overall data quality of processed event logs. Another promising area is exploring methods to instantiate and integrate domain knowledge derived from EVErPREP and process mining analysis back into the EKG. This could include incorporating consolidated activity-based descriptions or derived process models as additional annotations. Furthermore, EVErPREP could be enhanced by including semi-automated approaches for consolidation and aggregation using natural language processing techniques to improve the efficiency of event data preparation. Such enhancements to the EVErPREP workflow would further streamline the process mining workflow and reduces key challenges of process mining [24].

In conclusion, EVErPREP offers a promising approach for streamlining event data handling, pre-processing, and interpretation in knowledge-intensive domains. By addressing key challenges in event log preparation, it paves the way for more efficient and effective process mining analyses, particularly in complex environments like airport operations.

Author Contributions and Acknowledgements. Conceptualization, P.F. and R.D.; methodology, P.F. and R.D.; writing - original draft preparation, P.F. and R.D.; writing - review and editing, P.F. and R.D; supervision A.H.; funding acquisition, A.H.

This work was funded by the Bayerisches Verbundforschungsprogramm (BayVFP) des Freistaates Bayern through the KIWI project (grant no. DIK0318/03) and by the German Federal Ministry for Economic Affairs and Climate Action (BMWK) through the Antrieb 4.0 project (Grant No. 13IK015B).

References

1. Bozkaya, M., et al.: Process diagnostics: a method based on process mining. In: 2009 International Conference on Information, Process, and Knowledge Management (2009). https://doi.org/10.1109/eKNOW.2009.29
2. Choueiri, A.C.C., Santos, E.A.P.: Multi-product scheduling through process mining: bridging optimization and machine process intelligence. J. Intell. Manuf. **6** (2021). https://doi.org/10.1007/s10845-021-01767-2
3. de Medeiros, A.K.A., Pedrinaci, C., van der Aalst, W.M.P., Domingue, J., Song, M., Rozinat, A., Norton, B., Cabral, L.: An outlook on semantic business process mining and monitoring. In: Meersman, R., Tari, Z., Herrero, P. (eds.) OTM 2007. LNCS, vol. 4806, pp. 1244–1255. Springer, Heidelberg (2007). https://doi.org/10.1007/978-3-540-76890-6_52
4. Ehrlinger, L., Wöß, W.: Towards a definition of knowledge graphs. In: 1st International Workshop on Semantic Change & Evolving Semantics (2016)
5. Eichele, S., Hinkelmann, K., Spahic-Bogdanovic, M.: Ontology- driven enhancement of process mining with domain knowledge (2023)
6. Fahland, D.: Process mining over multiple behavioral dimensions with event knowledge graphs. In: Process Mining Handbook. Springer, Cham (2022). https://doi.org/10.1007/978-3-031-08848-3_9
7. Freund, M., Rott, J., Harth, A.: FAIR Internet of Things data: enabling process optimization at Munich airport. In: ESWC: Extended Semantic Web Conference. Hersonissos, Greece (2024). https://doi.org/10.1007/978-3-031-60626-7

8. Guan, S., et al.: What is event knowledge graph: a survey. IEEE Trans. Knowl. Data Eng. (2021)

9. Harris, S., Seaborne, A.: SPARQL 1.1 Query Language. W3C Recommendation. W3C (2013)

10. Issahaku, F.Y., et al.: An overview of semantic-based process mining techniques: trends and future directions. Knowl. Inf. Syst. (2024). https://doi.org/10.1007/s10115-024-02147-x

11. Khayatbashi, S., Hartig, O., Jalali, A.: Event knowledge graph to object-centric event logs: a comparative study for multi dimensional process analysis. In: Conceptual Modeling. Springer, Cham (2023). https://doi.org/10.1007/978-3-031-47262-6_12

12. Klijn, E.L., et al.: Event knowledge graphs for auditing: a case study. In: Process Mining Workshops. Springer, Cham (2024). https://doi.org/10.1007/978-3-031-56107-8_7

13. Lanthaler, M., Wood, D., Cyganiak, R.: RDF 1.1 Concepts and Abstract Syntax. W3C Recommendation. W3C (2014)

14. Mans, R.S., et al.: Process mining in healthcare: evaluating and exploiting operational healthcare processes. In: Springer Briefs in Business Process Management. Springer, Cham (2015). https://doi.org/10.1007/978-3-319-16071-9

15. Aali, M.N., et al.: Clinical event knowledge graphs: enriching healthcare event data with entities and clinical concepts - research paper. In: Process Mining Workshops. Springer, Cham (2024). https://doi.org/10.1007/978-3-031-56107-8_23

16. Nykänen, O., et al.: Associating event logs with ontologies for semantic process mining and analysis. In: Proceedings of the 19th International Academic Mindtrek Conference, Tampere, Finland (2015). https://doi.org/10.1145/2818187.2818273

17. Queralt-Rosinach, N., et al.: Applying the FAIR principles to data in a hospital: challenges and opportunities in a pandemic. J. Biomed. Semant. **1** (2022). https://doi.org/10.1186/s13326-022-00263-7

18. Rott, J., et al.: Breaking down barriers with knowledge graphs: data integration for cross-organizational process mining (2024). https://doi.org/10.1007/978-3-031-56107-8_38

19. Dani, V.S., et al.: Towards understanding the role of the human in event log extraction. In: Business Process Management Workshops. Springer, Cham (2022). https://doi.org/10.1007/978-3-030-94343-1_7

20. van der Aalst, W., et al.: Process mining manifesto. In: Business Process Management Workshops. Springer, Heidelberg (2012). https://doi.org/10.1007/978-3-642-28108-2_19

21. van der Aalst, W.M.P., et al.: Service interaction: patterns, formalization, and analysis. In: Formal Methods for Web Services. Springer, Heidelberg (2009). https://doi.org/10.1007/978-3-642-01918-0_2

22. van Eck, M.L., et al.: PM^2: a process mining project methodology. In: Advanced Information Systems Engineering. Lecture Notes in Computer Science. Springer, Cham (2015). https://doi.org/10.1007/978-3-319-19069-3_19

23. van Hage, W.R., et al.: Design and use of the simple event model (SEM). SSRN Electron. J. (2011). https://doi.org/10.2139/ssrn.3199512

24. Wynn, M.T., et al.: Rethinking the input for process mining: insights from the XES survey and workshop. In: Process Mining Workshops. Springer, Cham (2022). https://doi.org/10.1007/978-3-030-98581-3_1

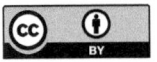

Representative Sampling in Process Mining: Two Novel Sampling Algorithms for Event Logs

Frederik Fonger[1]([envelope])[ID], Niclas Nebelung[1][ID], Arvid Lepsien[1][ID],
Milda Aleknonytė-Resch[1][ID], and Agnes Koschmider[1,2][ID]

[1] Department of Computer Science, Kiel University, Kiel, Germany
{ffo,ale,mar}@informatik.uni-kiel.de
[2] Chair of Business Informatics and Process Analytics, University of Bayreuth,
Bayreuth, Germany
agnes.koschmider@uni-bayreuth.de

Abstract. Process mining allows the discovery of business processes from an event log. However, event logs are rapidly increasing in size and process mining algorithms struggle with the computational load when efficient processing is required. This calls for methods that decrease the event log size while still preserving the representativeness of the event log. This paper presents two new algorithms for sampling event logs. The first algorithm called `RemainderPlus` chooses traces from an event log above a threshold and subsequently selects traces with underrepresented Directly Follows Relations. The second sampling algorithm called `AllBehavior` selects samples that have a high intersection of Directly Follows Relations with the original event log. Usually, `AllBehavior` is complemented with `RemainderPlus` for a more accurate sample representation. They perform well for conformance checking and excel in certain scenarios for process discovery. Thus, both algorithms outperform existing sampling algorithms.

Keywords: event log · sampling · algorithm · process mining · process analysis

1 Introduction

Process mining is a form of process analytics with a focus on discovering business processes from an event log, measuring the conformance between the as-is and to-be process behavior and for predictive monitoring. However, the increased volume of event log data challenges computational resources of process discovery algorithms and conformance checking [1,5]. Therefore, techniques which reduce the size of the event log to be processed while maintaining event log usefulness are necessary.

To overcome this challenge, a few sampling algorithms have been suggested [4, 14] aiming to find a representative subset of an event log. The naive approach to randomly select a subset of an event log is not an efficient solution, although

© The Author(s) 2025
A. Delgado and T. Slaats (Eds.): ICPM 2024 Workshops, LNBIP 533, pp. 44–56, 2025.
https://doi.org/10.1007/978-3-031-82225-4_4

some sampling algorithms exist following this approach [12,18]. These algorithms particularly struggle with smaller sample sizes, as the probability of excluding rare traces increases, potentially leading to an unrepresentative sample. Rather, algorithms which choose a subset of an event log that still maintains utility in terms of the quality dimensions of process mining are required. In fact, this is still an open challenge of existing sampling algorithms, which warrants further research. Therefore, this paper suggests two new sampling algorithms for event logs called RemainderPlus and AllBehavior.

Figure 1 shows how the RemainderPlus algorithm works. The algorithm initially extracts the trace variants of an event log and sorts them by occurrence. Then, traces are selected to be included in the sample by the following two steps. In the first step, the occurrence of each trace variant is counted and multiplied by the sample ratio to determine the trace frequency for the sample. In order not to exceed the sample size, the calculated occurrence of traces is rounded down. Afterwards, the traces are added to the sample according to the frequency of their occurrence. In the second step, a score is calculated to determine the number of underrepresented and overrepresented Directly Follows Pairs (DFPs). This means that the trace variants are ranked according to the frequency of their occurrence. The top-ranked variant is added to the sample and the ranking is reshuffled. This is repeated until the target sample size is reached. The AllBehavior algorithm aims to find an event log sample that has a high intersection of Directly Follows Relations with the original event log. Therefore, the AllBehavior algorithm ranks the traces by its unsampled DFPs and adds them to the sample. If there are no unsampled Directly Follows Relations left, the AllBehavior algorithm terminates and the RemainderPlus algorithms is used to complete the sample.

We evaluated both sampling algorithms on seven event logs (e.g., BPIC 2012 [6] and the Sepsis dataset [15], etc.). We also compared the evaluation results with existing approaches. The evaluation results show superiority in terms of quality measures on the sample level, like mean absolute error and coverage. Furthermore, both sampling algorithms perform well for conformance checking and process discovery, as the results closely match those derived from the original log.

The remainder of the paper is structured as follows. Section 2 summarizes the terms and notations to which we refer throughout the paper. Section 3 presents the sampling algorithms RemainderPlus and AllBehavior. The evaluation results are described and discussed in Sect. 4. Related works are summarized in Sect. 5. The paper ends in Sect. 6 with an outlook and future research directions.

2   Preliminaries

This section first introduces the basic notations to which we will refer throughout the paper. Subsequently, quality measures for evaluating event log samples are summarized.

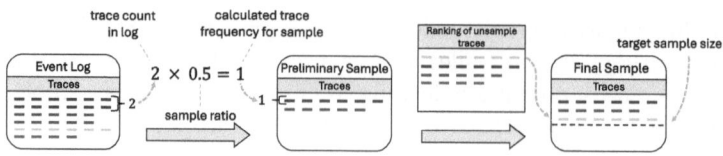

Fig. 1. A simplified representation of the RemainderPlus sampling algorithm applied on an event log.

2.1 Definitions

The basic notations are based on the definitions presented in [12]. Let X be a set. A *multiset* is a function $M : X \rightarrow \mathbb{N}_0$, where for $x \in X$, $M(x)$ denotes the number of occurrences of x in M. Multisets can also be denoted with square brackets, e.g., $M = [e_1^{k_1}, e_2^{k_2}, \ldots, e_n^{k_n}]$ where $k_i = M(e_i)$ for $1 \leq i \leq n$. $\mathbb{B}(X)$ is the set of all multisets over X. For any $x \in X$, inclusion is defined as $x \in M \Leftrightarrow M(x) > 0$. Another multiset S is a subset of M if $\forall_{x \in X} S(x) \leq M(x)$. $|M| = \sum_{x \in X} M(x)$ is the cardinality of a multiset. The union of two multisets is defined as $\forall_{x \in X} (M \uplus S)(x) = M(x) + S(x)$. A (finite) *sequence* over some set X is a function $\sigma : \{1, \ldots, n\} \rightarrow X$ with $\sigma(i) = x_i$ for $1 \leq i \leq n$. The sequence has length $|\sigma| = n$, the set of all possible sequences over X is denoted as X^*, and two sequences $\sigma, \rho \in X^*$ are equivalent if $|\sigma| = |\rho| \wedge \forall_{1 \leq i \leq |\sigma|} \sigma(i) = \rho(i)$. Next, an event log is defined as follows:

Definition 1 (Event log, sample). *The universe of activities is denoted as $\mathcal{A}$. Let $A \subseteq \mathcal{A}$ be a non-empty set of activities. Then, an event log is a multiset of sequences of activities $L \in \mathbb{B}(A^*)$. In an event log, a sequence of activities $\sigma \in L$ is called a trace. An occurrence of an activity in an event log is called an event. A subset $S_L \subseteq L$ is called a sample of L, with sample ratio $r_L(S_L) = \frac{|S_L|}{|L|}$.*

A *sampling algorithm* is any algorithm that takes a target sample ratio c and and event log L as input a produces a sample $S_L \subseteq L$. The actual sample ratio $r_L(S_L)$ should match the target sample ratio c closely. A small error range might be expected since traces cannot be partially included in a sample. Finally, the Directly Follows Relation, which is used as a basis of the algorithms and the sample quality measures, is defined.

Definition 2 (Directly Follows Relation [12]). *Let $A \subseteq \mathcal{A}$, and let $L \in \mathbb{B}(A^*)$ be an event log. For any $a, b \in A$, the Directly Follows Relation is defined via $a >_\sigma b :\Leftrightarrow \exists_{1 \leq i < |\sigma|} \sigma(i) = a \wedge \sigma(i+1) = b$ for traces, and $a >_L b :\Leftrightarrow \exists_{\sigma \in L} a >_\sigma b$ for event logs. The set of all Directly Follows Pairs (DFPs) present in an event log is defined as $\mathcal{B}(L) = \{(x, y) \in A \times A \mid x >_L y\}$. $f_\sigma(a, b) = |\{1 \leq i < |\sigma| \mid \sigma(i) = a \wedge \sigma(i+1) = b\}|$ is the frequency of a DFP (a, b) in a trace σ, and $f_L(a, b) = \sum_{\sigma \in L} L(\sigma) \cdot f_\sigma(a, b)$ the frequency in an event log L.*

2.2   Quality Measures

Plenty of process discovery and conformance checking algorithms consider the Directly Follows Relation essential [2] and various quality measures have been suggested for them [12, 18]. One common quality measure is the coverage $F_L(S_L)$, which calculates the ratio of DFPs of the original event log represented in the sample, i.e. [12]:

$$F_L(S_L) = \frac{|\mathcal{B}(S_L)|}{|\mathcal{B}(L)|}.$$ (1)

Definition 3 (Truly sampled, oversampled, undersampled and unsampled behavior [12]). *Let $A \subseteq \mathcal{A}$ and $L \in \mathbb{B}(A^*)$ be an event log, let $S_L \subseteq L$ be a sample of L, and let $t \in \mathbb{R}$ with $0 \le t \le 1$ be the truly-sampled-bandwidth. Let $\rho_L^{S_L}(a,b) = \frac{f_{S_L}(a,b)}{f_L(a,b)}$ be the (actual) sample ratio of a DPF (a,b). Then, we call $\mathcal{T}_L^{S_L} = \{(a,b) \in \mathcal{B}(L) \mid |\rho_L^{S_L}(a,b) - r_L(S_L)| \le t\}$ the truly sampled behavior, $\mathcal{O}_L^{S_L} = \{(a,b) \in \mathcal{B}(L) \mid \rho_L^{S_L}(a,b) - r_L(S_L) > t\}$ the oversampled behavior, $\mathcal{U}_L^{S_L} = \{(a,b) \in \mathcal{B}(L) \mid \rho_L^{S_L}(a,b) + t < r_L(S_L)\}$ the undersampled behavior, and $\mathcal{N}_L^{S_L} = \mathcal{B}(L) \setminus \mathcal{B}(S_L)$ the unsampled behavior. When context is clear, the sub- and superscripts are omitted.*

Based on this classification the percentages of truly sampled ($\mathcal{P}_\mathcal{T}$), oversampled ($\mathcal{P}_\mathcal{O}$), undersampled ($\mathcal{P}_\mathcal{U}$) and unsampled ($\mathcal{P}_\mathcal{N}$) DFPs are calculated as:

$$\mathcal{P}_\mathcal{T} = \frac{|\mathcal{T}|}{|\mathcal{B}(L)|}, \quad \mathcal{P}_\mathcal{O} = \frac{|\mathcal{O}|}{|\mathcal{B}(L)|}, \quad \mathcal{P}_\mathcal{U} = \frac{|\mathcal{U}|}{|\mathcal{B}(L)|}, \quad \mathcal{P}_\mathcal{N} = \frac{|\mathcal{N}|}{|\mathcal{B}(L)|}$$ (2)

Finally, the expected and actual frequency of each DFP are defined as follows:

Definition 4 (Expected and actual DFP frequency [18]). *Let $A \subseteq \mathcal{A}$ and $L \in \mathbb{B}(A^*)$ be an event log, let $S_L \subseteq L$ be a sample of L with sampling rate $c \in \mathbb{R}$. Then, the behavior of L is $\mathcal{B}(L) = \{b_1, b_2, \ldots, b_n\} \subseteq A \times A$ with $n = |\mathcal{B}(L)|$. The expected DFP frequency for a DFP $b_i = (x,y)$ is defined as $e_i = f_L(b_i) \cdot c$ and the actual DFP frequency in the sample as $s_i = f_{S_L}(b_i)$*

Relying on these definitions, a common statistical measure comparing the two distributions – the mean absolute error (MAE) – is calculated as follows [18]:

$$MAE = \frac{1}{n} \sum_{i=1}^{n} |s_i - e_i|$$ (3)

In our evaluation we also used further measures which are available online (GitHub[1]) like the normalized mean absolute error, coverage, the normalized root mean square error, the symmetric root mean square percentage error, the mean average percentage error and the symmetric mean average percentage error. For reference see Van der Werf et al. [18].

---

[1] https://github.com/Frederik-Fonger/Sampling_RP_AB_2024.

3   Method

This section presents two new algorithms for sampling event logs. RemainderPlus sampling aims to optimize the representativeness of a sample, while AllBehavior sampling aims to generate a sample with a high coverage. The code for both algorithms can be found on GitHub[2].

Algorithm 1: RemainderPlus sampling

Data: $L \in \mathbb{B}(A)$ *with* $A \subseteq \mathcal{A}$, $c \in (0,1]$, $S_{init} \subseteq L$
Result: $S_L \subseteq L$

// First phase: initialize preliminary sample
$S_p \leftarrow [\sigma^{\lfloor L(\sigma) \cdot c \rfloor - S_{init}(\sigma)} \mid \sigma \in L \wedge \lfloor L(\sigma) \cdot c \rfloor - S_{init}(\sigma) \geq 1]$
// Second phase
while $|S_p| < \lfloor |L| \cdot c \rfloor$ **do**

  $\hat{F} \leftarrow \emptyset$
  for $\sigma \in L$ **do**
   $f_e \leftarrow L(\sigma) \cdot c - S_p(\sigma)$ // Remaining expected variant
   frequency
   $sgn \leftarrow 1$ *if* $f_e \geq 0$ *else* -1
   $\hat{f} \leftarrow sgn \cdot \lfloor 10 \cdot (|f_e| - \lfloor |f_e| \rfloor) \rfloor$ // Signed first decimal
   $\hat{F} \leftarrow \hat{F} \cup (\sigma, \hat{f})$
  end
  $\Lambda \leftarrow \arg\max_{\sigma \in L} rem(\sigma)$ *with* $rem(\sigma) = \hat{f}$ $\forall (\sigma, \hat{f}) \in \hat{F}$

  $\Delta_{norm} \leftarrow \emptyset$
  for $\lambda \in \Lambda$ **do**
   $n_{\mathcal{U}} \leftarrow \sum_{b \in \mathcal{B}(\lambda) \cap \mathcal{U}_L^{S_p}} f_\lambda(b)$ // Frequency of undersampled
   Directly Follows Relations
   $n_{\mathcal{O}} \leftarrow \sum_{b \in \mathcal{B}(\lambda) \cap \mathcal{O}_L^{S_p}} f_\lambda(b)$ // Frequency of oversampled
   Directly Follows Relations
   $\delta_{norm} \leftarrow \frac{n_{\mathcal{U}} - n_{\mathcal{O}}}{\sum_{b \in \mathcal{B}(\lambda)} f_\lambda(b)}$ // Normalized difference
   $\Delta_{norm} \leftarrow \Delta_{norm} \cup (\lambda, \delta_{norm})$
  end

  $S_p \leftarrow S_p \uplus \arg\max_{\lambda \in \Lambda} normdiff(\lambda)$ *with*
   $normdiff(\lambda) = \delta_{norm}$ $\forall (\lambda, \delta_{norm}) \in \Delta_{norm}$
end
return S_p

3.1   RemainderPlus Sampling

The RemainderPlus algorithm aims to maintain the original event log's trace and behavior distribution, ensuring a representative sample. First, the occurrence of

---

[2] https://github.com/Frederik-Fonger/Sampling_RP_AB_2024

each trace variant is counted and multiplied by the sample ratio to determine the trace frequency for the sample. To avoid exceeding the sample size, the calculated frequency of traces for the sample is rounded down. Afterwards, the traces are added to the sample according to the frequency of their occurrence. When determining a preliminary sample, the expected frequencies are adjusted by subtracting the frequencies of variants already included in the preliminary sample. Next, the remaining variants (which have less then $1/r$ occurrences) are ranked based on the first decimal place of their expected frequencies relative to the original event log, considering that all expected frequencies are less than one. If two variants have the identical first decimal place, a secondary ranking criterion is applied. This criterion calculates and normalizes the difference between the number of already oversampled and currently undersampled DFPs in each variant. The variant with the highest ranking according to these criteria is then added to the sample. This ranking process is repeated, with the rankings reshuffled each time, until the target sample size is achieved. The pseudo code is provided in Algorithm 1.

3.2   AllBehavior Sampling

The second algorithm, `AllBehavior` sampling, aims to maximize the coverage of the final sample, i.e., it aims to cover as many DFPs of the original event log as possible. This algorithm follows two phases. Firstly, the variants are ranked by the cumulative frequencies of still unsampled DFPs. These are normalized by trace length to avoid a bias of traces with repeated DFPs due to loops. Next, a trace variant with the highest rank is added to the sample. This is repeated until there are no unsampled DFPs left. When the `AllBehavior` algorithm reaches optimal coverage (i.e., all DFPs are in the sample) but has not met the target sample size, it terminates and `RemainderPlus` sampling (see Sect. 3.1) is applied to complete the sample. If trace coverage is more essential than representativeness, then the `AllBehavior` sampling algorithm is a better alternative to the `RemainderPlus` algorithm. The pseudo code is provided in Algorithm 2.

4   Evaluation

To evaluate our sampling algorithms, we used seven event logs from the BPM community (see Table 1) and compared the results to three other sampling algorithms, namely, random, stratified and C-min [4] sampling. We only considered these three algorithms, because they do not need a discovery model prior to sampling. Therefore, we follow our goal to provide sampling algorithms for the general use in process mining including process discovery. We generated samples with target sampling ratios of $c \in \{0.001, 0.005, 0.01, 0.05, 0.1, 0.2, 0.3, 0.4, 0.5, 0.6, 0.7, 0.8\}$ for each of the seven event logs. We used the quality measures as presented in Sect. 2.2 for the first part of the evaluation (Sect. 4.1). Following this, we evaluated the algorithms for conformance checking (see Sect. 4.2) and process discovery (see Sect. 4.3). To evaluate

---

Algorithm 2: `AllBehavior` sampling

Data: $L \in \mathbb{B}(A)$ *with* $A \subseteq \mathcal{A}$, $c \in (0, 1]$, $S_{init} \subseteq L$
Result: $S_L \subseteq L$
`// First phase`
$S_p \leftarrow []$ `// Initialize preliminary sample`
while $\mathcal{N}_L^{S_p} \neq \emptyset$ **do**   `// See Def. 2`
  if $|S_p| = \lfloor |L| \cdot c \rfloor$ **then**
  | **return** S_p
  else
  | $\sigma_{max} \leftarrow \underset{\sigma \in L}{\arg \max} \ \frac{1}{|\sigma|} \sum_{b \in \mathcal{N}_L^{S_p} \cap \mathcal{B}(\sigma)} f_\sigma(b)$
  | $S_p \leftarrow S_p \uplus \sigma_{max}$
  end
end
`// Second phase`
return `RemainderPlus`$(L, \ c, \ S_p)$

---

the models we used the token based approach to calculate fitness and precision for the F1-score [17]. For non-deterministic (random and stratified) samplings, we repeated the sampling four times and calculated an average of the quality measures. The tables only show the results for a sample ratio of 0.3 due to space limitations. All evaluation results are available in the GitHub repository.[3]

4.1   Sample Quality Measures

For each sampling algorithm, we tested 84 combinations in total, stemming from 12 sample ratios for each of the 7 event logs.

Table 1. Event logs used for the evaluation.

Name	Traces	Trace Variant	Events	Activity
BPIC 2012 [6]	13087	4366	262200	24
DDLog (BPIC 2020) [7]	10500	99	56437	17
ID Log (BPIC 2020) [7]	6449	753	72151	34
Permit Log (BPIC 2020) [7]	7065	1478	86581	51
PTC Log (BPIC 2020) [7]	2099	202	18246	29
RfP Log (BPIC 2020) [7]	6886	89	36796	19
Sepsis Log [15]	1050	846	15214	16

---

[3] https://github.com/Frederik-Fonger/Sampling_RP_AB_2024.

Result Mean Absolute Error and Coverage. A small MAE (Eq. 3) value indicates a higher representativeness. `RemainderPlus` achieves the lowest values for MAE for all samplings compared to existing approaches. The `RemainderPlus` (`Allbehavior`) sampling algorithm achieved the best results in 67% (24%) of the evaluated combinations. The performance of the other algorithms depends on the properties of the event log (e.g., size, trace frequencies). For example, the random sample nearly matches the best results in the "BPI-Challenge 2012" log, but underperforms for the event logs "Domestic Declarations" or "Request for Payment". The `AllBehavior` algorithm achieves the highest *coverage* among all evaluated event logs for sample ratios of up to 0.5. The evaluation indicates that other sampling algorithms achieve similar coverage for sample ratio values above 0.6. Although the `AllBehavior` algorithm does not match the optimal *coverage* at a sample ratio of 0.01, it still outperforms all other algorithms. For additional details, see GitHub[4]. The evaluation results for `RemainderPlus` show that it ranks closely with other methods, usually slightly below the random sample, but superior to both C-min and stratified sampling. All algorithms tend to produce a higher *coverage* value when the sample size increases, which might be explained by the increasing probability of rare cases occurring.

Runtime. The runtime of each sampling iteration is shown in Table 2. The computation was performed on a processor with 6×3.7 GHz and 16 Gigabyte of memory. The random and the stratified sampling both rely on a randomized selection of traces. As a result, there is no additional calculation required for the selection of cases. That being considered, it is expected that they have the shortest runtime in comparison to other approaches. The increase in runtime for the `AllBehavior`, `RemainderPlus` and C-min sampling depends on the size and complexity of the event log to be sampled. The `RemainderPlus` algorithm is the fastest of the non-randomized algorithms in 92% of the evaluated combinations.

Table 2. The runtime of sampling iterations in seconds for a sample ratio of 0.3.

	AB	RP	Random	Stratified	C-min
BPIC 2012	149.8878	119.715	**0.0219**	0.9362	205.0922
DD Log	9.7479	9.8556	**0.0120**	0.2296	149.2675
ID Log	10.6056	7.7004	**0.0135**	0.2588	421.1549
Permit Log	29.8082	20.4941	**0.0434**	0.4446	35.3743
PTC Log	1.114	1.0612	**0.0045**	0.0900	5.5172
RfP Log	5.2101	5.3636	**0.0107**	0.1927	36.8803
Sepsis Log	2.1732	2.2789	**0.0037**	0.2045	3.7131

---

[4] https://github.com/Frederik-Fonger/Sampling_RP_AB_2024.

4.2   Sampling for Conformance Checking

To evaluate the sampling methods for conformance checking, the process model was discovered from the original event log and conformance checking was applied with and without sampling. We applied process discovery with the miner-threshold of $t \in \{0, 0.2, 0.4, 0.6, 0.9\}$. This evaluation was done for the aforementioned 84 combinations, resulting in 420 combinations. Conformance checking was also applied for the original event log to have a baseline. A score for comparing the sample algorithms was calculated by dividing the F1-score when sampling was applied by the baseline F1-score of the original event log, which we denote as $\lambda_{f_1} = |\frac{f_1^{sample}}{f_1^{originallog}} - 1|$. From here, we present the data for a sample ratio of $r = 0.01$ in the tables, as the differences for process discovery and conformance checking are more significant for smaller sample ratios. All results for other sample ratios can be found in the GitHub [3]. Overall, `AllBehavior` out-performs all other algorithms in terms of keeping the F1-score consistently close to the baseline. This is obvious since the algorithm focuses on high coverage and retaining the DFPs for smaller sample ratios (see Sect. 4.1). Most algorithms retain results close to the baseline for sample ratios larger than $r = 0.05$, as shown in Fig. 2. The `RemainderPlus` algorithm mostly achieves the second best results, as shown in Table 3. For the small sample ratio of $r = 0.001$, all algorithms significantly deviate from the baseline. The decreased processing time for the conformance checking calculation is significant. E.g., for the Permit Log, the calculation time decreases from 55 s on the original log to 23 s on a sample with $r = 0.5$ and to 1.9 s on a sample with $r = 0.01$.

Table 3. F1-score ratio λ_{f_1} between the sample and original log, with both F1-scores calculated against the model discovered from the original log (sample ratio $r = 0.01$, inductive miner with threshold set to 0)

	AB	RP	Random	Stratified	C-min
BPIC 2012	0.1478	0.2196	**0.0948**	0.1320	0.1325
DD Log	**0.0219**	0.1590	0.2275	0.1575	0.2090
Permit Log	**0.1667**	0.3833	0.3709	0.4159	0.3860
ID Log	**0.0573**	0.2695	0.2652	0.2853	0.2954
PTC Log	**0.2957**	0.3698	0.3735	0.4055	0.4486
RfP Log	**0.2024**	0.2175	0.3269	0.2358	0.4221
Sepsis Log	**0.6118**	0.6187	0.6274	1.0000	0.6621

4.3   Sampling Usage for Process Discovery

To evaluate the sampling algorithms for process discovery, the inductive and heuristic miners are applied to every sample. Afterwards, conformance checking

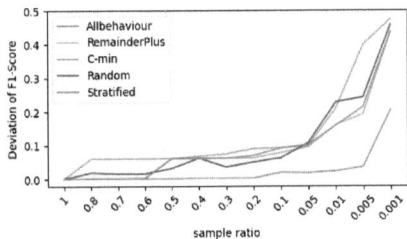

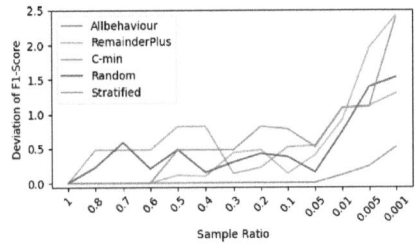

Fig. 2. F1-score ratio λ_{f_1} between the sample and original log with both F1-scores calculated against the model discovered from the original log (Domestic Declarations log, models discovered using the inductive miner with threshold set to 0)

Fig. 3. F1-score ratio λ_{f_1} between the model discovered from the sample and the model from the original log, with both F1-scores calculated against the original log (International Declarations log, models discovered using the inductive miner with threshold set to 0)

is applied to the original event log. The score is calculated by dividing the conformance checking results through the results from the original event log (λ_{f_1}). Due to runtime constraints, we only evaluated process models for 5 of the 7 event logs, as we stopped the conformance checking calculation for these models after 48 h. Therefore, the number of combinations decreased for this setting to 300 combinations. The results are shown in Table 4. The results vary depending on the configuration and event log quality. For example, for the International Declarations log, `AllBehavior` sampling is able to reach an equal F1-score to the baseline until a sample ratio of $r = 0.05$ (Fig. 3). With smaller sample ratios it still remains close to the baseline. On the other hand, for the Request for Payments log, the results are not fully convincing. Overall, in 66 % of the tested combinations, `AllBehavior` sampling's F1-score was closest to the baseline.

Table 4. F1-score ratio λ_{f_1} between the model discovered from the sample and the model from the original log with both F1-scores calculated against the original log (sample ratio $r = 0.01$, inductive miner with threshold set to 0)

	AB	RP	Random	Stratified	C-min
DD Log	0.3406	0.1078	**0.1068**	0.1378	0.6575
Permit Log	**0.0644**	1.034	0.9953	0.5118	0.5709
PTC Log	**0.0384**	1.7245	1.6028	2.9022	3.0264
RfP Log	0.3795	0.8021	**0.0859**	0.6859	0.5423
ID Log	**0.1155**	0.9129	0.7448	1.0847	1.0849

5   Related Work

Different random sampling approaches have been evaluated in the literature [4,12,14,18]. The C-min sampling algorithm aims to optimize the earth mover's distance between the original log and the sample [4]. The log-rank algorithm uses a graph-based ranking model for sampling, however, due to the lack of code availability it is not included in our evaluation [14]. Therefore, we compared `RemainderPlus` and `AllBehavior` against random sampling and C-min sampling algorithms and discussed the results above. However, to the best of our knowledge, no structured approach exist to compare sampling algorithms. While some algorithms compare metrics of event logs [4,12], others consider the process model as the indicator for quality [14]. Also, a direct comparison of existing approaches is difficult since the approaches were not evaluated using the same sample sizes [4,11,12,18]. To overcome these shortcomings in existing sampling evaluations, we evaluated the algorithms based on plenty of configurations to demonstrate the efficiency of our two algorithms. Sani et al. propose using different sampling approaches depending on the quality of event logs and use cases [10] as well as evaluate different sampling strategies [8,9,16].

Sampling strategies have also been suggested for conformance checking [3,11]. In [11], the authors suggest a conformance checking sampling algorithm that takes a log and a model as input and applies relevance-guided sampling of event logs [11] to decrease runtime processing. The approach of [3] decreases the runtime of optimal alignments. Additionally, Bauer et al. found that a subset of a log, sometimes with a size below 1% of the original log, is enough to assess its quality while significantly reducing processing times [3].

6   Conclusion

This paper introduces two novel event log sampling algorithms, `RemainderPlus` and `AllBehavior`. While `RemainderPlus` focuses on optimizing the representativeness of the sample, `AllBehavior` aims to maximize coverage. Both algorithms select traces for sampling deterministically, which means that the results are reproducible and not random. The evaluation results show that `RemainderPlus` outperforms existing algorithms in terms of sample representation to the original event log by demonstrating lower error values for MAE. It is therefore well-suited for general application where representative samples are required. The `AllBehavior` algorithm consistently produces samples with high coverage, but trades enhanced coverage for trace distribution accuracy. This trade-off is especially evident for smaller sample sizes. Surprisingly, while `RemainderPlus` performs better on the individual algorithm metrics on the model level, `AllBehavior` outperforms `RemainderPlus` for process discovery and conformance checking applications. This is most probably because `AllBehavior` focuses on covering as much behavior as possible. Generally, the evaluation results indicate different significance for process discovery and conformance checking for smaller sample ratios. The results for process discovery show that `AllBehavior` is more appropriate.

Potential validity threats to our methods and evaluation include the risk of overfitting from testing on specific event logs, which we countered by using a wide range of sample sizes and event log characteristics. Also, challenges arose with respect to a comparative analysis against existing approaches since some code implementations are not accessible. A promising direction for future research might be a holistic combination of sampling techniques that can be individually adjusted based on the characteristics of the event log and some specific requirements imposed by the data analysis. Both algorithms presented in this paper promise a more efficient analysis of large event logs for process mining, which allow novel insights in disciplines with high volume of data [13].

Acknowledgments. This project has received funding from the Federal Ministry for Economic Affairs and Climate Action under the Marispace-X project grant no. 68GX21002E and the State of Schleswig-Holstein under the Datencampus project grant no. 220 21 016. The project ProcessPig is funded by the European Union within the framework of the European Innovation Partnership (EIP-AGRI) and the state program rural areas of the state Schleswig-Holstein (LPLR) (www.eip-agrar-sh.de).

References

1. van der Aalst, W., et al.: Process mining manifesto. In: Daniel, F., Barkaoui, K., Dustdar, S. (eds.) BPM 2011. LNBIP, vol. 99, pp. 169–194. Springer, Heidelberg (2012). https://doi.org/10.1007/978-3-642-28108-2_19
2. van der Aalst, W.M.: Foundations of process discovery. In: Process Mining Handbook, pp. 37–75. Springer, Cham (2022). https://doi.org/10.1007/978-3-031-08848-3_2
3. Bauer, M., van der Aa, H., Weidlich, M.: Sampling and approximation techniques for efficient process conformance checking. Inf. Syst. **104**, 101666 (2022)
4. Bernard, G., Andritsos, P.: Selecting representative sample traces from large event logs. In: ICPM 2021, pp. 56–63. IEEE, Eindhoven, Netherlands (2021)
5. Carmona, J., van Dongen, B., Weidlich, M.: Conformance checking: foundations, milestones and challenges. In: Process Mining Handbook, pp. 155–190. Springer, Cham (2022). https://doi.org/10.1007/978-3-031-08848-3_5
6. van Dongen, B.: Bpi challenge 2012 (2012). https://data.4tu.nl/articles/dataset/BPI_Challenge_2012/12689204
7. van Dongen, B.: Bpi challenge 2020 (2020). https://data.4tu.nl/collections/_/5065541/1
8. Fani Sani, M., van Zelst, S.J., van der Aalst, W.M.P.: The impact of event log subset selection on the performance of process discovery algorithms. In: Welzer, T., et al. (eds.) ADBIS 2019. CCIS, vol. 1064, pp. 391–404. Springer, Cham (2019). https://doi.org/10.1007/978-3-030-30278-8_39
9. Fani Sani, M., van Zelst, S.J., van der Aalst, W.M.P.: The impact of biased sampling of event logs on the performance of process discovery. Computing **103**(6), 1085–1104 (2021)
10. Fani Sani, M., et al.: Event log sampling for predictive monitoring. In: International Conference on Process Mining, vol. 433, pp. 154–166 (2022)
11. Kabierski, M., et al.: Sampling what matters: Relevance-guided sampling of event logs. In: ICPM 2021. pp. 64–71 (2021)

12. Knols, B., van der Werf, J.M.E.M.: Measuring the behavioral quality of log sampling. In: ICPM 2019, pp. 97–104. IEEE, Aachen (2019)
13. Koschmider, A., et al.: Process mining for unstructured data: challenges and research directions. In: Modellierung 2024, pp. 119–136. GI, Bonn (2024)
14. Liu, C., et al.: Sampling business process event logs using graph-based ranking model. Concurr. Computat.: Pract. Exper. **33**(5), e5974 (2021)
15. Mannhardt, F., Blinde, D.: Analyzing the trajectories of patients with sepsis using process mining. In: RADAR+EMISA 2017, Essen, Germany, 12–13 June 2017, pp. 72–80. CEUR Workshop Proceedings, CEUR-WS.org (2017)
16. Sani, M., Van Zelst, S., Van Der Aalst, W.: Improving the performance of process discovery algorithms by instance selection. Comp. Sci. Inf. Syst. **17**(3), 927–958 (2020)
17. Van Der Aalst, W.: Process Mining. Springer, Heidelberg (2016)
18. van der Werf, J.M.E.M., et al.: All that glitters is not gold: four maturity stages of process discovery algorithms. Inf. Syst. **114**, 102155 (2023)

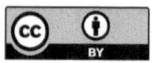

Root Cause Analysis Using Rule Mining on Object-Centric Event Logs

Benedikt Knopp$^{(\boxtimes)}$, Mahsa Pourbafrani, and Wil van der Aalst

Chair of Process and Data Science, RWTH Aachen University, Aachen, Germany
{knopp,mahsa.bafrani,wvdaalst}@pads.rwt-aachen.de

Abstract. In business processes, the behavior, evolution and interactions of objects influence the outcome of process instances, and thus the value that a business user may assign to them. For example, in an order-to-cash process, a complete and timely delivery of a package is desirable, but depends on what happens to other objects upstream, like production batches. Negative outcomes call for a Root Cause Analysis (RCA) on the process. While many approaches for RCA using process mining exist, none is native to object-centric frameworks and thus suitable for capturing dependencies across object types. This work presents a method for RCA that operates on object-centric event logs (OCELs). Given an OCEL, our method returns a set of association rules on the activity level. These rules associate descriptive patterns over the various object types occurring at events with patterns indicating the process outcome. The patterns are abstracted from the log with the help of a first-order logic based query engine. A case study confirmed that our method can identify problematic interactions across various object types in real-life business processes.

Keywords: Root Cause Analysis · Association Rule Mining · Object-Centric Process Mining · Process Querying

1 Introduction

A common goal in analyzing business processes is to understand operational problems. This endeavour is called *Root Cause Analysis (RCA)*. For the purpose of RCA, process mining techniques have been successfully deployed [1–3]. Existing approaches usually operate on event data that uses a fixed case notion, that is, logs in which each process instance relates to a unique object of a fixed type (e.g., a sales order or a delivery). The nature of processes, however, is not so simple, because objects of various types and their interactions constitute the processes of an organization. Hence, existing methods for RCA in process mining have to either neglect information from foreign case notions or flatten these information into the chosen case notion. This may cause issues of data redundancy, additional effort in maintaining data integrity, or information loss through aggregation.

A. Delgado and T. Slaats (Eds.): ICPM 2024 Workshops, LNBIP 533, pp. 57–69, 2025.
https://doi.org/10.1007/978-3-031-82225-4_5

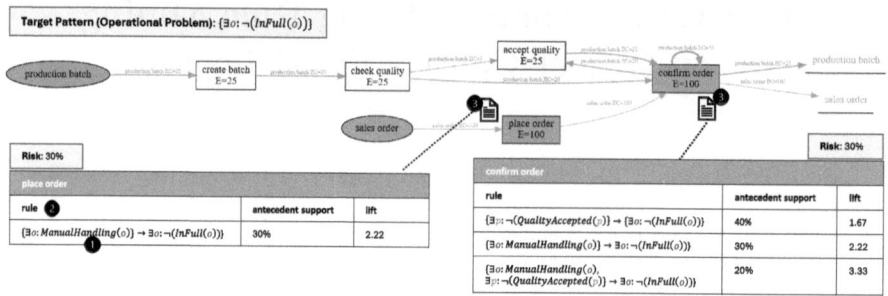

Fig. 1. Our method returns association rules on the event type level (3) that can be embedded into an object-centric process model. These rules (2) indicate which patterns are problematic with regards to an undesired process outcome. Patterns, in turn, are formulas over characteristics present at events, e.g., object characteristics (1).

To better account for the entangled nature of processes, object-centric process mining frameworks have been proposed [4,5]. The principle of these frameworks is to relate events not to a single case, but to arbitrarily many heterogeneously typed objects. While standard process mining utilities such as log standards [6] do exist for the object-centric setting, we are not aware of a designated RCA method. However, we argue that root causes of bad process outcomes may be found across interacting objects. For instance, in a company producing and selling goods, production of insufficient quality could be a cause for unfulfilled orders downstream. It is therefore the goal of the research presented here *(a)* to provide a method for RCA on object-centric process event logs and *(b)* to provide empirical evidence from real-life processes that the supposed root causes can in fact be found in object interactions, and that the method is able to discover this.

The output of our approach is illustrated in Fig. 1. Here, an exemplary order management process coupled to a production process is depicted as an object-centric process model [7]. On the one hand, *production batches* are created, undergo a quality check and are eventually released after accepting the quality. *Sales orders*, on the other hand, are placed by the customer and then confirmed by the company, at which point the order is assigned to supply from production units. In the process, it may happen that customer demands cannot be satisfied, causing the respective order to be not delivered *in full*. This is an operational problem that calls for an RCA. The process model is annotated with findings from applying our RCA approach, which is briefly described in the following.

We highlight three components that constitute our method, referring to the bullets in Fig. 1. *(1)* First, *patterns* are learned as descriptions of event characteristics. For this, a query language based on first-order logic is deployed in order to formulate these patterns across the objects occurring and interacting at the events. Since in object-centric processes, objects may occur at events in varying cardinalities, this query engine offers a means to precisely formulate properties across objects. *(2)* We mine for association rules [8] to identify among frequent combinations of patterns those that are likely to lead to the negative process outcome. This outcome is encoded in a *target pattern* on the object level. For example, here, the rule indicated at *(1)* expresses that if a newly placed order will be handled manually, the likelihood of an incomplete delivery is 2.22 times higher (*lift*), and 30% of the cases are handled manually (*antecedent support*). The third rule at *confirm order* exemplifies a rule that is a combination of patterns. *(3)* We suggest to embed mined rules into an object-centric process model [7]. This provides a map based on which business users could identify risky interactions and counteract as early as possible, given that rules provide actionable insights. To enable interpreting the output, we report on the model, as in Fig. 1, event counts and object flow counts. Also, the *risk* at each activity gives the a priori likelihood that an object interacting at an event will eventually have a negative outcome.

In describing the details of our approach in the following chapters, we will clarify some technical background concerning rule mining, and then rigorously formalize the method. Finally, we apply the approach to a real-life log and discuss the results in light of the research goals. We start by reviewing related work.

2 Related Work

In the simplest case, an RCA in process mining can be considered as a standard ML task, using a data set where each instance has its outcome encoded in a target attribute. Existing works use general classification methods [9, 10]. As in this work, rule mining has been applied for RCA [2, 11, 13]. Of course, instead of investigating negative outcomes, one can also foster positive process outcomes [12], in general, mine for deviances [13]. [14] proposes a general framework for analyzing process properties beyond RCA.

An important step to refine basic classification is to distinguish between correlation and causation. [3] uses structural equation models for estimating causality and assessing the impact of potential improvement actions. [1] follows a probabilistic approach with the intent to increase the robustness of findings towards spurious correlations. [12] distinguishes between controllable and non-controllable descriptive attributes in order to propose actionable treatments.

Closely related to our work are [2] and [13]. [2] clusters traces with regards to problematic attributes and extracts association rules from these clusters to discover problematic subgroups. [13] describes an approach to explain process deviances based on declarative rule and sequence mining, also taking into account the data perspective. As opposed to [2] and [13], our work focuses solely on the event-type level, but extends the scope to object-centricity. To the best of our knowledge, our work is the first to propose a pattern mining framework, as well as more specifically an RCA method on object-centric event logs.

3 Approach

In the following, we describe how we conduct this RCA. While our approach works on an object-centric log standard [6], we impose some assumptions on the structure of the input that we achieve through (semi-)automatic preprocessing. Thus, after listing preliminaries (Sect. 3.1), we give our custom specification of the input data (Sect. 3.2), before describing how this input is converted into a suitable format for rule mining (Sect. 3.3).

3.1   Preliminaries

Let X be a set. The powerset of X is denoted with $\mathcal{P}(X)$. With $\mathcal{B}(X)$, we denote the set of multisets over X. For example, $[a^4, b^1] \in \mathcal{B}(X)$ is a multiset over a set $X = \{a, b\}$ in which a occurs four times and b once. Given sets X, Y and a partial function $f : X \nrightarrow Y$, $dom(f) \subseteq X$ denotes the domain of f. *Bool* is the set of boolean values *true* and *false*.

We deploy concepts from association rule mining [8] as follows. Let again X be a set, in this context called a set of *patterns*. A *dataset* over X is $D = [T_1^{n_1}, ..., T_k^{n_k}] \in \mathcal{B}(\mathcal{P}(X))$, $k \geq 0$, where for each $i, 1 \leq i \leq k$, $T_i \subseteq X$ and $n_i \geq 1$. We call T_i the *transactions* in D. Let $X' \subseteq X$. The *support* of X' in D is defined as $supp_D(X') = \Sigma_{i=1,...,k, X' \subseteq T_i} n_i / \Sigma_{i=1,...,k} n_i$. Thus, the support of a pattern set is the fraction of transactions that include a pattern set. For $X_1, X_2 \subseteq X$, we call $r = X_1 \rightarrow X_2$ an *association rule* over X, with X_1 being the *antecedent* and X_2 the *consequent* of r. The *confidence* of r in D is defined as $conf_D(r) = supp_D(X_1 \cup X_2)/supp_D(X_1)$. The confidence of a rule gives the relative likelihood to observe the rule consequent given the antecedent. The *lift* of r is defined as $lift_D(r) = supp_D(X_1 \cup X_2)/(supp_D(X_1) \cdot supp_D(X_2))$. The lift of a rule is a measure for the positive correlation between antecedent and consequent; in other words, it quantifies how much more likely the consequent is to appear in the context of the antecedent, compared to an a priori observation.

3.2   Input

Single source of truth for our approach is an object-centric event log. As remarked previously, the basic difference between object-centric and traditional event logs is that in the former, events may relate to an arbitrary amount of objects instead of a fixed single case. To describe these object-centric logs, we assume the following universes to be given: $\mathbb{U}_{ev}$ are events, $\mathbb{U}_{etype}$ are event types, $\mathbb{U}_{obj}$ are objects, $\mathbb{U}_{otype}$ are object types, and $\mathbb{U}_{time}$ are timestamps. For each object, a given function $otype \in \mathbb{U}_{obj} \rightarrow \mathbb{U}_{otype}$ fixes an object type. Furthermore, $\mathbb{U}_{oattr}$ are object attributes. Object attributes are assumed to resemble properties of exactly one object type, again fixed by a type signature $oatype \in \mathbb{U}_{oattr} \rightarrow \mathbb{U}_{otype}$.

Log standards such as XES or OCEL capture the data perspective of a process through event or case attributes using standard data types such as strings, booleans, and numbers. In our work, aiming for an RCA, we analyze the interplay of objects and attributes via pattern mining. Therefore, we enforce a discretization of the process data, that is, properties have to be encoded as logical propositions. On the one hand, this may impose limitations to our approach, since the question how to convert data types into a propositional form is not trivial: for example, a naive handling of continuous attributes by converting each possible value assignment to a distinct pattern is neither feasible nor sensible for association rule mining. On the other hand, attributes with a propositional encoding offer a natural way to establish expressivity for describing the interplay of objects, namely by an embedding into a first-order logic framework. That is, we regard these encodings as *predicates* in the context of events. Event attributes are regarded as predicates of arity 0, since they take no input parameters (assuming the event gives the context and is thus not a parameter itself). Object attributes are predicates of arity 1, and relations between objects are predicates of arity 2. These predicates may be assembled to formulas to be evaluated over events: Firstly, event contexts restrict the domain of predicates to the set of objects occurring at the events. Secondly, event contexts provides an intuitive interpretation, assigning truth values by looking up event attributes, and object properties at the time of event occurrence.

We would like to choose this conceptualization as the backbone of our method, since such formulas also naturally translate to patterns in the context of rule mining. That is, a formula satisfied at an event could be considered as a pattern being part of the transaction defined by the event. In order to simplify matters, however, we restrict ourselves here to consider only object attributes, that is, predicates of arity 1, using from now on the terms *predicate* and *object attribute* interchangeably. Hence, we neglect object interrelationships and event attributes, but argue that an extension is straightforward. The following is an accordingly customized and restricted definition of object-centric event data.

Definition 1 (Object-Centric Event Log). An object-centric event log (in short, OCEL) is a tuple $L = (E, O, E2O, ET, evtype, time, oattr, F, \Gamma)$ where $E \subseteq \mathbb{U}_{ev}$, $E \neq \{\emptyset\}$, are events, $O \subseteq \mathbb{U}_{obj}$ are objects, $E2O \subseteq E \times O$ are event-object relations, $ET \subseteq \mathbb{U}_{etype}$ are event types, $evtype \in E \to ET$ are event types per event, $time \in E \to \mathbb{U}_{time}$ are event timestamps, $oattr \subseteq \mathbb{U}_{oattr}$ are object attributes (predicates), and furthermore

- $F \in ET \to \mathcal{P}(oattr)$ are predicates for each event type, and
- $\Gamma \in E \to (\mathcal{P}(oattr) \nrightarrow (O \nrightarrow Bool))$ such that for all $e \in E, et \in ET$, if $evtype(e) = et$, then $dom(\Gamma(e)) = F(et)$, and for all $oa \in dom(\Gamma(e))$, $dom(\Gamma(e)(oa)) = \{o \in O \mid otype(o) = oatype(oa) \land (e, o) \in E2O\}$, are predicate interpretations.

To sum up, an OCEL is a set of variously typed events (E, $evtype$) that are ordered with respect to time ($time$). Objects (O) can occur at these events ($E2O$), and the objects can carry data ($oattr$). In our approach, we treat event types as first-class citizens: at those, we investigate the interplay of objects with respect to root causes. Some attributes may hence be more or less interesting to be considered at specific event types, for example, the elapsed time of an object is uninteresting at an object creation event. Because of this, and also to restrict the set of candidates for a more efficient rule mining upfront, only a subset of the predicates describes each event type (F). Finally, an event is characterized by the selected attributes of objects that occur at these events (Γ).

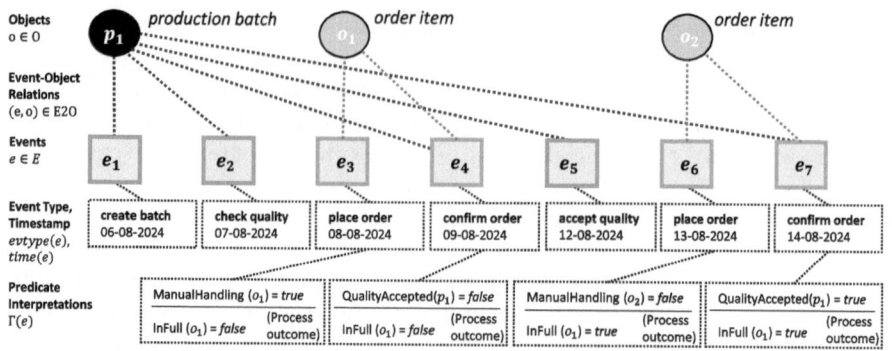

Fig. 2. An exemplary OCEL L_1.

Example 1. Figure 2 depicts an exemplary OCEL L_1. This log represents a process involving the object types *order items* and *production batches*. Here, we have:

- $E = \{e_1, ..., e_7\}$, $O = \{o_1, o_2, p_1\}$ with $otype(o_1) = otype(o_2) = order\ item$, $otype(p_1) = production\ batch$. $E2O = \{(e_1, p_1), (e_2, p_1), ...\}$, as indicated. $ET = \{create\ batch, check\ quality, accept\ quality, place\ order, confirm\ order\}$.
- Types and timestamps per event are, for example, $evtype(e_1) = create\ batch$ and $time(e_1) = 06\text{-}08\text{-}2024$, and for other events as indicated.
- $oattr = \{ManualHandling, QualityAccepted, InFull\} \subseteq \mathbb{U}_{oa}$, with $oatype(InFull) = oatype(ManualHandling) = order\ item$, and $oatype(QualityAccepted) = production\ batch$.
- $F(place\ order) = \{ManualHandling, InFull\}$,
- $F(confirm\ order) = \{QualityAccepted, InFull\}$, and
- $F(et) = \emptyset$ for $et \in \{create\ batch, check\ quality, accept\ quality\}$.
- Interpretations of predicates are, for example at e_3, $\Gamma(e_3) = \{(InFull, \{(o_1, false)\}), (ManualHandling, \{(o_1, true)\})\}$, and for other events as indicated.

The business scenario of L_1 is the same as the one for the example described in Sect. 1, depicted in Fig. 1 for a bigger underlying log. For an fexplanation on the business logic, we hence refer to the first section. Note that in L_1, *InFull* reflects an object attribute that we associate with the process outcome. For our RCA method, we impose two important assumptions on input logs. First, the categorization of process outcomes with regards to the business problem has to be encoded in such an attribute on the object level. Second, this outcome has to be known for each object and thus recorded (retrospectively) in the log.

In the following, we describe our approach to extract rules from such event logs that are useful for an RCA, using above log as a running example.

3.3 Pattern Mining

The artificial example L_1 reflects two explanations for negative outcomes in the process it describes. Firstly, orders that are assigned for manual instead of automatic handling are associated with more processing mistakes, e.g., picking wrong quantities. Secondly, orders assigned to unfinished production batches may face the issue that the supposed batch release date is not met. To unveil such correlations, we rely on mining association rules that encode the explanations (ideally, root causes reflecting real causality) in the rule antecedent and the process outcome in the consequent. To this end, input event data has to be transformed into a database for rule mining. For this, the concrete predicate interpretations observed in the log have to be abstracted into generic patterns. As mentioned, we proceed by constructing formulas over the predicates by means of common logical connectives. In the log context, these formulas are then interpreted at events with regards to the predicate interpretation qualifying the event.

In the following, *well-formed first-order logic formulas* over predicates can be constructed by means of the binary conjunction and disjunction operators $\wedge, \vee$, the unary negation operator $\neg$, and existential and universal quantifiers $\exists, \forall$.

Definition 2 (Pattern). Let L be an object-centric event log with events E, event types ET and predicates F. A *pattern* over L is a function $p \in E \nrightarrow Bool$. With P_L, we denote the set of all patterns over L. For each $et \in ET$, the *pattern formulas* $P_{L,et} \subseteq P_L$ are the well-formed first-order logic formulas over $F(et)$.

For example, $\exists o : InFull(o)$ and $\exists o : \neg(InFull(o))$[1] are pattern formulas at the event type *place order* in L_1. In the context of e_3, for instance, $\exists o : \neg(InFull(o))(e_3) = true$ because there exists an order o at the event, namely o_1, where the *InFull* predicate does not evaluate to true.

Since many different formulas, and usually also many non-equivalent formulas can be constructed over a set of predicates, we also need to make a *selection* of potentially interesting candidate patterns for conducting the RCA.

Definition 3 (Pattern Selection). Let L be an object-centric event log with event types ET and patterns $P_{L,et}$ for each $et \in ET$. A *pattern selection* is a function $psel \in ET \rightarrow \mathcal{P}(P_L)$, such that for all $et \in ET$, $psel(et) \subseteq P_{L,et}$.

Given this, we can transform an OCEL into datasets for rule mining.

Definition 4 (OCEL to Pattern Datasets). Let L be an object-centric event log with events E, event types ET and patterns P_L. Furthermore, let $psel \in ET \rightarrow \mathcal{P}(P_L)$ be a pattern selection. The pattern datasets $\mathcal{D}_{L,psel} \in ET \rightarrow \mathcal{B}(\mathcal{P}(P_L))$ corresponding to the event types in L are defined as $\mathcal{D}_{L,psel}(et) = [\{p \in psel(et) \,|\, p(e)\} \,|\, e \in E, evtype(e) = et]$.

Example 2. For L_1, Table 1 lists the pattern datasets $\mathcal{D}_{L_1,psel}(et)$ for $et \in \{place\ order, confirm\ order\}$. Here, $psel$ selects the indicated formulas (that is, patterns) over the predicates *ManualHandling, InFull* at *place order*, and at *confirm order* over *QualityAccepted, InFull*. Consider for example event e_3 (*place order*). Here, the two patterns $\exists o : ManualHandling(o), \exists o : (\neg InFull(o))$ are satisfied, yielding the corresponding transaction in the pattern dataset. Since no other *place order* event satisfies the very same patterns, the corresponding count is 1, as for all other listed transactions (indicated by set superscripts).

---

[1] We assume that variables are implicitly typed through the attribute typing *oatype*. For example, o is of type *sales order* because this is the *oatype* of *InFull*.

Table 1. Pattern datasets for activities in the exemplary log L_1.

Event Type et	Dataset $\mathcal{D}_{L_1,psel}(et)$
place order	$[\{\exists\, o\, :\, ManualHandling(o), \exists\, o\, :\, (\neg\, InFull(o))\}^1,$
	$\{\exists\, o\, :\, \neg\, (ManualHandling(o)), \exists\, o\, :\, InFull(o)\}^1]$
confirm order	$[\{\exists\, p\, :\, \neg(QualityAccepted(p)), \exists\, o\, :\, (\neg\, InFull(o))\}^1,$
	$\{\exists\, p\, :\, QualityAccepted(p), \exists\, o\, :\, InFull(o)\}^1]$

Consider now $D_1 = \mathcal{D}_{L,epat}(place\ order)$ and $D_2 = \mathcal{D}_{L,epat}(confirm\ order)$. Let $r_1 = \emptyset \rightarrow \{\exists\, o\, :\, (\neg\, InFull(o))\}$ be an association rule. In both datasets, we have the rule confidence (risk) $conf_{D_1}(r_1) = conf_{D_2}(r_1) = 0.5$. Speaking in terms of an RCA in the domain, this is the a priori probability that an order will eventually be rejected at the time when *place order* and *confirm order* happen, respectively. Consider now the rule $r_2 = \{\exists\, p\, :\, \neg\, QualityAccepted(p)\} \rightarrow \{\exists\, o\, :\, (\neg\, InFull(o))\}$. We have $lift_{D_2}(r_2) = 2$. This indicates that the risk value doubles (in absolute terms) if at the time when *confirm order* is executed, the quality of the production batch corresponding to the order has not yet been accepted.

Hence, the rationale of our approach is to analyze root causes of negative process outcomes *(a)* along the process, that is, for each activity of interest and *(b)* across all relevant object types of interest. For this, we deploy association rules where the problematic outcome is encoded in the rule consequent (in the following called *target pattern*), and the rule antecedents (in the following called *descriptive patterns*) reflect possible explanations. In the next chapter, we describe the implementation of our solution.

4 Implementation

We implemented facilities for the approach presented here, also provided via Github[2]. In the following, we describe the application pipeline of the tool **(1–2)**, describe how the results can be put into the context of a process model **(3)**, and give heuristics to select interesting rules from the mined rules **(4)**.

1) Log Preprocessing. Our tool accepts a log in the OCEL2.0 [6] standard. Upon upload, predicates are derived from the observations. As mentioned earlier, we are not restricted to capture only object attributes, but may also encode event attribute assignments and object relationships. Attributes are only regarded if the number of unique labels (values) does not exceed a user-defined threshold. This applies to attributes of any type, both nominal and non-nominal.

2) Pattern Search. By default, existentially quantified formulas are constructed over object attributes, comparable to the examples shown in the previous section. Also, formulas describing event attributes are constructed. Our tool

---

[2] https://github.com/beneknopp/interaction-pattern-mining

allows to specify custom formulas over the available predicate symbols. Besides a selection of descriptive patterns, the target pattern has to be specified. After selecting patterns for each event type of interest, association rules are mined [8], parametrized by a minimal support of individual patterns.

3) Presentation. In order to comprehensively report the mining results, we suggest to consider a frequency-annotated *object-centric directly-follows graph (OCDFG)* [7], as depicted in Fig. 1. An OCDFG is the generalization of a traditional DFG involving multiple object types. Each activity shows the frequency of occurrences, i.e., the number of events of that activity. Each typed edge between two activities is also annotated with the number of times this directly-follows relation was realized by an object of the respective type. Here, we report at each event type as *risk* the confidence of the rule $\emptyset \rightarrow \{p\}$, where p is the target pattern. That is the a priori likelihood that at event time, the process will eventually have a negative outcome. The annotated model may be helpful in putting the rules at event types into the context of the whole process.

5   Experiments

To show the usefulness our approach, we investigated the order-to-cash process of a globally acting food and drink processing company. The used (confidential) object-centric log describes a time span of 1.5 years and is based on SAP data from multiple dimensions. We focus here on the object types *sales order items, delivery items, delivery headers* and *production batches*. A sales order item is (transitively) linked to objects of other types. Namely, each item has one to many delivery items, each delivery item has exactly one header and draws supply from exactly one production batch. However, by filtering, we select only sales order items that are linked to exactly one delivery item. We choose this filter in order to facilitate interpreting the mined rules, since each existentially quantified formula in a rule, for each event, binds to an unambiguous reference object. Thus, measurements are not obfuscated by varying object type multiplicities.

As the use case, we investigated the *On-Time-In-Full (OTIF)* KPI of the order-to-cash process. OTIF measures the degree to which orders were delivered timely and completely to customers. On the level of object types, this KPI can by definition be decomposed into the *OnTime* property on delivery items and the *InFull* property on sales order items. We considered a binary representation of these subproperties, comparable to the *InFull* example presented in the previous sections, so each sales order item is either *InFull* or not and each delivery item is either *OnTime* or not. Findings for the *OnTime* property are shown in Table 2 and for the *InFull* property in Table 3.

The exemplary findings for *OnTime* in Table 2 are based on a sample of 10.000 delivery items and apply to instances at the time of the *perform batch split* activity, at which point production supply is assigned to the item. This activity usually happens shortly before the actual delivery. The first depicted rule shows that 25% of all batch splits are performed on a *Friday*, and in this case, the risk of an untimely delivery was 1.89 times higher. The other two depicted rules

Table 2. Rules for the *OnTime* property at the activity *perform batch split*, on a data set of 10.000 records (events). The risk of the target pattern $\exists i : \neg OnTime(i)$ is 0.64%. Variable i denotes the delivery item, o the sales order item and d the delivery header. The rules narrow down to a specific subset of delivery items that had a negative outcome because of inaccurate inventory slot availability forecasts for weekends.

Pattern	Support	Lift
$\{Friday()\}$ $\rightarrow \{\exists i : \neg OnTime(i)\}$	0.25	1.89
$\{Friday(),$ $\exists o : DaysSinceOrderCreation = 3(o)\}$ $\rightarrow \{\exists i : \neg OnTime(i)\}$	0.15	27.65
$\{Friday(),$ $\exists o : DaysSinceOrderCreation = 3(o),$ $\exists d : DaysUntilDeliveryDue = 0(s)\}$ $\rightarrow \{\exists i : \neg OnTime(i)\}$	0.01	39.91

Table 3. Rules for the *InFull* property at the activity *confirm order* across a segmentation of the process with regards to material types. Variable o denotes the sales order item and p the associated production batch. Each cell in a pattern row shows the support on top and the lift below. The rules show that root causes with respect to the production dimension are prevalent and vary across the different material types.

Material	1	2	3	4	5	6	7
Event (Object) Count	4.5k	1.5k	2.0k	800	700	1.7k	2.0k
Risk	1.7%	1.3%	2.7%	5.4%	7.8%	1.2%	2.2%
$\{\exists p : IssueOnTime(p)\}$ $\rightarrow \{\exists o : \neg InFull(o)\}$	0.01 0.00	0.12 1.57	0.01 4.06	0.06 0.77	0.08 0.87	0.00 0.00	0.05 2.45
$\{\exists p : Underproduction(p)\}$ $\rightarrow \{\exists o : \neg InFull(o)\}$	0.52 1.30	0.64 1.17	0.46 1.35	0.34 1.15	0.33 1.23	0.56 1.37	0.67 0.93
$\{\exists p : MotherBatchScrap(p)\}$ $\rightarrow \{\exists o : \neg InFull(o)\}$	0.10 0.37	0.04 6.50	0.08 1.80	0.01 3.1	0.01 0.00	0.05 1.56	0.05 1.42
$\{\exists p : PlantX(p)\}$ $\rightarrow \{\exists o : \neg InFull(o)\}$	0.32 0.12	0.0 0.0	0.61 1.06	0.01 0.00	0.01 0.0	0.05 1.91	0.05 2.00

show that this risk strongly increases in that context if also the associated order had been placed several days before, and furthermore, the delivery is due on the day of event time. Discussing the details of the affected process instances with domain experts, we found out that the negative outcomes were due to not enough inventory slots being available at the customers' side, which in turn was due to inaccurate forecasts of inventory availabilities several days in advance. In consequence, delivery had to be shifted past the originially requested date. While this true root cause is not - and, in fact, cannot be - represented by means of the object-centric patterns since the data is scoped intra-organizationally, the patterns provide a minimal discriminating description of the affected instances.

The rules in Table 3 are based on a segmentation of the process across various material types *1,...,7*, and associate the *InFull* outcome of sales order items of these material types with various patterns on related production batches at time of *confirm order*. Again, there is a one-to-one correspondence between observations (events) and objects (sales order items). The descriptive patterns comprise: indicators that the batch had an on-time issue in production (*IssueOnTime*), that less was produced than planned (*Underproduction*), that there is a related mother batch that was scrapped (*MotherBatchScrap*), and that the batch was produced at a specific plant (*PlantX*). As compared to the *OnTime* rules in Table 2, the findings for *InFull* do not pinpoint to specific instances; rather, they give a broad overview on how different factors in production upstream might have an influence on the order fulfillment. Here, we remark that threads to validity partly exist due to rather low risk and support values of some of the rules.

6   Discussion

The experimental results show the strength of the approach and, in particular, the added value of the surrounding object-centric framework, in conducting an RCA. This is exemplified by all rules depicted in Tables 2 and 3, since they relate the outcome captured on the level of one object type to descriptive patterns at other object types. In particular, the rules of greater length in Tables 2, by linking together multiple patterns, show the usefulness of mining for sets of patterns for the RCA. Furthermore, note that information across several object types (sales order items, delivery headers and items) was required here to find a description of minimal length for the set of problematic instances. In summary, we argue that we have found evidence that bad process outcomes can in fact be explained via interacting objects, as aimed for in our research goal.

A limitation of the approach is that rules can be hard to interpret if formulas refer to object types of varying cardinalities. This challenge is inherent to the object-centric framework that allows for this variability. As stated, we dispelled such ambiguities in our experiments by pre-filtering the input. Another shortcoming of our approach follows from the inherent limitation of itemset mining to discretized attributes. Here, we see potential for refinement in future work, for example by adapting the mechanisms of the C4.5 algorithm well-known from decision tree learning for discretizing numerical and continuous attributes.

7   Conclusion

In this paper, we have introduced a novel method for root cause analyses (RCA) on object-centric logs using association rule mining. The experiments have substantiated the usefulness of that method. In our opinion, the results suggest a synergy between pattern mining and object-centric process mining.

The first-order logic based query engine implemented here is not restricted in its use to RCA. We argue that other use cases are possible, as long as these can be formulated on the event level. For example, one could validate constraints at event types using arbitrary complex formulas. In future work, we would like to explore via case studies whether complex root causes can be found in real processes that further leverage the presented logical query engine. Also, we would like to improve the extent to which the object-centric rules can provide operational support by embedding them into a causal inference framework [3,12]. Finally, we would like to explore whether pattern-based descriptions can be used for creating more realistic discrete event simulation models [15].

References

1. Van Houdt, G., Depaire, B., Martin, N.: Root cause analysis in process mining with probabilistic temporal logic. In: Munoz-Gama, J., Lu, X. (eds.) ICPM 2021. LNBIP, vol. 433, pp. 73–84. Springer, Cham (2022). https://doi.org/10.1007/978-3-030-98581-3_6
2. Fani Sani, M., van der Aalst, W., Bolt, A., García-Algarra, J.: Subgroup discovery in process mining. In: Abramowicz, W. (ed.) BIS 2017. LNBIP, vol. 288, pp. 237–252. Springer, Cham (2017). https://doi.org/10.1007/978-3-319-59336-4_17
3. Qafari, M.S., van der Aalst, W.: Root cause analysis in process mining using structural equation models. In: Del Río Ortega, A., Leopold, H., Santoro, F.M. (eds.) BPM 2020. LNBIP, vol. 397, pp. 155–167. Springer, Cham (2020). https://doi.org/10.1007/978-3-030-66498-5_12
4. van der Aalst, W.: Object-centric process mining: unraveling the fabric of real processes. Mathematics **11**(12), 2691 (2023)
5. Fahland, D.: Process mining over multiple behavioral dimensions with event knowledge graphs. In: Process Mining Handbook. Springer, Cham (2022). https://doi.org/10.1007/978-3-031-08848-3_9
6. Koren, I., Adams, J.N., Berti, A.: OCEL 2.0 Resources–www. ocel-standard. org. arXiv preprint arXiv:2403.01982 (2024)
7. Berti, A., van der Aalst, W.: Extracting multiple viewpoint models from relational databases. In: Ceravolo, P., van Keulen, M., Gómez-López, M.T. (eds.) SIMPDA 2018-2019. LNBIP, vol. 379, pp. 24–51. Springer, Cham (2020). https://doi.org/10.1007/978-3-030-46633-6_2
8. Agrawal, R., Imieliński, T., Swami, A.: Mining association rules between sets of items in large databases. In: Proceedings of the 1993 ACM SIGMOD International Conference on Management of Data (1993)
9. Gupta, N., Anand, K., Sureka, A.: Pariket: mining business process logs for root cause analysis of anomalous incidents. In: Chu, W., Kikuchi, S., Bhalla, S. (eds.) DNIS 2015. LNCS, vol. 8999, pp. 244–263. Springer, Cham (2015). https://doi.org/10.1007/978-3-319-16313-0_19
10. Suriadi, S., Ouyang, C., van der Aalst, W.M.P., ter Hofstede, A.H.M.: Root cause analysis with enriched process logs. In: La Rosa, M., Soffer, P. (eds.) BPM 2012. LNBIP, vol. 132, pp. 174–186. Springer, Heidelberg (2013). https://doi.org/10.1007/978-3-642-36285-9_18
11. Böhmer, K., Rinderle-Ma, S.: Mining association rules for anomaly detection in dynamic process runtime behavior and explaining the root cause to users. Inf. Syst. **90**, 101438 (2020)
12. Bozorgi, Z.D., Teinemaa, I., Dumas, M., La Rosa, M., Polyvyanyy, A.: Process mining meets causal machine learning: discovering causal rules from event logs. In: 2nd International Conference on Process Mining (ICPM). IEEE (2020)

13. Bergami, G., di Francescomarino, C., Ghidini, C., Maggi, F.M., Puura, J.: Exploring business process deviance with sequential and declarative patterns. arXiv preprint arXiv:2111.12454 (2021)
14. de Leoni, M., van der Aalst, W.M.P., Dees, M.: A general framework for correlating business process characteristics. In: Sadiq, S., Soffer, P., Völzer, H. (eds.) BPM 2014. LNCS, vol. 8659, pp. 250–266. Springer, Cham (2014). https://doi.org/10.1007/978-3-319-10172-9_16
15. Knopp, B., Pourbafrani, M., van der Aalst, W.: Discovering object-centric process simulation models. In: 5th International Conference on Process Mining (ICPM). IEEE (2023)

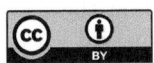

The Jensen-Shannon Distance for Stochastic Conformance Checking

Tian Li[1,2(✉)], Sander J. J. Leemans[1,3(✉)], and Artem Polyvyanyy[2(✉)]

[1] RWTH Aachen University, Aachen, Germany
{t.li,s.leemans}@bpm.rwth-aachen.de
[2] The University of Melbourne, Melbourne, Australia
artem.polyvyanyy@unimelb.edu.au
[3] Fraunhofer FIT, Sankt Augustin, Germany

Abstract. A sub-field of process mining, conformance checking, quantifies how well the process behavior of a model represents the observed behavior recorded in a log. A stochastic-aware perspective that accounts for the probability of behavior in both model and log is necessary to support conformance checking. However, existing stochastic conformance checking measures are not comparable for a broad framework that includes log-to-log (L2L), log-to-model (L2M), and model-to-model (M2M) comparison settings. Therefore, we propose a stochastic conformance checking measure based on the Jensen-Shannon Distance (JSD), which interprets models and logs as probability distributions over traces. It can be applied to perform L2L, L2M, and M2M conformance, while the latter requires approximation. Notably, it is the only known stochastic conformance measure that is a metric. JSD has been implemented and is publicly available. Our quantitative evaluations show the feasibility of computing JSD over real-life event logs, and that it provides diagnostic results different from those of existing measures. Moreover, experiments in the M2M setting confirm that our measure can be approximated using unbiased sampling.

Keywords: Stochastic process mining · Stochastic conformance checking

1 Introduction

Information systems in modern organizations record process executions performed by employees, managers, and customers as event data. Such data can be extracted as an event log, which is a collection of recorded traces, where each trace is a sequence of activities observed in a process execution. By leveraging the historical event data in event logs, process mining studies ways to optimize real-world processes [1].

In process mining, process models are used to better understand the process and identify issues. *Conformance checking* relates events in the event log to

A. Delgado and T. Slaats (Eds.): ICPM 2024 Workshops, LNBIP 533, pp. 70–83, 2025.
https://doi.org/10.1007/978-3-031-82225-4_6

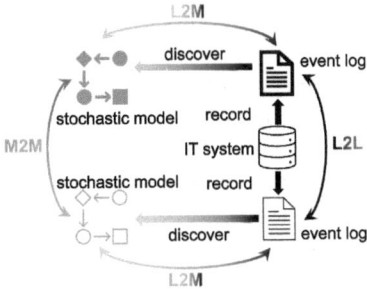

Fig. 1. Three settings of stochastic conformance checking: L2L, L2M, and M2M.

activities in the process model to identify commonalities and differences between them, i.e., log-to-model comparison (L2M). For example, the results of L2M conformance checking can be used to inform auditing efforts. Additionally, conformance checking may involve model-to-model comparisons (M2M) [1, p265], for instance, to compare models discovered from event logs recorded in geographically different regions. Furthermore, log-to-log conformance checking (L2L) compares two logs directly with one another. L2L conformance checking can be used for detecting process drift [28], which refers to the problem of finding changes in a process over time.

In real-life processes, certain behavior can occur more frequently than the other. Consider two event logs $[\langle a,b\rangle^{50}, \langle b,a\rangle^{50}]$ and $[\langle a,b\rangle^{80}, \langle b,a\rangle^{20}]$, which have the same trace variants but differ in the frequency of observations of these variants. As these logs are different, this should be reflected in conformance checking measurements. As for M2M conformance checking, one can detect and quantify changes in stochastic behavior by comparing the latest discovered model with a previous version of the model. Similarly, event logs that cover long periods or merge data from multiple organizations may contain different versions of process behavior. By applying stochastic conformance for L2L settings, one can avoid misleading conclusions when addressing process drift. We illustrate these settings of stochastic conformance checking in Fig. 1.

None of the existing stochastic conformance checking techniques support all of L2L, L2M and M2M, or the measure results in values that are incomparable across the three settings [20,22,25]. In this paper, we propose a stochastic conformance checking metric based on the Jensen-Shannon Distance (JSD) [13]. This metric interprets process behavior in an event log or a stochastic process model as a probability distribution over traces. JSD can be applied for stochastic conformance checking across three settings: i) L2L setting, ii) L2M setting where the stochastic model has a finite state space, and iii) M2M setting that relies on unbiased sampling.

The JSD metric has been implemented and is publicly available[1]. We compared it quantitatively with existing stochastic conformance techniques on sev-

---

[1] https://bpm.rwth-aachen.de/ebi.

eral real-life event logs and stochastic process models, which demonstrated that JSD measurements can lead to different conclusions. Moreover, for the M2M setting, we evaluated the influence of the sample size and confirmed that the approximation converges with the growth of simulated event logs.

The remainder of the paper proceeds as follows. We first discuss related work in Sect. 2 and introduce preliminaries in Sect. 3. In Sect. 4, we discuss how JSD can be applied in L2L, L2M, and M2M settings, after which we evaluate it in Sect. 5. Finally, Sect. 6 concludes the paper.

2   Related Work

Recently, several techniques for stochastic process discovery have been proposed, including the weight estimation techniques that discover a stochastic labeled Petri net (SLPN) from the input event log and control flow model [6,7,18], and techniques that directly construct a stochastic model from an input event log [3,26].

Conformance checking for non-stochastic models has been extensively discussed [8]. Van der Aalst [2] emphasized the importance of considering probabilities in conformance checking. Entropic Relevance (ER) [25] computes the average number of bits to compress each log trace by leveraging the trace likelihood information in a stochastic model. Entropy Recall (E-Recall) and Entropy Precision (E-Precision) [20] quantifies frequent and rare deviations between an event log and a stochastic model by treating both log and model as stochastic automata, and comparing the entropy of these automata with the entropy of a third automaton that represents the joint behavior. Probabilistic Alignments [4] consider the frequencies of traces in logs and calculate the likelihood of a move being synchronous or not in the stochastic process model. Bogdanov et al. [5] proposed an alignment-based algorithm that computes the conformance cost between a model and a stochastically known log [14]. Alpha Precision [10] uses the stochastic language of the model and the event log, and inferences about the underlying system that generated the log. Another recent work proposed unit Earth Movers' Stochastic Conformance (uEMSC) and Earth Movers' Stochastic Conformance (EMSC) [16] that measure the effort of transforming the distribution of traces in the log to that described in the stochastic model. Although EMSC can be applied to compute L2M and M2M conformance, it relies on a biased truncation to sample traces from models.

These stochastic conformance checking techniques either only support L2M settings, or the measures provide values that are incomparable across the L2L, L2M, and M2M settings.

3   Preliminaries

Given a set of elements S, a multiset $X : S \to \mathbb{N}$ maps the elements of S to the natural numbers, such that X allows for multiple instances for each of its elements. For example, $X = [a, b^4, c^5]$ is a multiset with ten elements: one

a, four b's, and five c's. The union of two multisets X_1 and X_2 is denoted as $X_1 \uplus X_2$. Multiset subset $X_1 \subseteq X_2$ denotes $\forall_{s \in S} X_2(s) \geq X_1(s)$. If $X_1 \subseteq X_2$, then $X_3 = X_2 \setminus X_1$ is the multiset difference, such that $\forall_{s \in S} X_3(s) = X_2(s) - X_1(s)$.

An *event log* is a collection of *traces*, which are sequences of activities. We can transform an event log into a stochastic language by dividing the frequency of each trace by the total number of traces.

Definition 1 (Stochastic Languages). *Let Σ be a finite set of* activities *and let Σ^* be the set of all finite sequences of activities (*traces*) over Σ. Then, a* stochastic language *l is a function that maps each trace in Σ^* to a probability, that is, $l : \Sigma^* \to [0, 1]$ such that $\sum_{\sigma \in \Sigma^*} l(\sigma) = 1$.*

A stochastic language assigns probabilities to traces so that the assigned probabilities sum up to one. Inherently, an event log denotes a finite stochastic language. For instance, given two event logs $L_1 = [\langle a, b \rangle^3, \langle b, a \rangle^2]$ and $L_2 = [\langle a, b \rangle^{80}, \langle a, b, b \rangle^{20}]$, their finite stochastic languages are $l_1 = [\langle a, b \rangle^{0.6}, \langle b, a \rangle^{0.4}]$ and $l_2 = [\langle a, b \rangle^{0.8}, \langle a, b, b \rangle^{0.2}]$, respectively.

A stochastic process model is a model that describes a stochastic language. We introduce two types of stochastic process models: stochastic labeled Petri nets and stochastic deterministic finite automata.

Definition 2 (Stochastic Labeled Petri Nets). *Let Σ be a finite set of activities, a* stochastic labeled Petri net *(SLPN) is a tuple (P, T, F, w, ρ, m_0) where P is a finite set of places, T is a finite set of transitions such that $P \cap T = \emptyset$, $F \subseteq (P \times T) \cup (T \times P)$ is a flow relation, $w : T \to \mathbb{R}^0$ is a weight function, $\rho : T \to \Sigma \cup \{\tau\}$ is a labeling function, and m_0 is the initial marking.*

A marking in an SLPN is a multiset of places. An SLPN starts its execution from its initial marking. Let ${}^\bullet t = [p \mid (p, t) \in F]$ be the set of places directly before transition t, $t^\bullet = [p \mid (t, p) \in F]$ be the set of places directly after t, and $T_m = \{t \mid {}^\bullet t \subseteq m\}$ denote all *enabled* transitions in marking m. An enabled transition $t \in T_m$ can *fire* with probability $\mathrm{p}(t \mid m) = \frac{w(t)}{\sum_{t' \in T_m} w(t')}$, which results in a new marking $m' = m \uplus t^\bullet \setminus {}^\bullet t$.

A *path* is a sequence of transitions $\langle t_1, \ldots, t_n \rangle$ that are fired along with a sequence of markings $\langle m_0, \ldots, m_n \rangle$, such that $\forall_{1 \leq i \leq n} {}^\bullet t_i \subseteq m_{i-1} \wedge m_i = m_{i-1} \uplus t_i^\bullet \setminus {}^\bullet t_i$ and $T_{m_n} = \emptyset$ for m_n. That is, a path brings the model from its initial marking m_0 to a deadlock marking, in which no marking is enabled. The probability of the path $\langle t_0, \ldots, t_n \rangle$ is $\prod_{0 \leq i \leq n} \mathrm{p}(t_i \mid m_{i-1})$. A transition t with $\rho(t) = \tau$ is unobservable, or silent. The projection of a path by labeling function ρ on the non-τ transitions is a trace, and there may be several (even countably-infinite many [19]) paths that project to the same trace.

For instance, M_1 in Fig. 2 is an SLPN with two silent transitions τ_1 and τ_2 and three transitions with labels a, b, and c. $\langle a, \tau_1, \tau_2, \tau_1, b \rangle$ and $\langle a, \tau_1, b \rangle$ are two paths that correspond to the trace $\langle a, b \rangle$. M_1 can generate infinitely many different traces, thus its stochastic language is infinite.

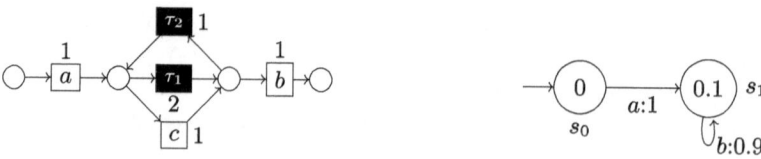

Fig. 2. SLPN M_1.   **Fig. 3.** SDFA M_2.

Definition 3 (Stochastic Deterministic Finite Automaton). *A stochastic deterministic finite automaton (SDFA) $A = (S, Q, \delta, p, s_0)$ consists of a finite set of states S, with $s_0 \in S$ the initial state, a set of actions $Q \subseteq V$, a transition function $\delta : S \times Q \to S$, and a transition probability function $p : S \times Q \to [0, 1]$ such that for each state $s \in S$, it holds that $\sum_{q \in Q} p(s, q) \leq 1$.*

For example, Fig. 3 shows an SDFA using graphical notation. The states and transition function are visualized as circles and arcs, respectively. It has two states, s_0 and s_1. The initial state is s_0, and its transition function is defined by $\{(s_0, a, s_1), (s_1, b, s_1)\}$. Arc from s_0 to s_1 with label $a{:}1$ specifies that $(s_0, a, s_1) \in \delta$ and $(s_0, a, 1) \in p$. Likewise, arc from s_1 to s_1 with label $b{:}0.9$ specifies that $(s_1, b, s_1) \in \delta$ and $(s_1, b, 0.9) \in p$.

By converting event logs and stochastic models to stochastic languages, we reduce stochastic conformance to the problem of computing the similarity of two stochastic languages. Given two stochastic languages, the Kullback-Leibler Divergence quantifies the difference between the probability distributions over traces in these languages.

Definition 4 (Kullback-Leibler Divergence [9]). *Let Σ be a finite set of activities, Σ^* be the set of all finite sequences of activities (traces) over Σ, and l and l' be two stochastic languages over Σ. The Kullback-Leibler Divergence (KLD) of l with respect to l' is defined as:*

$$\mathrm{kld}(l, l') = \sum_{\sigma \in \Sigma^*} l(\sigma) \log_2 \frac{l(\sigma)}{l'(\sigma)}.$$

We accept that $0 \log_2 0 = 0$. KLD is not symmetric, as $\mathrm{kld}(l, l')$ may not equal $\mathrm{kld}(l', l)$. If one trace has a zero probability in l' and a non-zero probability in l, $\mathrm{kld}(l, l')$ is undefined. The Jensen-Shannon Distance (JSD) overcomes this limitation by comparing two stochastic languages based on their average stochastic language.

Definition 5 (Average Stochastic Languages). *Let Σ be a finite set of activities, Σ^* be the set of all finite sequences of activities (traces) over Σ, and l and l' be two stochastic languages. The stochastic languages l'' for which it holds that $\forall_{\sigma \in \Sigma^*} l''(\sigma) = 0.5(l(\sigma) + l'(\sigma))$, is the average stochastic language of l and l' denoted by $avg(l, l')$.*

For example, $avg(l_1, l_2) = [\langle a, b \rangle^{0.7}, \langle b, a \rangle^{0.2}, \langle a, b, b \rangle^{0.1}]$ is the average stochastic language of l_1 and l_2. Given two stochastic languages, their Jensen-Shannon Distance is defined as follows.

Definition 6 (Jensen-Shannon Distance [13]). *Let l and l' be two stochastic languages. The* Jensen-Shannon Distance *(JSD) between l and l' is defined as:*

$$\mathrm{jsd}(l, l') = \sqrt{\frac{\mathrm{kld}(l, avg(l, l')) + \mathrm{kld}(l', avg(l, l'))}{2}}$$

JSD is bound between 0 and 1. Moreover, JSD using a square root is a metric [13], thus for any stochastic languages l, l' and l'', we have: i) Reflexivity: $\mathrm{jsd}(l, l') = 0 \Leftrightarrow l = l'$, ii) Symmetricity: $\mathrm{jsd}(l, l') = \mathrm{jsd}(l', l)$, and iii) Triangle inequality: $\mathrm{jsd}(l, l') + \mathrm{jsd}(l', l'') \geq \mathrm{jsd}(l, l'')$.

4   Stochastic Conformance Checking with JSD

In this section, we discuss how to compute JSD in L2L, L2M, and M2M settings.

4.1   Log-to-Log Conformance

In the L2L setting, given that a log induces a finite stochastic language, and the average stochastic language of two logs is also finite, one can directly apply Definition 6. Let l and l' be the stochastic languages of two event logs, $L_{>0} = \{\sigma \mid l(\sigma) > 0\}$ and $L'_{>0} = \{\sigma \mid l'(\sigma) > 0\}$, it holds that:

$$\mathrm{jsd}(l, l') = \sqrt{\frac{\mathrm{kld}(l, avg(l, l')) + \mathrm{kld}(l', avg(l, l'))}{2}}, \text{ where:} \qquad (1)$$

$$\mathrm{kld}(l, avg(l, l')) = \sum_{\sigma \in L_{>0}} l(\sigma) \log_2 \frac{l(\sigma)}{avg(l, l')(\sigma)} \text{ and,}$$

$$\mathrm{kld}(l', avg(l, l')) = \sum_{\sigma \in L'_{>0}} l'(\sigma) \log_2 \frac{l'(\sigma)}{avg(l, l')(\sigma)}$$

As l and l' for both event logs are finite, the terms in Eq. (1) are finite. We adopt $l(\sigma) \log_2 \frac{l(\sigma)}{avg(l,l')(\sigma)} = 0$ if $l(\sigma) = 0$, and $l'(\sigma) \log_2 \frac{l'(\sigma)}{avg(l,l')(\sigma)} = 0$ if $l'(\sigma) = 0$.

For instance, given the stochastic languages l_1, l_2, for logs L_1 and L_2, we have: $\mathrm{kld}(l_1, avg(l_1, l_2)) = 0.6 \log_2 \frac{0.6}{0.7} + 0.4 \log_2 \frac{0.4}{0.2} \approx 0.267$ and $\mathrm{kld}(l_2, avg(l_1, l_2)) = 0.8 \log_2 \frac{0.8}{0.7} + 0.2 \log_2 \frac{0.2}{0.1} \approx 0.354$. Hence, the JSD between L_1 and L_2 is $\mathrm{jsd}(l_1, l_2) = \sqrt{\frac{0.267 + 0.354}{2}} \approx 0.575$.

4.2   Log-to-Model Conformance

The definition of JSD relies on the average stochastic language of two input stochastic languages. Hence, the average stochastic language may be infinite. However, as an event log always corresponds to a finite stochastic language, we can avoid explicitly constructing the potentially infinite average stochastic language of an event log and a stochastic model with a finite state space by rewriting Definition 6.

Let l and m be the stochastic language of the input event log and the stochastic language of the stochastic model, respectively. Based on Definition 4 and Definition 5, we have:

$$\text{jsd}(l,m) = \sqrt{\frac{\sum_{\sigma \in \Sigma^*} n(\sigma)}{2}}, \text{ where:} \tag{2}$$

$$n(\sigma) = l(\sigma) \log_2 \frac{2l(\sigma)}{l(\sigma) + m(\sigma)} + m(\sigma) \log_2 \frac{2\,m(\sigma)}{l(\sigma) + m(\sigma)}.$$

Let $\Sigma_0^* = \{\sigma \mid l(\sigma) = 0 \wedge m(\sigma) = 0\}$ denote the set of traces that are in neither the log nor the model. For all $\sigma \in \Sigma_0^*$, we have $n(\sigma) = 0$. Hence, we only consider the traces in $\Sigma^* \backslash \Sigma_0^*$, i.e., traces that are observed in l or m.

It holds that $\Sigma^* \backslash \Sigma_0^* = \Sigma_1^* \cup \Sigma_2^* \cup \Sigma_3^*$ where $\Sigma_1^* = \{\sigma \mid l(\sigma) > 0 \wedge m(\sigma) > 0\}$, $\Sigma_2^* = \{\sigma \mid l(\sigma) > 0 \wedge m(\sigma) = 0\}$, and $\Sigma_3^* = \{\sigma \mid l(\sigma) = 0 \wedge m(\sigma) > 0\}$. By splitting set $\Sigma^* \backslash \Sigma_0^*$ into the union of three subsets, $n(\sigma)$ in Eq. (2) can be written as a piecewise function:

$$n(\sigma) = \begin{cases} l(\sigma) \log_2 \frac{2l(\sigma)}{l(\sigma) + m(\sigma)} + m(\sigma) \log_2 \frac{2\,m(\sigma)}{l(\sigma) + m(\sigma)}, & \text{if } \sigma \in \Sigma_1^* \\ l(\sigma), & \text{if } \sigma \in \Sigma_2^* \\ m(\sigma), & \text{if } \sigma \in \Sigma_3^* \end{cases}$$

Then, one can rewrite Eq. (2) as follows:

$$\text{jsd}(l,m) = \sqrt{\frac{j_1(l,m) + j_2(l,m) + j_3(l,m)}{2}}, \text{ where:} \tag{3}$$

$$j_1(l,m) = \sum_{\sigma \in \Sigma_1^*} l(\sigma) \log_2 \frac{2l(\sigma)}{l(\sigma) + m(\sigma)} + m(\sigma) \log_2 \frac{2\,m(\sigma)}{l(\sigma) + m(\sigma)},$$

$$j_2(l,m) = \sum_{\sigma \in \Sigma_2^*} l(\sigma) = 1 - \sum_{\sigma \in \Sigma_1^*} l(\sigma), \text{ and}$$

$$j_3(l,m) = \sum_{\sigma \in \Sigma_3^*} m(\sigma) = 1 - \sum_{\sigma \in \Sigma_1^*} m(\sigma).$$

First, we query the model for the probability of each log's trace leveraging the technique discussed in [19] for $j_1(l,m)$. Note that this step is non-trivial, as there can be an infinite number of SLPN paths corresponding to one trace. Therefore, we avoid explicitly computing an infinite average stochastic language for l and m. For instance, for L_2 and M_1, we first calculate the probability of each trace from L_2 in model M_1, that is, $m_1(\langle a,b \rangle) = 0.5$, $m_1(\langle b,a \rangle) = 0$. Given that $l_2(\langle a,b \rangle) = 0.8$, we have: $j_1(l_2,m_1) = 0.8 \log_2 \frac{0.8}{0.65} + 0.5 \log_2 \frac{0.5}{0.65} \approx 0.050$.

Then, the second term $j_2(l_2,m_1) = 1 - 0.8 = 0.2$, as trace $\langle b,a \rangle$ is only observed in log. The third term $j_3(l_2,m_1) = 1 - 0.5 = 0.5$ is the probability sum of traces generated by M_1 while not observed in L_2. Finally, the JSD between L_2 and M_1 is $\text{jsd}(l_2,m_1) = \sqrt{\frac{0.050+0.2+0.5}{2}} \approx 0.613$.

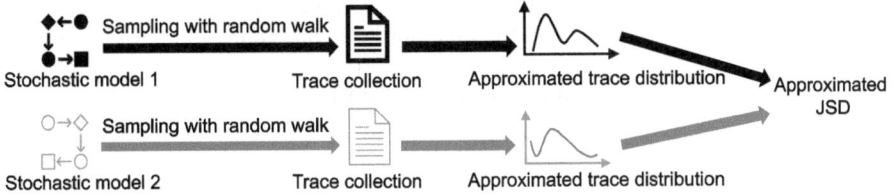

Fig. 4. JSD approximation for the M2M setting.

4.3   Model-to-Model Conformance

In the M2M setting, given two SDFAs, if their average stochastic language is an SDFA, then it is possible to transform the computation of JSD by leveraging Definition 5. Let m, m', m'' be three SDFAs, such that m'' is the SDFA that induces the average stochastic language of m and m'. The JSD of m and m' is:

$$\text{jsd}(m, m') = \sqrt{\frac{\text{kld}(m, m'') + \text{kld}(m', m'')}{2}}. \tag{4}$$

Applying Eq. (4) relies on the average SDFA for two input SDFAs. However, such an SDFA does not always exist [27]. Hence, in this paper, we do not attempt to find a general strategy to construct an average SDFA for two input SDFAs. Instead, we approximate the true value of JSD by sampling, as illustrated in Fig. 4. For each model, we generate a collection of traces that represent the model's process behavior. In each sampling iteration, a random walk is performed to generate a trace from the model. During a random walk in an SLPN, the probability of firing an enabled transition depends only on the current marking. In an SDFA, the probability of taking the next action depends only on the current state. The walk continues until it reaches the final marking for SLPN or the final state for SDFA, and a trace is generated. Furthermore, each trace is generated independently. Subsequently, the collection of sampled traces is used to construct a finite stochastic language.

The difference between our approach and the truncation technique in [22] is that traces are generated by their probability rather than length, as the truncation approach favors shorter traces over lengthier ones. Thereby, an approximated JSD value can be computed following Eq. (1) using event logs sampled from the models.

5   Evaluation

JSD has been implemented and is publicly available [23]. First, we compare JSD with existing stochastic conformance checking measures. Then, we study the implication of sample size when approximating JSD in the M2M setting.

Table 1. Experiment results of different stochastic conformance values with row-wise ranking. The errors for E-Recall and E-Precision were due to an unknown exception.

Event Log	Measure	d-uemsc	d-er	d-freq	d-align	d-scale
Road [24]	uEMSC	0.408 (1)	0.221 (2)	0.010 (5)	0.219 (3)	0.112 (4)
	EMSC	0.731 (3)	0.758 (1)	0.641 (5)	0.735 (2)	0.658 (4)
	ER	8.302 (4)	6.685 (1)	23.296 (5)	6.698 (2)	7.731 (3)
	E-Recall	0.909 (1)	0.909 (1)	Error	0.909 (1)	0.836 (4)
	E-Precision	0.783 (1)	0.692 (3)	Error	0.707 (2)	0.512 (4)
	JSD	0.338 (1)	0.389 (3)	0.818 (5)	0.387 (2)	0.514 (4)
Offer [12]	uEMSC	0.656 (1)	0.583 (2)	0.539 (4)	0.581 (3)	0.581 (3)
	EMSC	0.916 (1)	0.910 (2)	0.901 (5)	0.910 (2)	0.910 (2)
	ER	3.363 (4)	3.209 (1)	8.429 (5)	3.210 (2)	3.214 (3)
	E-Recall	0.996 (1)	0.996 (1)	0.996 (1)	0.996 (1)	0.923 (5)
	E-Precision	1.000 (1)	1.000 (1)	1.000 (1)	1.000 (1)	1.000 (1)
	JSD	0.114 (4)	0.108 (1)	0.208 (5)	0.108 (1)	0.109 (3)
Request [11]	uEMSC	0.778 (1)	0.766 (2)	0.005 (5)	0.712 (3)	0.418 (4)
	EMSC	0.886 (2)	0.885 (3)	0.457 (5)	0.897 (1)	0.644 (4)
	ER	8.465 (2)	8.368 (1)	28.471 (5)	8.604 (3)	11.389 (4)
	E-Recall	0.764 (1)	0.764 (1)	0.764 (1)	0.764 (1)	0.000 (5)
	E-Precision	1.000 (1)	1.000 (1)	0.003 (4)	0.814 (3)	0.000 (5)
	JSD	0.091 (2)	0.072 (1)	0.995 (5)	0.118 (3)	0.582 (4)

5.1 Quantitative Comparison

In this experiment, we compare the result of JSD with other stochastic conformance checking measures using three publicly available event logs [11,12,24]. First, given an event log, Inductive Miner [17] is used to construct a control-flow model. Next, we discover a stochastic model (SLPN) using stochastic discovery techniques, including d-uemsc, d-er, d-freq, d-align, and d-scale [7,18]. Finally, different measures have been applied to evaluate the stochastic conformance between each log and SLPNs, namely uEMSC, EMSC, ER, E-Recall, E-Precision, and JSD. The results are presented in Table 1. Note that for uEMSC, EMSC, E-Recall, and E-Precision, a higher value indicates better stochastic conformance. For distance measures ER and JSD, a lower value denotes a better conformance.

Overall, a model with a good uEMSC, EMSC, and ER also ranks higher for JSD. Although there is no unanimous agreement across JSD and other measures on the best stochastic models, there is partial agreement on the worst models. Stochastic models discovered using d-freq and d-scale have lower stochastic quality, as indicated by their ranks of JSD and other conformance measures.

When using the Spearman Correlation to examine the relationship between JSD and other conformance measures, JSD does not present a strong positive

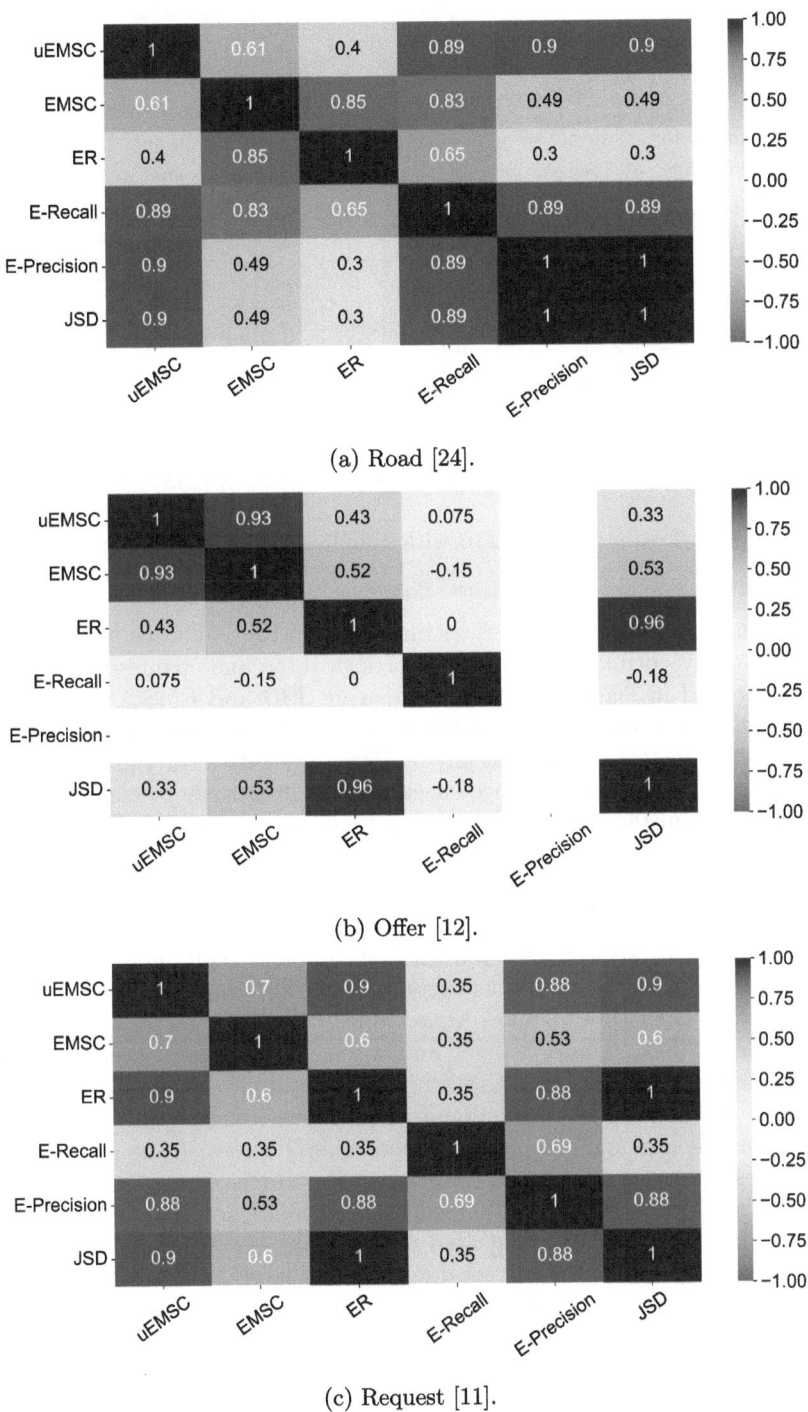

(a) Road [24].

(b) Offer [12].

(c) Request [11].

Fig. 5. Spearman correlation for stochastic conformance measures over different logs.

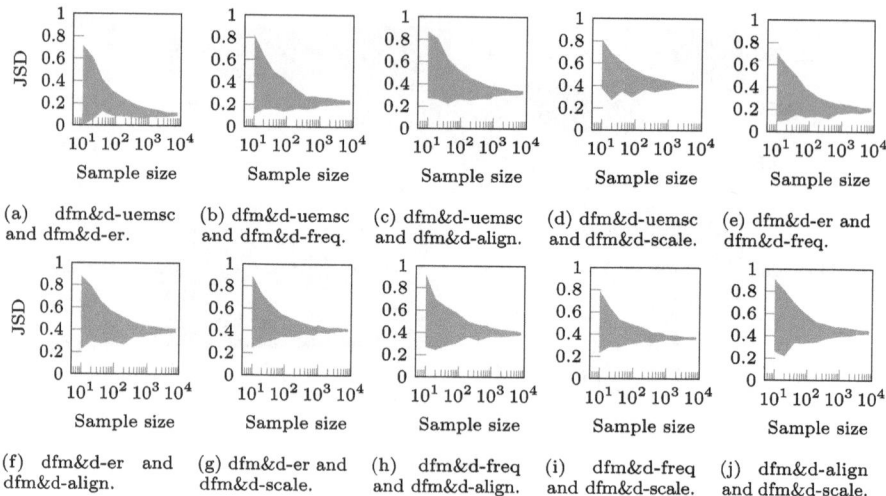

Fig. 6. Approximated JSD with sampling in the M2M settings.

correlation with existing measures, as illustrated in Fig. 5. For instance, although JSD is strongly correlated to uEMSC for logs Road and Request, this pattern is not observed in log Offer. When comparing JSD and EMSC, a medium to high correlation is observed in all three logs. As E-Precision for log Offer is 1 for all models, it does not present any positive or negative correlation with JSD. Therefore, stochastic conformance checking with JSD leads to conclusions that are different from those of existing stochastic conformance measures.

5.2   Influence of Sample Size

In this evaluation, we study the influence of sample size on approximating JSD between two SLPNs. We first constructed control-flow models with loops for log Domestic [11] using Direct-Follow Miner (dfm) [21], and then discovered SLPNs with d-uemsc, d-er, d-freq, d-align, and d-scale. We increased the number of traces sampled from 10 to 8000 to study how the sample size influences returned values. To reduce the effect of randomness, we repeat the computation 500 times for each sample size and compute the average JSD across all the repetitions.

The results are shown in Fig. 6, in which the x-axis represents the sampled trace size and the y-axis is the JSD value. The blue region represents the range of JSD values obtained from repeated experiments. As the number of sampled traces increases, the blue region gradually converges. Specifically, if the sample size is small and insufficient traces are generated, the JSD values vary considerably.

JSD shows expected behavior with an increasing number of sampled traces. The sampling we use is unbiased, i.e., it does not favor shorter traces over longer ones like the truncation technique used in EMSC [22]. With a larger sample size, loops are unfolded in the model with more traces generated, and the stochastic language approaches the true trace distribution of the model.

6   Conclusion

This paper studies the applicability of Jensen Shannon Distance for stochastic conformance checking. JSD is a metric that compares the trace distributions of two stochastic languages with that of their average language. This distance measure can be applied for log-to-log, log-to-model, and model-to-model conformance checking, the latter setting in general requiring an approximation using, for instance, an unbiased sampling presented in this work.

We evaluated the feasibility of JSD for conformance checking using real-life event logs and stochastic process models discovered from these logs. The comparison with existing stochastic conformance measures demonstrated that JSD measurements may lead to different conclusions, an observation deserving of further exploration in future works. In addition, we confirmed empirically that the proposed approximation of model-to-model conformance converges with the growth of simulated event logs.

The metric property of JSD can be useful in applications like searching for similar models [15]. Another interesting direction for future work is to identify the explicit construction of an average stochastic language, i.e., extend the measure for accurate computation for subclasses of models (M2M). Finally, one can assess whether JSD satisfies desired properties for stochastic conformance measures, such as properties designed for stochastic recall and precision measures [20].

References

1. van der Aalst, W.M.P.: Process Mining - Data Science in Action, 2nd Ed. Springer, Heidelberg (2016)
2. van der Aalst, W.M.P.: Relating process models and event logs - 21 conformance propositions. In: ATAED@Petri Nets/ACSD. CEUR Workshop Proceedings, vol. 2115, pp. 56–74. CEUR-WS.org (2018)
3. Alkhammash, H., Polyvyanyy, A., Moffat, A.: Stochastic directly-follows process discovery using grammatical inference. In: CAiSE. LNCS, vol. 14663, pp. 87–103. Springer, Heidelberg (2024)
4. Bergami, G., Maggi, F.M., Montali, M., Peñaloza, R.: Probabilistic trace alignment. In: ICPM, pp. 9–16. IEEE (2021)
5. Bogdanov, E., Cohen, I., Gal, A.: Conformance checking over stochastically known logs. In: BPM (Forum). LNBIP, vol. 458, pp. 105–119. Springer, Heidelberg (2022). https://doi.org/10.1007/978-3-031-16171-1_7
6. Brockhoff, T., Uysal, M.S., van der Aalst, W.M.P.: Wasserstein weight estimation for stochastic petri nets. In: ICPM, pp. 81–88. IEEE (2024)
7. Burke, A., Leemans, S.J.J., Wynn, M.T.: Stochastic process discovery by weight estimation. In: ICPM Workshops. LNBIP, vol. 406, pp. 260–272. Springer, Heidelberg (2020). https://doi.org/10.1007/978-3-030-72693-5_20

8. Carmona, J., van Dongen, B.F., Solti, A., Weidlich, M.: Conformance Checking - Relating Processes and Models. Springer, Heidelberg (2018). https://doi.org/10.1007/978-3-319-99414-7
9. Carrasco, R.C.: Accurate computation of the relative entropy between stochastic regular grammars. RAIRO Theor. Inf. Appl. **31**(5), 437–444 (1997)
10. Depaire, B., Janssenswillen, G., Leemans, S.J.J.: Alpha precision: Estimating the significant system behavior in a model. In: BPM (Forum). Lecture Notes in Business Information Processing, vol. 458, pp. 120–136. Springer, Heidelberg (2022). https://doi.org/10.1007/978-3-031-16171-1_8
11. van Dongen, B.: Bpi challenge 2020 (2020)
12. van Dongen, B.: Bpi challenge 2017 - offer log (2021)
13. Endres, D.M., Schindelin, J.E.: A new metric for probability distributions. IEEE Trans. Inf. Theory **49**(7), 1858–1860 (2003)
14. Gal, A.: Everything there is to know about stochastically known logs. In: ICPM. IEEE (2023)
15. Kunze, M., Weidlich, M., Weske, M.: Behavioral similarity - a proper metric. In: BPM. LNCS, vol. 6896, pp. 166–181. Springer, Heidelberg (2011). DOI: https://doi.org/10.1007/978-3-642-23059-2_15
16. Leemans, S.J.J., van der Aalst, W.M.P., Brockhoff, T., Polyvyanyy, A.: Stochastic process mining: earth movers' stochastic conformance. Inf. Syst. **102**, 101724 (2021)
17. Leemans, S.J.J., Fahland, D., van der Aalst, W.M.P.: Discovering block-structured process models from incomplete event logs. In: Ciardo, G., Kindler, E. (eds.) PETRI NETS 2014. LNCS, vol. 8489, pp. 91–110. Springer, Cham (2014). https://doi.org/10.1007/978-3-319-07734-5_6
18. Leemans, S.J.J., Li, T., Montali, M., Polyvyanyy, A.: Stochastic process discovery: can it be done optimally? In: CAiSE. Lecture Notes in Computer Science, vol. 14663, pp. 36–52. Springer, Heidelberg (2024). https://doi.org/10.1007/978-3-031-61057-8_3
19. Leemans, S.J.J., Maggi, F.M., Montali, M.: Enjoy the silence: analysis of stochastic petri nets with silent transitions. Inf. Syst. **124**, 102383 (2024)
20. Leemans, S.J.J., Polyvyanyy, A.: Stochastic-aware precision and recall measures for conformance checking in process mining. Inf. Syst. **115**, 102197 (2023)
21. Leemans, S.J.J., Poppe, E., Wynn, M.T.: Directly follows-based process mining: exploration & a case study. In: ICPM. IEEE (2019)
22. Leemans, S.J.J., Syring, A.F., van der Aalst, W.M.P.: Earth movers' stochastic conformance checking. In: Hildebrandt, T., van Dongen, B.F., Röglinger, M., Mendling, J. (eds.) BPM 2019. LNBIP, vol. 360, pp. 127–143. Springer, Cham (2019). https://doi.org/10.1007/978-3-030-26643-1_8
23. Leemans, S.J., Li, T., van Detten, J.N.: Ebi - a stochastic process mining framework. In: ICPM Doctoral Consortium and Demo Track. CEUR Workshop Proceedings. CEUR-WS.org (2024)
24. de Leoni, M.M., Mannhardt, F.: Road traffic fine management process (2015)
25. Polyvyanyy, A., Moffat, A., García-Bañuelos, L.: An entropic relevance measure for stochastic conformance checking in process mining. In: ICPM, pp. 97–104. IEEE (2020)
26. Rogge-Solti, A., van der Aalst, W.M.P., Weske, M.: Discovering stochastic petri nets with arbitrary delay distributions from event logs. In: Lohmann, N., Song, M., Wohed, P. (eds.) BPM 2013. LNBIP, vol. 171, pp. 15–27. Springer, Cham (2014). https://doi.org/10.1007/978-3-319-06257-0_2

27. Vidal, E., Thollard, F., de la Higuera, C., Casacuberta, F., Carrasco, R.C.: Probabilistic finite-state machines-part I. IEEE Trans. Pattern Anal. Mach. Intell. **27**(7), 1013–1025 (2005)
28. Yeshchenko, A., Di Ciccio, C., Mendling, J., Polyvyanyy, A.: Comprehensive process drift detection with visual analytics. In: Laender, A.H.F., Pernici, B., Lim, E.-P., de Oliveira, J.P.M. (eds.) ER 2019. LNCS, vol. 11788, pp. 119–135. Springer, Cham (2019). https://doi.org/10.1007/978-3-030-33223-5_11

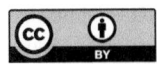

A Dynamic Programming Approach for Alignments on Process Trees

Christopher T. Schwanen[1][(✉)] , Wied Pakusa[2] ,
and Wil M. P. van der Aalst[1]

[1] Chair of Process and Data Science (PADS), RWTH Aachen University,
Aachen, Germany
{schwanen,wvdaalst}@pads.rwth-aachen.de
[2] Federal University of Applied Administrative Sciences, Brühl, Germany
wied.pakusa@hsbund.de

Abstract. A fundamental task in conformance checking is to compute optimal alignments between a given event log and a process model. In general, it is known that this unavoidably incurs high computational costs which, in turn, leads to poor scalability in practice. One angle to attack the complexity is to develop alignment algorithms that exploit particular syntactic restrictions of the underlying process models. In this article, we study alignments for process trees with unique labels. These models are the output of the Inductive Miner, a family of state-of-the-art process discovery algorithms also used by the leading process mining tools. Our main contribution is a novel algorithm that constructs optimal alignments for process trees with unique labels efficiently, i.e., in polynomial time. This is in contrast with general process trees where the problem is NP-complete and general workflow nets where the problem is PSPACE-hard. We give a proof-of-concept implementation of our algorithm in PM4Py and evaluate it on a collection of real-life event logs.

Keywords: Process Mining · Conformance Checking · Alignments · Process Trees · Dynamic Programming

1 Introduction

Constructing optimal alignments between a trace and a process model is a key task in conformance checking. Unfortunately, the algorithmic complexity of alignments is a major bottleneck in practice. It can be shown that computing optimal alignments on safe and sound workflow nets is PSPACE-complete. One approach to overcome the intractability is to consider (syntactic) restrictions on the process models and to make use of the additional structure to speed up the alignment computation. Along these lines, we recently showed that computing optimal alignments on *process trees* is in NP and we gave a novel Mixed Integer Linear Programming (MILP) formulation which outperforms the state-of-the-art alignment algorithms in PM4Py [20]. In this work, we reconsider process trees,

© The Author(s) 2025
A. Delgado and T. Slaats (Eds.): ICPM 2024 Workshops, LNBIP 533, pp. 84–97, 2025.
https://doi.org/10.1007/978-3-031-82225-4_7

but with the further restriction that each activity label occurs at most once in the process tree (i.e., *process trees with unique labels*).

In many real-life scenarios, process models have a tree-like structure, meaning that the full process decomposes into subprocesses that are interconnected in a tree-like fashion. In process mining, this kind of process models has been formalized as the concept of *process trees*. Process trees have gained quite some popularity in the process mining community, most importantly, since they form the basis for a widely used family of mining algorithms, the so-called *Inductive Miner* [15]. It is fair to say that process trees provide a good trade-off between expressiveness and computational efficiency.

But there is more to the story: the structure of process trees that come out of the Inductive Miner have *unique* activity labels, meaning that each activity label occurs at most once in the process tree. This clearly is a strong restriction, but it really is this assumption which makes the Inductive Miner tractable in practice. For us, it was reason enough to reconsider the alignment problem on process trees and ask if it is possible to exploit the *unique label property* to speed up the alignment computations even further, in particular: can alignments on process trees with unique labels be computed in polynomial time?

In this paper, we answer this question affirmatively. We give a new efficient (polynomial-time) dynamic programming algorithm to compute optimal alignments between a trace and a process tree with unique labels. This places the alignment problem for process trees with unique labels in P. Our key observation is that the unique label property allows us to handle the *parallel operator* in an efficient manner. The parallel operator models independent parallel computation and corresponds to a *parallel gateway* in BPMN or to the *shuffle operator* in formal languages. In fact, without the restriction to unique labels, the parallel operator requires the exploration of an exponential number of possible alignments which brings us to the realm of NP for general process trees. Besides the parallel operator, we further make use of the unique label property to speed-up computations of the sequence operator. We show how we can restrict the set of possible splits of a trace with respect to an optimal alignment. This saves a high number of recursive calls in the dynamic programming algorithm. We implemented our new algorithmic approach in form of a proof-of-concept based on the PM4Py ecosystem [4] and also evaluated it on a set of real-life benchmark logs. Our experiments show that the dynamic programming algorithm is competitive with the state-of-the-art alignment algorithms in PM4Py and even outperforms them in some cases. This underlines our belief that the structure of process models should be better taken into account when solving the alignment problem in practice.

2   Related Work

Alignments [3] are the state-of-the-art technique for conformance checking [7,8]. Besides the (textbook) algorithm based on A^*, several algorithmic approaches have been explored to compute alignments, e.g., see [5,11,16] for a technique based on Linear Programming (LP) to improve the A^*-heuristics, or [21] for an approximative scheme based on Mixed Integer Linear Programming (MILP). Other approaches use decomposition techniques to tackle large process model instances, e.g., see [1].

Process trees were first applied by [2,6] in the context of genetic process discovery. Since then, process trees have proven to be a modeling language with a great balance between expressiveness and algorithmic simplicity. In particular, they form the basis of one of the most popular process discovery algorithms, the so-called *Inductive Miner* [13–15]. Thus, optimized algorithms for alignment computations on process trees have been studied. Most notably, [19] proposed an approximation algorithm which performs well on many process trees, but which does not guarantee optimality in all cases. We also like to point to our MILP formulation for the alignment problem on process trees [20].

Finally, alignments for process trees have been studied much earlier in the context of the *error correction problem* for regular languages with shuffle operator, e.g., see [18] (under a different term). Our new algorithmic approach can be transferred into this field as well where, by the best of our knowledge, the unique label property has not been studied before.

3   Preliminaries

Let $\mathbb{N}$ ($\mathbb{N}_0$) be the set of natural numbers excluding 0 (including 0). For an n-tuple $a \in A_1 \times \cdots \times A_n$, $\pi_i(a)$ denotes the *projection* on its ith element, i.e., $\pi_i \colon A_1 \times \cdots \times A_n \to A_i, (a_1, \ldots, a_n) \mapsto a_i$.

Definition 1 (Alphabet). An *alphabet* Σ is a finite, non-empty set of *labels* (also referred to as *activities*).

Definition 2 (Sequence). *Sequences* with index set I over a set A are denoted by $\sigma = \langle a_i \rangle_{i \in I} \in A^I$. The *length* of a sequence σ is written as $|\sigma|$ and the set of all finite sequences over A is denoted by A^*. For a sequence $\sigma = \langle a_i \rangle_{i \in I} \in A^I$, $\sum \sigma$ is a shorthand for $\sum_{i \in I} a_i$. The restriction of a sequence $\sigma \in A^*$ to a set $B \subseteq A$ is the subsequence $\sigma|_B$ of σ consisting of all elements in B. A function $f \colon A \to B$ can be applied to a sequence $\sigma \in A^*$ given the recursive definition $f(\langle\rangle) := \langle\rangle$ and $f(\langle a \rangle \cdot \sigma) := \langle f(a) \rangle \cdot f(\sigma)$. For a sequence of tuples $\sigma \in (A^n)^*$, $\pi_i^*(\sigma)$ denotes the sequence of every ith element of its tuples, i.e., $\pi_i^*(\langle\rangle) := \langle\rangle$ and $\pi_i^*(\langle(a_1, \ldots, a_n)\rangle \cdot \sigma) := \langle \pi_i(a_1, \ldots, a_n) \rangle \cdot \pi_i^*(\sigma) = \langle a_i \rangle \cdot \pi_i^*(\sigma)$. As an important extension of π_i^* we write π_i^B for the composition of π_i^* with the restriction to B, i.e. $\pi_i^B := \pi_i^*|_B$.

We identify languages of traces $\mathcal{L} \subseteq \Sigma^*$ with sets of (observed) behavior of a (business) process. Each trace corresponds to a single process execution (also known as a *case*). The symbols in the trace correspond to the *events* or *activities* that occurred. In this article, we study *process trees* as a modeling mechanism for business processes. Each process tree T defines a language $\mathcal{L}(T) \subseteq \Sigma^*$ of possible process behaviors. Before we give the definition, we recall a central operator which captures independent parallel computations.

Definition 3 (Shuffle $\sqcup\!\sqcup$). For $x, y \in \Sigma^*$, the *shuffle* $x \sqcup\!\sqcup y$ of x and y is

$$x \sqcup\!\sqcup y := \{v_1 w_1 \ldots v_k w_k \mid x = v_1 \ldots v_k, y = w_1 \ldots w_k, v_i, w_i \in \Sigma^*, 1 \leq i \leq k\}.$$

Let $\mathcal{L}_1, \mathcal{L}_2 \subseteq \Sigma^*$. The shuffle of $\mathcal{L}_1$ and $\mathcal{L}_2$ is defined as

$$\mathcal{L}_1 \sqcup\!\sqcup \mathcal{L}_2 := \bigcup \{w_1 \sqcup\!\sqcup w_2 \mid w_1 \in \mathcal{L}_1, w_2 \in \mathcal{L}_2\}.$$

Definition 4 (Process Trees). Let Σ be an alphabet and let $\tau \notin \Sigma$ be the silent activity. The set of *process trees* (over Σ) is defined recursively:

- each activity $a \in \Sigma$ and the silent activity τ is a process tree,
- $\rightarrow(T_1, \ldots, T_n)$, $\times(T_1, \ldots, T_n)$, $\circlearrowleft(T_1, T_2)$, and $\wedge(T_1, \ldots, T_n)$ are process trees with $T_1, \ldots, T_n$, $n \in \mathbb{N}$ being process trees as well.

The symbols $\rightarrow$ (sequence), $\times$ (exclusive choice), $\circlearrowleft$ (loop), and $\wedge$ (parallel) are *process tree operators*. The *language* of a process tree T is denoted by $\mathcal{L}(T)$ and is also recursively defined where

- $\mathcal{L}(\tau) = \{\langle\rangle\}$ and $\mathcal{L}(a) = \{\langle a\rangle\}$,
- $\mathcal{L}(\rightarrow(T_1, \ldots, T_n)) = \mathcal{L}(T_1) \cdot \ldots \cdot \mathcal{L}(T_n)$,
- $\mathcal{L}(\times(T_1, \ldots, T_n)) = \mathcal{L}(T_1) \cup \ldots \cup \mathcal{L}(T_n)$,
- $\mathcal{L}(\circlearrowleft(T_1, T_2)) = \mathcal{L}(T_1) \cdot (\mathcal{L}(T_2) \cdot \mathcal{L}(T_1))^*$, and
- $\mathcal{L}(\wedge(T_1, \ldots, T_n)) = \mathcal{L}(T_1) \sqcup\!\sqcup \ldots \sqcup\!\sqcup \mathcal{L}(T_n)$.

In order to simplify notation in this article, from now on, we consider the process tree operators $\{\rightarrow, \times, \circlearrowleft, \wedge\}$ in their binary form only. This also allows us to use infix notation, e.g., $T_1 \rightarrow T_2$ instead of $\rightarrow(T_1, T_2)$. This is no restriction, since the general n-ary version can easily be rewritten in form of binary operators (all operators are associative). For a process tree T, let *Letters*$(T) \subseteq \Sigma$ denote the set of all labels occurring in T. Inductively, *Letters*(T) is defined as: *Letters*$(\tau) = \emptyset$, *Letters*$(a) = \{a\}$ for $a \in \Sigma$, and for all binary operators we have

$$Letters(T_1 \rightarrow T_2) = Letters(T_1 \times T_2) = Letters(T_1 \wedge T_2) =$$
$$Letters(T_1 \circlearrowleft T_2) = Letters(T_1) \cup Letters(T_2).$$

A process tree T has *unique labels* if for all binary operators op $\in \{\rightarrow, \times, \wedge, \circlearrowleft\}$ and all subtrees $(T_1 \text{ op } T_2)$ that occur in T we have *Letters*$(T_1) \cap$ *Letters*$(T_2) = \emptyset$. Note that the silent activity τ can occur multiple times in process trees T with unique labels.

Definition 5 (Moves, Alignments). Let Σ be an alphabet and let $\gg$ be a fresh symbol not in Σ. We use $\gg$ to indicate a *skip* in the trace or model and define $\Sigma_\gg := \Sigma \cup \{\gg\}$ as the alphabet extended by the skip-symbol $\gg$. We define *Moves*$(\Sigma) \subseteq \Sigma_\gg \times \Sigma_\gg$ as the set of all *moves* over Σ given by

$$Moves(\Sigma) := \quad \{(a,a) \mid a \in \Sigma\} \qquad \qquad synchronous\ moves$$
$$\cup \{(a,\gg) \mid a \in \Sigma\} \qquad \qquad model\ moves$$
$$\cup \{(\gg,a) \mid a \in \Sigma\} \qquad \qquad log\ moves.$$

An *alignment* $\gamma \in Moves(\Sigma)^*$ between $w \in \Sigma^*$ and a process tree T is a sequence of moves $\gamma = \langle m_1, \ldots, m_n \rangle$ such that $\pi_1^{\Sigma}(\gamma) = w$ and $\pi_2^{\Sigma}(\gamma) \in \mathcal{L}(T)$.

In other words, γ forms an alignment if the first components of each move in γ yield the trace w (when we remove all skip symbols $\gg$) and the second components yield a trace in the language of the process tree T (again without skip symbols). Intuitively, we aim to modify the trace w (the first component) such that it becomes a trace in the language of the process tree T (the second component). From this point of view, a log move $(a, \gg)$ deletes the symbol a from w while a model move $(\gg, b)$ inserts the symbol b into the trace w.

We determine the *costs* $c(\gamma)$ of an alignment γ by summing up the costs $c(m)$ of the individual moves m in γ where synchronous moves have cost 0 and, with respect to the standard cost function, log and model moves have cost 1 (other cost functions are possible). The set of all alignments between a trace w and a process tree T is denoted by $\Gamma(w, T)$. An *optimal alignment* $\gamma_{opt} \in \Gamma(w, T)$ is an alignment with minimal costs $\sum c(\gamma_{opt})$ among all alignments in $\Gamma(w, T)$.

4   Structure of Process Tree Alignments

Process trees have an inductive definition which lends itself to recursive algorithms. We next show that this inductive structure carries over to the set of alignments as well.

For a trace $w \in \Sigma^*$ of length n, $w = \langle w_1, w_2, \ldots, w_n \rangle$, we call a mapping $\varphi \colon \{1, \ldots, n\} \to \{1, 2\}$ a *factorization* of w. For a factorization φ of w we define $\varphi_1 \in \Sigma^*$ as the trace that results by concatenating all symbols w_i with $\varphi(i) = 1$. Likewise, $\varphi_2 \in \Sigma^*$ denotes the trace that results by concatenating all symbols w_i with $\varphi(i) = 2$. For the special case where $n = 0$, we only have a single factorization $\varphi = \emptyset$ with $\varphi_1 = \varphi_2 = \langle \rangle$. We write $\Phi(w)$ to denote the set of all factorizations of w. Note the connection between factorizations and the shuffle operator: for $w, w_1, w_2 \in \Sigma^*$ we have $w \in w_1 \sqcup\!\sqcup w_2$ if and only if there exists a factorization φ of w such that $\varphi_1 = w_1$ and $\varphi_2 = w_2$. In this sense, the *factorization* can be seen as a kind of inverse of the *shuffle* operator.

Theorem 1 (Structure of Alignments over Process Trees). *Let T_1 and T_2 be process trees and $w \in \Sigma^*$ be a trace. Then the following holds.*

$$\Gamma(w, T_1 \to T_2) = \bigcup_{w_1 \cdot w_2 = w} \Gamma(w_1, T_1) \cdot \Gamma(w_2, T_2) \tag{1}$$

$$\Gamma(w, T_1 \times T_2) = \Gamma(w, T_1) \cup \Gamma(w, T_2) \tag{2}$$

$$\Gamma(w, T_1 \wedge T_2) = \bigcup_{\varphi \in \Phi(w)} \{\gamma \in \Gamma(\varphi_1, T_1) \sqcup \Gamma(\varphi_2, T_2) \mid \pi_1^{\Sigma}(\gamma) = w\} \tag{3}$$

$$\Gamma(w, T_1 \circlearrowleft T_2) = \bigcup_{k \in \mathbb{N}_0} \{\Gamma(w_0, T_1) \cdot \Gamma(y_1, T_2) \cdot \Gamma(z_1, T_1) \cdots \Gamma(y_k, T_2) \cdot \Gamma(z_k, T_1) \mid$$
$$w = w_0 y_1 z_1 \ldots y_k z_k, w_0, y_i, z_i \in \Sigma^*, 1 \leq i \leq k\} \tag{4}$$

Proof. Ad (1): Let $T = T_1 \to T_2$ and $w \in \Sigma^*$ be a trace. We show that $\Gamma(w, T) = \bigcup_{w_1 \cdot w_2 = w} \Gamma(w_1, T_1) \cdot \Gamma(w_2, T_2)$. The direction $\supseteq$ is obvious, so let us focus on the direction $\subseteq$. Let $\gamma \in \Gamma(w, T)$. Since $T = T_1 \to T_2$, we find $y_1 \in \mathcal{L}(T_1)$ and $y_2 \in \mathcal{L}(T_2)$ such that $\pi_2^{\Sigma}(\gamma) = y_1 \cdot y_2$. Hence, we can write $\gamma = \gamma_1 \cdot \gamma_2$ with $\pi_2^{\Sigma}(\gamma_1) = y_1$ and $\pi_2^{\Sigma}(\gamma_2) = y_2$. Define $w_1 = \pi_1^{\Sigma}(\gamma_1)$ and $w_2 = \pi_1^{\Sigma}(\gamma_2)$. Then we have $w = w_1 \cdot w_2$ and $\gamma_1 \in \Gamma(w_1, T_1)$ and $\gamma_2 \in \Gamma(w_2, T_2)$.

Ad (2): Straightforward.

Ad (3): For $\supseteq$, observe that for a projection operator π and sequences x, y we have $\pi(x \sqcup y) = \pi(x) \sqcup \pi(y)$. For the direction $\subseteq$, let $\gamma \in \Gamma(w, T)$. Let $y = \pi_2^{\Sigma}(\gamma)$. Since $T = T_1 \wedge T_2$, we find a factorization φ of y such that $y_1 := \varphi_1 \in \mathcal{L}(T_1)$ and $y_2 := \varphi_2 \in \mathcal{L}(T_2)$. We lift this factorization to a factorization of γ by assigning to each log move m in γ the value 2 (the choice of 2 is arbitrary and we could have chosen 1 as well). Call the resulting factorization ψ and let $\gamma_1 = \psi_1$ and $\gamma_2 = \psi_2$. Let $w_1 = \pi_1^{\Sigma}(\gamma_1)$ and $w_2 = \pi_1^{\Sigma}(\gamma_2)$. Then, $w \in w_1 \sqcup w_2$ since $w = \pi_1^{\Sigma}(\gamma)$. Moreover, $\gamma_1 \in \Gamma(w_1, T_1)$ and $\gamma_2 \in \Gamma(w_2, T_2)$ since $\pi_2^{\Sigma}(\gamma_1) = y_1$ and $\pi_2^{\Sigma}(\gamma_2) = y_2$ (we have only assigned new log moves to the second component of the alignment). This concludes the argument for the parallel operator.

Ad (4): We can get a decomposition analogously as for the sequence operator (1) using the semantics of the loop operator $T_1 \circlearrowleft T_2$ as $\mathcal{L}(T_1) \cdot (\mathcal{L}(T_2) \cdot \mathcal{L}(T_1))^*$. $\square$

From Theorem 1 we can derive a recursive algorithm for computing an optimal alignment between a trace w and a process tree T. Let $Cost(w, T)$ denote the minimal costs of an alignment in $\Gamma(w, T)$, i.e.,

$$Cost(w, T) = \min\{\textstyle\sum c(\gamma) \mid \gamma \in \Gamma(w, T)\}.$$

Then, we have the following recursive procedure for computing $Cost(w, T)$.

Theorem 2 (Recursive Computation of Alignment Costs). *Let T_1 and T_2 be process trees and $w \in \Sigma^*$ a trace. Then the following holds.*

$$Cost(w, T_1 \to T_2) = \min_{w_1 \cdot w_2 = w} \{Cost(w_1, T_1) + Cost(w_2, T_2)\}$$

$$Cost(w, T_1 \times T_2) = \min\{Cost(w, T_1), Cost(w, T_2)\}$$

$$Cost(w, T_1 \wedge T_2) = \min_{\varphi \in \Phi(w)} \{Cost(\varphi_1, T_1) + Cost(\varphi_2, T_2)\}$$

$$Cost(w, T_1 \circlearrowleft T_2) = \min_{k \in \mathbb{N}_0} \left\{ Cost(w_0, T_1) + \sum_{i=1}^{k} Cost(y_i, T_2) + Cost(z_i, T_1) \right.$$

$$\left. w = w_0 y_1 z_1 \ldots y_k z_k, w_0, y_i, z_i \in \Sigma^*, 1 \leq i \leq k \right\}$$

Proof. This follows immediately from Theorem 1. Note that for the case of the parallel operator (3) we have dropped the condition $\pi_1^\Sigma(\gamma) = w$. This can be justified as follows. If $\varphi \in \Phi(w)$ and $\gamma \in \gamma_1 \sqcup\!\sqcup \gamma_2$ with $\gamma_1 \in \Gamma(\varphi_1, T_1)$ and $\gamma_2 \in \Gamma(\varphi_2, T_2)$, then the costs of *all* alignments in $\gamma_1 \sqcup\!\sqcup \gamma_2$ are the same (they consist of the same moves) *and* at least for one $\gamma \in \gamma_1 \sqcup\!\sqcup \gamma_2$ we have $\pi_1^\Sigma(\gamma) = w$. $\square$

The missing base cases for $Cost(w, T)$ can be determined easily.

Theorem 3 (Alignment Costs for Base Cases). *Let $w \in \Sigma^*$ be a trace and $a \in \Sigma$. Then $Cost(w, \tau) = |w|$. Moreover, $Cost(w, a) = |w| + 1$ if a does not occur in w and $Cost(w, a) = |w| - 1$ otherwise.*

5   A Dynamic Programming Algorithm

The recursive computation of the optimal alignment costs $Cost(w, T)$ can be turned into a dynamic programming algorithm. We use the formulae from Sect. 4 and avoid recomputation for identical subproblems by storing the results of $Cost(w, T)$ in a table which we denote by *CostTable*, see Algorithm 1.

As presented, Algorithm 1 has exponential runtime. First, the number of recursive calls required for the *loop operator* $T_1 \circlearrowleft T_2$ corresponds to the (exponential) number of decompositions of w into subtraces $w = w_0 y_1 z_1 \ldots y_k z_k$. However, this blowup can be avoided. Consider a graph on the positions of w, $n := |w|$, with an edge from position $0 \leq p \leq n$ to position $n \geq q \geq p$ with costs

$$\min_{p \leq r \leq q} \{Cost(w[p, r], T_2) + Cost(w[r, q], T_1)\}.$$

These are the costs of aligning the subtrace $w[p, q]$ of w against the process tree $T_2 \to T_1$. In turn, a *path* from p to $n := |w|$ corresponds to a *partition* of the suffix $w[p, n]$ of w into segments (each edge yields one segment) where each segment is aligned against $T_2 \to T_1$. Specifically, the costs of a *cost-minimal* path from p to n are the costs of an optimal alignment of $w[p, n]$ against $(\mathcal{L}(T_2) \cdot \mathcal{L}(T_1))^*$.

Algorithm 1. Dynamic Programming Algorithm to Compute $Cost(w, T)$

$CostTable := \emptyset$
function COST(w, T)
   if $(w, T) \in$ CostTable **then return** CostTable(w, T)
   if $T = a$ **then** cost $\leftarrow |w| - 1$ if a occurs in w, else cost $\leftarrow |w| + 1$
   else if $T = \tau$ **then** cost $\leftarrow |w|$
   else if $T = T_1 \rightarrow T_2$ **then**
      for all $w_1 \cdot w_2 = w$ **do**
         cost $\leftarrow$ min$\{$cost, COST(w_1, T_1) + COST$(w_2, T_2)\}$
   else if $T = T_1 \times T_2$ **then** cost $\leftarrow$ min$\{$COST(w, T_1), COST$(w, T_2)\}$
   else if $T = T_1 \wedge T_2$ **then**
      for all $\varphi \in \Phi(w)$ **do**
         cost $\leftarrow$ min$\{$cost, COST(φ_1, T_1) + COST$(\varphi_2, T_2)\}$ (see improvements below)
   else if $T = T_1 \circlearrowleft T_2$ **then**
      for all $w_0 y_1 z_1 \ldots y_k z_k = w$ with $w_0, y_i, z_i \in \Sigma^*, 1 \le i \le k, k \in \mathbb{N}_0$ **do**
         cost $\leftarrow$ min$\{$cost, COST(w_0, T_1) + COST(y_1, T_2) + COST(z_1, T_1) + $\cdots$ +
COST(y_k, T_2) + COST$(z_k, T_1)\}$ (see improvements below)
   CostTable$(w, T) \leftarrow$ cost
   return cost

Hence, these costs can be determined efficiently with a shortest-path algorithm. This yields polynomial runtime for the loop operator.

The second problematic case is the *parallel operator* $T_1 \wedge T_2$. Here, we have to consider all factorizations of the trace w into two subtraces w_1 and w_2 which is an exponential number (in the length of w). In contrast to the loop operator, this exponential search cannot be avoided in general (unless P = NP). However, for process trees with *unique labels*, the situation is different.

Process Trees with Unique Labels. Let us reconsider the case $T = T_1 \wedge T_2$ where

$$Cost(w, T) = \min_{\varphi \in \Phi(w)} \{Cost(\varphi_1, T_1) + Cost(\varphi_2, T_2)\},$$

from Theorem 2 for process trees with *unique labels*. Let $L_1 = Letters(T_1)$ and $L_2 = Letters(T_2)$ be the sets of labels occurring in T_1 and T_2, respectively. We claim that we can restrict the set of factorizations to a singleton. Indeed, each letter w_i of w either belongs to L_1 or L_2 (or to none of them). For example, if $w_i = a$, and we know that $a \in L_1$, then it cannot reduce the alignment costs if we assign a to T_2. In fact, in T_2 we have to delete a anyway (log move $(a, \gg)$) and we could do exactly the same in T_1 (without increasing costs). In other words, without loss of generality we can assume that $\varphi(i) = 1$. We can argue analogously for letters in L_2. If the letter a at position i does neither belong to L_1 nor to L_2, then we can assign it to T_1 or T_2 without changing the alignment costs (in both cases, a deletion move $(a, \gg)$ is unavoidable). Arbitrarily, we assign such letters to T_2. In conclusion, for the *single* factorization $\varphi^\star$ with $\varphi^\star(i) = 1$ if $w_i \in L_1$

and $\varphi^*(i) = 2$ otherwise, we have:

$$Cost(w, T) = Cost(\varphi_1^\star, T_1) + Cost(\varphi_2^\star, T_2).$$

With these adaptations, Algorithm 1 becomes polynomial-time. To see this, let w be the input trace, and let T denote the input tree. Let $n = |w|$. A first observation is that the total number of entries in *CostTable* is bounded by $\mathcal{O}(|T| \cdot n^2)$. This is because each entry (v, T') in *CostTable* is determined by T' together with a segment $w[i, j]$, $1 \leq i \leq j \leq n$, of the original input trace w (indeed, v either is the segment $w[i, j]$ itself or the restriction of $w[i, j]$ to letters that occur in T'). This is in contrast to the case of process trees with *non-unique* labels where the shuffle operator would produce an exponential number of recursive calls for its subtrees (and the corresponding traces v could not easily be described as segments of the original input trace). With the same argument, $\mathcal{O}(|T| \cdot n^2)$ is a bound on the number of recursive calls of the function $\mathrm{COST}(w, T)$.

Secondly, we bound the runtime for each call of $\mathrm{COST}(w, T)$ (besides the recursive calls). By going through the different cases, it can be seen that the most expensive step is the shortest path computation for the loop operator. Here, we compute a cost-minimal path on a graph with $\mathcal{O}(|v|)$ nodes. Since $|v| \leq n$, and since shortest paths can be computed in quadratic time in the number of vertices (e.g., by using Dijkstra), the total runtime for a call of $\mathrm{COST}(w, T)$ is bounded by $\mathcal{O}(n^2)$ (not considering the runtime for the sparked recursive calls, of course). Altogether this yields a runtime bound of $\mathcal{O}(|T| \cdot n^4)$.

Theorem 4 (Dynamic Programming Algorithm for Process Trees with Unique Labels). *The costs $Cost(w, T)$ of an optimal alignment between a process tree T with unique labels and a trace w can be computed efficiently in time $\mathcal{O}(|T| \cdot |w|^4)$.*

6   Evaluation

We implemented our novel alignment algorithm in Python[1] and compared its runtime against the available algorithms in PM4Py [4] on a set of real-life event logs. We like to discuss one further algorithmic idea which lead to a significant speed-up on the benchmarks. Consider the sequence operator $T_1 \rightarrow T_2$ and recall that

$$Cost(w, T) = \min_{w_1 \cdot w_2 = w} \{ Cost(w_1, T_1) + Cost(w_2, T_2) \}.$$

Implemented naively, we need to check n splits of w into subtraces w_1 and w_2 where $n = |w|$. Let $L = Letters(T_1)$ and $R = Letters(T_2)$ be the sets of labels occurring in the (left) subtree T_1 and the (right) subtree T_2, respectively. Because of the unique label property, $L \cap R = \emptyset$. Let us label the letters in w with L if they belong to L and with R if they belong to R. Call the resulting $\{L, R\}$-trace $decomp(w)$. Of course, w could contain letters that neither belong to L nor to R. Such letters a can be removed in a preprocessing step (they incur deletion costs

---

[1] https://github.com/christopher-schwanen/process-tree-alignments.

anyway). Hence, we can assume that $decomp(w)$ and w have the same length. We claim that it is sufficient to check only the following split positions of the trace w: $seg = \{1, n\} \cup \{i : decomp(w)_i = L \wedge decomp(w)_{i+1} = R\}$.

To see why, let $i \in seg$ be a position with a flip from L- to R-labels. Then, by definition, this position is followed by R-labels. The alignment costs can only *increase* for a split within the upcoming R-segment. This is because to handle R-labels in the left subtree T_1 we need to delete them. Moreover, if the R-part is followed by an L-segment, then it makes sense to include as many L-labels for the next split as possible (since L-labels will necessarily incur deletion costs in the right subtree T_2). Hence, the next optimal split can only be after the last L-label (either at the end of the trace or right before the next R-label).

We compared our algorithm (*Dynamic*) against the standard (A*-based) algorithm for computing alignments in PM4Py (*Standard*) and an approximation algorithm in PM4Py tailored for process trees (*Approx*). For each algorithm and trace variant, we took the best out of 5 repetitions (meaning the minimum required time for computing the costs of an optimal alignment). To visualize the results, we computed the *performance factors* for each trace variant, i.e., we took the best runtime and divided the runtime of all three algorithms by this optimal runtime (trace-variant-wise). For instance, a performance factor of 2 indicates, that the algorithm took twice as long as the best algorithm for the given trace. We set a timeout of 65 s (instead of say 60 s) to compensate for overhead and to give each algorithm the safe chance to finish its computation in one minute. If a computation hits the timeout in one of the repetitions, the algorithm is considered to have failed on the trace/model pair. In the chart below, we plotted the empirical CDF of the performance factors for each of the three algorithms. The frequencies of performance factors of some algorithms do not sum up to 1; this indicates, that the algorithms ran into timeouts on a certain fraction of instances.

Log Data and Results. The general picture is that our algorithm (*Dynamic*) is *very* close to the approximation algorithm (*Approx*) and, in almost all cases, clearly outperforms the standard algorithm (*Standard*). Let us start with the BPI Challenge 2019 event log [12]. We used the *Inductive Miner* [15] to discover process trees with different noise thresholds (0 %, 10 %, 25 % and 50 %) and aligned 1000 randomly chosen trace variants from the log against the resulting process trees. The CDF of the performance factors is depicted in Fig. 1. The analogous graph for the Hospital Billing event log [17] can be found in Fig. 2.

On the BPI Challenge 2017 event log [10], our algorithm is slightly superior to Approx for noise thresholds of 10 % and 50 %, while it is slightly below the performance of Approx for thresholds of 0 % and 25 %. On the BPI Challenge 2012 event log [9], our algorithm is slightly superior to Approx for noise thresholds of 0 % and 10 %, while it is slightly below the performance of Approx for thresholds of 25 % and 50 %. This is with respect to the CDF of performance factors. To give some further results, Table 1 depicts the median computation times of the three algorithms for the runs on the BPI Challenge 2012 and 2017 event logs with respect to the different noise thresholds (0 %, 10 %, 25 %, 50 %).

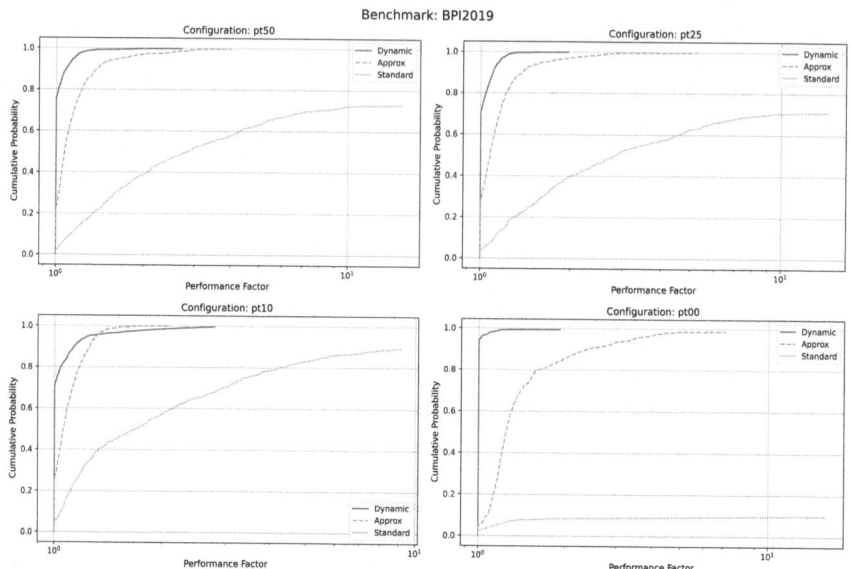

Fig. 1. CDF of the performance factors of *Dynamic, Approx, Standard* in `PM4Py` on the *BPI Challenge 2019* event log [12] with different noise thresholds.

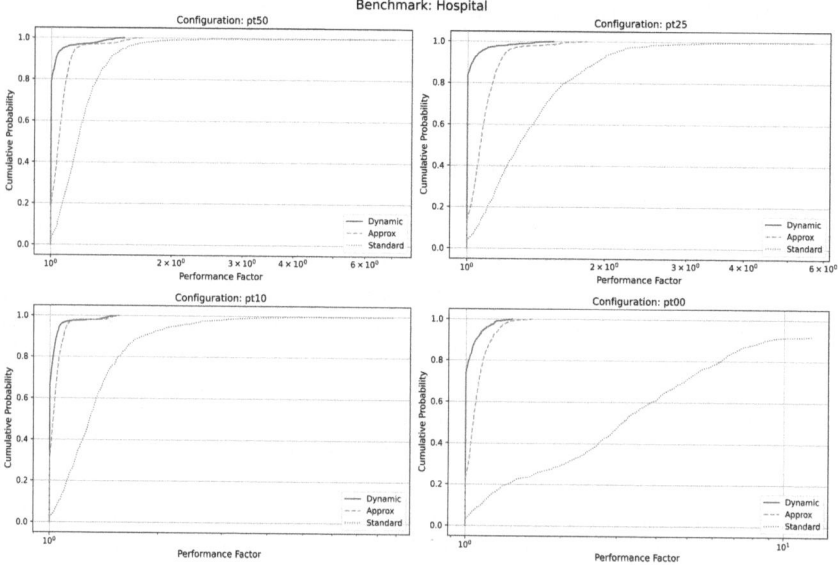

Fig. 2. CDF of the performance factors of *Dynamic, Approx, Standard* in `PM4Py` on the *Hospital Billing* event log [17] with different noise thresholds.

Table 1. Median computation times (in seconds) of *Dynamic*, *Approx*, and *Standard* in PM4Py for the BPI Challenge 2012 and 2017 event logs with different noise thresholds.

Threshold	BPI Challenge 2012 [9]				BPI Challenge 2017 [10]			
	50 %	*25 %*	*10 %*	*0 %*	*50 %*	*25 %*	*10 %*	*0 %*
Dynamic	5.69	**5.24**	**4.86**	**4.91**	**4.92**	8.24	**4.88**	6.00
Approx	**5.68**	5.25	5.48	5.51	5.37	**6.18**	5.29	**5.91**
Standard	21.40	22.49	7.91	8.48	17.44	40.07	9.87	37.56

7   Conclusion

We proved that the alignment problem for process trees with unique labels can be solved in polynomial time using dynamic programming. A proof-of-concept implementation in Python demonstrates that our algorithm is competitive with (and in some cases outperforms) the existing techniques of the PM4Py library. We discussed ideas how the algorithm can be further optimized in practice.

This article is part of a broader research agenda where we try to understand better the structure and algorithmic complexity of the alignment problem. We saw an interesting, and practically relevant, class of process models, where the alignment problem can be solved in polynomial time. This is rather the exception than the rule, since the alignment problem has high complexity in general (PSPACE-hard for sound workflow nets). Our work leads to many questions for future research. For example, it would be interesting to study relaxations of the *unique label* property and study the influence of these parameters on the complexity. Also, it would be interesting to see how restrictive the *unique label* property really is. Can we get a characterization of the event logs that can be defined using process trees with unique labels? And, as sound workflow nets with unique labels are more powerful than process trees with unique labels (in terms of modeling power), what is the complexity of the alignment problem for sound workflow nets with unique labels?

Acknowledgement. The research of the first author is funded by the IGF project 22485 N by the Federal Ministry for Economic Affairs and Climate Action (BMWK) on the basis of a decision of the German Bundestag. The first and third author thank the Alexander von Humboldt (AvH) Stiftung for supporting their research.

References

1. van der Aalst, W.M.P.: Decomposing petri nets for process mining: a generic approach. Distrib. Parallel Datab. **31**(4), 471–507 (2013). https://doi.org/10.1007/s10619-013-7127-5
2. van der Aalst, W.M.P., Buijs, J.C.A.M., van Dongen, B.F.: Towards improving the representational bias of process mining. In: Aberer, K., Damiani, E., Dillon, T. (eds.) SIMPDA 2011. LNBIP, vol. 116, pp. 39–54. Springer, Heidelberg (2012). https://doi.org/10.1007/978-3-642-34044-4_3

3. Adriansyah, A.: Aligning observed and modeled behavior. Ph.D. dissertation, Technische Universiteit Eindhoven (2014). https://doi.org/10.6100/IR770080
4. Berti, A., van Zelst, S.J., Schuster, D.: PM4Py: a process mining library for Python. Softw. Impacts **17**, 100556 (2023). https://doi.org/10.1016/j.simpa.2023.100556
5. Bloemen, V., van de Pol, J., van der Aalst, W.M.P.: Symbolically aligning observed and modelled behaviour. In: Application of Concurrency to System Design, pp. 50–59. IEEE Computer Society (2018). https://doi.org/10.1109/ACSD.2018.00008
6. Buijs, J.C.A.M., van Dongen, B.F., van der Aalst, W.M.P.: A genetic algorithm for discovering process trees. In: 2012 IEEE Congress on Evolutionary Computation, pp. 1–8 (2012). https://doi.org/10.1109/CEC.2012.6256458
7. Carmona, J., van Dongen, B.F., Solti, A., Weidlich, M.: Conformance Checking, Relating Processes and Models. Springer, Cham (2018). https://doi.org/10.1007/978-3-319-99414-7
8. Carmona, J., van Dongen, B.F., Weidlich, M.: Conformance checking: foundations, milestones and challenges. In: Process Mining Handbook, LNBIP, vol. 448, pp. 155–190. Springer, Cham (2022). https://doi.org/10.1007/978-3-031-08848-3_5.
9. van Dongen, B.F.: BPI challenge 2012. Eindhoven University of Technology (2012). https://doi.org/10.4121/UUID:3926DB30-F712-4394-AEBC-75976070E91F
10. van Dongen, B.F.: BPI challenge 2017. Eindhoven University of Technology (2017). https://doi.org/10.4121/UUID:5F3067DF-F10B-45DA-B98B-86AE4C7A310B
11. van Dongen, B.F.: Efficiently computing alignments. In: Weske, M., Montali, M., Weber, I., vom Brocke, J. (eds.) BPM 2018. LNCS, vol. 11080, pp. 197–214. Springer, Cham (2018). https://doi.org/10.1007/978-3-319-98648-7_12
12. van Dongen, B.F.: BPI challenge 2019, 4TU.Centre for Research Data (2019). https://doi.org/10.4121/uuid:d06aff4b-79f0-45e6-8ec8-e19730c248f1.
13. Leemans, S.J.J.: Robust Process Mining with Guarantees, Process Discovery, Conformance Checking and Enhancement (LNBIP), vol. 440. Springer, Cham (2022). https://doi.org/10.1007/978-3-030-96655-3.
14. Leemans, S.J.J., Fahland, D., van der Aalst, W.M.P.: Discovering block-structured process models from event logs containing infrequent behaviour. In: Lohmann, N., Song, M., Wohed, P. (eds.) BPM 2013. LNBIP, vol. 171, pp. 66–78. Springer, Cham (2014). https://doi.org/10.1007/978-3-319-06257-0_6
15. Leemans, S.J.J., Fahland, D., van der Aalst, W.M.P.: Discovering block-structured process models from incomplete event logs. In: Ciardo, G., Kindler, E. (eds.) PETRI NETS 2014. LNCS, vol. 8489, pp. 91–110. Springer, Cham (2014). https://doi.org/10.1007/978-3-319-07734-5_6
16. de Leoni, M., Marrella, A.: Aligning real process executions and prescriptive process models through automated planning. Expert Syst. Appl. **82**, 162–183 (2017). https://doi.org/10.1016/j.eswa.2017.03.047
17. Mannhardt, F.: Hospital billing - event log. Eindhoven University of Technology (2017). https://doi.org/10.4121/uuid:76c46b83-c930-4798-a1c9-4be94dfeb741
18. Mayer, A.J., Stockmeyer, L.J.: The complexity of word problems - this time with interleaving. Inf. Comput. **115**(2), 293–311 (1994). https://doi.org/10.1006/inco.1994.1098
19. Schuster, D., van Zelst, S.J., van der Aalst, W.M.P.: Alignment approximation for process trees. In: Leemans, S., Leopold, H. (eds.) ICPM 2020. LNBIP, vol. 406, pp. 247–259. Springer, Cham (2021). https://doi.org/10.1007/978-3-030-72693-5_19
20. Schwanen, C.T., Pakusa, W., van der Aalst, W.M.P.: Process tree alignments. In: Enterprise Design, Operations, and Computing. LNCS. Springer, Cham (2024), forthcoming. https://doi.org/10.1007/978-3-031-78338-8_16

21. Taymouri, F., Carmona, J.: A recursive paradigm for aligning observed behavior of large structured process models. In: La Rosa, M., Loos, P., Pastor, O. (eds.) BPM 2016. LNCS, vol. 9850, pp. 197–214. Springer, Cham (2016). https://doi.org/10.1007/978-3-319-45348-4_12

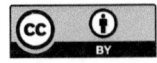

3rd International Workshop on Education Meets Process Mining (EduPM 2024)

Preface

3rd International Workshop Education Meets Process Mining (EduPM 2024)

The relation between process mining and education is twofold: (1) the best way to drive the adoption of process mining is to teach the core process mining principles to children, students, consultants, process owners, and managers, and (2) process mining provides a powerful tool to analyze and improve educational processes (e.g., learning analytics applied to Moodle or Coursera data). The International Workshop "Education meets Process Mining" series, embedded in the International Conference on Process Mining (ICPM) series, provides a meeting place for researchers, educators, and practitioners to discuss the relationship between the two fields.

The 2024 edition of the Process Mining for Education (EduPM 2024) workshop took place in Copenhagen (Denmark) on October 14, 2024. The call for papers solicited again two types of contributions: regular papers and Show&Tell submissions. Regular papers should make a research contribution to one of the topics listed above. They were evaluated on the basis of their significance, originality, technical quality, and potential to generate relevant discussion. Show&Tell submissions are non-research contributions that give authors the opportunity to present an item or initiative of interest to the EduPM community. They include experiential cases, educational resources, innovative tools, and lightning presentations for tentative or preliminary work, ideas, and collaborative opportunities.

The third edition of EduPM received 13 submissions, of which there were 12 regular papers and one Show&Tell contribution. After thorough reviewing by the program committee members, five regular submissions were accepted for full-paper presentation. The Show&Tell submission was also accepted. EduPM 2024 also featured a keynote by Daniel Spikol, who provided an external perspective on learning analytics using multi-modal data. Below, we briefly describe the papers included in these proceedings.

The paper *Assessing the impact of exam preparation process on students' careers* by Domenico Potena, Laura Genga, Lorenzo Galeazzi, Gianmarco Vigano, and Claudia Diamantini examines the relationship between a student's exam-taking behavior in their first year of university and their graduation performance, specifically their graduation time. The authors propose a methodology to predict student performance (early vs. late graduation) based on their exam-taking patterns, analyzing data from over 700 graduated students from an Italian university. The study finds that incorporating exam-taking patterns as features significantly improves the prediction accuracy of Decision Tree and XGBoost models. The study highlights the value of process mining techniques in understanding and predicting student performance based on their exam-taking behavior. This paper received the EduPM 2024 Best Paper award.

The paper *Understanding Student Behavior using Active Window Tracking and Process Mining* by Mahendrawathi Er, Wouter Van Der Waal, Iris Beerepoot, Moch. Aqmal

Rasyadan Reza Putra, and Hardhika Propitadewa presents a novel approach to under-standing student behavior by combining Active Window Tracking (AWT) with process mining techniques. The aim is to investigate Media MultiTasking (MMT) among stu-dents and its impact on academic performance. Correlation analysis indicated no direct correlation between MMT and assignment scores, suggesting that students could man-age multitasking without significant performance detriment on the given assignments. However, MMT was found to extend the duration of work, leading students to work closer to deadlines and often late into the night, potentially impacting their well-being. The findings highlight the need for educators to address the potential negative impacts of MMT on time management and well-being.

The paper *Measuring Skill Acquisition and Retention: A Case Study of Math Fluency* by Gert Janssenswillen, Seppe Van Daele, and Marc Van Daele investigates the use of process-oriented data analysis to understand math fact fluency development in primary school students. The study uses data from Automatus, an arithmetic practice platform, to answer two main questions: (1) the practice time required to master arithmetic operations and (2) the impact of different learning characteristics on skill retention. The authors define metrics for measuring the regularity, focus, and stability of student practice, as well as a method for determining when a pupil reaches a "mastery skill level" based on their accuracy and speed on exercises. A total of 203,309 scores were computed based on the activity data extracted from Automatus. The analysis identifies key learning characteristics that influence the time to reach mastery, such as the pupil's initial skill level and their reliance on accuracy vs. speed. Students with a higher reliance on accuracy tend to take longer to reach mastery but exhibit better skill retention.

The paper *Evaluation of Study Plans using Partial Orders* by Christian Rennert, Mahsa Pourbafrani, and Wil van der Aalst proposes a novel approach using partial orders and process mining techniques to evaluate the effectiveness of study plans in higher education. The goal is to identify deviations between the proposed study plan and the actual order in which students take courses. Study plans are mapped onto workflow nets, allowing for courses to be taken concurrently (i.e., courses are partially ordered and are expected to take place in a specific semester). Partial-order alignments are used to compare the study plan model with the student's course-taking behavior, highlighting deviations in both the order of courses and the terms in which they are taken. The approach was applied to data from 1,162 RWTH Aachen University Computer Science Bachelor's graduates. Initial results show that the approach can be used to analyze the impact of changes to study plans and to identify areas where students may need additional support. Partial-order alignments provide a more robust and informative method for evaluating study plans compared to traditional sequence-based approaches.

The paper *Constructive Alignment in Process Mining* by Mitchel Brunings, Dirk Fahland, and Boudewijn van Dongen argues that process mining projects can be improved by applying the principles of constructive alignment, a concept from the field of education. Constructive alignment emphasizes aligning intended learning outcomes, teaching/learning activities, and assessment methods to ensure that students are actively engaged in learning and can demonstrate their understanding of the material. The PM^2 process mining methodology is used as a reference and two main types of problems are identified. The authors argue that process mining can benefit from the insights of the field of education, and that process mining itself can be seen as a form of education.

The Show & Tell contribution *Celonis - Making OCPM available for everyone (in academia)* by Angela-Sophia Gebert, Keisha Glori Natalia, and Clemens Drieschner presented new teaching resources to learn Object-Centric Process Mining (OCPM). OCPM is rapidly changing the process mining landscape, but only a few data sets and tools are available. OCPM is now available in the academic version of the Celonis software, which includes Object-Centric Event Data (OCED) and lecture slides. This triggered a discussion about whether teaching should start with Object-Centric Process Mining (OCPM) or still first introduce traditional case-centric techniques.

The workshop closed with the keynote presentation *Challenges and Opportunities of LA, with a focus on Multimodality* by Daniel Spikol from the University of Copenhagen. The goal of the keynote was to provide an external perspective from someone working on Learning Analytics (LA), but not using process mining. In his keynote, Spikol focused on collaborative multimodal learning analytics, physical computing, and technologies that enhance learning, play, and reflection. He described various projects where learning processes are closely observed in a controlled physical setting and highlighted the practical challenges when doing this. Moreover, he suggested incorporating social signal processing and ambient computing to develop tools that inspire computational tinkering and thinking in educational settings.

We would like to thank all the members of the EduPM 2024 Program Committee for their efforts in reviewing the papers. Our sincere thanks go to all the authors and the workshop participants, who contributed with their work and the lively discussions on the workshop day. A special note of gratitude goes also to the organizing committee and workshop chairs of ICPM 2024 for this successful edition of the conference.

November 2024

Jorge Munoz-Gama
Francesca Zerbato
Gert Janssenswillen
Wil van der Aalst

Organization

Workshop Chairs

Jorge Munoz-Gama	Pontificia Universidad Católica de Chile, Chile
Francesca Zerbato	Eindhoven University of Technology, The Netherlands
Gert Janssenswillen	Hasselt University, Belgium
Wil van der Aalst	RWTH Aachen University, Germany

Program Committee

Wil van der Aalst	RWTH Aachen University, Germany
Iris Beerepoot	Utrecht University, The Netherlands
Mitchel Brunings	Eindhoven University of Technology, The Netherlands
Daniel Calegari	Universidad de la República, Uruguay
Ronan Champagnat	Université de la Rochelle, France
Jochen De Weerdt	Katholieke Universiteit Leuven, Belgium
Boudewijn van Dongen	Eindhoven University of Technology, The Netherlands
Luciano Hidalgo	Pontificia Universidad Católica de Chile, Chile
Richard Hobeck	TU Berlin, Germany
Gert Janssenswillen	Hasselt University, Belgium
Manuel Lama	University of Santiago de Compostela, Spain
Sander Leemans	RWTH Aachen University, Germany
Felix Mannhardt	Eindhoven University of Technology, The Netherlands
Niels Martin	Hasselt University, Belgium
Jorge Munoz-Gama	Pontificia Universidad Católica de Chile, Chile
Cristobal Romero	Universidad de Córdoba, Spain
Marcos Sepúlveda	Pontificia Universidad Católica de Chile, Chile
Pnina Soffer	University of Haifa, Israel
Emilio Sulis	University of Turin, Italy
Francesca Zerbato	Eindhoven University of Technology, The Netherlands

Constructive Alignment in Process Mining

Mitchel Brunings[✉][iD], Dirk Fahland[iD], and Boudewijn van Dongen[iD]

Eindhoven University of Technology, Eindhoven, The Netherlands
{m.d.brunings,d.fahland,b.f.v.dongen}@tue.nl

Abstract. Constructive alignment is a well-established concept in education that helps teachers design courses and modules. When we look at constructive alignment as engineers, we can interpret it as a set of axioms for setting up successful process mining projects. While in process mining we have several useful methodologies (e.g. PM^2), they cover some, but not all aspects of constructive alignment. In this paper we translate the ideas from constructive alignment to terms in process mining. We exploit the key similarity between process mining and teaching, which is that there is someone who wants to learn something. From the analysis of PM^2, we identify two main types of problems and discuss these in a bit more detail before concluding the paper with ideas for future work.

Keywords: Constructive alignment · design · process mining projects · methodologies

1 Introduction

In Chap. 1.2 of his book "Quality in Business Process Modeling" [8], John Krogstie describes Process Thinking; In "Principle 5: You get what you measure", he writes about the relationship between goals and measures. As educators, we known that the alignment between goals and assessment is important, as this is one of the things that constructive alignment teaches us.

In this paper we explore how constructive alignment can be useful to process mining. We give a short explanation of constructive alignment and the axioms it sets in Sect. 2. We look at a successful process mining methodology in Sect. 3. In Sect. 4 we compare the axioms from Sect. 2 and the methodology from Sect. 3. We explain and support our view that constructive alignment should be applied in process modeling in Sect. 5 before finishing this paper with our conclusions in Sect. 6.

2 Constructive Alignment

2.1 What Is Constructive Alignment?

Constructive alignment [2] is the combination of two important concepts in education: constructivist learning [9] and instructional design [6].

© The Author(s) 2025
A. Delgado and T. Slaats (Eds.): ICPM 2024 Workshops, LNBIP 533, pp. 105–116, 2025.
https://doi.org/10.1007/978-3-031-82225-4_8

For any given course/program/module/assignment ("unit"), instructional design [6] tells us to align our intended learning outcomes, our teaching/learning activities, and our assessment. Intended learning outcomes should specify in what ways a student should be able to perform by the end of the unit. They are a set of statements carefully constructed to formulate the knowledge and skills the student should gain by following the unit. There are several criteria one could set for these statements; a common requirement is that each statement uses a single verb from Bloom's taxonomy [3]. Teaching/learning activities serve to elicit the desired behavior from students as specified in the intended learning outcomes. Finally the assessment is there to grade students based on how well they perform the intended learning outcomes.

Constructivist learning [9] states that everyone has their own mental model of the world. When learning new concepts or skills, these have to fit onto and expand this existing mental model. Teaching/learning activities are ideally a mix of different instructional methods (such as lectures, group work, and self-study) that activate the students. By making the students active, they already start showing the desired behavior during the unit, preparing them well for the assessment.

Together, that means for any unit, we should clearly state the subjects and skills we want our students to master, design our teaching/learning activities so that students engage with these materials without involving (too much) out-of-context material, and in our assessment ensure we cover all of the stated intended learning outcomes and nothing else.

2.2 Related Work

Most work building on Constructive Alignment discusses how this is applied in specific educational design settings (for example group work [14] or medicine [4]). We could find only one paper that tried to augment constructive alignment: Tepper [10] proposed a method to measure the alignment of a course. In their effort to develop an alignment metric, they use four elements: teaching/learning activities, assessment tasks, learning outcomes, and learning objectives. However, they also mention that Biggs [2] does not differentiate between learning outcomes and learning objectives. In this paper we go with the three elements as defined in [2]. Furthermore, [10] relates all these four elements to each other, either directly or indirectly. However, in the mathematics in the paper, they make assumptions on the completeness of mappings that are not supported by the original work of [2]. For example, that assessment happens on all levels of Bloom's taxonomy [3] that are part of the learning objectives, while it is only necessary to test at the highest level.

2.3 Constructive Alignment Axioms

Biggs ([2], page 361) writes: "the curriculum or unit objectives are clearly stated in terms of content specific levels of understanding that imply appropriate performances, the teaching methods require students to be placed in contexts that will likely elicit those performances, and the assessment tasks address those same performances." In other words, all three elements (intended learning outcomes, teaching/learning activities, and assessment) of constructive alignment are focused on the same performances. We take this to mean that the intended learning outcomes define performances that are elicited by teaching/learning activities, and the teaching/learning activities elicit performances that are defined by the intended learning outcomes, and that similar relationships hold between all three elements.

Based on this, we believe that constructive alignment can be seen as a set of axioms that each properly developed course should adhere to. While they have never been stated explicitly, constructive alignment consists of seven axioms. In these axioms, we are treating intended learning outcomes, teaching/learning activities, and assessment as atomic terms with an intuitive interpretation. While we could also formulate axioms for these terms, that is beyond the scope of this paper, i.e. we limit our scope to the axioms that are added by constructive alignment.

1. The student is central in the design, i.e. the design includes intended learning outcomes, teaching/learning activities, and assessment, all set up in a constructivist manner ([2], page 349, 360–361).
2. For each intended learning outcome, there is an element in the assessment that measures the achievement of this outcome.
3. For each element in the assessment, there is an intended learning outcome of which the achievement is measured by this element.
4. For each intended learning outcome, there is a teaching/learning activity that helps the student achieve this outcome.
5. For each teaching/learning activity, there is an intended learning outcome that is taught or trained by this activity.
6. For each teaching/learning activity, there is an element in the assessment that tests the performance of this activity.
7. For each element in the assessment, there is a teaching/learning activity that teaches the student (how) to perform well.

Axioms 2–7 are a translation of [2], page 361.

3   Process Mining Methodologies

There are several process mining methodologies in literature (e.g. PM^2 [13], L* [12], PDM [5], PMPM [7], PMM [1]). In this section, we consider one of the more successful methodologies: PM^2 [13] defines 6 stages (shown in Fig. 1) through which a process mining project should move to be successful.

In Stage 1, *planning*, a process is chosen to work on, research questions are defined, and a team is picked to work on this project. The team may consist of one or more business owners, business experts, system experts, and/or process analysts. Stage 2, *extraction*, tells us to define a scope for the project, then

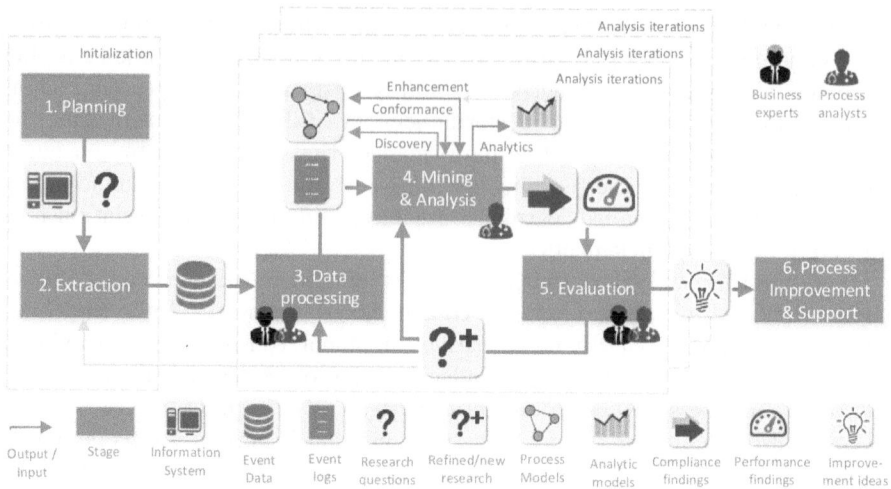

Fig. 1. An overview of the PM^2 methodology. (Source: [13])

extract event data and transfer process knowledge. This last activity involves process analysts interviewing business experts and/or brainstorming with them.

Stage 3, *data processing*, is focused on transforming the raw data obtained in Stage 2 into event logs for further analysis through creating views, aggregating events, enriching logs, and/or filtering logs. Stage 4, *mining and analysis*, tries to answer the research questions from Stage 1 using the event logs from Stage 3. Activities in this stage are process discovery, conformance checking, enhancement, and process analytics. The first three of these work with process models, but through 'process analytics' other data mining techniques or visual analytics may also be used.

In Stage 5, *evaluation*, the results from Stage 4 are diagnosed and/or verified and validated. PM^2 further mentions that process experts are essential for verification and validation, and they should ideally already be involved during Stage 4. Either way, after Stage 5, it may not be time to go to Stage 6 yet, as it may be necessary to iterate over stages 3 and 4 for follow-up research questions.

Finally, Stage 6, *process improvement and support*, aims to use the newly gained knowledge. Implementing improvements may require launching an entirely new project, after which another process mining project should be launched to measure the effect. Supporting operations may also be possible, but can be very challenging.

4 Comparing Constructive Alignment and Process Mining

In education, a course about a subject is a methodological way to learn about that subject. In process mining, a process mining project is a methodological way to learn about a process. Hence, successfully following a course is not very different from successfully executing a process mining project. In both cases, the aim is to learn (Fig. 2).

In education, course design methodologies define how to design courses. Similarly, in process mining, methodologies define how to design a process mining project. However, where in education constructive alignment gives axioms for course design methodologies, such axioms do not exist for the design of process mining methodologies.

In this section we translate the terms and axioms of constructive alignment to process mining, thereby providing axioms for process mining methodologies. Then, we analyze how PM² does or does not follow these design axioms. In Sect. 5 we discuss the two main types of problems identified during this analysis.

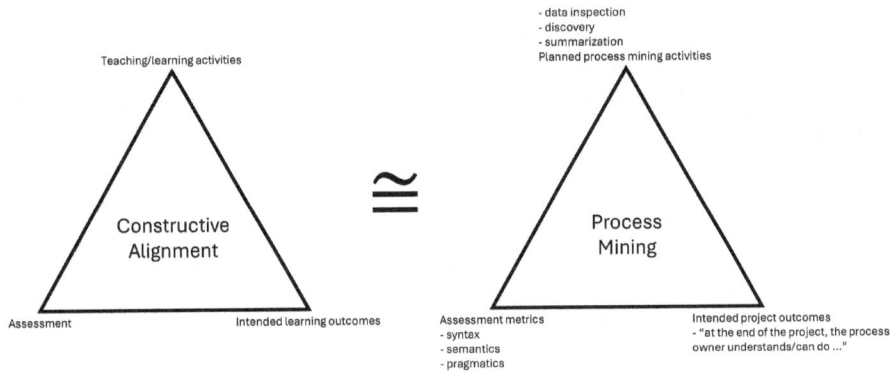

Fig. 2. Comparing constructive alignment with process mining.

4.1 Translating Constructive Alignment Terms to Process Mining

There are several terms in Constructive Alignment that we need to translate to Process Mining. In this paper, we make the following choices:

Student (or Learner): *Process owner.* Each methodology defines their own terms for the people involved in the project. In this paper, we use the term 'process owner' for the people who absorb the knowledge created by process mining techniques. Doing a process mining project is analogous with learning about that process where the process owner is the learner. This works because in the end *they* need to learn about their process, whether it is for conformance/compliance checking, for making improvements, or for some other reason.

The notion that the process owner is the learner is further supported by PM² [13] (there called 'business expert'). In their discussion section, they explain that adding the business expert to all phases of the project was essential to achieving the project goals. They also explicitly mention it was necessary to educate the business expert in process mining.

Teacher: *A whole team.* This includes those who help the process owner in their efforts to learn about their process. For example: an instructor teaching the basics of process mining, or the engineers that prepare the data (similar to how an assistant might prepare chemicals in a lab for class) because it is too dangerous/complex/time consuming for the process owner to do themself.

Intended Learning Outcomes: *Intended project outcomes.* The needs of the process owner to learn about their process (whether it is for conformance/compliance checking, for making improvements, or for some other reason) form the basis of the intended project outcomes for a process mining project. When writing these down, it is important to keep the process owner in focus, just like the student is in focus when writing intended learning outcomes. Research questions could, for example, be rewritten to formulate skills or knowledge that the process owner needs to gain.

Teaching/Learning Activities: *Planned process mining activities.* These activities should focus on bringing the process owner from where they are to where they want to be: a series of process mining activities that build up from the knowledge that the process owner already has to the level that they need.

Assessment: *Assessment metrics.* The assessment metrics of a process mining project should reflect the goals: When the goal was for the process owner to improve the process, the success could for example be measured through achieving certain KPI improvements, or a dashboard that meets expectations. Alternatively, in more exploratory projects, the goal could be for the process owner to come up with ideas for process improvement.

Looking at process mining, we also have the role of a client, which we should map to education to complete the analogy. While education management is not explicitly part of constructive alignment, it is in charge of organizing educational activities, learning outcomes, and assessment of all students over a longer period of time. As such, you could see the education management to be translated to a "client" in process mining within a company.

Other choices for these translations are also possible. However, we have to make sure these translations follow constructive alignment. For example, one cannot translate students to process mining experts, as it is not required for them to gain knowledge about the process. Process mining experts may move on to other projects on other processes, while the process owner stays behind where they may use their newly gained knowledge.

4.2   Axiom 1

In constructive alignment, Axiom 1 states: "The student is central in the design, i.e. the design includes intended learning outcomes, teaching/learning activities, and assessment, all set up in a constructivist manner."

Translated to process mining, this means: The process owner is central in the set up. There must be intended project outcomes, assessment metrics, and planned process mining activities, all set up in a constructivist manner.

In a bit more detail: As intended project outcomes, we expect something along the lines of "at the end of the project, the process owner understands/can do [something]." The assessment metrics should measure the degree of success of these intended project outcomes. And the planned process mining activities may cover a wide array of activities such as data inspection, process discovery, and summarization. Constructivism, in this context, requires that the project should be set up in such a way that each new bit of knowledge for the process owner is added to the knowledge that they already possess and can contribute to the intended outcomes of the project.

In PM^2 we see all elements: Intended project outcomes are set through research questions in Stage 1, assessment metrics are applied in stages 4 and 5, and the majority of planned process mining activities can be found in stages 3 and 4. Stages 3, 4 and 5 can be repeated to build the process owner's knowledge of the process. However, we also notice that the evaluation criteria are not set together with the goal and the plan, but this takes place only after the main process mining activities have been carried out.

Furthermore, the most important element of Axiom 1 is missing, namely: a clear learner that is central to all these parts. From the discussion section of [13] it is clear that the business expert is the learner in PM^2. However, they are not central to the methodology. Instead, in [13] the business expert is sometimes an educator and sometimes a learner. Therefore, it is unclear which activities aim to help the business expert learn about the process and which activities aim at the business expert teaching others. The latter may be important, but should not be part of the methodology and should be considered as a separate teaching and learning activity, analogous to courses having prerequisites.

4.3   Axiom 2

Axiom 2 states: "For each intended learning outcome, there is an element in the assessment that measures the achievement of this outcome."

Translated to process mining, this means: For each intended project outcome, there is an assessment metric that measures the achievement of this outcome.

In a bit more detail: This makes sense, and in practice also happens a lot; SMART goals and similar techniques are well known and applied. This axiom further adds that it must be done for *each* intended project outcome.

In Stage 1 in PM^2, the intended project outcomes are defined as initial research questions. At the end of Stage 5, these questions may be refined, new questions may be added and questions may even be lost. After several iterations, it is therefore not guaranteed that the original intended outcomes are achieved before Stage 6, nor that they can be measured. In this sense, PM^2 does not adhere fully to Axiom 2.

We consider PM^2 as a single project with a start and an end, but one could take a more detailed view and address the iterative "loop" through stages 3,

4, and 5. For this specific view, we might make the analogy with personalized learning, as described in [11]. However, this does not mean that there should be a moving goalpost in the form of changing intended project outcomes and/or assessment.

4.4 Axiom 3

Axiom 3 states: "For each element in the assessment, there is an intended learning outcome of which the achievement is measured by this element."

Translated to process mining, this means: For each assessment metric, there is an intended project outcome of which the achievement is measured by this metric.

In a bit more detail: KPIs for measures like process throughput or sojourn time make sense. When we see measures like fitness and precision, though, we should wonder if they really measure what we want to measure. They are not always valid substitutes for model quality. This is not the point of this paper, but a good thing to keep in mind when deciding on assessment metrics nonetheless.

In Stage 5 of PM^2, it is made explicit that the findings from Stage 4 should be related to the project's goals. That means that each element in the evaluation is (or at least should be) related to a project goal. This is in line with Axiom 3.

4.5 Axiom 4

Axiom 4 states: "For each intended learning outcome, there is a teaching/ learning activity that helps the student achieve this outcome."

Translated to process mining, this means: For each intended project outcome, there is a planned process mining activity that helps the process owner achieve this outcome.

In a bit more detail: When we set goals for a project, we should already think about how we want to achieve those goals. Constructivism adds to this that not every intended project outcome may be achievable in one step. This may require setting intermediate goals.

In Stage 5 of PM^2, it is possible to refine or specify some research questions before iteration over stages 3 and 4. However, it does not make explicit that each and every research question should get attention. In this sense, PM^2 does not adhere fully to Axiom 4.

4.6 Axiom 5

Axiom 5 states: "For each teaching/learning activity, there is an intended learning outcome that is taught or trained by this activity."

Translated to process mining, this means: For each planned process mining activity, there is an intended project outcome that this activity contributes to.

In a bit more detail: There are many tools for process mining, from manual inspection to machine learning. We should make sure that the methods we use fit with the goals we want to achieve. If our work is not helping to achieve our goals, we should not be doing it or we did not set our goals right.

In PM^2, each stage builds on the stage that came before, right back down to Stage 1. This ensures that all work that is done in any stage is based on one of the initial project goals set in Stage 1. This is in line with Axiom 5.

4.7 Axiom 6

Axiom 6 states: "For each teaching/learning activity, there is an element in the assessment that tests the performance of this activity."

Translated to process mining, this means: For each planned process mining activity, there is an assessment metric that tests the performance of this activity.

In a bit more detail: We need to check that all the process mining activities that were carried out were done correctly to ensure that the quality of the results is satisfactory. Anything left untested is prone to error.

Stage 5 of PM^2 makes clear that the work done in Stage 4 needs to be tested. This is in line with Axiom 6.

4.8 Axiom 7

Axiom 7 states: "For each element in the assessment, there is a teaching/learning activity that teaches the student (how) to perform well."

Translated to process mining, this means: For each assessment metric, there is a planned process mining activity that helps the process owner to achieve success.

In a bit more detail: All of the assessment metrics that we use should measure (the effect of) some process mining activity that was carried out. Testing elements that were not touched by the work done in the project is irrelevant. We should either be doing the thing we are testing for, or not do the test.

Similar to Axiom 5, PM^2's sequential structure between the stages ensures that there is no evaluation of work that was not done. That means PM^2 also satisfies Axiom 7.

Table 1. A summary of the findings for PM^2's adherence to the axioms of constructive alignment.

Axiom	1	2	3	4	5	6	7
PM^2	✗	✗	✓	✗	✓	✓	✓

To conclude, PM^2 does not adhere to all the axioms of constructive alignment, shown in Table 1. In the following section, we discuss the two main types of problems that arise from this in more detail.

5   Discussion

PM^2 has all the required parts (intended project outcomes, assessment metrics, and planned process mining activities) to be able to check for constructive alignment. When we do this check, we notice two kinds of 'defects': (1) instead of planning for all of these parts up front, most plans are generated on the fly and (2) there is not a clear learner central to all these parts.

(1) By generating required parts on the fly, we lose some grip on the final outcome of the project. If we do not determine up front how to test results or what level of results would be acceptable, we could end up in undesirable situations. E.g. if we are given a research question and a budget, but no indication of an acceptable outcome, we may end up producing something that is not good enough. If we had the indication beforehand, an experienced educator (e.g. process analyst) could already say up front that the provided resources would not be enough. Of course overspending could also happen.

(2) We believe it is important to specify a clear learner that is central to all parts. As we mentioned before, the authors of PM^2 also make note of this in the discussion section of their paper [13]. The project went a lot better once the business experts were involved in all steps and were educated in the basics of process mining. If we take from this that the business expert is the learner in PM^2, we can set much clearer intended project outcomes, appropriate assessment metrics, and set up a good plan for various process mining activities for the business expert to try.

The learner can go through all this on their own, but it is often much more beneficial to have an educator present to help them. If we take the process analysts as educators, we see them keeping the business expert on track, preventing them from wasting time on work that will not yield meaningful results, providing input on likely methods that would work, etc.

Process mining is not a one-step solution. Automated process discovery is misleading. Feeding data from a process into an algorithm that produces a single process model is not enough. Process mining is learning about the process, and there is a person doing the learning. We need to keep this in mind, and start treating process mining projects as education. We should apply constructive alignment to process mining projects.

6   Conclusion

Education has been around for millennia, while process mining has only been around for decades. It would be a mistake to not recognize the immense amount of knowledge gathered before us. In this paper, we took one element of this knowledge, constructive alignment, and saw what it could do for process mining.

This work is limited in some respects. First, we limited our set of axioms to those introduced by constructive alignment. Exploring axioms for intended learning outcomes, teaching/learning activities, and assessment could yield additional valuable insights. Second, we limited ourselves in this work to analyzing PM²'s adherence to the axioms. Expanding the analysis to include other process mining project methodologies would be useful to further our understanding. Finally, we only consider only one possible translation of roles and axioms from constructive alignment to process mining. There may be other valid translations.

Of course, in this paper, we took only a first step. We should continue looking into each of the axioms and how they can be applied to process mining while keeping a critical eye on their effect. We should also invest more into educating ourselves on education, as we have shown that process mining is a form of education.

Acknowledgments. We thank the reviewers for their constructive feedback. It was instrumental in improving this paper.

References

1. Aguirre, S., Parra, C., Sepúlveda, M.: Methodological proposal for process mining projects. Int. J. Bus. Process. Integr. Manag. **8**(2), 102–113 (2017)
2. Biggs, J.: Enhancing teaching through constructive alignment. High. Educ. **32**(3), 347–364 (1996)
3. Bloom, B.S.: Taxonomy of educational objectives: the classification of educational goals. In: Benjamin, S.B. (ed.) Handbook I, Cognitive Domain. McKay; Longman, New York (1956)
4. Bogomolova, K., et al.: The effect of stereoscopic augmented reality visualization on learning anatomy and the modifying effect of visual-spatial abilities: a double-center randomized controlled trial. Anat. Sci. Educ. **13**(5), 558–567 (2020)
5. Bozkaya, M., Gabriels, J., Van der Werf, J.M.: Process diagnostics: a method based on process mining. In: 2009 International Conference on Information, Process, and Knowledge Management, pp. 22–27. IEEE (2009)
6. Cohen, S.A.: Instructional alignment: searching for a magic bullet. Educ. Res. **16**(8), 16–20 (1987)
7. Van der Heijden, T.: Process mining project methodology: developing a general approach to apply process mining in practice. Master of Science in Operations Management and Logistics. TUE. School of Industrial Engineering, Netherlands (2012)
8. Krogstie, J.: Quality of Business Process Models. Springer, Heidelberg (2016)
9. Steffe, L., Gale, J.: Constructivism in Education. Lawrence Erlbaum, Hillsdale (1995)
10. Tepper, J.: Measuring constructive alignment: an alignment metric to guide good practice. Innov. Learn. Teach. J. (2005)
11. U.S. Department of Education, Office of Educational Technology: Reimagining the role of technology in education: 2017 national education technology plan update (2017)
12. van der Aalst, W., et al.: Process mining manifesto. In: Daniel, F., Barkaoui, K., Dustdar, S. (eds.) BPM 2011. LNBIP, vol. 99, pp. 169–194. Springer, Heidelberg (2012). https://doi.org/10.1007/978-3-642-28108-2_19

13. van Eck, M.L., Lu, X., Leemans, S.J.J., van der Aalst, W.M.P.: PM^2: a process mining project methodology. In: Zdravkovic, J., Kirikova, M., Johannesson, P. (eds.) CAiSE 2015. LNCS, vol. 9097, pp. 297–313. Springer, Cham (2015). https://doi.org/10.1007/978-3-319-19069-3_19
14. Vanhove, A., Opdecam, E., Mestdagh, S., Haerens, L.: Catme-b in secondary education: exploring the perceptions of students and teachers. Eur. J. Educ. e12751 (2024)

Understanding Student Behavior Using Active Window Tracking and Process Mining

E. R. Mahendrawathi[1(✉)] ⓘ, Wouter van der Waal[2] ⓘ, Iris Beerepoot[2] ⓘ,
M. Aqmal R. R. Putra[1] ⓘ, and Hardhika Propitadewa[1] ⓘ

[1] Institut Teknologi Sepuluh Nopember, Surabaya, Indonesia
mahendra_w@is.its.ac.id, aqmal2009@gmail.com,
propitadewa@gmail.com
[2] Utrecht University, Utrecht, The Netherlands
{w.g.vanderwaal,i.m.beerepoot}@uu.nl

Abstract. This paper proposes a new way of collecting and processing event logs using Active Window Tracking (AWT) to investigate media multitasking (MMT) among students in higher education institutions in Indonesia. Students recorded their computer windows while doing assignments and midterms. Data from the students were preprocessed and structured into event logs. Correlation analysis indicated that MMT has no direct correlation with performance. The PM results revealed that students engaging in MMT frequently switch between assignments, social media, and multimedia. High-scoring students focused more on assignment-related activities, while low-scoring students started late, multitasked extensively, and submitted their work close to the deadline. While these results indicate that MMT does not directly affect the student's performance for the type of assignment, MMT extends work duration. Students tend to work closer to the deadline, so they often work very late into the night, negatively impacting their well-being. Recommendations are provided to mitigate these issues.

Keywords: media multitasking · student behavior · active window tracking · event log · process mining

1 Introduction

The learning process has dramatically changed with the advancement of technology. Learning Management Systems (LMS) allow all students' learning activities and academic achievements to be documented in an integrated system, providing valuable data for lecturers [7]. Educational Data Mining (EDM) is a field aimed at extracting and analyzing this data. However, understanding the learning process requires a more comprehensive, process-centric approach called Education Process Mining (EPM). EPM uses algorithms to find patterns in event log data from educational systems, providing insights into actual learning activities [1, 6].

The ability of students to manage tasks and focus affects their academic performance and mental health [18, 23]. Students often face multiple tasks within limited time frames,

A. Delgado and T. Slaats (Eds.): ICPM 2024 Workshops, LNBIP 533, pp. 117–128, 2025.
https://doi.org/10.1007/978-3-031-82225-4_9

making it hard to focus, especially with increased media access and multitasking [17, 21]. Media multitasking (MMT), used as a coping strategy, burdens working memory and cognitive function, reducing focus and academic performance [16, 17, 20]. The theory of attention highlights that individuals have limited cognitive resources, and multitasking increases cognitive load, hindering information retention and understanding [22]. It is suggested that focusing on one task can improve learning outcomes by reducing the working memory load and enhancing effective learning [11].

Recent studies have analyzed student behavior using process mining (PM) [9, 13–15]. However, no study has explored the use of media multitasking during the learning process, such as doing assignments or taking exams, which is an interesting area to explore. The investigation of MMT behavior requires a new approach to collecting and creating an event log. This study will use Active Window Tracking (AWT) [5] to gain insights into students' media multitasking behavior during assignments and midterms. AWT records user interactions to create detailed event logs, which will be analyzed with PM and correlation analysis to understand student behavior and its impact on academic performance.

The remainder of this paper is structured as follows. Relevant literature on media multitasking and EPM is discussed in Sect. 2. Section 3 presents the method used in the paper to collect and process the event log from the AWT records. Results from the PM and correlation analysis are presented in Sect. 4. A discussion on the implications of our study for educators in Sect. 5 follows this. Concluding remarks are given in the final section.

2   Related Work

2.1   Educational Data Mining and Educational Process Mining

Educational Data Mining (EDM) develops methods to explore educational data, applying data mining techniques to address key questions in education [4, 20]. Studies show EDM's value in extracting insights into student behavior and learning effectiveness, including predicting performance, detecting unwanted behavior, and grouping students [3, 12, 19]. Educational Process Mining (EPM) is an emerging area within Educational Data Mining (EDM) that aims to reveal implicit knowledge and enhance understanding of educational processes. EPM uses log data from educational environments to uncover, analyze, and visually describe these processes [6]. Specifically, EPM applies Process Mining (PM) techniques to raw educational data [6]. Several studies have investigated student behavior in the learning process with PM. For example, PM has been used to analyze student behavior in completing quizzes on the LMS [13]. Student behavior in accessing the LMS has also been examined by [9], as well as the relationship between LMS log data and student achievement [14]. However, using LMS data alone does not allow for analyzing the full breadth of student behavior, e.g., other tools they are using while doing assignments. In this study, we will record this behavior using AWT, allowing for extended behavioral analysis, for example exploring multitasking behavior.

2.2   Multitasking and Media Multitasking

Multitasking involves performing multiple tasks simultaneously through rapid attention switching, dividing attention, or task planning, which is common in daily activities like meeting deadlines or managing chores [8]. Media multitasking (MMT), a subset, involves using multiple digital media streams at once, such as texting while watching TV or checking social media while gaming. This behavior, especially prevalent among adolescents and young adults, has increased with smartphone use.

Despite its perceived benefits, MMT negatively affects cognitive performance. It increases cognitive load due to frequent attention switching, disrupts memory and learning, and impairs executive functions like planning and self-regulation. Long-term effects are still under study, but MMT is linked to mental health issues such as depression and anxiety and may impact cognitive development in children and adolescents [20]. The impact of MMT on homework and academic performance has been studied by [15]. To our knowledge, Active Window Tracking has not been used to study multimedia multitasking, and no study has utilized PM to observe MMT behavior during assignments or midterms.

3   Method

3.1   Context

Data is taken from the students' activities in two different batches that took a Business Process Modeling course at a public university in Surabaya, Indonesia. The students are in their fourth semester. Batch 1 consists of class 1, with 30 students, and class 2, with 31 students. Batch 2 has two classes with 17 students each. The BPM course is supported by a Learning Management System (LMS). The lecturer used the LMS to provide course materials, announce and collect assignments and conduct assessments.

3.2   Event Log Collection and Processing

Three learning activities, including two assignments and a midterm, are used as datasets from each batch. Students must create BPMN models based on textual descriptions for assignments 1 (A1) and 2 (A2). The assignments are delivered via the LMS, and students are given certain deadlines to submit them. The students can do the assignments outside the class hours. For batch 1, A1 is announced on 18/09/2023, 6.00 AM and the deadlines for the two classes are on 20/09/2023, 6.00 AM, while A2 is announced on 26/09/2023, 6.00 AM, and the deadlines are 2/10/2023, 6:00 AM. Only A2 in batch 2 has different deadlines. Details about the assignments and deadlines can be found in supplementary materials. After the submission deadline, the lecturers discussed the assignments during the class. The mid-term is conducted during in-person meetings to assess their modeling skills.

To collect the event log, students in the four classes are asked to record their windows using the Active Window Tracking application, tockler.io, while doing their assignments and mid-term. The experiments are conducted in line with the ethical procedure of Institut Teknologi Sepuluh Nopember. Students' involvement in the experiment is voluntary, and the students who volunteer fill in a formal consent form. Even after volunteering, students can opt-out (i.e., deciding not to submit their tockler.io recording) whenever they feel uncomfortable. Students who continue the experiments submit their Tockler log results in the LMS.

After all data was collected, we started event log processing. Python scripts were used for the data pre-processing stage, which involved tagging and labeling the window titles recorded on Tockler based on pre-defined keywords. For example, if the window title contains keywords related to Spotify (a music player application), the code will be "multimedia". Labeling was done to make it easier for the researchers to identify the activities carried out by participants while completing the assignment or midterm. The complete list of labels and labeling process can be found in the supplementary materials.

Data cleaning is also done to eliminate double logging generated by preprocessing. To facilitate participant identification and analysis with PM, a new attribute called User ID is added to each participant's log data file. Each User ID uniquely identifies the log data associated with each participant. After adding the User ID attribute, each participant's activity recording data is combined into one event log. The event log workflow will combine the three core attributes for each recorded activity: (1) *Case ID*: An attribute that acts as a *unique identifier* for each participant (in this case, the User ID), (2) *Activity*: represents a label assigned based on the content of the window title (e.g., "Social Media", "Modeling tools"), and (3) *Timestamp*: Records the specific time when each activity occurs. An example of a log event structure from results preprocessing activity recording log data for one participant (one Case ID) can be found in supplementary material.

3.3 Correlation Analysis and Process Mining

To help identify interesting patterns for our process mining analysis, we first conducted a correlation analysis on several variables: the number of activities, the duration students take to do the assignment or midterm, and the score/grade. The activities are classified into those related to assignments (related) and those unrelated (unrelated) to assignments, such as doing other assignments, accessing social media, zoom, or other tasks. An additional variable called MMT density is calculated by dividing the number of activities by the duration. MMT measures the intensity of the windows switching within a certain period. Additionally, we analyze two temporal variables to calculate the intervals when students submit their assignment with 1) the official submission deadline and 2) midnight preceding the deadline. These variables offer critical insights into student behavior, potentially highlighting trends in time management and last-minute work habits that eventually correspond to their well-being. For the correlation analysis, we used Spearman correlations, as most individual variables were not normally distributed. We used a Bonferroni-Holm correction to account for the high number of comparisons. PM with the Apromore tool is then used to investigate interesting patterns based on correlation analysis.

4   Results

4.1   Media Multitasking and Its Impact

The correlation analysis result in Fig. 1 reports only the statistically significant correlations, all with a rounded p-value of 0.000. First, we look at the student's behavior related to activities and MMT density. For both assignments, **the duration is negatively correlated with the MMT, positively with the number of related activities**, and **strongly correlated with the number of unrelated activities**. Then, we also found correlations between the number of related activities to the number of unrelated activities within both assignments. Students who perform more relevant activities also tend to perform more irrelevant ones. Although the effect is weak, students who perform more relevant activities for A1 also tend to do that for A2. A1's unrelated activities seem to be weakly correlated with the number of both types of activities in A2. These results indicate that students tend to have the same behavior while doing both assignments. Using PM, we further investigate the connection between these related and unrelated tasks in Sect. 4.2.

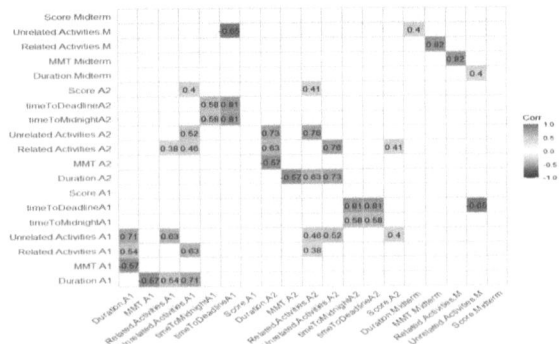

Fig. 1. Correlation results. Only the statistically significant correlation values are shown.

We also want to know whether students' MMT affects their performance. With A2, we find that the more relevant activities a student performs, the higher their expected score. Interestingly, nothing indicates that MMT has a clear relation with scores. The relationship between MMT and performance for A1 is close to significant. For A2 and the midterm, we find nothing close to significance with low correlation. The strongest correlation is between the midterm's MMT and the number of related activities. As this observation does not align with the established theory about MMT, we investigate the relationship between MMT and performance with process mining in Sect. 4.2.

The time to midnight for A1 is weakly correlated with the hand-in times of A2. We find a much stronger effect if we check the same correlation for the time to the deadline of A1 and the hand-in times of A2. Finally, we found a moderately strong negative effect between the time to the deadline of A1 and the number of unrelated activities of the midterm. Students who handed in their work closer to the deadline seemed to perform more unrelated activities during the midterm.

4.2   Insights from Process Mining (PM)

Results from the correlation analysis help us identify how the variables relate to one another, which needs to be investigated further. We use PM to provide deeper insights into some of the strong correlations and unexpected findings to understand students' media multitasking.

Activities, Duration and Media Multitasking Intensity

The correlation analysis result indicates that students who spend more time on an assignment perform more activities, especially those unrelated to the task. They switch less between screens, as the negative correlation with MMT shows. This could mean students who take more time are more focused or may have been idle or not actively involved with the assignment.

To investigate these correlations, we filter one case from Batch 1 with the longest duration during assignment one from Class 1. As shown in Fig. 2, this student activates Tockler for two days, with several idle times in between. This may be because, in the first assignment, the student was unfamiliar with AWT and did not change the setting. Tockler is immediately launched whenever the student activates their laptops. This way, the students continuously recorded their activities.

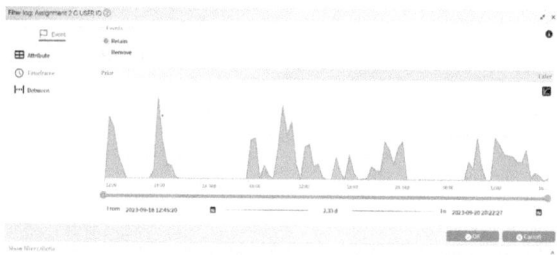

Fig. 2. Timeframe of Student from Batch 1 with the Longest Duration

To exclude those students who continuously recorded their activities, we focused on Batch 1, Class 1 while doing A2, as the students should be more familiar with operating AWT. We then drilled down on students who could finish in less than 2 hours, assuming that these students deliberately recorded their activities when they were about to do their assignments. There are 12 out of 30 students that belong to this category. The process map is shown in Fig. 3.

Most students in these categories switch between doing related activities (modeling tools, course MPB: view assignments, see materials, assignment completion, MPB materials) with unrelated activities (others, other assignments and social media). **Students with shorter durations switch across many applications, which explains the negative correlation of duration with the MMT.**

MMT and its Effect on Scores

The correlation analysis indicates that MMT and assignment scores are mostly unrelated. Related activities do not predict scores any better than unrelated activities. This is most likely linked to the nature of the assignment. A1 and A2 instructed the students to create a BPMN model from a certain process description, and they were given approximately two days to submit. No correlation is found between the intensity of MMT with the student's assignment scores, showing that students can still manage the assignment while working with something else.

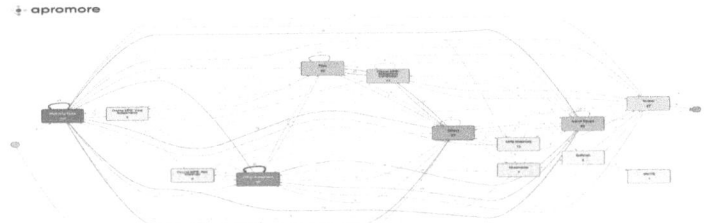

Fig. 3. Students from Batch 1, Class 1 with Less than 2 h Duration

The course is designed so students learn and practice during assignments to prepare for the midterm. So, those who are not focused, seen from the high intensity of MMT and prolonged work on the assignments, may find it difficult to do the midterm as it forces them to be more focused within a shorter timeframe. Thus, the lack of statistical significance between students' behavior during assignments, their assignment scores and the midterm results need to be investigated further.

For our analysis, we selected three students (U5 and U24) from Batch 1, Class 2, with relatively low A2 scores compared to their peers. User 24 only started working at midnight before the assignment deadline (Fig. 4). For almost six hours, U24 switched between working on the assignment with another assignment and spending more time on unrelated activities than assignment-related activities. The process map of U5 can be found in the supplementary material.

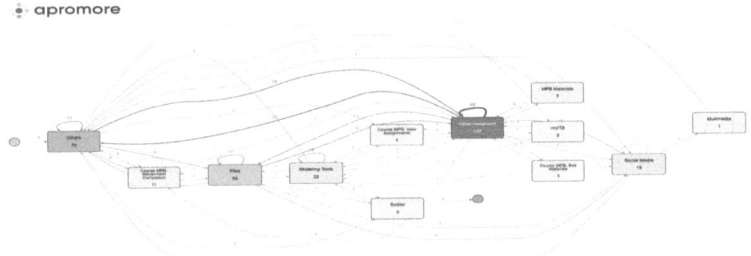

Fig. 4. Process Map of User 24 from Batch 1 while Doing A2 (abstract by case frequency, 100 nodes and arcs)

Then, we compared user 11 (U11) from batch 1, which scored very high for A2 and midterm. While doing A2, U11 did more related than unrelated activities, indicating more focus on the assignment (Fig. 5).

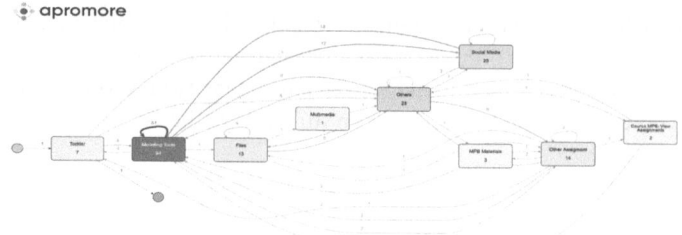

Fig. 5. Process Map of User 11 from Batch 1 while Doing A2 (abstract by case frequency, 100 nodes and arcs)

Correlation Analysis Found the Strongest Correlation Between the Midterm's MMT and the Number of Related Activities. Unlike assignments, during midterm, students are only given two hours and cannot open other unrelated applications or windows. Figure 6 shows the process map of U9 (Batch 1 Class 2), during midterms that clearly shows the user switch between activities related to the test. **The correlation analysis also found a weak correlation between the duration of the test and the number of unrelated activities**. This is evident in the process map of U30 (Batch 1 Class 2) shown in Fig. 7. U30 finished the midterm in 1.88 hours but spent more time with activities unrelated to the midterm. U30 also violated the rules by accessing social media applications and files from the tryout.

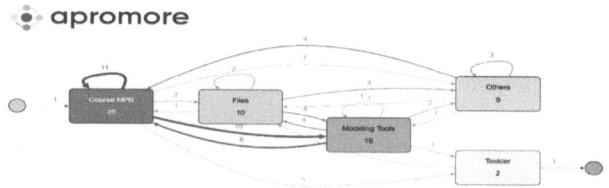

Fig. 6. Process Map of User 9 from Batch 1 During Midterm (abstract by case frequency, 100 nodes and arcs)

Submission Time

We also use PM to investigate the students' behavior toward the submission deadline. A strong correlation is found between the time to the deadline of A1 and the hand-in times of A2, indicating that students tend to work similarly for subsequent assignments. We infer from the correlation analysis that students mostly determine their hand-in time based on the deadline, not their schedule. This can be shown in Batch 2, where A1 for class 1 has a different submission time than class 2.

Figure 8 shows the timeframe of users from Class 1 in Batch 2 while doing A1. The deadline is 25 March 2024 at 10 PM, and we can see that most students started working on the assignment after midnight before the deadline. Figure 9 shows the timeframe of users from Class 2 in Batch 2 while doing A1. For this class, the deadline is 25 March

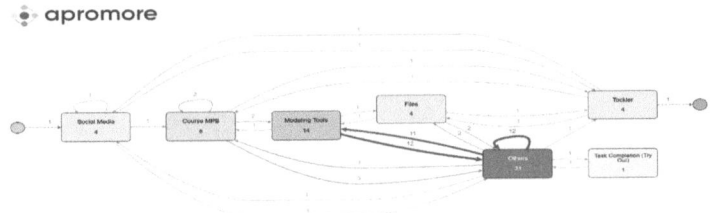

Fig. 7. Process Map of User 30 Batch 1 Class 2 During Midterm (Abstract by case frequency, 100% nodes & arcs)

2024 at 07 AM. Most students started working on the assignment on 24 March at 3 PM until midnight, and some even worked until just two hours before the submission time.

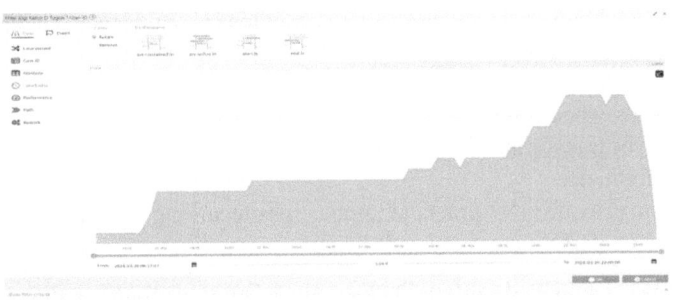

Fig. 8. Timeframe of Users from Class 1, Batch 2 while Doing A1

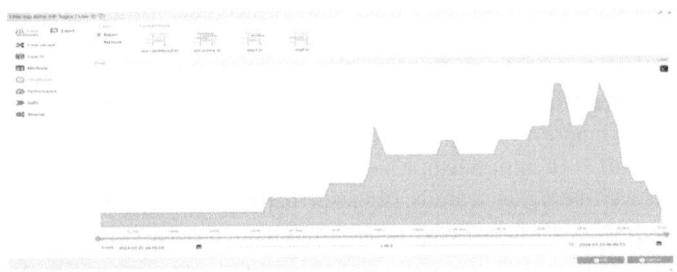

Fig. 9. Timeframe of Users from Class 2, Batch 2 while Doing A1

Finally, we found a moderately strong negative effect between the time to the deadline of A1 and the number of unrelated activities of the midterm. Students who handed in their work closer to the deadline seemed to perform more unrelated activities during the midterm. We chose U2 from Batch 1, Class 1, which handed in A1 at 05.24 AM. The process map of the same student during the midterm is shown in Fig. 10. U2 conducted many unrelated activities and even violated the rule by accessing social media and files from course material (tryout). This result shows that students who hand in their assignments close to the deadline have lower time management skills and most likely face difficulties during the midterm.

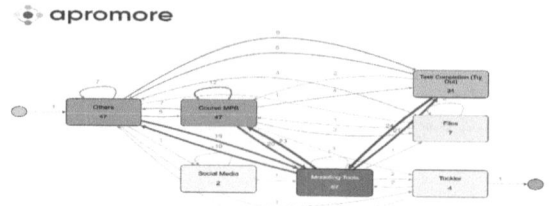

Fig. 10. Process Map of U2, Batch 1, Class 1 during Midterm (abstract by case frequency, 100 nodes and arcs)

5   Implications

This paper has two main implications. First, for researchers in PM and EPM, we propose a new way of collecting and processing event logs using Active Window Tracking (AWT). This paper demonstrates that AWT can provide rich insights into students' media multitasking while doing their learning activities. This can be applied to similar digital environments where users perform certain tasks while accessing other media. The recordings can be transformed into event logs and used to investigate the impact of MMT on users' performance.

Second, we provide more practical implications regarding students' MMT behavior and its impact on performance and well-being.

I1. Student MMT and Assignment Performance. Our study found no direct correlation between MMT and students' scores, unlike [14], which reported negative effects. The difference may stem from the assignment type. Process mining shows both high and low scorers multitasked, but low scorers started and finished late, while high scorers focused more on assignment-related tasks.

I2. Student MMT, Last-Minute Habit and Well-being. Correlation analysis indicates a relation of students' hand in time between assignments. PM reveals that students adjust their time of working on the assignment closer to the deadline and often work very late into the night, even until dawn. This highlights their last-minute habit, potentially affecting their well-being, as a study suggests that individuals with an earlier, regular, consistent sleep schedule have better health examination results [10].

Several recommendations can be made to address the issues:

R1. Timed Assignments: To reduce students' last-minute habits, lecturers can set timed assignments, ensuring students have the necessary skills and defining a standard completion time. The submission period should match this standard time.

R2. Adjusted Deadlines: Instead of early morning deadlines, instructors can set submission times during normal working hours to help students manage their time better.

R3. Balanced Workload: Course coordinators and lecturers should consider students' overall workload by coordinating assignment schedules and course deadlines.

6   Concluding Remark

This paper proposes a new way to collect and process event logs using Active Window Tracking (AWT) to investigate media multitasking (MMT) among students in higher education institutions in Indonesia. Correlation analysis revealed students' consistent behavior across assignments, no direct correlation between MMT and performance, and close to the deadline submission. The PM results revealed that students engaging in MMT frequently switch between assignments, social media, and multimedia. High-scoring students focused more on assignments, while low-scoring students started late, multitasked extensively, and submitted their work close to the deadline. While these results indicate that MMT does not directly affect the performance for the type of assignment, MMT extends work duration. Students tend to work closer to the deadline, so they often work very late into the night, negatively impacting their wellbeing. Recommendations are provided to mitigate these issues.

Appendix: Supplementary Material

Supplementary material for this article is available online at https://bit.ly/3XUzPPC.

References

1. van der Aalst, W.: Data science in action. In: Process Mining, pp. 3–23 Springer, Heidelberg (2016)
2. van der Aalst, W.M.P., Weijters, A.J.M.M.: Process mining: a research agenda. Comput. Ind. **53**(3), 231–244 (2004)
3. Alshareef, F., et al.: Educational Data Mining Applications and Techniques. (2020)
4. Bakhshinategh, B., et al.: Educational data mining applications and tasks: a survey of the last 10 years. Educ. Inf. Technol. (Dordr). **23**(1), 537–553 (2018)
5. Beerepoot, I., et al.: A window of opportunity: active window tracking for mining work practices (2023)
6. Bogarín, A. et al.: A survey on educational process mining. Wiley Interdisc. Rev. Data Min. Knowl. Disc. **8** (2018)
7. Bradley, V.M.: Learning management system (LMS) use with online instruction. Int. J. Technol. Educ. **4**(1), 68 (2020)
8. Buser, T., Peter, N.: Multitasking. Exp. Econ. **15**(4), 641–655 (2012)
9. Cenka, B.A.N., et al.: Analysing student behaviour in a learning management system using a process mining approach. Knowl. Manag. E-Learn. **14**(1), 62–80 (2022)
10. Chaput, J.-P., et al.: Sleep timing, sleep consistency, and health in adults: a systematic review. Appl. Physiol. Nutr. Metab. **45**(10), S232–S247 (2020)
11. Cotton, K., et al.: The effects of mind-wandering, cognitive load, and task engagement on working memory performance in remote online experiments. Exp. Psychol. **70**(5), 271–284 (2023)
12. Farrah Siddiqui, I., Ali Arain, Q.: Analyzing students' academic performance through educational data mining. In: 3C Tecnología. Glosas de innovación aplicadas a la pyme. Edición Especial, pp. 402–421 (2019)
13. Juhaňák, L., et al.: Using process mining to analyze students' quiz-taking behavior patterns in a learning management system. Comput. Human Behav. **92**, 496–506 (2019)

14. Lerche, T., Kiel, E.: Predicting student achievement in learning management systems by log data analysis. Comput. Human Behav. **89**, 367–372 (2018)
15. de las Martín-Perpiñá, M., et al.: Media multitasking impact in homework, executive function and academic performance in spanish adolescents. Psicothema. **31**(1), 81–87 (2019)
16. Maslovat, D., et al.: Evidence for a response preparation bottleneck during dualtask performance: effect of a startling acoustic stimulus on the psychological refractory period. Acta Psychol. (Amst) **144**(3), 481–487 (2013)
17. May, K.E., Elder, A.D.: Efficient, helpful, or distracting? a literature review of media multitasking in relation to academic performance (2018)
18. Miller, L.A., Schmidt, J.R.: The effects of online assignments and weekly deadlines on student outcomes in a macroeconomics course. Am. Econ. **66**(1), 46–60 (2021)
19. Ray, S., Saeed, M.: Applications of educational data mining and learning analytics tools in handling big data in higher education. In: Applications of Big Data Analytics: Trends, Issues, and Challenges, pp. 135–160 Springer, Heidelberg (2018)
20. Van Der Schuur, W.A., et al.: The consequences of media multitasking for youth: a review (2015)
21. Uncapher, M.R., et al.: Media multitasking and memory: differences in working memory and long-term memory. Psychon. Bull. Rev. **23**(2), 483–490 (2016)
22. Wickens, C.: Attention: theory, principles, models and applications. Int. J. Hum. Comput. Interact. **37**(5), 403–417 (2021)
23. Yadav, C.S., Monga, S.: The effect of time management on subjective well-being among university students. Int. J. Manag. (IJM). **11**(12), 1642–1651 (2020)

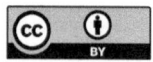

Measuring Skill Acquisition and Retention: A Case Study of Math Fluency

Gert Janssenswillen[1,2](✉)(iD), Seppe Van Daele[3], and Marc Van Daele[3]

[1] Faculty of Business Economics, UHasselt - Hasselt University,
3590 Diepenbeek, Belgium
`gert.janssenswillen@uhasselt.be`
[2] UHasselt, EDM - Expertise Centre for Digital Media, 3950 Diepenbeek, Belgium
[3] Wijsr, 3590 Diepenbeek, Belgium
`{seppe,marc}@wijsr.com`

Abstract. This study examines the application of process-oriented techniques to analyse learning stages in primary education, specifically developing math fact fluency. Utilizing data from an arithmetic practice platform used in primary schools, this research addresses three primary questions: the amount of practice time required to master arithmetic operations, the learning characteristics influencing this duration, and the impact of different learning characteristics on skill retention. The analysis reveals significant variability in the time and effort needed for a pupil to master a skill, influenced by initial skill levels and whether students prioritise accuracy or speed. Students leaning towards accuracy tend to achieve steady progress, attaining higher accuracy before enhancing their speed, whereas those leaning towards speed may reach mastery more quickly but risk inconsistencies in accuracy resulting in a lower skill retention. The findings highlight the effectiveness of process-oriented methodologies in education, in providing more nuanced insights into student learning phases. The case study underscores the necessity for adaptive learning platforms and personalised educational strategies that accommodate diverse learning behaviours and needs. It furthermore highlights that gamification tactics should facilitate these diverse learning behaviours, rather than counteract them.

Keywords: Process Mining · Learning Analytics · Math Fact Fluency

1 Introduction

In recent years, the application of process mining techniques has proved valuable in various education contexts, from analysing learning behaviours on online learning platforms to analysing student trajectories in higher education programs [5]. Advances in Educational Process Mining were initially fuelled by the availability of large datasets from Massive Open Online Course (MOOC) platforms [10,13], and techniques were subsequently also applied in more traditional higher-education institutions [7]. The use of process-oriented methodologies and techniques enables an holistic view of student trajectories that goes

© The Author(s) 2025
A. Delgado and T. Slaats (Eds.): ICPM 2024 Workshops, LNBIP 533, pp. 129–141, 2025.
https://doi.org/10.1007/978-3-031-82225-4_10

beyond momentary pass rates and graduation times, allowing for more detailed diagnostic observations.

The increasing prevalence of PC's and tablets in primary and secondary school classrooms now enables us to get novel data-driven insights into foundational learning processes, such as arithmetic, reading and writing [9]. Student performance in these areas, as measured for 15-year-olds by PISA-scores, OECD's Programme for International Student Assessment, have been showing negative trends in many countries, notably in Europe, North-America and Australia [8,12]. Inadequate levels of support provided by teachers and school staff, as well as the lacking of sufficient resources for student assistance have been identified as possible causes [6].

In this paper, we showcase the use of process-oriented data analysis to provide novel insights about learning in a primary education context. Specifically, we use data from an arithmetical practice platform to measure and analyse different stages of learning in math fact fluency. Math fact fluency, or the *automation* of mental arithmetic, is a crucial formation step for pupils at the age of 6 and beyond, where they practice to perform arithmetic operations both *correctly* and *quickly* [3]. The case study aims to answer two main questions,

- **RQ1:** What is the required practice time to master arithmetic operations, and which learning characteristics influence this?
- **RQ2:** Do different learning characteristics result in better skill retention?

The remainder of this paper is structured as follows. Section 2 provides necessary background information related to math fact fluency and learning stages. Section 3 describes the scope and working of the platform and the resulting data, along with some descriptive statistics. In Sect. 4 the findings for the research questions are presented, which are further discussed in Sect. 5. Section 6 concludes the paper.

2   Background

Math Fact Fluency. Math fact fluency refers to the ability to accurately and quickly answer basic arithmetic facts, such as 5×6 or $12 + 4$. While these exercises might feel quite easy and redundant, especially with technology at our fingertips, they remain crucial for mathematical development. Research shows that students with better math fact fluency retain more working memory for complex exercises [16], are less likely to develop math anxiety, show higher self-confidence in their abilities [1], and tend to outperform their less fluent peers in both academic success [4] and future income levels [14].

Learning Stages. A common framework to conceptualise different stages of learning is the Conscious Competence Learning (CCL) Model [2]. According to the CCL-model, learning starts with *unconscious incompetence*, a phase in which learners are *ignorant* of their lack of knowledge. This is followed by *conscious incompetence*, also known as *awareness*. At this point, they are aware of the lack of knowledge or skills, but not yet proficient. Once learners have developed the necessary skills, they move to a phase of *conscious competence*, also known as *learning*. In this stage, learners know how to do it, but it still requires considerable conscious effort, and mistakes are still made. Finally, in the stage of *unconscious competence*, also known as *mastery*, the skill becomes a second nature. At this point, the learners are able to conduct the operations without conscious effort or attention, i.e. the skill has become automated.

3   Data Understanding

The data analysed in this case study originates from the online platform *Automatus*.[1] Using *Automatus*, pupils learn to automate basic arithmetic operations in a playful and adaptive manner, both in their classroom and at home. While Automatus is a novel tool, it has seen a steady increase of usage in Belgian and Dutch schools, for pupils from 1st to 6th grade.[2]

Each exercise series performed by a pupil typically consists of 20 exercises (configurable by the teacher), where each exercise requires solving a single arithmetic operation. All arithmetic operations in a series are of a specific type, which is referred to as a *brick*. The definition of bricks, and the order in which they are practised, are defined in line with applicable primary school curricula. Figure 1 shows how each of these *bricks* together form an arithmetic *wall*. The higher the location of a brick in the wall, the more difficult the operations get.

Once pupils have practised at least 20 exercises belonging to a specific brick, that brick will get a colour-code in their wall that represents their attained skill-level (cf. further). Teachers can inspect the individual wall of each pupil to evaluate their progress over time. When a pupil's attained skill-level for a brick is sufficient, next series will contain exercises of more advanced bricks.[3]

3.1   Scope

In this paper, two types of data recorded by the platform are used. On the one hand, we consider *activity* data, which records all the exercises that students have conducted. On the other hand, we consider *scoring* data, which indicate the level of understanding the pupil has of a specific *brick* at a specific point in time. The scoring data is directly derived from the activity data, and is updated whenever a pupil has performed an additional 20 exercises concerning the brick in question. The data used in this paper was recorded between September 1, 2023 and May 21, 2024. Only pupils who were active over a period of 4 weeks or more were considered for the analysis, in order to focus on pupils for which we can measure progress over time. Finally, 5 827 pupils were analysed, belonging to 446 different classes from 220 different schools.

---

[1] https://automatus.be/.

[2] In this paper, we use Belgian terminology, meaning that 1st grade refers to 6-year-olds and 6th grade to 12-year-olds.

[3] In practice, this depends on whether a teacher follows Automatus' predefined learning paths. A teacher can choose to practice other specific (successions of) bricks.

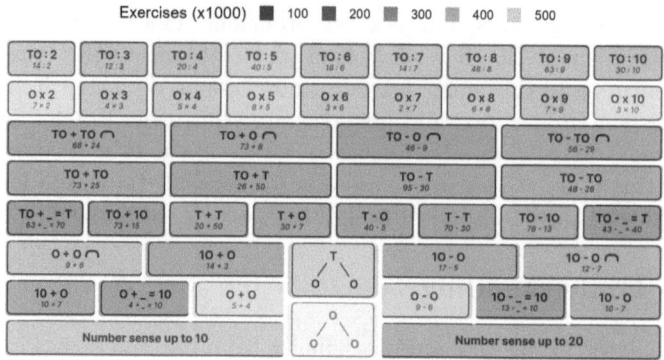

Fig. 1. Arithmetic wall used by Automatus, coloured by number of exercises. (Color figure online)

3.2 Activity Data

Table 1 lists descriptive statistics about the activities of pupils. A total of 8 765 500 exercises were made, divided over 380 525 exercise series. In total, the pupils under consideration on average spend 1.54 h on the platform, although the entire period over which this activity took place on average measured 115 days. If the time between exercises was less than 10 min, they were considered to belong to the same practice *session*, resulting in 69 118 sessions. An average practice session took 10.37 min, containing 5.51 series with an average total of 126.82 exercises.

Table 1. Descriptive statistics activities per pupil.

	Total	Per pupil			
		Q1	Median	Mean	Q3
Period with activity (days)		57.88	112.06	115.01	160.02
Time spent (hours)	8 955.17	0.59	1. 07	1.54	1.84
Nr. of exercises	8 765 500	414	828	1504.29	1707
Nr. of series	380 525	19	37	65.30	76
Nr. of sessions	69 118	5	8	11.86	13

As is shown in Fig. 1, some bricks were practised more than others. Naturally, these numbers are related to the demographic characteristics of the pupils: 15.5% are first graders, which are mostly focused on number sense, addition and subtraction. Pupils from second until fourth grade (68.1%) also practice addition and subtraction, but predominantly focus on multiplication and addition. The final 16.4% of pupils are fifth and sixth graders, which only practised these 2 upper levels of the wall.

3.3 Scoring Data

After each 20 exercises of a specific brick, a score is calculated. This score reflects both the accuracy and the speed of the pupil. Both characteristics are scaled to a number between zero and 100. For a pupil of which the accuracy on the last 20 exercises was below 50%, the accuracy score is zero. Accuracy's higher than 50% are scaled to the interval (0,100). For duration, a predefined target duration is considered for each brick. If the average duration spent is higher than 5 times this target time, the speed score is zero. Any average duration between 5 and zero times the target duration is again scaled to the interval (0,100).

A total of 203 309 scores were computed based on the activity data described above, of which the spread according to accuracy and speed is shown in Fig. 2. Because the original accuracies are multiples of 0.05, the accuracy score has a discrete nature. In the figure, some random noise was added to the points to better visualise the mass of the data points.

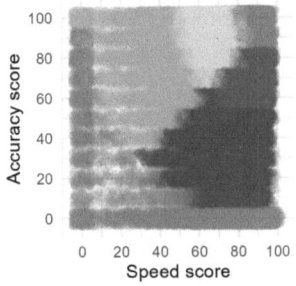

Fig. 2. Distribution of scores.

Table 2. Frequency of scores.

Tier	Score		Perc.	Total
1	Green			47 715
2	Yellow	50 971	53.6%	95 104
	Blue	44 133	46.4%	
3	Orange	13 529	30.8%	43 991
	Purple	30 462	69.2%	
4	Red			16 499

As can be seen in this figure, Automatus attaches one of six colour labels to each score, which are organized in four tiers. In the upper right green tier, pupils score good on both accuracy and speed.[4] In the lowest red tier, pupils score poorly on both aspects. Both intermediate tiers are further divided along the diagonal. Above the diagonal, the orange and yellow scores represent pupils that score relatively better on accuracy than on speed. The purple and blue scores represent pupils that score relatively better on speed.

From the frequencies listed in Table 2, it can be seen that in the second tier, slightly more scores are above the diagonal (yellow, accuracy > speed). This can be explained by the fact that the blue area is in fact smaller than the yellow area, given that a perfect score on speed is unlikely. In contrast, in

---

[4] Note that while an accuracy score of 100 is quite frequent, the speed score will always be strictly less than 100. By the scaling Automatus uses as outlined above, a speed score of 100 means that the pupil would perform exercises instantaneously. Nonetheless, if a pupil receives a green score, it means that they were able to perform the exercises below the predefined target time of the brick.

the third tier, considerably more scores fall below the diagonal (purple, speed > accuracy), emphasising that pupils tend to score much better on speed than accuracy. This is because the scores on the speed scale are highly centralised, with 50% of scores lying between 70 and 87, whereas there is somewhat more variance on the accuracy scale. Presumably, this is because pupils tend to be more motivated by the speed aspect, as this is part of the gamification on the platform. As such, the mass of scores is mostly situated in the area towards the right of the space, stretching from the yellow to purple segment.

4   Results

In the following paragraphs, we present the results in answering the research questions outlined above. Firstly, Sect. 4.1 defines a way to measure the regularity of practice, which will be one of the learning characteristics used in the further analysis. Section 4.2 describes the approach used to define when a pupil obtains a *mastery* skill level. Section 4.3 will then analyse the time it takes to reach this skill level, including the influence of learning characteristics, while Sect. 4.4 describes differences in skill-retention.

4.1   Measuring Regularity of Practice

In order to measure the regularity of practice, we examine whether pupils tends to cluster their practice one a specific day of the week (*focused*), or spread it out over multiple days a week (*unfocused*). Furthermore, we investigate whether their focus is *stable* from one week to the next, or *unstable*. Focus and stability are measured both w.r.t. the day-of-the-week and the time of day.

In order to measure the degree of focus for day-of-the-week, we compute the Shannon entropy [15] for each pupil in each week, based on the distribution of their practised exercises. An entropy of one indicates the activity is equally spread over the seven days of the week, while an entropy of zero indicates all activity happened on a single day. We subsequently define *focus* as 1 - entropy.

In order to measure the *stability* of the focus over a period of n weeks, we use the Jensen-Shannon divergence JSD [11] for measuring the difference between multiple distributions, which is defined as the difference between the overall Shannon entropy[5], and the average entropy. As the upper bound of JSD depends on the number of distributions, we divide by the normalising constant $log_7(n)$—base 7 because of the number of days—so that the final values lie between 0 and 1. The higher the difference in distribution from one week to the other, the higher JSD. The stability is thus defined as the 1 - JSD, so that a high divergence corresponds with a low stability.

Table 3 shows an example in which the pupil has a focus varying between 0.67 and 0.85 over the course of three weeks, which is relatively high as his activity

---

[5] Entropy calculated over the distribution M which is the average over all distributions.

is always spread over just 2 days. The average focus for this pupil is 0.75. The JSD equals $(0.60–0.25)/0.56 = 0.62$, where 0.6 is the overall entropy, 0.25 the average weekly entropy, and 0.56 the normalising constant $log_7(3)$.

Table 3. Example measurement of focus and stability.

Week	Mon	Tue	Wed	Thu	Fri	Sat	Sun	Entropy		Mean entropy	0.25
1	0	0	0	0.91	0.09	0	0	0.15		Focus	0.75
2	0.67	0	0	0.33	0	0	0	0.33			
3	0.23	0	0.77	0	0	0	0	0.28		JSD	0.62
M	0.3	0	0.26	0.41	0.03	0	0	0.60		Stability	0.38

In a similar way, focus and stability was measured for the time-of-day, dividing exercises between morning (-8am), before noon (8am-12pm), afternoon (12pm-4pm) and evening (4pm-). The distribution of the computed metrics is shown in Fig. 3. It can be seen that for both aspects, the mass of the distribution for focus is situated near the upper bound, indicated that pupils tend to practice on one specific day of the week, and during one specific moment of that day. The stability is much higher when considering the time-of-day, i.e. pupils tend to practice on a fixed moment. The same is not true for the day of the week, where the stability averages 0.5. I.e. while pupils practice on a single day in the week, for many pupils, the specific day is flexible over the course of multiple weeks.

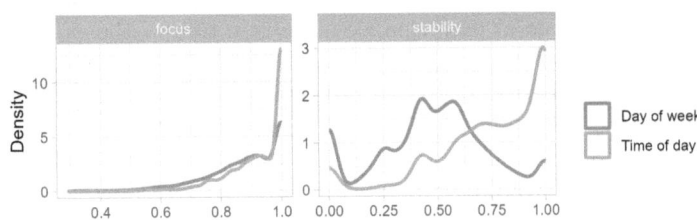

Fig. 3. Distribution of the focus and stability of practice.

4.2   Mastery Skill Level

As its name suggest, the goal of *Automatus* is to automate solving mathematical operations, not to teach them. We can thus assume that pupils using the platform have already encountered the math facts during classes. As a result, when considering the CCL-model, even the *red* scores refer to pupils who have at least some *awareness* of the skill. Pupils which solve the exercises fast and accurately—i.e. a green score—can be considered to have reached *mastery*, and the intermediary scores are various representations of the *learning* stage.

In order to analyse the different stages of learning, we define the *score* data as an event log, where each *pupil+brick* is a case, and every score is an event with the corresponding colour as event type. The resulting log contains 43 604 different cases. In Fig. 4, the coloured dots show the history of an example pupil+brick pair. The *aggregated* line shows the *active* colour.

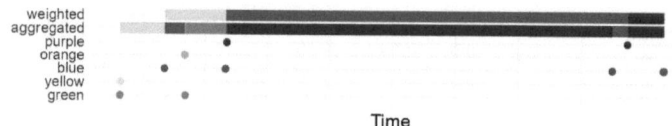

Fig. 4. Example case showing both detailed, aggregated and weighted scores. (Color figure online)

The example shows that there can be a high diversity in the sequence of scores. In this example, the pupil consecutively gets a green, yellow, blue, orange, and green score, followed by alternating blue and purple scores. While this pupil obtained several green scores, it seems that their level of learning has not reached *mastery*. In order to properly measure the achievement of a mastery skill level, we therefore calculate a weighted moving average which takes into account the scaled speed and accuracy of the last 3 scores, where the last score has a weight of 3, the penultimate score a weight of 2, etc. Based on the weighted accuracy and speed, the weighted score is defined. It can be seen that for this pupil, the moving average never reaches green, which aligns with the conclusion that—notwithstanding some good performance at certain times—the skill level of the pupil falls short of *mastery*.

Of the 43 604 pupil+brick cases, 21 801 obtained at least one weighted average score, meaning they practised at least 60 exercises. Of those, 7 258 (33%) were able to reach a green weighted average score. If we consider a green weighted average score as mastery level, we can divide both activities and scores in a *pre-mastery* and *post-mastery* interval. In the following sections, we investigate 1) how long it takes to reach a mastery score, and by which factors this is influenced? and 2) how the different learning characteristics influence skill-retention.

4.3   Time till Mastery

Among the 7 258 cases with a weighted green score, 53% reached it immediately—indicating that pupils coming to the platform often already have had considerable practice. In only 17 cases, the pupil starts with a red weighted average score—indicating pupils who are merely aware of skill at hand, which is clearly lacking. Given the small amount of data on these kinds of pupils, we will not consider them further in this analysis.

For the remaining 3 390 cases, we take into account the *starting tier*—the tier to which their first weighted average score belongs (i.e. tier 2 for blue and orange, tier 3 for purple and yellow)—as a proxy for the initial level of a pupil's skill. Furthermore, we define *reliance* as a pupils tendency to score better in terms of speed or accuracy. In order to quantify the reliance, we compute the difference between the scaled accuracy score and the scaled speed score for every received score in the pre-mastery period, and take the average distance for each case. This average difference is then compared with the median average difference over all cases, so that cases are divided into two equal-size groups. Note that the median difference is 3.16, indicating that there is a slight overall tendency towards accuracy among these cases.

In order to illustrate both groups, Fig. 5 shows the directly-follow probabilities as well as relative frequencies of different scores in both groups. It can be seen that pupils with a reliance on accuracy most often obtain yellow scores, while those leaning towards speed most often obtain blue scores. This is apparent both when looking at the relative frequencies of scores and the directly follows relationships. For example, for a pupil with an accuracy-lean, the most-likely next score will almost always be yellow, while for a pupil with a reliance on speed it will almost always be blue. Given the definition of yellow and blue in Fig. 2, this aligns indeed with an accuracy or speed reliance, respectively.

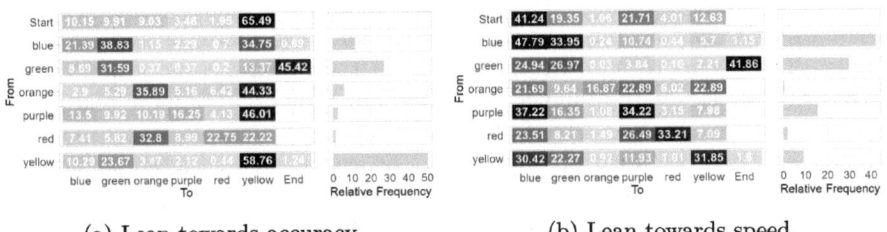

(a) Lean towards accuracy. (b) Lean towards speed.

Fig. 5. Directly-follows relations and relative score frequencies pre-mastery.

The time needed to reach mastery, can be expressed both as exercises performed, and as active time spent practising. Table 4 (a) shows that for the 3 390 cases under consideration, the median required number of exercises is 160, and the median time spent is 6.93 min. According to Table 4 (b), much more time and exercises are needed for cases that start in the lower tier 3, as expected. If we look at differences according to reliance (Table 4 (c)) for each starting tier, we see some important difference. Pupils starting in tier 2 are quite similar, whether they rely on accuracy or speed. The only (logical) difference is that pupils leaning towards speed perform the exercises in less time, and make more mistakes. The story is different for pupils starting in tier 3. For these cases, pupils who lean towards accuracy tend to need much more exercises before they obtain mastery, as well as more practice time. Even when taking into account that the data on this group of pupils is smaller (only 379 cases), the differences in both exercises and practice time are large.

Table 4. Median nr. of (correct) exercises and practice time from start to reaching mastery, in total (a), by starting tier (b) and by starting tier and lean (c).

Start tier	Reliance	Nr. of cases	First practice ↓ mastery (days)	Nr. of correct exercises	Nr. of exercises	Time spent (min)
(a)		3390	30.87	137.00	160.00	6.93
(b) 2		2994	27.11	128.00	140.00	6.34
3		379	55.08	246.00	300.00	16.19
(c) 2	speed	1423	28.00	127.00	140.00	5.39
	accuracy	1571	26.12	131.00	140.00	7.38
3	speed	260	42.61	210.50	260.00	11.78
	accuracy	119	71.91	377.00	420.00	37.35

The group focused on accuracy also required a longer period before they reach mastery (median 71.91 days vs 42.61 days). When investigating behavioural characteristics of pupils in both groups, we did not find important differences in terms of focus nor stability, as defined in Sect. 4.1. Direct correlations between the focus and stability measures, and the required practice time and exercises, where found to be negligible. In terms of behaviour, both reliance groups were found to be slightly different in terms of the number of sessions (more for speed-focused pupils) and average exercises per session (also more for speed-focused pupils). This seems to indicate that pupils in the speed-focused group do not necessarily practice with a higher regularity, but they do have more and longer practice sessions, leading to a faster achievement of a mastery skill level. A possible explanation of this lower intensity of practice among accuracy-leaning pupils might be a demotivating feeling when being too slow, as the gamification elements on the platform are more organised around speed rather than accuracy.

4.4   Skill Retention

Figure 6 shows the relative frequency of obtaining different scores *after* a pupil reaches a weighted green score, i.e. indicating a level of mastery, as well as the directly-follows matrices, based on their reliance on speed or accuracy *before* mastery. It can be seen that pupils that showed more dependence on speed are less likely to keep their green score. It is in fact almost equally likely that the pupil obtains a blue score, indicating a lack of accuracy. For pupils with a focus on accuracy pre-mastery on the other hand, the percentage of green scores is the largest by a significant margin.

While some caution in interpreting these results is needed, they seem to indicate that—while requiring more practice time—pupils with a lean towards accuracy tend to build up more robust skills. It should be noted that the average trace length post-mastery (i.e. the number of scores) equals 7.90, which is comparable to the average trace length pre-mastery (7.63). Overall, there were 25 859 recorded scores pre-mastery and 22 478 post-mastery. As such, for both periods the insights are supported by a similar amount of data.

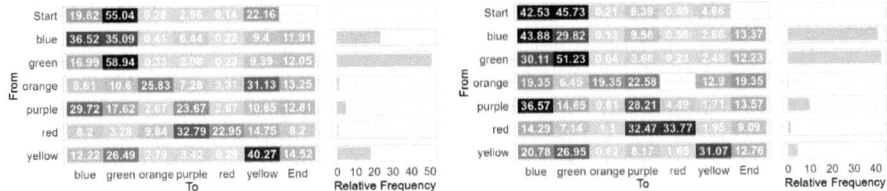

(a) Lean towards accuracy.   (b) Lean towards speed.

Fig. 6. Directly-follows relations and relative score frequencies post-mastery.

5   Discussion

Our analysis reveals that specific learning behaviours, particularly the lean towards accuracy or speed, play a crucial role in the progression towards mastery. Pupils who prioritise accuracy tend to progress through different learning stages more gradually, often achieving higher accuracy scores before improving their speed. Conversely, those who focus on speed might reach mastery more quickly but are at a higher risk of regressing. This suggests that educational tools like Automatus should balance the emphasis on speed and accuracy, ensuring that pupils are not stimulated to compromise one for the other. Gamification elements that reward both accurate and quick responses might encourage a more balanced development of skills.

While no relationship between regularity of practice and learning progress became apparent, some caution is needed. As most of the pupils in this study showed a high degree of focus, and a relatively high stability, especially with respect to the time-of-day aspect, it might be the case that no relationship was found because the data showed little variation.

One of the limitations of the current study is that the context of pupils is missing, as we do not know f.e. when they started learning the specific skills under analysis. Nor do we have information on teaching methods that were used, or the precise context and goal for which the pupils used Automatus. While these aspects can be considered for a more controlled future case study, there are privacy and ethical considerations to address.

In terms of skills, the current analysis mostly approached different bricks in isolation, and did not analyse the connections between different math fact skills. Future research could extend towards a more comprehensive analysis of the arithmetic wall and its interconnections, and also analyse pupil's progress over a period of multiple years.

6   Conclusion

This study explored the application of process-oriented analysis to examine learning stages in primary education, specifically math fluency. By leveraging data from the Automatus platform, we were able to provide insights into the time required to master arithmetic operations, the characteristics that influence this progress, and the impact of different learning behaviours on skill retention.

The study demonstrates the value of using process-oriented methodologies in educational contexts, gaining a deeper understanding of how pupils learn and the stages they progress through to achieve fluency in essential skills. This approach contributes to the broader field of education, presenting a powerful tool for enhancing our understanding of learning processes.

References

1. Boaler, J., Williams, C., Confer, A.: Fluency without fear: research evidence on the best ways to learn math facts. Reflections **40**(2), 7–12 (2015)
2. Curtiss, P.R., Warren, P.W.: The dynamics of life skills coaching. Prince Albert, Sask.: Training Research and Development Station, Department (1973)
3. Fuchs, L.S., et al.: The role of cognitive processes, foundational math skill, and calculation accuracy and fluency in word-problem solving versus prealgebraic knowledge. Dev. Psychol. **52**(12), 2085 (2016)
4. Geary, D.C.: Cognitive predictors of achievement growth in mathematics: a 5-year longitudinal study. Dev. Psychol. **47**(6), 1539 (2011)
5. Ghazal, M.A., Ibrahim, O., Salama, M.A.: Educational process mining: a systematic literature review. In: 2017 European Conference on Electrical Engineering and Computer Science (EECS), pp. 198–203. IEEE (2017)
6. Harper, D.: European education slips downward, according to PISA report by OECD. Euronews (2023). Accessed 30 July 2024
7. Hobeck, R., Pufahl, L., Weber, I.: Process mining on curriculum-based study data: a case study at a German university. In: International Conference on Process Mining, pp. 577–589. Springer, Heidelberg (2022). https://doi.org/10.1007/978-3-031-27815-0_42
8. Jerrim, J.: The reliability of trends over time in international education test scores: is the performance of England's secondary school pupils really in relative decline? J. Soc. Policy **42**(2), 259–279 (2013)
9. Kovanovic, V., Mazziotti, C., Lodge, J.: Learning analytics for primary and secondary schools. J. Learn. Anal. **8**(2), 1–5 (2021)
10. Maldonado, J.J., Palta, R., Vázquez, J., Bermeo, J.L., Pérez-Sanagustín, M., Munoz-Gama, J.: Exploring differences in how learners navigate in moocs based on self-regulated learning and learning styles: a process mining approach. In: 2016 XLII Latin American Computing Conference (CLEI), pp. 1–12. IEEE (2016)
11. Menéndez, M.L., Pardo, J., Pardo, L., Pardo, M.: The Jensen-Shannon divergence. J. Franklin Inst. **334**(2), 307–318 (1997)
12. Morsy, L., Khavenson, T., Carnoy, M.: How international tests fail to inform policy: the unsolved mystery of Australia's steady decline in pisa scores. Int. J. Educ. Dev. **60**, 60–79 (2018)
13. Mukala, P., Buijs, J., Van Der Aalst, W.: Exploring students' learning behaviour in moocs using process mining techniques, pp. 179–196. Department of Mathematics and Computer Science, University of Technology, Eindhoven, The Netherlands (2015)
14. Parsons, S., Bynner, J.: Does numeracy matter more? (2005)

15. Shannon, C.E.: A mathematical theory of communication. Bell Syst. Tech. J. **27**(3), 379–423 (1948)
16. Sweller, J.: Cognitive load during problem solving: effects on learning. Cogn. Sci. **12**(2), 257–285 (1988)

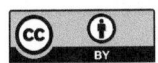

Assessing the Impact of Exam Preparation Process on Students' Careers

Domenico Potena[1], Laura Genga[2(✉)], Lorenzo Galeazzi[1], Gianmarco Vigano[1], and Claudia Diamantini[1]

[1] Università Politecnica delle Marche, Ancona, Italy
[2] Eindhoven University of Technology, Eindhoven, The Netherlands
l.genga@tue.nl

Abstract. Educational Process Mining techniques leverage educational data to gather relevant insights on the corresponding processes, ultimately supporting the development of evidence-based strategies for their improvement. In this work, we analyze students' exam preparation process to i) uncover process patterns describing students' behaviors and ii) develop predictive models capable of predicting students' performance regarding graduation times. The results of the analysis can be employed both to formulate improvements to the study curricula and to enable the early detection of students who are likely to struggle in their career, to support them at an early stage of their studies.

Keywords: Educational process mining · Curriculum Mining · Student performance analysis

1 Introduction

A major challenge for today's universities is enhancing their educational programs. This effort is especially crucial for Italian universities, where around 40% of students do not complete their studies on time, and of those, only 20% graduate within a year of the expected timeframe[1]. The increasingly widespread use of digital platforms to support university processes boosted the development of evidence-based techniques to support this effort in recent years. Among those, a discipline which is gaining increasing attention is *Educational Process Mining* (EPM). The goal of EPM is to uncover patterns and trends within educational data to understand how educational processes are carried out and identify improvement opportunities [4]. In this study, we focus on a specific branch of EPM, the so-called "curriculum mining", whose goal consists in analyzing data related to students' *careers*, i.e. the sequence of registrations of credits-bearing

---

[1] https://www2.almalaurea.it/cgi-php/universita/statistiche/visualizza.php?
anno=2023&corstipo=tutti&ateneo=tutti&facolta=tutti&gruppo=tutti&
livello=tutti&area4=tutti&classe=tutti&postcorso=tutti&isstella=0&
presiui=tutti&disaggregazione=&LANG=it&CONFIG=profilo.

A. Delgado and T. Slaats (Eds.): ICPM 2024 Workshops, LNBIP 533, pp. 142–153, 2025.
https://doi.org/10.1007/978-3-031-82225-4_11

Table 1. Percentage of early and late students for each academic year

Year	Early	Late
2010	0%	100%
2011	37.14%	62.86%
2012	35.71%	64.29%
2013	38.36%	61.64%
2014	47.54 %	52.46%
2015	40.00%	60.00%
2016	42.86%	57.14%
2017	50.60%	49.40%
2018	64.21%	35.79%
2019	69.23%	30.77%
2020	100%	0%

activities, to determine valuable insights on the curricula chosen by students. Previous studies show how these techniques can facilitate understanding behaviors that characterize students' academic performance, e.g., graduation times.

Our study showcases the application of these techniques to answer the following research question: "How does a student's exam-taking behavior in the first year impact their graduation performance¿' The "exam taking behaviour" consists of the sequences of activities modelling each exam's successful or unsuccessful taking. This task is inherently challenging due to the heterogeneity of the pathways followed by students, which stems from the lack of constraints in the examination process, as will be elaborated upon later in this paper. Nevertheless, our goal is to investigate whether there exists some regularities or patterns in the exam-taking behaviour among different students, which may provide a reliable estimate of whether a given student is likely to graduate on time or not. Identifying these behaviours is beneficial both to develop improvements in the overall study curricula and to spot-on students who are expected to struggle at an early stage of their career, to support them and mitigate the probabilities of graduation delays or dropping.

The rest of this manuscript is organized as follows. Section 2 describes the case study and the research design. Section 3 illustrates the obtained results. Section 4 provides an overview of relevant related work, while Sect. 5 draw some conclusions and delineates future work.

2   Study Design

2.1   Case Study: Bachelor Program of an Italian University

Our study focuses on a 3-year Bachelor's Degree program from an Italian university. The dataset comprises over 700 graduated students spanning 11 academic years (from 2010/2011 to 2020/2021). Table 1 reports the percentage of *early* students, i.e., students who took their degree within the standard duration of the degree programme, and *late* students who experienced one or more years of delays in their graduation. For the year 2010, we only have a small portion of students, all of whom graduated late. As for the students enrolled in 2020, since we have information up to 2023, we only have those who took less than three and a half years and, therefore, are considered early. While Table 1 shows a consistent improvement in students' performance over time, we observe that at least 30% of students graduated later than expected. As mentioned in Sect. 1, our analysis aims to assess the impact of students' exam-taking behaviors on their graduation performance. This question can be modeled in terms of a classification problem. Namely, we aim to develop a robust classifier that can learn the relation between a set of input features modeling different characteristics of students' exam-taking behaviors in the first year and a target variable corresponding to students' graduation performance. Note that we are interested in studying both the impact of students' overall performance (e.g., the average grades of passed exams) and the impact of *process-related* features, modeling the order in which exams have been taken by students. The latter enables the development of evidence-based recommendations on *when* students should strive to take one or more exams, as well as to identify which (combinations of) exam(s) have a critical impact on students' careers. Given the high variability of students' careers, we focus on extracting patterns (or subprocesses) modeling relevant combinations of exam-taking events.

Consequently, we identify the following sub-questions that must be addressed to answer the overarching one.

- **RQ1** Which common patterns in exam-taking behaviors arise from the students' career paths?
- **RQ2** How do exam-taking behaviors patterns in the first year affect students' graduation performance?

Dataset. We merged the information from two datasets that record the students' academic pathways to create the event log. In the first dataset, each row corresponds to an exam passed by a student, and the following information is provided: the student's identification code, the name of the exam, the date when the exam was passed, the grade obtained, the weight in CFU, and whether the exam is mandatory. The second dataset extends the information found in the first dataset by including unsuccessful exam attempts for each student together with reasons for not passing the exam, such as student absence, failure/withdrawal, or an insufficient mark. The resulting event log consists of one trace for each student, where each event tracks the outcome of an attempt for a specific exam, enriched with the corresponding attributes. To gain a better understanding of when activities are carried out w.r.t. the academic year, we have inserted in the log four artificial activities as a time reference to indicate the end of each semester and year: "End first semester", "End first year", "End third semester" and "End second year".

The next subsection delves into the methodology applied for each subquestion.

2.2 Methodology

RQ1: Extracting Exam-Taking Patterns. Several techniques have been proposed in the literature to extract process patterns from an event log. Our analysis employs the strategy devised by [10], since it considers the potential *concurrency* among process activities. They propose a pipeline where first, each sequential log trace is converted in a so-called *Instance Graph* (IG), which is a direct acyclic graph where each graph corresponds to an event in the trace and edges model dependency relation among the corresponding process activities. Then, they apply *subgraph mining* techniques to extract the most important subgraphs from the IG set which, in this setting, correspond to the most important process patterns.

We applied an ad-hoc procedure to build the IG set to reflect the concept of concurrency in our case study. From our discussions with stakeholders from the University, we derived the assumption that two different exams for which an attempt is made within one month can be considered concurrent, intended as exams that the student is preparing simultaneously.

In the following, we illustrate our procedure to build an IG for a trace in the event log, using the trace $\sigma = \langle start, A, B, efs, C_1, C_2, D, E, efy \rangle$ as an example. A, B, C, D, E correspond to an exam; C_1 and C_2 correspond to two attempts of taking the exam C, indicating that the exam has been failed the first time. The artificial activities have been marked as "start," "efs" (end first semester) and "efy" (end first year). First, we create one node for each exam and each artificial activity (Step 1 in Fig. 1). The colors in Fig. 1 (Step 1) illustrate the concurrency between the activities under the assumption previously introduced. To connect the nodes, we iterate through each pair of nodes, and we create an edge connecting them as follows:

a) If the pair contains at least one artificial activity, the pair is connected based on chronological order. In Fig. 1 (Step 2), "start," "efs," and "efy" are connected to every node.
b) If the pair does not contain artificial activities but the nodes are concurrent, no edges are added unless the pair represents two attempts for the same subject. For example, in Fig. 1, even though C_1 and C_2 were concurrent, they are not considered as such.
c) If the pair does not contain artificial activities and the nodes are not concurrent, edges are created based on chronological order.

Once the graph is created, we apply a transitive reduction to remove superfluous edges while maintaining reachability. In our example, edges removed by the transitive reduction are the dotted ones (Fig. 1 Step 3).

One the IG set has been created, we leverage the SUBDUE algorithm [15] to derive the most important subgraphs. SUBDUE iteratively analyzes the input

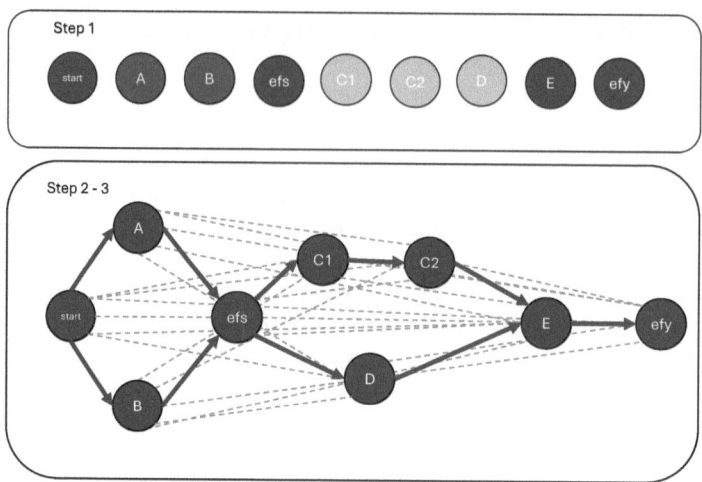

Fig. 1. Steps for Instance Graphs creation

graphs to extract at each step the subgraph that best compresses the graphs set. This subgraph is then used to compress the graph set by replacing each occurrence of the substructure with a single node. The compressed graphs are presented to SUBDUE again to repeat these steps until no more compression is possible. The algorithm returns a hierarchy of subgraphs with different levels of abstraction. Top-level subgraphs are defined only through elements belonging to input graphs (i.e., nodes and arcs). Lower-level subgraphs contains also upper-level subgraphs as nodes, defining a lattice structure. Descending the hierarchy, we pass from subgraphs that are very common in input graphs (i.e., frequently occurring, with a high support) to subgraphs specific of few input graphs (i.e., with low support). Since the top-level subgraphs are the most relevant, we used those for our analysis.

RQ2: Assessing the Impact of the Exam-Taking Patterns on Students' Graduation Performance. To evaluate the usefulness of subgraphs in predicting student performance, we first develop different predictive models using a set of variables extracted from the original event logs: **High school grade, First year mean grades, Consistency in votes, Exam passed first year, Credits given first year, Exams given first semester, Credits given first semester, Exams given second semester, Credits given second semester, Replayed fitness, Aligned fitness, Mean temporal interval between exams, Temporal consistency** and **First year failures**, which is the amount of times the student failed an exam in the first year. **Consistency in votes** and **Temporal consistency** correspond to the standard deviation of, respectively, the exam grades and the temporal intervals between consecutive exams.

The fitness measures presented earlier were calculated by implementing conformance checking with the first event log, which contains only exams passed, on the Petri net representing the ideal process model for the first year. This model

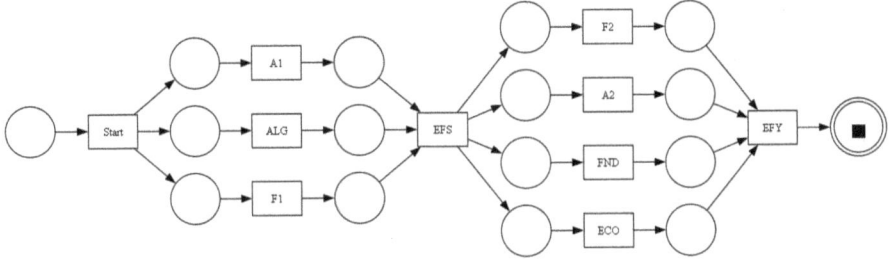

Fig. 2. Path definied by Univerity's manifesto

Table 2. Classification models and their corresponding parameters

Model	Parameters
SVM	'C', 'gamma', 'kernel'
Decision Tree	'criterion', 'splitter', 'max depth', 'min samples split', 'min samples leaf'
Random Forest	'n° estimators', 'criterion', 'max depth', 'min samples split', 'min samples leaf', 'bootstrap'
XGBOOST	'colsample bytree', 'learning rate', 'max depth', 'n estimators', 'subsample'

is considered the standard path defined by the university's manifesto, with the addition of "artificial" activities, as illustrated in Fig. 2. A value between 0 and 1 is assigned to each student based on their level of conformance to that ideal path.

All categorical variables were encoded through one-hot encoding, while the numerical variables were normalized using a standard scaler, that subtract to each value the mean and divide it by the standard deviation, transforming the data to have a mean of 0 and a standard deviation of 1. Four classifiers frequently mentioned in the literature were used for prediction: SVM, Decision Tree, Random Forest, and XGBoost. We used 70% of the dataset for the train set, and 30% for the test set.

For all classifiers and feature sets (i.e., without and with subgraphs), we performed hyperparameter tuning using Grid-Search with 5-fold cross-validation and maximizing accuracy. The parameters we combined for each model through grid search are shown in Table 2.

After finding the best hyperparameters, we evaluated the model on the test set. Due to the inherent randomness of Decision Tree, Random Forest, and XGBoost we trained these models 20 times using the same dataset and parameters while iterating the random seed every time. For these stochastic models, we evaluated 20 different values for accuracy to enhance the robustness of the results and then calculated the mean accuracy and the standard deviation of the accuracy. To evaluate performance, we considered accuracy because the two classes are balanced. After comparing the results of the models with all the sub-

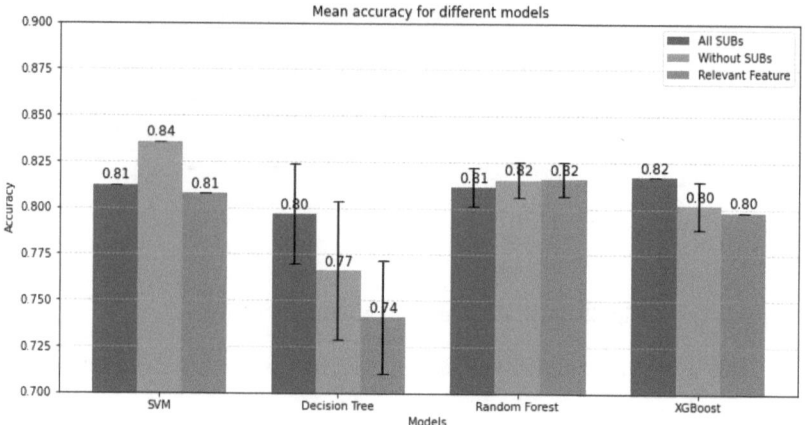

Fig. 3. Classification results

graphs and without them, we implemented a feature selection wrapper method for each model to identify the best set of features specific to each model and observe if the results improved.

Once we identified the best classifier, we employed Explainable AI (XAI) techniques to elucidate which features had the most significant impact among those used in our model. In particular, we employed SHAP (Shapley Additive exPlanations) [17], a widely used XAI technique based on game theory that uses Shapley values to fairly distribute the "credit" for a model's prediction among its input features.

3   Results

This section discusses the results of our study. First, we compare the results obtained with and without including the exam-taking patterns. Then, we show results obtained applying wrapper methods for each classifier. Finally, we discuss the importance of different features obtained with SHAP.

3.1   Impact of Exam-Taking Patterns on Classification Performance

First, we made predictions using a feature set composed only of the initial variables listed in Sect. 2.2. The results, in terms of accuracy for each classifier, are represented by the orange bars in Fig. 3. The most performant classifier is the SVM, which is also the most consistent with respect to the varying seed.

The blue bars show the accuracy obtained when all the exam-taking patterns are considered. Overall, including the patterns lead to the same or worse classification performance. This is possibly due to the increase in dataset features and, therefore, the sparsity of the obtained data.

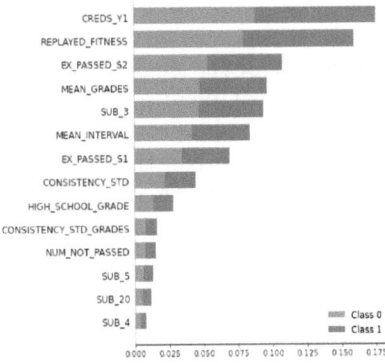

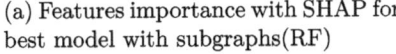

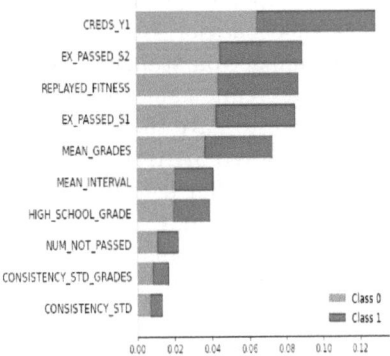

(a) Features importance with SHAP for best model with subgraphs(RF)

(b) Features importance with SHAP for the best overall model (SVM)

Fig. 4. Features importance with SHAP

After comparing the results of the classifiers with and without subgraphs, we proceed to calculate the accuracy using only the relevant features. These features are identified for each classifier based on wrapper methods of feature selection specific to each classifier. The results are presented in Fig. 3, in green. The SVM performs similarly to the situation with all subgraphs, thus also lower than the case without subgraphs. The decision tree keeps obtaining the worst performance, with a low average accuracy and high variability. The random forest remains the best among the stochastic models, with a stable average accuracy across all three scenarios and a much lower variability compared to the decision tree. Finally, XGBoost's performance remains similar to the situation where the dataset contains only the initial variables, and consequently, it is inferior compared to when we also consider all subgraphs.

3.2 Importance of Subgraphs

The results show that the model that best predicts student performance based on first-year information is the SVM, which considers only the initial variables. Although other models improve their accuracy by utilizing student behavior patterns, the results do not provide evidence supporting the usefulness of these features in the predictive model.

To delve deeper into the relation between the occurrence of the extracted subgraphs and the student's performance, we applied SHAP to the Random Forest model since it is the best-performing model when subgraphs are considered. The results are illustrated in Fig. 4a.

After selecting the best features for the Random Forest, only 4 of the 18 subgraphs features were retained. In Fig. 4a, we can see that only SUB_3 significantly impacted the model's output. This subgraph represents the absence of exam attempts in the first semester, which is reasonable to consider important as it indicates a total lack of engagement, thereby predicting a negative outcome due to this behavior. However, no other exam-taking patterns have shown a significant impact on students' performance. Instead, the figure suggests that the amount of credits gained during the first year and the compliance with the student manifesto have the strongest impact on students' graduation performance.

We employed SHAP to highlight the impact of the features for the best overall model as well, that is the SVM when subgraphs are not considered. The results depicted in the Fig. 4b indicate that the most impactful features are similar to those previously highlighted for the random forest when considering subgraphs. The credits earned in the first year remain the most important feature, significantly outpacing the second feature, which is no longer replayed fitness but rather the exams passed in the second semester.

Discussion. The results show that the exam-taking process does not demonstrate a predictive capacity that confirms its usefulness. This may be due to several factors. The first factor concerns the variability in student behavior. Each student can choose which exams to take, the order to take them, and how many times to retake them. This results in the creation of behavior patterns that pertain to a small number of students, compared to the total population. Another factor is that the common behaviors analyzed are only the "root" subgraphs, meaning they are the subgraphs that do not contain other subgraphs. Consequently, some potentially relevant behaviors were not considered in our analysis. Nevertheless, our analysis was able to derive robust and well-performing classifiers leveraging aggregated indicators of students' behaviors, such as the total number of credits earned in the first year, the level of conformity with the standard path, the grade point average, and so on. Such classifiers can be used to spot students' in need of help early in their careers, when there is still time to intervene and support them to improve their performance.

4   Related Work

Educational Data Mining (EDM) is an emerging discipline that aims to understand and improve students' learning process [19,22]. Our work is mainly related to EDM approaches that analyze students' academic performance and their failure. A popular trend in this respect consists in modeling students according to predefined features and applying machine learning to predict student's performance [9,11–13,16,23]. Many of these studies provide a perspective complementary to the one provided by our analysis, taking into account factors external to the graduation process itself. Even studies centered on the graduation process usually perform a data-oriented analysis, in which students' behaviors are encoded in terms of features without considering the study program's underlying structure. In this respect, our work is similar to the one in [8], which proposes to model and analyze students' careers. They introduce the notion of *ideal career* that corresponds to the career of a graduated student who took each exam just after the end of the corresponding course. Different metrics are used to measure the distance between each student's career and the ideal one (e.g., the Bubblesort distance). Compared to our approach, the work in [8] does not exploit the potentialities of process-based analysis in modeling students' behaviors. In particular, they do not infer any model representing the overall students' behaviors. In contrast, we exploit process formalisms to model the manifesto of study programs that explicitly accounts for parallelisms, thus allowing us to obtain a more accurate evaluation of the difference between single careers and the ideal path.

The application of process mining techniques to educational data, referred to as *Educational Process Mining* (EPM) [4], is a subject that has been recently gaining increasing interest. EPM has been applied to deal with different educational problems, such as on-line learning environments [5,18,25], computer-supported collaborative learning tools [3,21], professional training [2,6]. However, only a few works investigated the applications of EPM to curriculum mining. [24] propose a set of patterns modeling typical constraints of academic curricula and use these patterns to analyze the graduation process. However unlike the present work, they do not infer the process model representing students' careers and do not focus on delay analysis. Our approach is similar to [14], in analyzing the exam-taking process and program study compliance. However, [14] do not consider differences between early and late students.

In [1], authors apply process mining techniques to analyze event log data generated within educational information systems, with the purpose of understanding students' behavior during online learning. The work differs from ours in two main ways: (i) it is based on the concept of digital twin for the representation of students' activities and (ii) its focus is on the single course while ours is on the entire career. To the best of our knowledge, [7,20] are the only work considering the entire student's career. The former applies process discovery techniques to curriculum event logs with the purpose of characterizing behaviors of students that performed best/worst in terms of years required to complete the graduation process and final grade. The latter shifts the focus to classes of early and late students, similar to our study. However, they did not consider the potential impact of exam-taking patterns on students' performance in their analysis.

5 Conclusion and Future Works

This study focused on the analysis of the students' behaviors during their first year. The goal was to determine if and how these behaviors influenced graduation times. Our results show the feasibility of leveraging these properties to estimate students' performance early during their careers, though the extracted exam-taking pattern behaviors did not show a significant impact on the classification performance. These results call for additional research on the subject. In future work, first we intend to investigate the use of alternative process pattern discovery techniques, as the kind of extracted patterns are likely to have a strong influence on their predictive capabilities. Furthermore, we aim to explore how to transform the insights gained from this analysis into practical recommendations. These recommendations will help students identify the best career paths at various stages, considering their current progress.

References

1. Azeta, A., Agono, F., Adesola, F., Nwaocha, V., Tjiraso, S.: A process mining framework for analysing students' behaviours using digital twin (2022). Available at SSRN 4331450
2. Bergenthum, R., Desel, J., Harrer, A., Mauser, S.: Learnflow mining. In: DeLFI 2008: Die 6. e-Learning Fachtagung Informatik, pp. 269–280. Gesellschaft für Informatik eV (2008)
3. Bergenthum, R., Desel, J., Harrer, A., Mauser, S.: Modeling and mining of learnflows. In: Transactions on Petri Nets and Other Models of Concurrency V, pp. 22–50. Springer (2012)
4. Bogarín, A., Cerezo, R., Romero, C.: A survey on educational process mining. Wiley Interdisc. Rev. Data Min. Knowl. Discov. **8**(1), e1230 (2018)
5. Bogarín, A., Romero, C., Cerezo, R., Sánchez-Santillán, M.: Clustering for improving educational process mining. In: Proceedings of International Conference on Learning Analytics and Knowledge, pp. 11–15. ACM (2014)
6. Cairns, A.H., Gueni, B., Assu, J., Joubert, C., Khelifa, N.: Analyzing and improving educational process models using process mining techniques. In: Proceedings of International Conference on Advances in Information Mining Management, pp. 17–22 (2015)
7. Cameranesi, M., Diamantini, C., Genga, L., Potena, D.: Students' careers analysis: a process mining approach. In: Proceedings of International Conference on Web Intelligence, Mining and Semantics, p. 26. ACM (2017)
8. Campagni, R., Merlini, D., Sprugnoli, R., Verri, M.C.: Data mining models for student careers. Expert Syst. Appl. **42**(13), 5508–5521 (2015)
9. Dekker, G.W., Pechenizkiy, M., Vleeshouwers, J.M.: Predicting students drop out: a case study. Int. Working Group Educ. Data Min. (2009)
10. Diamantini, C., Genga, L., Potena, D.: Behavioral process mining for unstructured processes. J. Intell. Inf. Syst. **47**(1), 5–32 (2016). https://doi.org/10.1007/s10844-016-0394-7
11. Gowda, S.M., Baker, R.S.J.D., Pardos, Z., Heffernan, N.T.: The sum is greater than the parts: Ensembling student knowledge models in assistments. In: Proceedings of KDD Workshop on Knowledge Discovery in Educational Data (2011)
12. Guruler, H., Istanbullu, A., Karahasan, M.: A new student performance analysing system using knowledge discovery in higher educational databases. Comput. Educ. **55**(1), 247–254 (2010)
13. Herzog, S.: Measuring determinants of student return vs. dropout/stopout vs. transfer: a first-to-second year analysis of new freshmen. Res. High. Educ. **46**(8), 883–928 (2005)
14. Hobeck, R., Pufahl, L., Weber, I.: Process mining on curriculum-based study data: a case study at a German university. In: International Conference on Process Mining, pp. 577–589. Springer (2022)
15. Jonyer, I., Cook, D.J., Holder, L.B.: Graph-based hierarchical conceptual clustering. J. Mach. Learn. Res. **2**(Oct), 19–43 (2001)

16. Why do higher education students drop out? Evid. Spain. Educ. Econ. **16**(1), 89–105 (2008)

17. Lundberg, S.M., Lee, S.I.: A unified approach to interpreting model predictions. In: Advances in Neural Information Processing Systems, pp. 4766–4775 (2017)

18. Mukala, P., Buijs, J.C.A.M., Leemans, M., van der Aalst, W.: Learning analytics on coursera event data: a process mining approach. In: Proceedings of International Symposium on Data-Driven Process Discovery and Analysis, pp. 18–32 (2015)

19. Peña-Ayala, A.: Educational data mining: a survey and a data mining-based analysis of recent works. Expert Syst. Appl. **41**(4), 1432–1462 (2014)

20. Potena, D., Genga, L., Basta, A., Mercati, C., Diamantini, C.: Evidence-based student career and performance analysis with process mining: a case study. In: International Conference on Process Mining, pp. 349–360. Springer (2023)

21. Reimann, P., Frerejean, J., Thompson, K.: Using process mining to identify models of group decision making in chat data. In: Proceedings of International Conference on Computer Supported Collaborative Learning, pp. 98–107. International Society of the Learning Sciences (2009)

22. Romero, C., Ventura, S.: Educational data mining: a survey from 1995 to 2005. Expert Syst. Appl. **33**(1), 135–146 (2007)

23. Romero, C., Ventura, S., Espejo, P.G., Hervás, C.: Data mining algorithms to classify students. In: Proceedings of International Conference on Educational Data Mining, pp. 8–17 (2008). www.educationaldatamining.org

24. Trcka, N., Pechenizkiy, M.: From local patterns to global models: towards domain driven educational process mining. In: Proceedings of International Conference on Intelligent Systems Design and Applications, pp. 1114–1119. IEEE (2009)

25. Vidal, J.C., Vázquez-Barreiros, B., Lama, M., Mucientes, M.: Recompiling learning processes from event logs. Knowl. Based Syst. **100**, 160–174 (2016)

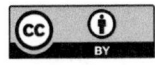

Evaluation of Study Plans Using Partial Orders

Christian Rennert$^{(\boxtimes)}$, Mahsa Pourbafrani , and Wil van der Aalst

Chair of Process and Data Science (PADS), RWTH Aachen University,
Aachen, Germany
{rennert,mahsa.pourbafrani,wvdaalst}@pads.rwth-aachen.de

Abstract. In higher education, data is collected that indicate the
term(s) that a course is taken and when it is passed. Often, study plans
propose a suggested course order to students. Study planners can adjust
these based on detected deviations between the proposed and actual
order of the courses being taken. In this work, we detect deviations by
combining (1) the deviation between the proposed and actual course
order with (2) the temporal difference between the expected and actual
course-taking term(s). Partially ordered alignments identify the deviations between the proposed and actual order. We compute a partial order
alignment by modeling a study plan as a process model and a student's
course-taking behavior as a partial order. Using partial orders in such
use cases allows one to relax the constraints of strictly ordered traces.
This makes our approach less prone to the order in which courses are
offered. Further, when modeling course-taking behavior as partial orders,
we propose distinguishing intended course-taking behavior from actual
course-passing behavior of students by including either all terms in which
a course is attempted or only the term that a course is passed, respectively. This provides more perspectives when comparing the proposed
and actual course-taking behavior. The proposed deviation measuring
approach is evaluated on real-life data from RWTH Aachen University.

Keywords: Educational Process Mining · Conformance Checking ·
Event Data · Partial Order · Campus Management System

1 Introduction

In Germany, universities must provide students with the knowledge, skills,
and methods required for their subjects.[1] Furthermore, regulations state that
(1) every degree program must offer a study plan completable within the degree's
standard duration, and (2) universities must create individual study plans for
students if required.[2] In this work, a study plan comprises several courses whose

---

[1] In Germany, states regulate higher education. For example, North Rhine-Westphalia
defines the purpose of study plans in §58 (1) Hochschulgesetz (HG) NRW.
[2] According to §58 (3) Hochschulgesetz (HG) NRW.

A. Delgado and T. Slaats (Eds.): ICPM 2024 Workshops, LNBIP 533, pp. 154–166, 2025.
https://doi.org/10.1007/978-3-031-82225-4_12

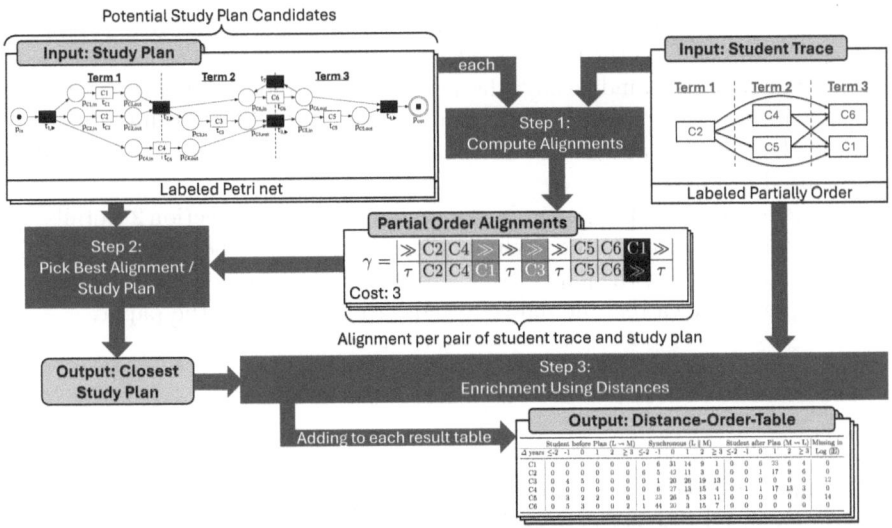

Fig. 1. Framework for the evaluation of study plans using partial orders.

completion is assessed by examination activities. Here, only the passing of final exams is considered as such activities, although this is not a general restriction.

Across all study programs offered in 2022 in Germany, nearly 247,000 students received their bachelor's degree[3]. First-time graduates received their degree on average after around 4 years of studies[4]. However, the standard period of study for bachelor's degree courses in Germany is three years. This indicates an average extension of studies by around one year in 2022.

In [8], potential reasons for an individual to extend the duration of their study are categorized. In detail, they identify (1) study conditions, (2) individual characteristics and entry requirements, and (3) personal living conditions and context factors as categories of reasons. Although there are many reasons for an extended study duration, if possible, study planners should implement measurements to avoid an extended study duration. Therefore, a systematic analysis of student data and study plans helps identify and improve study plan shortcomings such that study conditions are improved.

One approach is to use process mining to understand students' interactions with their study plan. In detail, we model study plans as process models and store exam data in event logs to allow for systematic analysis.

The complete approach presented in this work is the following. Workflow nets are used to model all study plans for a given time period, as there may be multiple study plans available due to changes applied to a degree over time. Partial orders are used to model the student's course-taking order. Both are compared using partial order alignments. The alignment with the lowest cost is

---

[3] https://www.statista.com/statistics/584454/bachelor-and-master-degrees-number-universities-germany/, 2024, last access 2024-07-05.

[4] https://www.statista.com/statistics/584277/average-study-duration-graduates-germany/, 2023, last access 2024-07-05.

then identified. For its study plan and all its courses, we aggregate counts for each combination of (1) the course's relative position between the log and model parts of the alignment, indicating whether a course is moved forward, backward, or if it is in the right position in the study plan, and (2) the absolute difference between the expected and actual terms that the course is taken. This procedure is visualized in Fig. 1.

The remainder of this paper is structured as follows. Section 2 details the related work, Sect. 3 gives the preliminaries for this work, Sect. 4 describes the approach introduced in the paper, Sect. 5 evaluates the results obtained by applying the approach to a real-life dataset, and Sect. 6 concludes the paper.

2   Related Work

Process mining in the context of education, also known as Educational Process Mining (EPM), is the subject of several papers. An extensive survey by Bogarín et al. [4] discusses educational process mining as an educational data mining (EDM) technique. Here, the authors show that there are some works using conformance checking techniques to identify the agreement between students' exam histories as event traces and their study plans as process models. Alternatively, the authors in [4] also discuss that conformance checking can be applied using rule modeling for expected student behavior, which is another conformance checking technique not investigated in this paper. For more details on EPM, we refer to the survey in [4]. We limit our scope to works that target the course-taking process of students and their interactions with the study plan.

Hobeck et al. [6] apply process mining and in particular the PM^2 methodology on exam data from the university information system of the TU Berlin. For a group of students, the authors investigate the question of whether students follow their study plan by comparing its conformance with the full student's exam history. In the work of Bendatu and Yahya [3], they also compare exam histories with a single study plan by computing the temporal distance between the expected and actual point in time when an exam is taken. We use the general idea and extend the study plan to allow for several expected terms.

In [5], Diamantini et al. model study plans as blocks of exams to be taken to compare the ordering of exams in the student's exam history and in the study plan. They use their approach to understand bottlenecks and to make a distinction between successful and non-successful students. Similar to abstracting study plans into course blocks, some works model student exam histories as blocks, using a set abstraction per term. In [9], Priyambada et al. use this approach to compare and cluster students by detecting course patterns for the relative term course sets. In [10], Rafiei et al. exploit atomic ordering and educational KPI information in exam data to derive labels for rule extraction with the aim to assist study planners. In their work, they derived partial orders by considering DFGs to directly represent a partial order.

Usually in process mining, the ordering based on timestamps between events and a suggested ordering of activities in process models can be compared using alignments as first introduced by Adriansyah [2]. Later, in [7], Lu et al. extended alignments to also be applicable for partial orders. Nevertheless, so far no existing work incorporates partial order alignments in its research or case study. Therefore, this is among the first works to incorporate partial orders.

In the following section, we discuss the preliminaries of this work.

3 Preliminaries

Basic Notations. A *multiset* generalizes the concept of a set and allows for multiple occurrences of the same element, e.g., $[x, y, y, x, x, z]$ $= [x^3, y^2, z]$. The set of all multisets over a set X is $\mathbb{M}(X)$. Similarly to a multiset, a *sequence* can contain multiple occurrences of the same element. However, within a sequence, all elements are *totally ordered*, e.g., $\sigma = \langle x, y, y, x, z \rangle$ is a sequence over the set $X = \{x, y, z\}$ and thus it is in its *Kleene closure* X^*, i.e., $\sigma \in X^*$. Given a sequence σ and a value $i \in \mathbb{N}$ with $1 \leq i \leq |\sigma|$, we denote by $\sigma(i)$ the element at the i-th position of the sequence σ, e.g., for $\sigma = \langle x, y, z \rangle$ it holds that $\sigma(3) = z$. Given an

Table 1. Example educational event log L_1.

Student	Course	Term	State
S1	C2	1	1
S2	C1	2	1
S1	C4	2	1
S2	C4	2	0
S2	C4	2	1
S1	C5	2	1
S1	C6	3	1
S1	C1	3	1

n-tuple $(a_1, a_2, \ldots, a_n)$, we define π_i to be the selector function that returns the i-th entry, e.g., $\pi_2((a, b, c)) = b$. We define that applying a single element function $f : X \rightarrow Y$ to a sequence $\sigma \in X^*$, applies the function f to each element in the sequence, i.e., $f(\sigma) = \langle f(x) \mid x \in \sigma \rangle$. The domain of a function f is described by $dom(f)$, e.g., $dom(f) = \{1, 2, 3\}$ for $f(1) = 4$, $f(2) = 5$, and $f(3) = 3$.

Educational Event Log. In process mining, *event data* are used to observe and keep track of *behavior*. In our use case, an event exists for each exam try of a student. Therefore, we first introduce the universe of student matriculation numbers $\mathcal{U}_{Mat}$ and the universe of course IDs $\mathcal{U}_{cid}$. An event $e \in \mathcal{U}_{Mat} \times \mathcal{U}_{cid} \times \mathbb{N} \times \{0, 1\}$ is a quadruple of a student's matriculation number, a course ID of a taken course, a natural representing the term in which the event occurred relative to the start of the student's studies, and a state indicating whether the exam attempt is passed (1) or failed (0). We may also refer to the matriculation number as student ID. The universe of events is denoted by $\mathcal{U}_e$. An example of an event is $e_1 = (S2, C4, 2, 1) \in \mathcal{U}_e$ which shows that the course C4 is passed by the student S2 in its second term of studies. An event log $L \in \mathbb{M}(\mathcal{U}_e)$ is a multiset of events, as there can be several exam attempts within a term.

Given an event e, for better readability, we define $\pi_{mat}(e) = \pi_1(e)$, $\pi_{cid}(e) = \pi_2(e)$, $\pi_{term}(e) = \pi_3(e)$, and $\pi_{pass}(e) = \pi_4(e)$, e.g., $\pi_{cid}(e_1) = $ C4. In this work, we restrict each educational event log L to only contain courses that are eventually passed, i.e., $\forall_{e \in L} \exists_{e' \in L} : ((\pi_{cid}(e) = \pi_{cid}(e')) \wedge (\pi_{pass}(e') = 1))$. An example of an educational event log L_1 is given in Table 1 where $e_1 \in L_1$ holds.

Partial Orders. We use *partial orders* to model temporal relations between student events, these are used because multiple events an occur for the same term and we do not consider the order within a term. In detail, labeled partial orders are used, as we may have to model students who took several courses with

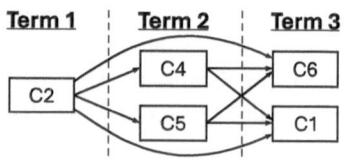

Fig. 2. Labeled partial order lpo_{S1} of passed courses for the student with student ID S1.

the same course ID. This might be the case for a student that is required to take distinct seminars with the same course ID. A labeled partial order *lpo* is a quadruple $lpo = (V, \prec, A, l)$ where V is a set of nodes, $\prec$ is a partial order relation, A is a set of activities, and $l: V \to A$ is a labeling function. Figure 2 shows the labeled partial order for the student with Student ID S1 from event log L_1. The next section describes how to derive labeled partial orders from an event log. First, we introduce labeled Petri nets as process models so that we can model study plans.

Petri and Workflow Nets. A *labeled Petri net* N is a quintuple $N = (P, T, F, A, l)$, where P is a finite set of *places*, T is a finite set of *transitions* such that $P \cap T = \emptyset$, $F \subseteq (P \times T) \cup (T \times P)$ is a set of directed arcs, the so-called *flow relation*, A is a set of activities, and $l: T \to A \cup \{\tau\}$ is a *labeling function* with $\tau \notin A$ being a reserved silent activity label corresponding to no activity being performed.

A *workflow net* is a labeled Petri net $N = (P, T, F, A, l)$ for which there is exactly one input place $in \in P$ such that $\{(p, in) \in F \mid p \in P\} = \emptyset$, one output place $out \in P$ such that $\{(out, p) \in F \mid p \in P\} = \emptyset$, and for which modifying it to be short-circuited makes it strongly connected. An example workflow net is shown in Fig. 3. For more details on Petri nets as process models and their semantics, we refer to [1]. Workflow nets and labeled partial orders describing observed behavior can be checked for conformance using alignments.

Alignments. A partial order alignment $\gamma(lpo, N)$ relates the behavior described by a labeled partial order *lpo* with the behavior of a workflow net N. Therefore, an alignment consists of several moves that distinguish whether the behaviors agree and are in synchronization or whether they disagree and deviate. In detail, we distinguish the following four move types. (1) *Synchronous moves* (lightgray) indicate no deviation, (2) *log moves* (black) indicate a deviation such that a move was taken on the log side but not on the model side, (3) *model moves* (gray) indicate a deviation such that a move was taken on the log side but not on the model side, and (4) *invisible model moves* indicated by τ specify that a not observable model move is taken and that a misalignment on the log side is not required. In a deviation, the misalignment is denoted by "$\gg$", to indicate that either the log or the model does not have any matching behavior.

An alignment that best matches the model and partial order is the so-called *optimal alignment* because it has a minimal number of mismatches. In Table 2,

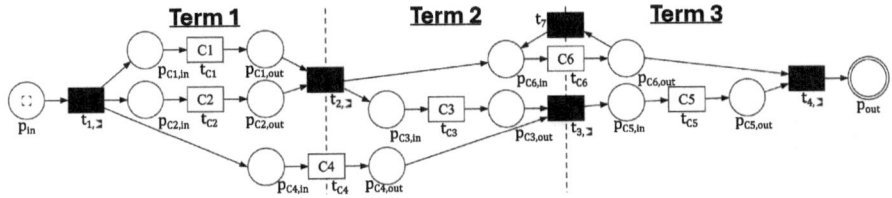

Fig. 3. Example workflow net N_1.

an optimal alignment $\gamma(lpo_{S1}, N_1) = \langle (\gg, \tau), (C2, C2), \ldots, (\gg, \tau) \rangle$ between the labeled partial order lpo_{S1} and the workflow net $N1$ is given. The optimal alignment $\gamma(lpo_{S1}, N_1)$ has three misalignments, i.e., one log and two model moves. The upper row indicates the log behavior, while the lower row indicates the model behavior. For an alignment γ, we define $\gamma_L = \pi_1(\gamma)$ and $\gamma_M = \pi_2(\gamma)$, e.g., $\gamma_L(lpo_{S1}, N_1) = \langle \gg, C2, C4, \gg, \gg, \gg, \gg, C5, C6, C1, \gg \rangle$ and $\gamma_M(lpo_{S1}, N_1) = \langle \tau, C2, C4, C1, \tau, C3, \tau, C5, C6, \gg, \tau \rangle$ for the behavior on the log and model side, respectively. We can now consider the impact of using labeled partial orders instead of ordering courses within a term. Consider a labeled partial order lpo'_{S1} that requires $C4$ and $C6$ to always occur before $C5$ and $C1$, respectively, although events $(S1, C4, 2, 1)$ together with $(S1, C5, 2, 1)$ and $(S1, C6, 3, 1)$ together with $(S1, C1, 3, 1)$ each have the same term, which otherwise indicates no strict ordering. Computing an optimal alignment $\gamma(lpo'_{S1}, N_1)$, as shown in Table 3, between lpo'_{S1} and N_1 results in a worse alignment than the alignment $\gamma(lpo_{S1}, N_1)$, since its cost is higher by a value of two. Therefore, abstracting course orderings within the same term affects alignment computation. For details on the computation of partial order alignments, we refer to [7].

Table 2. An optimal alignment $\gamma(lpo_{S1}, N_1)$ for lpo_{S1} and N_1.

Table 3. An optimal alignment $\gamma(lpo'_{S1}, N_1)$ for lpo'_{S1} and N_1.

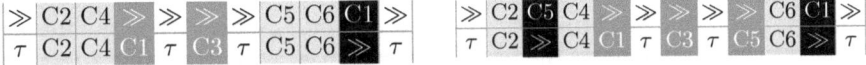

4 Approach

Study Plan. For each degree program, study planners provide a study plan. It organizes the degree program into terms, stating when each course should be taken. In addition, it differentiates between mandatory courses, required to complete a degree program, and elective courses, of which only a subset must be taken. We take electives into account by mapping all elective course IDs to a reserved placeholder elective course ID $C_{el} \notin \mathcal{U}_{cid}$. A study plan process model should allow for the elective course ID C_{el} to reoccur multiple times, modeling an unknown number of electives to be taken by an individual student. Formally, we define a study plan SP as $SP: (\mathcal{U}_{cid} \cup \{C_{el}\}) \to \mathbb{N} \times \mathbb{N}$ mapping a course

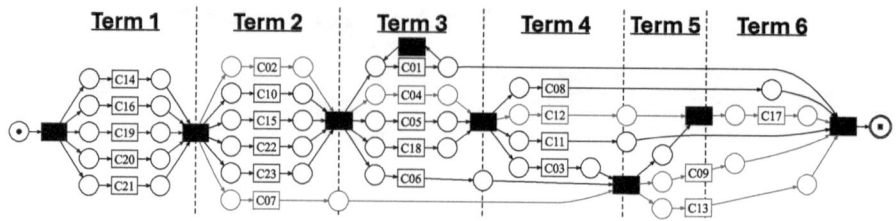

Fig. 4. Workflow net N_{10} from the study plan SP_{10}.

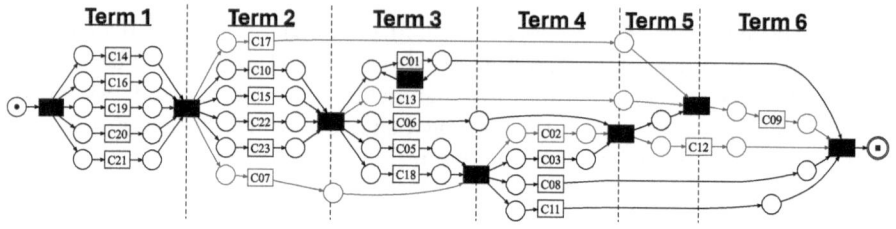

Fig. 5. Workflow net N_{18} from the study plan SP_{18}.

ID $cid \in (\mathcal{U}_{cid} \cup \{C_{el}\})$ to its first expected term T_{start} and its last expected term T_{end}, i.e., $SP(cid) = (T_{start}, T_{end})$. Next, we create a workflow net from a study plan to compute labeled partial orders.

Study Plan to Workflow Net. A workflow net $N_{SP} = (P, T, F, A, l)$ is constructed from a study plan SP as follows. **Introducing term start and end synchronizing silent transitions:** For each term $term \in \mathbb{N}$ with $1 \leq term \leq k$ contained in the study plan SP, with $k = max(\{\pi_2(SP(cid)) \mid cid \in dom(SP)\})$ being the highest term where max is the maximum function, we add a silent transition $t_{(term, \blacktriangleright)}$ with $l(t_{(term, \blacktriangleright)}) = \tau$ starting each term. We define that each transition $t_{(term, \blacktriangleright)}$ starting a term $term$ is the transition $t_{((term-1), \blacktriangleright)}$ that closes the previous term, i.e., $\forall_{term \in [2,k]} : t_{((term-1), \blacksquare)} = t_{(term, \blacktriangleright)}$. Since there is a missing silent transition that closes the term k, we add $t_{(k, \blacksquare)}$ with $l(t_{(k, \blacksquare)}) = \tau$ to the set of transitions T. We connect the transition that starts the first term with the input place $in \in P$ and the transition that ends the last term with the output place $out \in P$, i.e., $\{(in, t_{(1, \blacktriangleright)}), (t_{(k, \blacksquare)}, out)\} \subseteq F$. **Adding and connecting course transitions:** The set of activities is identical to the set of course IDs contained in the study plan, i.e., $A = dom(SP)$. Finally, we add a transition t_{cid} with $l(t_{cid}) = cid$ for each $cid \in dom(SP)$ and connect them by their start and end term in the study plan, i.e., we add places $\{p_{(cid,in)}, p_{(cid,out)} \mid cid \in dom(SP)\} \subseteq P$ and arcs $\{(t_{(T_{start}, \blacktriangleright)}, p_{(cid,in)}), (p_{(cid,in)}, t_{cid}), (t_{cid}, p_{(cid,out)}), (p_{(cid,out)}, t_{(T_{end}, \blacksquare)}) \mid cid \in dom(SP) \wedge (T_{start}, T_{end}) = SP(cid)\} \subseteq F$. Additionally, we make the transition with the elective course ID $C_{el} \in dom(SP)$ repeatable, i.e., $\{(p_{(C_{el},out)}, t_{C_{el}}), (t_{C_{el}}, p_{(C_{el},in)})\} \subseteq F$, e.g., C01 in Fig. 4.

We obtained two study plans SP_{10} and SP_{18} from the 2010 and 2018 study regulations for the RWTH Aachen University Computer Science B.Sc. program. In Fig. 4 and Fig. 5, we show the workflow nets N_{10} and N_{18} constructed from the study plans SP_{10} and SP_{18}, respectively. We highlight transitions labeled with course IDs missing in either study plan or differing in start/end terms in both workflow nets, i.e., $\{t_{cid} \mid (cid \in ((dom(SP_{10}) \setminus dom(SP_{18})) \cup (dom(SP_{18}) \setminus dom(SP_{10}))) \vee (cid \in (dom(SP_{10}) \cup dom(SP_{18})) \wedge SP_{10}(cid) \neq SP_{18}(cid)))\}$. The reserved elective course ID is C01 in both workflow nets.

Deriving Labeled Partial Orders. Next, we introduce how to derive labeled partial orders from an event log L. We derive two types of labeled partial orders: life-cycle-aware and atomic. Life-cycle-aware modeling considers all exam attempts for a course ID, including failed attempts, while atomic modeling only considers the passed attempt. This allows us to differentiate between students' intended conformance in exam-taking behavior and their actual conformance based only on passed attempts.

Let $L \in \mathbb{M}(\mathcal{U}_e)$ be an event log and $mat \in \mathcal{U}_{Mat}$ be a student ID. The filtered event log L_{mat} of all exam attempts by a student with student ID mat is the multiset $L_{mat} = [e \in L \mid \pi_{Mat}(e) = mat]$. For each course ID $cid \in \{\pi_{cid}(e) \mid e \in L_{mat}\}$ in the student's event data, we calculate the start term $t_{\blacktriangleright}(L, mat, cid)$ and the end term $t_{\blacksquare}(L, mat, cid)$. The end term is the passing term, i.e., $t_{\blacksquare}(L, mat, cid) = \pi_{term}(e)$ with $e \in L_{mat} \wedge \pi_{cid}(e) = cid \wedge \pi_{pass}(e) = 1$. The start term differs between life-cycle-aware and atomic modeling: atomic modeling uses a single point in time, i.e., $t_{\blacktriangleright}(L, mat, cid) = t_{\blacksquare}(L, mat, cid)$, whereas life-cycle-aware modeling uses the term of the first exam attempt, i.e., $t_{\blacktriangleright}(L, mat, cid) = min(\{\pi_{term}(e) \mid e \in L_{mat} \wedge \pi_{cid}(e) = cid\})$ with min being the minimum function.

Let $N = (P, T, F, A, l)$ be a workflow net constructed from a study plan SP. A labeled partial order $lpo_{mat} = (V_{mat}, \prec_{mat}, A_{mat}, l_{mat})$ for a student ID $mat \in \mathcal{U}_{Mat}$ that agrees with the workflow net N is derived as follows. First, we ensure that the workflow net N and the labeled partial order lpo agree by sharing the same activities, i.e., $A_{mat} = A$. Next, we add a node $v_{mat,cid} \in V$ for each course ID $cid \in \{\pi_{cid}(e) \mid e \in L \wedge \pi_{mat}(e) = mat\}$ in the event log L_{mat}. During labeling, we differ between mandatory and elective courses, i.e., $\forall_{v_{cid} \in V}: l(v_{mat,cid}) = cid$ if $cid \in (A \setminus \{C_{el}\})$ and $l(v_{mat,cid}) = C_{el}$ otherwise. Any two partial order nodes $v_{mat,cid}, v_{mat,cid'} \in V$ share an edge if one course's start term $t_{\blacktriangleright}(L, mat, cid')$ follows another course's end term $t_{\blacksquare}(L, mat, cid)$, i.e., $\forall_{v_{mat,cid}, v_{mat,cid'} \in V}: (t_{\blacksquare}(L, mat, cid) < t_{\blacktriangleright}(L, mat, cid')) \Rightarrow ((v_{mat,cid}, v_{mat,cid'}) \in \prec)$. Next, we define a function to calculate term distances between the courses in the event log and their expected times in the study plan.

Term Distance. Let SP be a study plan, L an event log, mat a student ID, and cid a course ID. For better readability, we conclude (1) $exp(\blacktriangleright) = \pi_1(SP(cid))$ if $cid \in dom(SP)$ and $exp(\blacktriangleright) = \pi_1(SP(C_{el}))$ otherwise, and (2) $exp(\blacksquare) = \pi_2(SP(cid))$ if $cid \in dom(SP)$ and $exp(\blacksquare) = \pi_2(SP(C_{el}))$ otherwise, the expected start and end term in the study plan, respectively. The term $act = t_{\blacksquare}(L, mat, cid)$ is the actual term in which the student with the student ID mat passed a course. We define the distance function $\Delta_t(SP, L, mat, cid)$ as follows:

$$\Delta_t(SP, L, mat, cid) = \begin{cases} 0, & \text{if, } exp(\blacktriangleright) \leq act \leq exp(\blacksquare), & \text{(in time)} \\ act \text{ - } exp(\blacktriangleright), & \text{if, } act < exp(\blacktriangleright), \text{ and} & \text{(early)} \\ act \text{ - } exp(\blacksquare), & \text{if, } act > exp(\blacksquare). & \text{(late)} \end{cases}$$

Thus, the distance function $\Delta_t(SP, L, mat, cid)$ indicates if a course was taken on time, early, or late, showing the distance to the expected start or end term(s). In our example, we know that all terms are semesters in the study plans and in the event log. Thus, we simplify the distance function to a year distance $\Delta_y(SP, L, mat, cid) = \left\lceil \frac{\Delta_t(SP,L,mat,cid)}{2} \right\rceil$, summarizing two terms as up to one year. Next, we align each course ID in the study plan and the labeled partial orders by their relative positions. Both are combined later to derive insights.

Alignment Order Relation. Let $\gamma(lpo, N)$ be a partial order alignment between a labeled partial order $lpo = (V, \prec, A', l')$ and a workflow net $N = (P, T, F, A, l)$. By construction, all activities in the labeled partial order lpo are contained in the workflow net N, i.e., $A' \subseteq A$, and each workflow net activity occurs at least once on the model side γ_M of the alignment γ. Thus, for each activity, or more precise course ID $cid \in \mathcal{U}_{cid}$, on the log side γ_L, we can determine its position relative to its position on the model side γ_M of the partial order alignment γ.

We distinguish four cases: (1) A course ID occurs at the same position in the alignment and therefore the student's behavior and the study plan are aligned ($L \parallel_{cid} M$). (2) A course ID occurs first on the log side then on the model side, indicating that the course is moved forward compared to the study plan ($L \leadsto_{cid} M$). (3) A course ID occurs first on the model side and then on the log side, indicating that the course is moved back compared to the study plan ($M \leadsto_{cid} L$). (4) A missing entry on the log side ($\mathbb{Z}_{cid}$).

Formally, for $i \in [1, |\gamma|]$ a position in the alignment where the i-th entry on the model side is a course ID $cid \in \mathcal{U}_{cid}$, i.e., $\gamma_M(i) = cid$, we define:

- $L \parallel_{cid} M,$ if $\gamma_L(i) = cid,$ (Synchronous)
- $L \leadsto_{cid} M,$ if $\exists_{j \in [1, i-1]} : \gamma_L(j) = cid,$ (Student before Plan)
- $M \leadsto_{cid} L,$ if $\exists_{j \in [i+1, |\gamma|]} : \gamma_L(j) = cid,$ and   (Student after Plan)
- $\mathbb{Z}_{cid},$ if $\forall_{j \in [1, |\gamma|]} : \gamma_L(j) \neq cid.$ (Missing in Log)

Next, we apply our approach to a real-life data set to demonstrate its applicability and gain insights.

5   Evaluation

We conducted the evaluation using PM4Py[5], an open-source Python library for process mining. For evaluation, we used a real-life data from three German universities collaborating in the BMBF-funded joint research project "AIStudy-Buddy". As part of the project, two software tools are being developed to assist

---

[5] https://github.com/pm4py/pm4py-core.

students in organizing their studies and study planners in analyzing study programs. The data includes 1,162 RWTH Aachen University Computer Science Bachelor's graduates who began earliest in 2010 and have at least 150 ECTS. As mentioned in Sect. 4, in Fig. 4 and Fig. 5 the corresponding plans for 2010 and 2018 are modeled as workflow nets N_{10} and N_{18}. For each student from the event log, a labeled partial order is created using the life-cycle-aware and atomic approach. The code for modeling study plans and translating educational event logs is publicly available on GitLab[6]. In addition, the published code includes mock student data and the two study plans used in this work. We computed alignments for both workflow nets using both, the atomic or life-cycle-aware labeled partial orders, and selected the study plan with the lower alignment cost for further result aggregation. We determined the expected study plan based on whether a student started before or from 2018 onward. Table 4 shows a confusion matrix for the expected and the most conforming study plan.

Of the 860 students, 237, or around 27.5%, expected to follow the 2010 study plan conform most to the 2018 plan. In contrast, only a fraction of around 13.2% of those expected to follow the 2018 plan conform most to the 2010 plan. An explanation may be that in an educational setting, students may adopt to a new study plan within their studies. It is to note, that the confusion matrix does not alter between the life-cycle-aware and atomic partial order modeling approach.

Table 4. Confusion matrix between expected study plans and most conforming study plans.

		Most conforming		
		2010	2018	Σ
Expected	2010	623	237	860
	2018	40	262	302
	Σ	663	499	1162

The alignment of the most conforming study plan is used to compute the alignment order relation and year distance for each course. We count the frequency of each combination for the two study plans. Tables 5 and 6 show the results for both study plans, respectively. Complete and further tables are available on Gitlab[7], showing all distances in terms and years and all courses being included as both life-cycle-aware and atomic. Although present, the difference between atomic and life-cycle-based modeling is marginal in our results. However, we expect that this may vary when future experiments are applied, and therefore requires further investigation. In the following, we focus only on life-cycle-aware modeling.

Next, we analyze the results to derive some potentially interesting insights for study planners. We select representatives from two groups of courses represented in both the 2010 and 2018 study plans: (1) Courses moved in the 2018 study plan compared to 2010, i.e., courses with course IDs C12, C13, and C17, and (2) courses not moved between the 2010 and 2018 study plans, i.e., courses with course IDs C05, C16, and C18.

---

[6] https://git.rwth-aachen.de/christian.rennert/po-based-SP-eval.
[7] See Footnote 6.

Table 5. Distance in years for the 2010 study plan and life-cycle-aware student courses.

Δ years	Student before Plan ($L \leadsto_{cid} M$)						Synchronous ($L \parallel_{cid} M$)						Student after Plan ($M \leadsto_{cid} L$)						Missing in Log ($\mathbb{L}_{cid}$)
	≤-2	-1	0	1	2	≥3	≤-2	-1	0	1	2	≥3	≤-2	-1	0	1	2	≥3	
C05	0	9	29	1	1	0	1	2	570	27	5	2	0	0	0	11	3	2	0
C12	13	0	1	0	0	0	2	16	493	100	25	6	0	0	3	4	0	0	0
C13	0	2	4	5	0	0	2	20	428	138	34	20	0	0	0	0	0	0	10
C16	0	0	0	0	0	0	4	7	530	13	3	1	0	0	0	60	22	23	0
C17	77	21	3	2	0	1	0	119	111	65	10	4	0	0	0	0	0	0	250
C18	0	3	3	0	1	0	1	2	456	21	7	1	0	0	1	69	57	41	0

Table 6. Distance in years for the 2018 study plan and life-cycle-aware student courses.

Δ years	Student before Plan ($L \leadsto_{cid} M$)						Synchronous ($L \parallel_{cid} M$)						Student after Plan ($M \leadsto_{cid} L$)						Missing in Log ($\mathbb{L}_{cid}$)
	≤-2	-1	0	1	2	≥3	≤-2	-1	0	1	2	≥3	≤-2	-1	0	1	2	≥3	
C05	2	3	25	2	1	0	1	6	371	46	9	1	0	0	3	19	6	4	0
C12	7	54	32	8	7	2	1	52	260	53	16	7	0	0	0	0	0	0	0
C13	0	0	0	0	0	0	0	1	250	160	51	33	0	0	0	0	0	0	-4
C16	0	0	0	0	0	0	6	5	326	16	2	0	0	0	1	75	44	24	0
C17	3	3	2	0	0	0	1	14	262	50	13	11	0	0	0	0	0	0	140
C18	0	4	3	1	0	0	0	6	282	37	5	4	0	1	1	87	30	38	0

For the former, we use our method to check if the changes are supported from results of the original 2010 study plan and if conformance improves. Therefore, we detail every change, describe the evidence, and evaluate the change in conformance. In the 2010 study plan, Course C12 is taken in the fourth to fifth term, but in 2018, it shifts to the fifth to sixth term. We do not identify direct results supporting this change. After the change, instances of students taking a course earlier than its expected position increased from 14 to 110. This holds even in relative counts, with more students conforming to the 2010 study plan than to the 2018 study plan. This suggests the change may need more time to take effect or may be impractical for students. For Course C17, the opposite holds. In the 2010 plan, it is expected in the sixth term only, but in the 2018 plan, in the second to fifth term. There is evidence of students taking the course earlier than planned and typically over 2 years ahead. Additionally, more events are missing in the logs for the 2010 study plan than for the 2018 study plan, strengthening the finding. Thus, we expect the change to positively impact conformance, as shown in the 2018 study plan results. Course C13 moves from the fifth and sixth terms to the third to fifth terms. There is minimal evidence of students taking the course early before the change and none after. In conclusion, we expect our approach to be usable for detecting and evaluating potential changes effectively using the available evidence.

For the second group, we investigate the general misalignment quota and its stability after other course changes. The misalignment quota may assess the course conformance as shown in the following. Courses C16 and C18, preliminary courses in the first and third term, are often delayed due to their difficulty. Life-cycle-aware course modeling together with "student after plan" counts shows individual delays of first exam attempts, i.e., for course C16, 75 students postpone by 1 year, 44 by two years, and 24 by three years. This information is relevant to study planners because preliminary courses contain essential knowledge for other courses and may lead to a longer study duration, which planners aim to avoid. We expect this method to provide study planners with a measurement of the frequency and role of delayed courses, serving as a basis for countermeasures like improved mentoring. Toward stability, the relative frequency of students taking courses C16 and C18 has increased, from 105 out of 558 to 143 out of 355 students. This may highlight the increasing importance of individual study planners' countermeasures and how to find them.

Future Work. We plan to apply the approach to more study plans and event data to further investigate the insights from the proposed method. In addition, an adaptation is to cluster students by key performance indices such as GPA or study duration to explore their relation to (non)conforming behavior. Finally, we plan to add the relative alignment positions to the event data to identify frequent itemsets of mismatched courses.

6 Conclusion

This work contributes to the field of educational process mining by combining conformance checking methods to account for the relation between course order and the difference between expected and actual course passing terms. We model study plans with workflow nets and student course-taking behavior with labeled partial orders, providing a basis for further experiments in educational process mining. Partial order alignments are used to compare expected and actual course orders. Using real-life data, initial experiments show our contribution's usability and may suggest valuable insights for study planners.

Acknowledgments. We thank the Alexander von Humboldt (AvH) Stiftung for supporting our research (grant no. 1191945). The authors gratefully acknowledge the financial support by the Federal Ministry of Education and Research (BMBF) for the joint project AIStudyBuddy (grant no. 16DHBKI016). Further, we thank all reviewers for their valuable feedback.

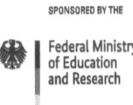

References

1. van der Aalst, W.M.P.: Process Mining - Data Science in Action, 2nd edn. Springer, Heidelberg (2016)
2. Adriansyah, A.: Aligning observed and modeled behavior. Phd thesis 1 (research tu/e / graduation tu/e), Mathematics and Computer Science (2014)
3. Bendatu, L.Y., Yahya, B.N.: Sequence matching analysis for curriculum development. Jurnal Teknik Industri **17** (2015)

 4. Bogarín, A., Cerezo, R., Romero, C.: A survey on educational process mining. WIREs Data Mining Knowl. Discov. **8**, e1230 (2018)
 5. Diamantini, C., Genga, L., Mircoli, A., Potena, D., Zannone, N.: Understanding the stumbling blocks of Italian higher education system: a process mining approach. Expert Syst. Appl. **242**, 122747 (2024)
 6. Hobeck, R., Pufahl, L., Weber, I.: Process mining on curriculum-based study data: a case study at a German University. In: Montali, M., Senderovich, A., Weidlich, M. (eds.) Process Mining Workshops - ICPM 2022. LNBIP, vol. 468, pp. 577–589. Springer, Cham (2022). https://doi.org/10.1007/978-3-031-27815-0_42
 7. Lu, X., Fahland, D., van der Aalst, W.M.P.: Conformance checking based on partially ordered event data. In: Fournier, F., Mendling, J. (eds.) BPM 2014. LNBIP, vol. 202, pp. 75–88. Springer, Cham (2015). https://doi.org/10.1007/978-3-319-15895-2_7
 8. Penthin, M., Fritzsche, E.S., Kröner, S.: Gründe für die überschreitung der regelstudienzeit aus studierendensicht (Reasons for exceeding the standard period of study from a student perspective). Beiträge zur Hochschulforschung **39**(2) (2017)
 9. Priyambada, S.A., ER, M., Yahya, B.N., Usagawa, T.: Profile-based cluster evolution analysis: identification of migration patterns for understanding student learning behavior. IEEE Access **9** (2021)
10. Rafiei, M., et al.: Extracting rules from event data for study planning. In: Process Mining Workshops - ICPM 2023. LNBIP, vol. 503. Springer (2023)

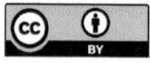

3rd International Workshop on Collaboration Mining for Distributed Systems (CoMinDS 2024)

Preface

3rd International Workshop on Collaboration Mining for Distributed Systems (CoMinDS 2024)

Business processes are becoming increasingly distributed and collaborative, involving heterogeneous participants, including people, robots, software components, organizations, and business units. These participants strive to share information, react to external changes, and cooperate to create new forms of business. Collaborative process mining aims to define customized approaches to identify and address issues typical of distributed systems. Key challenges include ensuring confidentiality and privacy, managing data heterogeneity, and dealing with different case notions. Additionally, there is a significant gap in the availability of discovery algorithms, conformance techniques, and enhancement methods tailored to these collaborative scenarios.

The Third Workshop on Collaboration Mining for Distributed Systems (CoMinDS 2024) aimed to address these challenges by fostering the exchange of research findings, ideas, and experiences related to new process mining techniques and practices for analyzing collaborative processes. CoMinDS 2024 explored advanced topics such as integrating artificial intelligence and machine learning in process mining, developing robust frameworks for real-time monitoring and analysis, and creating scalable solutions that can handle the vast amounts of data generated by distributed systems. The workshop also emphasized the importance of interdisciplinary collaboration, bringing together experts from various fields to tackle the multifaceted challenges of collaboration mining. By addressing these issues, CoMinDS 2024 aimed aims to facilitate more efficient and effective monitoring and analysis of collaborative processes. This will ultimately contribute to the advancement of distributed business models and the creation of innovative solutions that meet the evolving needs of today's dynamic business environment.

Among the submissions received by the workshop, five were accepted for presentation: two as full papers (selected for inclusion in the post-proceedings) and three as extended abstracts. Each submission followed a strict peer-review process involving three to four program committee members. The workshop opened with the keynote entitled "Applications of Collaborative Process Mining: From Compliance to Change Management" from a Stefanie Rinderle-Ma and continued with the presentation of the accepted papers. The articles are briefly summarized below.

The paper by J. Benzin and S. Rinderle-Ma proposes a standardized model class for collaboration process discovery to address inconsistencies across various techniques and model types used in collaboration processes. Using labeled Petri nets, the authors develop a formal approach to show that synchronous collaboration can represent message exchanges through a weak bisimulation equivalence. They conclude that a standard CPD model should prioritize synchronous collaboration as a core element.

The paper by A. Giacché et al. presents an approach to reveal one-to-many relations between process events in an Event Knowledge Graph. This approach defines these causal relations by examining object correlations and event order without relying solely on temporal proximity, addressing potential inaccuracies. Their contribution enables the discovery of causal relations between activities of collaborating processes.

The extended abstract by C. Rubensson et al. explores how process mining can analyze inter-organizational work patterns, specifically focusing on coordination, cooperation, and collaboration. These patterns help clarify inter-organizational activities and resource interactions within process mining, extending beyond traditional resource allocation views. The authors plan to create a coordination, cooperation, and collaboration framework for process mining, validate it with experts, and develop a data-driven model for real-world application.

The extended abstract by D. Calegari and A. Delgado explores the challenges of predictive process monitoring in collaborative processes. This paper proposes extending traditional predictive monitoring methods to handle the complexities of collaborative processes. The authors propose new prediction types specific to collaborative processes, such as predicting the next participant or message, demonstrating that traditional predictive monitoring techniques can be extended to collaborative processes.

The extended abstract by P. M. Kwantes discusses how existing algorithms for discovering Petri net models of business processes from local event logs can be adapted to discover models of cross-organizational processes. The extended abstract proposes using message logs, which record communication between local processes, as occurrences of local actions, resulting in a global event log that can be used to discover a collaboration model.

November 2024

Lorenzo Rossi
Mahsa Pourbafrani
Laura González

Organization

Workshop Chairs

Lorenzo Rossi   University of Camerino, Italy
Mahsa Pourbafrani   RWTH Aachen University, Germany
Laura González   Universidad de la República, Uruguay

Program Committee

Cristina Cabanillas   University of Seville, Spain
Marco Comuzzi   Ulsan National Institute of Science and
                             Technology, South Korea
Patrick Delfmann   University of Koblenz, Germany
Chiara Di Francescomarino   University of Trento, Italy
Dirk Fahland   Eindhoven University of Technology,
                             The Netherlands
Fabrizio Maria Maggi   Free University of Bozen-Bolzano, Italy
Pascal Poizat   Université Paris Nanterre, France
Daniel Calegari   Universidad de la República, Uruguay
Flavio Corradini   University of Camerino, Italy
Andrea Delgado   Universidad de la República, Uruguay
Marco Franceschetti   University of St. Gallen, Switzerland
Meroni Giovanni   Technical University of Denmark,
                             Denmark
Daniela Grigori   Université Paris Dauphine-PSL, France
Orlenys López Pintado   University of Tartu, Estonia
Majid Rafiei   RWTH Aachen University, Germany
Barbara Re   University of Camerino, Italy
Stefanie Rinderle-Ma   Technical University of Munich, Germany
Francesco Tiezzi   Università di Firenze, Italy
Mathias Weske   Hasso-Plattner-Institut, Germany
Andrea Vandin   Scuola Superiore Sant'Anna di Pisa, Italy

Additional Reviewers

Jonas Blatt   University of Koblenz, Germany
Ernest Ivanaj   Scuola Superiore Sant'Anna di Pisa, Italy

Towards Standardized Modeling of Collaboration Processes in Collaboration Process Discovery

Janik-Vasily Benzin[✉][iD] and Stefanie Rinderle-Ma[iD]

Technical University of Munich, TUM School of Computation,
Information and Technology, Garching, Germany
{janik.benzin,stefanie.rinderle-ma}@tum.de

Abstract. Collaboration processes represent behavior of collaborating cases within multiple process orchestrations that interact via collaboration concepts such as organizations, agents, objects, and services. The heterogeneity of collaboration concepts and types such as message exchange and synchronous collaboration has led to different models targeted by collaboration process discovery (CPD) techniques, but a standard model class is lacking. In this paper, in order to reduce heterogeneity among model classes and to reveal similarities between CPD techniques, we prove that the synchronous collaboration type simulates message exchanges, but not vice versa. This constitutes a step towards a standard CPD model class that achieves comparability between CPD techniques, enables approach and property transfer, and is a condition for a standardized collaboration mining pipeline similar to process mining.

Keywords: Collaboration Process Discovery · Collaboration Process Models · Standardization of Nets · Bisimulation · Collaboration Mining

1 Introduction

Business processes define the control-flow of business activities, i.e., what work has to be done in what order [13]. Process discovery [1], so far, has mostly discovered process orchestrations represented by, e.g., Petri nets, from a set of process instances correlated by similar cases [6]. *Collaboration processes* define the control-flow for similar *collaborating cases* [3]. As a collaboration process consists of multiple process orchestrations that collaborate to achieve a common business goal, its collaborating cases consist of multiple cases each corresponding to one of the process orchestrations. Hence, a collaborating case is a single collaboration process instance that consists of multiple process orchestration instances. *Collaboration process discovery* (CPD) techniques such as [2,5,15] aim at discovering a process model from a set of collaboration process instances grouped by collaborating cases.

Each collaboration occurs via various types of *collaboration concepts* such as a hospital's departments [15] or a company's agents [24]. Also, collaboration

© The Author(s) 2025
A. Delgado and T. Slaats (Eds.): ICPM 2024 Workshops, LNBIP 533, pp.171–183 2025.
https://doi.org/10.1007/978-3-031-82225-4_13

between collaboration concepts can be classified into four *collaboration types* Υ: υ_m is the *message exchange* (e.g., hospital department d_1 sends a health record to d_2), υ_h is the *handover-of-work* (e.g., d_1 sends a message to d_2 such that d_2 can only start working on the patient as soon as the message is received), υ_r is the *resource sharing* (e.g., both departments use the same information system), and υ_s is the *synchronous collaboration* (e.g., both departments consult together on how to treat the patient) [3,16,27]. Hence, a collaboration process consists of multiple collaboration concepts whose behavior is modeled as a process orchestration that collaborate with each other.

Although different proposals exist to represent the discovered collaboration processes, e.g., *composed RM_WF_nets* [15,16] and *BPMN collaboration diagrams* [4,20], a standard model class is missing [3]. Similar to the de-facto standard of *workflow nets* to model process orchestrations in process mining, a standard for collaboration processes achieves comparability between techniques, enables transfer of approaches and properties, and lays the foundation for a standardized and modular collaboration mining pipeline. To delineate a potential standard model class for CPD techniques, we consider existing model classes and aim to prove similarities between them. Hence, our research question is: **How can we reduce heterogeneity among existing model classes of collaboration process discovery by proving similarities towards standardization?**

In this work, we use Petri nets as notation, as either Petri nets or BPMN diagrams are targeted by CPD techniques and BPMN diagrams can be transformed into an equivalent Petri net, e.g., [4]. Overall, we reduce heterogeneity among existing model classes by proving that the synchronous type simulates message exchanges, but not vice versa. We repeat basic definitions and notations in Sect. 2. In Sect. 3, we introduce model classes for collaboration processes that are discovered by CPD techniques. In Sect. 4, we show that models with message exchanges are similar to models with synchronous collaboration and present the impact of our result. Lastly, we conclude and give an outlook in Sect. 5.

2   Labeled Petri Nets, Reachability, Language, WF-Net

In the following, we shortly repeat definitions and notation.

A *labeled Petri net* is a 5-tuple $N = (P, T, F, l, \Lambda_{\{\tau\}})$, where P is the set of *places*, T is the set of *transitions* with $P \cap T = \emptyset$, $F \subseteq ((P \times T) \cup (T \times P))$ is the *flow* relation, $l : T \to \Lambda_{\{\tau\}}$ is the *labeling* function, and Λ a finite set of *activity labels* with the *silent activity* τ. We define the *preset* of $x \in P \cup T$ by $\bullet x = \{y \mid (y, x) \in F\}$ and the *postset* of x by $x\bullet = \{y \mid (x, y) \in F\}$. A multiset of places $m \in \mathcal{B}(P)$ is called a *marking*. Given a marking m, $m(p)$ specifies the number of tokens in place p. The tuple (N, m) is called a *marked Petri net*. The *transition enabling* $(N, m)[t\rangle$ for $t \in T$ is defined by $(N, m)[t\rangle$ iff $m(p) \geq 1$ for all $p \in \bullet t$. An enabled transition $(N, m)[t\rangle$ can fire, which removes a token from each of it's input places, adds a token to each of it's output places, and executes an activity $\alpha \in \Lambda_{\{\tau\}}$ represented by $l(t)$. We define this behavior in the *firing rule*:

$(N, m) \xrightarrow{l(t)} (N, m')$ iff $(N, m)[t\rangle$ and $m' + \bullet t = m + t\bullet$.[1] We omit the labelled Petri net N, if the context is clear. A trace $\sigma = \langle \alpha_1, \dots, \alpha_n \rangle \in \Lambda_{\{\tau\}}^*$[2] is a *firing trace* of (N, m_0) iff $m_0 \xrightarrow{\alpha_1} \dots \xrightarrow{\alpha_n} m'$, in short $m_0 \xrightarrow{\sigma} m'$. We define the set of *reachable markings* by $\mathcal{R}(N, m_0) = \{m' \mid \exists_{\sigma \in \Lambda_{\{\tau\}}^*} m_0 \xrightarrow{\sigma} m'\}$ and the *language* given final marking $m_f \in \mathcal{B}(P)$ by $\mathcal{L}(N, m_0, m_f) = \{\sigma \in \Lambda_{\{\tau\}}^* \mid m_0 \xrightarrow{\sigma} m_f\}$. N is a *workflow net* (WF-net) iff (i) there exists a single source place $i \in P$ such that its preset is empty: $\bullet i = \emptyset$; (ii) there exists a single sink place $o \in P$ such that its postset is empty: $o\bullet = \emptyset$; and (iii) every node $x \in P \cup T$ is on a directed path from i to o.

3 Model Classes in Collaboration Process Discovery

This section gives an overview on existing model classes targeted by CPD techniques. In the past 16 years, research on collaboration mining has proposed 15 CPD techniques as depicted in Table 1. Each of the 15 CPD techniques target a different model class to represent the discovered collaboration process model. 12 techniques target Petri nets and 3 techniques target BPMN models. The four different collaboration types (Υ): message exchange (v_m), handover-of-work (v_h), resource sharing (v_r), and synchronous collaboration (v_s) are discovered by CPD techniques with varying degree. Most techniques discover message exchange and synchronous collaboration. Note that if a CPD technique discovers v_m, it also discovers v_h, because v_h is a special case of v_m. v_h corresponds to the "message start" BPMN element, i.e., handover-of-work is a message exchange in which the sent message enables the "first" activity in the receivers process [4,15,16].

Table 1. Overview of existing CPD techniques and their model classes.

CPD	Year	Model	Col. Types	Comm. Model	Net
[10]	2008	WF-nets	v_m	-	Labeled
[27]	2013	Integrated RM_WF_nets	v_m, v_r, v_s	P2P	Labeled
[19,21]	2013/15	Artifact-centric models	v_s	-	NA
[23]	2019	Communication nets	v_m, v_h	P2P	Higher
[1]	2020	Object-centric Petri nets	v_s	-	Higher
[26]	2020	Top-level process model	v_m, v_h	P2P	Higher
[12]	2021	BPMN Choreography	v_m, v_h	P2P	Higher
[14]	2022	Industry net	v_m, v_h	P2P	Labeled
[9]	2022	System net	v_m, v_h, v_s	P2P	Higher
[15,16]	2020/23	Composed RM_WF_nets	v_m, v_h, v_s, v_r	P2P	Labeled
[24]	2023	Multi-agent system net	v_h	P2P	Labeled
[2]	2023	Typed Jackson nets	v_s	-	Higher
[18]	2023	Generalized WF-nets	v_m, v_h, v_s	P2P	Labeled
[20]	2023	BPMN collab. diagram without signals	v_m, v_h	P2P	Labeled
[4,5]	2022/24	BPMN collab. diagram	v_m, v_h	P2P, Pub/Sub	Higher

---

[1] Addition, subtraction etc. are lifted to multisets in the common way.

[2] The universe of traces over alphabet $\Lambda_{\{\tau\}}$ is denoted as $\Lambda_{\{\tau\}}^*$.

Interestingly, almost all CPD techniques represent a message exchange by a place, a shared resource by a place, and a synchronous collaboration by a (fused via equal labels) transition. The only exception for message exchanges is [4] due to supporting a *Pub/Sub* communication model. In contrast to a *point-to-point* (P2P) communication in which a single message is only sent and received once, a Pub/Sub communication model allows that a sent message *msg* is received as often as there are receivers *subscribed* (Sub) to a *published* (Pub) message *msg*. In Table 1, any extension or change to the labeled Petri net definition in Sect. 2 is considered a *higher* Petri net. For example, the Pub/Sub communication cannot be represented in a labeled Petri net [11] such that the Petri net that is equivalent to the BPMN collab. diagram of [4] is classified as a higher Petri net. In the next section, we show how the different model classes targeted by CPD techniques can be brought closer together.

4   Simulating Collaboration Types

In the following, we bring the various model classes closer together by showing that synchronous collaboration suffices to also model message exchanges, but not vice versa. To that end, we state prerequisites of our proof in Sect. 4.1. Next, we introduce a simulation relation on collaboration types to state and prove our claim in Sect. 4.2. Lastly, we discuss the impact of our results in Sect. 4.3.

4.1   Prerequisites

We focus on labeled Petri nets for two reasons. First, quality metrics that measure the quality of discovered models , e.g., alignment-based metrics, are mostly defined on this "basic" formalism [7] such that a standard model class within labeled Petri nets enables use of the majority of quality metrics. Second, labeled Petri nets allow us to balance the complexity of the proof in the next section and the extent to which our results impact CPD (there exists a 50/50 split between labeled and higher in Table 1). As a consequence, we restrict message exchanges to the P2P communication model.

Next, we introduce the *collaboration composition* (CC) as an abstract model class that concisely represents the process orchestrations of n collaboration concepts collaborating via message exchange, handover-of-work, and synchronous collaboration in a collaboration process.

Definition 1 (Collaboration Composition). *Let $V = \{N_c \mid c \in \{1, \ldots, n\}\}$ be a set of n disjoint[3] WF-nets and let P_{AC} be a set of message types with sending* send $: P_{AC} \to \mathcal{P}(T_{\not\tau}^n)$[4] *and receiving transitions* rec $: P_{AC} \to \mathcal{P}(T^n)$ *for $T_{\not\tau}^n = T^n \backslash \{t \in T^n \mid l(t) = \tau\}, T^n = \bigcup_{c \in \{1,\ldots,n\}} T_c$. The collaboration composition (CC) is a labeled Petri net $\mathcal{C}(V, P_{AC}, \text{send}, \text{rec}) = (P, T, F, l, \Lambda_{\{\tau\}})$ defined by:*

---

[3] Two WF-nets N_1, N_2 are *disjoint* iff their place names $P_1 \cap P_2 = \emptyset$ and transition names $T_1 \cap T_2 = \emptyset$ are disjoint.

[4] Given set X, $\mathcal{P}(X) = \{X' \mid X' \subseteq X \land X' \neq \emptyset\}$.

1. $P = \bigcup_{c \in \{1,\ldots,n\}} P_c,$
2. $l' : T^n \rightarrow \Lambda_{\{\tau\}}, l'(t) = l_c(t)$ with $c \in \{1, \ldots, n\}$ and $t \in T_c,$
3. $T = \bigcup_{c \in \{1,\ldots,n\}} r(T_c),$ with r a renaming function: $r(x) = t_s$ if there exists $T_s \in ET$ such that $x \in T_s$ and $t_s \in T_s$ a fixed transition with $ET = \{T_s \subseteq T^n \mid \forall_{t,t' \in T_s} l'(t) = l'(t') \wedge l'(t) \neq \tau\}$ the set of equally-labeled (synchronous) transition subsets, otherwise $r(x) = x,$
4. $F = \{(r(x), r(y)) \mid (x, y) \in \bigcup_{c \in \{1,\ldots,n\}} F_c\} \cup$
   $\{(r(t), p_{ac}), (p_{ac}, r(t')) \mid p_{ac} \in P_{AC} \wedge t \in \text{send}(p_{ac}) \wedge t' \in \text{rec}(p_{ac})\},$ and
5. $l(t) = l'(t)$ for $t \in T.$

A CC $\mathcal{C}(V, P_{AC}, \text{send}, \text{rec})$ can only have initial markings $m_0 \in \mathcal{B}(P)$ that specify non-zero tokens $m_0(p) \neq 0$ for source places $p = i_c, c \in \{1, \ldots, n\}$ of its $N_c.$

Figure 1 depicts a marked CC $(\mathcal{C}(V, P_{AC}, \text{send}, \text{rec}), m_0)$ with $V = \{N_1, N_2\}, P_{AC} = \{p_{ac,1}, p_{ac,2}\},$ send $= \{(p_{ac,1}, \{t_4\}), (p_{ac,2}, \{t_2\})\},$ and rec $= \{(p_{ac,1}, \{t_1\}), (p_{ac,2}, \{t_5\})\}.$ Note that ts in Fig. 1 embodies the fused transition as defined in (3), i.e., $t_3, t_6 \in T^2$ with $l_1(t_3) = l_2(t_6) = c.$

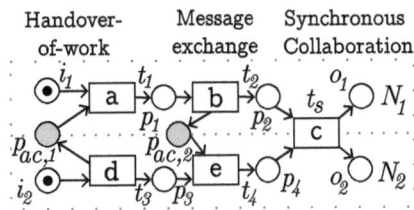

Fig. 1. Collaboration composition $\mathcal{C}(V, P_{AC}, \text{send}, \text{rec})$ with initial marking and two collaboration concepts collaborating via $\upsilon_h, \upsilon_m,$ and $\upsilon_s.$

Since resource sharing υ_r is modeled as marked *self-loop* places by CPD techniques [15, 16, 27], we deliberately left υ_r out of a CC. Self-loop places marked with a token can be removed without changing the behavior of labeled Petri nets due to imposing no restriction on enabling their respective transition [17], e.g., the language does not change. As υ_h is a special case of υ_m (cf. Sect. 3 and Fig. 1), we do not need to represent it in a CC on its own. Overall, we focus on collaboration types $\Upsilon_{ms} = \{\upsilon_m, \upsilon_s\}.$ We say collaboration type υ_s is *contained* in $\mathcal{C}(V, P_{AC}, \text{send}, \text{rec})$ iff $ET \neq \emptyset.$ Likewise, we say collaboration type υ_m is *contained* in $\mathcal{C}(V, P_{AC}, \text{send}, \text{rec})$ iff $P_{AC} \neq \emptyset.$ For example, the CC in Fig. 1 contains both υ_m and $\upsilon_s.$

In the next section, we apply the *weak bisimulation* equivalence [25] on collaboration types Υ_{ms} (cf. Definition 2) to show that message exchanges are "syntactic sugar" for synchronous collaborations (cf. Theorem 1), but not vice versa (cf. Theorem 2). Because the silent activity is typically "disregarded" for the purpose of analyzing a discovered Petri net, e.g., by conformance checking using alignments, the weak bisimulation equivalence that also "disregards" silent activities comes with a suitable granularity of differentiating labeled Petri nets. We define weak bisimulation as follows.

A *labeled transition system* (LTS) is a 4-tuple $\Gamma = (S, \Lambda_{\{\tau\}}, s_0, \longrightarrow)$, where S is a set of states, $\Lambda_{\{\tau\}}$ is the set of labels, $s_0 \in S$ is the *initial state*, and $\longrightarrow \subseteq S \times \Lambda_{\{\tau\}} \times S$ the set of labeled edges. Note that we overload the notation of $\longrightarrow$ similar to the firing rule in Sect. 2. We write $s_1 \xrightarrow{\sigma} s_{n+1}$ iff there exists $\sigma = \langle \alpha_1, \ldots, \alpha_n \rangle \in \Lambda_{\{\tau\}}^*$ and $s_1, \ldots, s_{n+1} \in S$ such that $s_1 \xrightarrow{\alpha_1} s_2 \ldots s_n \xrightarrow{\alpha_n} s_{n+1}$. We define the *weak transition relation* $\overset{\alpha}{\Longrightarrow} \subseteq S \times \Lambda_{\{\tau\}} \times S$ with $\alpha \in \Lambda_{\{\tau\}}$ by (i) $s (\xrightarrow{\tau})^* s_1 \xrightarrow{\alpha} s_2 (\xrightarrow{\tau})^* s'$, if $\alpha \neq \tau$, and (ii) $s (\xrightarrow{\tau})^* s'$, if $\alpha = \tau$, where $(\xrightarrow{\tau})^*$ is the reflexive, transitive closure of $\xrightarrow{\tau}$. We lift the notation of the weak transition relation to traces in the same manner as for $\longrightarrow$. We define the *weak bisimulation equivalence* on the set of all LTS with labels $\Lambda_{\{\tau\}}$. Let $\Gamma_1 = (S_1, \Lambda_{\{\tau\}}, s_{0,1}, \longrightarrow_1)$ and $\Gamma_2 = (S_2, \Lambda_{\{\tau\}}, s_{0,2}, \longrightarrow_2)$ be two LTSs. A relation $R \subseteq S_1 \times S_2$ is a *weak simulation*, denoted by $\Gamma_1 \preceq_R \Gamma_2$, iff

i $(s_{0,1}, s_{0,2}) \in R$, i.e., the initial states are related; and

ii for every $(p, q) \in R$ and $\alpha \in \Lambda_{\{\tau\}}$ it holds that: if $p \xrightarrow{\alpha}_1 p'$, then $\alpha = \tau$ and $(p', q) \in R$, or there exists $q' \in S_2$ such that $q \overset{\alpha}{\Longrightarrow}_2 q'$ and $(p', q') \in R$.

If R is symmetric, it is a *weak bisimulation equivalence*, written $\Gamma_1 \approx_R \Gamma_2$. We also say Γ_1 is weakly bisimilar to Γ_2. Two marked Petri nets $(N, m_0), (N', m_0')$ are weakly bisimilar, written $(N, m_0) \approx (N', m_0')$, iff the two LTSs $\Gamma_{N,m_0} = (\mathcal{B}(P), \Lambda_{\{\tau\}}, m_0, \longrightarrow), \Gamma_{N',m_0'} = (\mathcal{B}(P'), \Lambda_{\{\tau\}}, m_0', \longrightarrow')$ are weakly bisimilar[5].

4.2 Synchronous Collaboration Simulates Message Exchange

By means of the weak bisimulation equivalence, we state the two theorems of this paper as follows. First, any CC that only contains v_m is weakly bisimilar to another CC that only contains v_s (cf. Theorem 1). Second, any CC that only contains v_s does not have a CC that only contains v_m such that both are weakly bisimilar (cf. Theorem 2). To formalize both statements, we introduce our notion of *simulating* collaboration types.

Definition 2 (Simulating Collaboration Types). *A type $v_1 \in \Upsilon_{ms}$ simulates type $v_2 \in \Upsilon_{ms}$ with $v_1 \neq v_2$ iff for any marked collaboration composition $(\mathcal{C}(V, P_{AC}, \text{send}, \text{rec}), m_0) = (N, m_0)$ that contains type v_2, there exists a marked collaboration composition $(\mathcal{C}(V', P_{AC}', \text{send}', \text{rec}'), m_0') = (N', m_0')$ that only contains type v_1 such that $V' = V \cup \{N_c \mid c \in \{n+1, \ldots\}\}$ and $(N, m_0) \approx (N', m_0')$.*

In the construction of a (N', m_0') that simulates (N, m_0), it is important to prohibit changes to the WF-nets V except than extending to V', as other changes to V would mean that we allow simulating collaboration types by a collaboration concept's internal WF-net and not by some other collaboration

---

[5] $\longrightarrow$ is the firing rule for (N, m_0) and $\longrightarrow'$ the firing rule for (N', m_0') (cf. Sect. 2).

type. In the following, we show that synchronous collaboration v_s simulates message exchanges v_m , under three conditions: neither τ-labeled skipping nor τ-labeled loop for sending messages of type $p_{ac} \in P_{AC}$ exist and there does not exist a token generator [8] that can infinitely often send a message of type p_{ac}. A τ-labeled skipping for sending p_{ac} exists iff $\sigma \in \Lambda^*_{\{\tau\}}$, $m_1 \in \mathcal{R}(N, m_0)$ exist such that $m_1 \xrightarrow{\sigma} m_2$, $m_1 \xRightarrow{\tau} m_2$, and sending activity $l(t)$ occurs in σ, i.e., $l(t) \in \sigma^6$ for $t \in \text{send}(p_{ac})$. A τ-labeled loop in (N, m_0) for sending messages of type p_{ac} exists iff $m_1 \xrightarrow{l(t)} m_2$, $m_1 \in \mathcal{R}(N, m_0)$ and $m_2 \xRightarrow{\tau} m_3$ such that $(N, m_3)[t'\rangle$ for some $t, t' \in \text{send}(p_{ac})$. A token generator results in unbounded states of the coverability graph (ω-states) [17] and is characterized by: There exists $m \in \mathcal{R}(N, m_0), \sigma \in \Lambda^*_{\{\tau\}}, m' \in \mathcal{B}(P)$ such that $|m'| > 0$ and $m \xrightarrow{\sigma} m+m'$.

Theorem 1 (Synchronous execution simulates message exchange). v_s *simulates* v_m, *if for all* $p_{ac} \in P_{AC}$ *in* $\mathcal{C}(V, P_{AC}, \text{send}, \text{rec})$: *no* τ-*labeled skipping, no* τ-*labeled loop, and no token generator exist.*

Proof. Let $(\mathcal{C}(V, P_{AC}, \text{send}, \text{rec}), m_0) = (N, m_0)$ be a marked CC that contains message exchanges v_m. We prove the statement by constructing a new WF-net $N_{p_{ac}}$ for each message type $p_{ac} \in P_{AC}$ such that the new marked CC $(\mathcal{C}(V', \emptyset, \emptyset, \emptyset), m'_0) = (N', m'_0)$ with $V' = V \cup \{N_{p_{ac}} \mid p_{ac} \in P_{AC}\}$ is weakly bisimilar to the CC (N, m_0). Our construction is structured into four steps: Distinguishing three cases of how message exchanges occur (**step 1**), determining respective transition sets for two of the cases through analyzing the coverability graph (**step 2**), constructing a new WF-net $N_{p_{ac}}$ given the transition sets (**step 3**), and defining a weak bisimulation $Q \subseteq \mathcal{R}(N, m_0) \times \mathcal{R}(N', m'_0)$ to complete the proof (**step 4**).

Step 1. Given $p_{ac} \in P_{AC}$, either ① message type p_{ac} is *dead*, ② p_{ac} is *optional*, or ③ p_{ac} is *compulsory*. First, message type p_{ac} is *dead* iff for all $t \in \text{send}(p_{ac})$ there is no reachable marking $m \in \mathcal{R}(N, m_0)$ such that $(N, m)[t\rangle$, i.e., the message exchange via type p_{ac} can never occur. Second, p_{ac} is *optional* iff there exist at least two firing traces $\sigma_\neg, \sigma \in \mathcal{L}(N, m_0, m_f)$ such that $\forall_{\alpha \in l(\text{send}(p_{ac}))} \alpha \notin \sigma_\neg$ (i.e., no sending activity occurs in $\sigma_\neg$) and $\exists_{\alpha \in l(\text{send}(p_{ac}))} \alpha \in \sigma$ (i.e., a sending activity occurs in σ). The final marking m_f specifies that as many tokens are on a WF-nets N_c's sink place o_c, as the initial marking specifies for a N_c's source place i_c, i.e., for $c \in \{1, \ldots, n\}$: if $m_0(i_c) = x$, then $m_f(o_c) = x$. The final marking specifies $m_f(p) = 0$, if $p \in P$ is not a sink place, i.e., $p\bullet \neq \emptyset$. Third, p_{ac} is *compulsory* iff for every firing trace $\sigma \in \mathcal{L}(N, m_0, m_f)$ it holds that $\exists_{\alpha \in l(\text{send}(p_{ac}))} \alpha \in \sigma$ (i.e., at least one sending activity always occurs).

Step 2. Figure 2 depicts the WF-net $N_{p_{ac}}$ that is constructed in this and the next step. For ②, we ensure that the WF-net $N_{p_{ac}}$ that "simulates" optional message type p_{ac} with synchronous collaboration is able to skip all transitions with sending activities, as otherwise the corresponding markings would be missing in $\mathcal{R}(N', m'_0)$. Skipping has to occur synchronously with transitions $T_{p_{ac}, \times}$

---

[6] For $\sigma = \langle \alpha_1, \ldots, \alpha_n \rangle \in \Lambda^*_{\{\tau\}}$ and $\alpha \in \Lambda_{\{\tau\}}$, we write $\alpha \in \sigma$ iff $\exists_{i \in \{1, \ldots, n\}} \alpha_i = \alpha$.

"after" which sending cannot occur anymore (cf. Fig. 2). Also, sending activities may be repeated in the firing trace σ (cf. ② and ③) by traversing a loop. Hence, our construction must ensure that the transitions $T_{pac,\circlearrowright}$ "after" which sending occurs again and $T_{pac,\emptyset,\times}$ "after" which repeated sending stops are also copied to N_{pac} (cf. Fig. 2). In the following, we determine the necessary transition sets by sets of markings in the coverability graph.

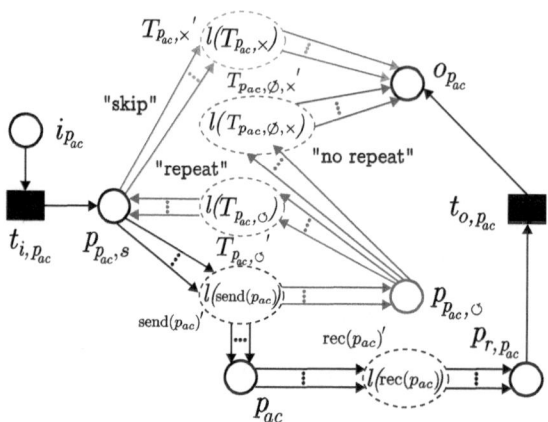

Fig. 2. WF-net N_{pac} constructed for message type $pac \in P_{AC}$ and its sending send(pac) and receiving activities rec(pac). Conditional parts of the WF-net that are only constructed in certain cases are highlighted in blue and green. (Color figure online)

Determine by breadth-first search for each $pac \in P_{AC}$ a unique set of markings $M_\times \subseteq \mathcal{R}(N, m_0)$ and set of markings $M_\circlearrowright \subseteq \mathcal{R}(N, m_0)$ in the coverability graph. $M_\times$ is characterized by the following formula that identifies the markings from which activities "decide" whether a message is sent or never sent. For each $m_\times \in M_\times$ it holds that $m_\times$ is reachable by paths in the coverability graph in which no sending activities $\alpha \in l(\text{send}(pac))$ have occurred and formula $\gamma(m_\times)$ holds. $\gamma(m)$ holds iff there exist two sets of activities $A_0, A_1 \subseteq \Lambda$ with $m \xrightarrow{\alpha_0} m_\neg$, $\alpha_0 \in A_0$ such that for all $m' \in \mathcal{R}(N, m_\neg)$ sending activities cannot occur $\neg(N, m')[t\rangle$ for all $t \in \text{send}(pac)$ and $m \xrightarrow{\alpha_1} m_1$, $\alpha_1 \in A_1$ such that there exists $m' \in \mathcal{R}(N, m_1)$ that enables sending activities $(N, m')[t\rangle$ for some $t \in \text{send}(pac)$. Note that A_0, A_1 exist iff ② holds or ③ with repeated sending, as sending and receiving transitions cannot be labeled with the silent activity (cf. Definition 1) and no τ-labeled skipping exists. Thus, the activities A_0 and A_1 represent the choice between not executing optional asynchronous collaboration pac and executing asynchronous collaboration pac.

Let $A_\times = \bigcup_{m_\times \in M_\times} A_{0,m_\times}$ be the union of activities $A_{0,m_\times}$ that are computed to satisfy $\gamma(m_\times)$. Define $T_{pac,\times} = \{t \in T^n \mid l(t) \in A_\times\}$. Note that l is a bijection for $l(t) \in \Lambda$, i.e., transitions are uniquely determined by their observable label. If a transition in $T_{pac,\times}$ fires, no sending activity for messages of type pac can occur anymore. Observe that $T_{pac,\times} = \emptyset$ in case ③.

To "simulate" loops, determine $M_\circlearrowleft$ whose markings are characterized by the following formula that identifies the markings from which activities "decide" whether a message will be sent again or not. For each $m_\circlearrowleft \in M_\circlearrowleft$ it holds that $m_\circlearrowleft$ is reachable by paths in the coverability graph in which some sending activity $\alpha \in l(\text{send}(p_{ac}))$ has occurred and $\gamma(m_\circlearrowleft)$ holds. If a sending activity is repeated, the set $M_\circlearrowleft$ cannot be empty, since the CC does not contain any τ-*labelled loops* for all $p_{ac} \in P_{AC}$.

Let $A_\circlearrowleft = \bigcup_{m_\circlearrowleft \in M_\circlearrowleft} A_{1,m_\circlearrowleft}$ be the union of activities $A_{1,m_\circlearrowleft}$ that are computed to satisfy $\gamma(m_\circlearrowleft)$. These activities indicate that sending activities are executed again. Let $T_{p_{ac},\circlearrowleft} = \{t \in T \mid l(t) \in A_\circlearrowleft\}$ be the set of transitions for message exchange p_{ac} that, if executed, result in firing traces with repeated sending activities. Observe that $T_{p_{ac},\circlearrowleft} = \emptyset$, if there are no loops involving sending activities. We refer to $T_{p_{ac},\circlearrowleft} = \emptyset$ with $\oslash$ and to the opposite with $\circlearrowleft$. Since $T_{p_{ac},\times}$ only covers transitions that indicate no message of type p_{ac} is sent at all for ②, it misses transitions that indicate no message of type p_{ac} is sent after a message has been sent already, i.e., a loop of repeated sending activities is not "traversed" again. Let $A_{0,m_\circlearrowleft}$ for $m_\circlearrowleft \in M_\circlearrowleft$ be the sets of activities that were computed to satisfy $\gamma(m_\circlearrowleft)$, i.e., an activity $\alpha \in A_{0,m_\circlearrowleft}$ indicates that after some sending activity has occurred, it will not occur again. Next, $A_{\oslash,\times} = \bigcup_{m_\circlearrowleft \in M_\circlearrowleft} A_{0,m_\circlearrowleft}$, and similarly: $T_{p_{ac},\oslash,\times} = \{t \in T \mid l(t) \in A_{\oslash,\times}\}$. Observe that $T_{p_{ac},\oslash,\times} \neq \emptyset$ if $\circlearrowleft$, because no token generator exists, no place $p \in \{p \mid p \in \bullet t \wedge t \in T_{p_{ac},\oslash,\times}\}$ is a sink place, and N is composed of WF-nets.

Step 3. If either ② or ③, construct WF-net $N_{p_{ac}} = (P_{p_{ac}}, T_{p_{ac}}, F_{p_{ac}}, l_{p_{ac}}, \Lambda_{\{\tau\}})$ as depicted in Fig. 2. Note that if we say $N_{p_{ac}}$ contains a part of Fig. 2, the renamed transitions depicted by a dotted oval with their labeling depicted inside the oval are added to $T_{p_{ac}}$ and $l_{p_{ac}}$ along with the places in their depicted pre- and postset to $P_{p_{ac}}$ and depicted arcs to $F_{p_{ac}}$. For example, the green part in Fig. 2 consists of renamed transitions $T'_{p_{ac},\times}$ with respective labels $l(T'_{p_{ac},\times})$, i.e., $T_{p_{ac}} = T_{p_{ac}} \cup T'_{p_{ac},\times}$ and $l_{p_{ac}}(t') = l(t)$ for $t' \in T'_{p_{ac},\times}$. Also, the green part adds the depicted arcs to $F_{p_{ac}}$. We distinguish four cases from the combination of ② and ③ with $\oslash$ and $\circlearrowleft$. All four constructed WF-nets include the black parts in Fig. 2 that represent a WF-net with sending and receiving transitions of p_{ac}.

Case ②, $\oslash$: In addition to the black part in Fig. 2, $N_{p_{ac}}$ contains the green part to skip sending messages.

Case ②, $\circlearrowleft$: In addition to the black part in Fig. 2, $N_{p_{ac}}$ contains the green parts to skip sending messages and the blue part to repeat and stop repeating sending messages. Hence, $N_{p_{ac}}$ is equal to all depicted parts in Fig. 2.

Case ③, $\oslash$: $N_{p_{ac}}$ contains the black part in Fig. 2 only.

Case ③, $\circlearrowleft$: In addition to the black part in Fig. 2, $N_{p_{ac}}$ contains the blue part to repeat and stop repeating sending messages.

Step 4. Define $V' = V \cup \{N_{p_{ac}} \mid p_{ac} \in P_{AC}\}$ with $N_{p_{ac}}$ as constructed in **step 3**. Then, $(\mathcal{C}(V', \emptyset, \emptyset, \emptyset), m'_0) = (N', m'_0)$. Define m'_0 similar to m_0 for source places i_c of WF-nets $N_c \in V$, additionally $m'_0(p) = 1$ if $p = i_{p_{ac}}$, and $m'_0(p) = 0$ otherwise. Observe that the set of equally-labeled transitions ET' includes for each p_{ac} the following transitions:

Case ③, ⌀: Because $N_{p_{ac}}$ only contains the black part in Fig. 2 in this case, ET' includes only renamed, equally-labeled sending and receiving transitions. Formally, for each $t \in ET'$ such that $t \in \text{send}(p_{ac}), t \in T^n$ another $t' \in ET'$ exists such that $t' \in \text{send}(p_{ac})', t' \in T_{p_{ac}}$ with $l(t) = l_{p_{ac}}(t')$. Similarly, ET' includes for each $t \in \text{rec}(p_{ac}), t \in T^n$ another $t' \in \text{rec}(p_{ac})', t' \in T_{p_{ac}}$ with $l(t) = l_{p_{ac}}(t')$. The remaining three cases are analogous.

Define relation $Q \subseteq \mathcal{R}(N, m_0) \times \mathcal{R}(N', m_0')$ such that $(m, m') \in Q$ iff $m(p') \leq m'(p')$ for all places $p' \in P'$ of N'[7]. Then, $(N, m_0) \approx_Q (N', m_0')$, since with the exception of new τ-labelled transitions in $N_{p_{ac}}$ for a message type p_{ac}, all transitions of the constructed WF-nets $N_{p_{ac}}$ are fused with their original counterparts in N, exactly the same flow relation is encoded in $\bullet p_{ac}$ and $p_{ac}\bullet$ as is defined by (4) in Definition 1, and optional and repeating behavior is exactly encoded. ∎

To illustrate the construction in the last theorem's proof, Fig. 3 depicts the marked CC $(\mathcal{C}(V \cup \{N_{p_{ac,1}}, N_{p_{ac,2}}\}, \emptyset, \emptyset, \emptyset), m_0')$ that only contains synchronous collaboration and that is weakly bisimilar to the CC in Fig. 1. Except for fused transitions, $N_{p_{ac,1}}$ and $N_{p_{ac,2}}$ are highlighted in grey in Fig. 3.

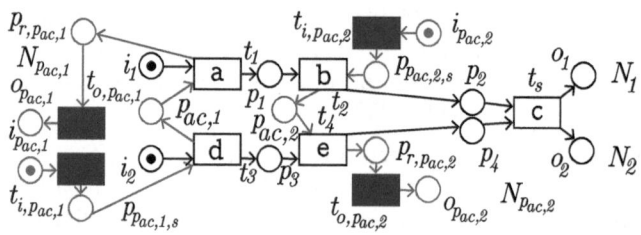

Fig. 3. Marked collaboration composition $(\mathcal{C}(V \cup \{N_{p_{ac,1}}, N_{p_{ac,2}}\}, \emptyset, \emptyset, \emptyset), m_0')$ constructed to simulate v_m in $\mathcal{C}(V, P_{AC}, \text{send}, \text{rec})$ (Fig. 1) by v_s as shown in Theorem 1.

Although v_s simulates v_m under three conditions, all three conditions are not realistic in many real-world collaboration processes, as τ-labeled skipping would mean that a collaboration concept can skip a collaboration without notifying the other collaborating concepts, the τ-labelled loop condition excludes arbitrary, non-observable sending of messages, and the existence of a token generator excludes arbitrarily creating collaboration concept instances.

The next theorem proves that synchronous collaboration v_s cannot be simulated by message exchange v_m.

Theorem 2 (Synchronous collaboration cannot be simulated). v_m *does not simulate* v_s.

Proof. We prove by contradiction. Assume v_m simulates v_s. Let $(\mathcal{C}(V, \emptyset, \emptyset, \emptyset), m_0) = (N, m_0)$ be a marked CC that contains v_s and $(\mathcal{C}(V', P_{AC}, \text{send}, \text{rec}), m_o') = (N', m_0')$ be a marked CC that contains only v_m such that $(N, m_0) \approx$

---

[7] If $p' \notin P$, $m(p') = 0$.

(N', m_0'). Observe that collaboration type v_m is represented by P_{AC}, send, and rec. From Definition 1 (3) and (4), it follows that no transitions with different labels are merged or changed for exchanging messages of type $p_{ac} \in P_{AC}$. Hence, from Definition 2 it follows that all transitions $t \in T_s, T_s \in ET$ are still merged in (N', m_0') (changing V is prohibited) such that $ET \neq \emptyset$ and v_s is contained in $(N', m_0')^8$.   ∎

Overall, our theory on collaboration types in labeled Petri nets demonstrates that modulo weak bisimilarity, message exchange can be simulated by synchronous collaboration, but not vice versa. In the next section, we elaborate on the implications.

4.3   Impact on Collaboration Process Discovery

The impact of the two theoretical results on simulating collaboration types on collaboration process discovery is twofold.

1. Since all CPD techniques in Table 1 that discover v_s share the design choice to represent v_s by fusing transitions similar to a CC (cf. Definition 1 (3)), the following statement holds at least for CPD techniques [14,20,24] that target labeled Petri net-based classes. If a CPD technique targets a model class that does not represent synchronous collaboration v_s, the CPD technique can only be advanced to discover v_s by both a structural change to the targeted model class and an algorithmic change to the technique. The statement is conjectured to also hold for CPD techniques [4,5,12,23,26] that target higher Petri net-based classes (cf. next section). Moreover, CPD techniques that can only discover v_s can be tweaked to also discover v_m by mirroring the construction of Theorem 1 in the event log, i.e., these techniques do not need to be changed.

2. Considering labeled Petri nets for a start, the standard model class for CPD must represent synchronous collaboration, but does not have to represent message exchanges, as it is "syntactic sugar". Interestingly, our result is supported by [22] that proposes an abstraction-based technique for discovering collaboration process models in a privacy-sensitive setting using the synchronous type only. Also, the two theorems indicate that the model classes of [9,15,16,27] (incl. v_s) are indistinguishable modulo weak bisimilarity. Additionally, models in these classes (incl. v_s) can weakly simulate models from model classes [14,20,24] (excl. v_s), but not vice versa.

All in all, the apparent heterogeneity in model classes among CPD techniques is misleading, as their models have more in common than is obvious.

---

[8]   The statement still holds, if we enable synchronizing arbitrary transitions in a CC, which is rarely done. Message exchange does not merge transitions and requires non-silent sending and receiving transitions, so we can never construct a single label out of at least a sending and receiving label.

5   Conclusion and Outlook

In this paper, we prove two statements that show to what extent heterogeneity in modeling collaboration by CPD techniques can be reduced to achieve a more standardized model class in collaboration mining. The first statement means that message exchanges are non-essential for discovering collaboration processes, while the second statement means that synchronous collaborations are essential. Hence, both a standard model class and a standard collaboration mining pipeline must be built with synchronous collaboration at their core. In the future, we will analyze how we can transfer the two statements to also hold for higher Petri nets with the aim of delineating a standard model class for all CPD techniques. Furthermore, we will apply the theoretical results in designing a standard benchmark for CPD techniques. Moreover, we will extend the scope of standardizing collaboration mining towards quality metrics as proposed in conformance checking.

References

1. van der Aalst, W.M.P., Berti, A.: Discovering object-centric Petri nets. Fundamenta informaticae **175**(1–4), 1–40 (2020)
2. Barenholz, D., Montali, M., Polyvyanyy, A., Reijers, H.A., Rivkin, A., van der Werf, J.M.E.M.: There and back again. In: PETRI NETS 2023, pp. 37–58 (2023)
3. Benzin, J.V., Rinderle-Ma, S.: Petri net classes for collaboration mining: assessment and design guidelines. In: Process Mining Workshops. ICPM 2023 (2024)
4. Corradini, F., Pettinari, S., Re, B., Rossi, L., Tiezzi, F.: A technique for discovering BPMN collaboration diagrams. SoSyM (2024)
5. Corradini, F., Re, B., Rossi, L., Tiezzi, F.: A technique for collaboration discovery. In: Enterprise, Business-Process and Inf, Syst. Modeling, pp. 63–78 (2022)
6. Diba, K., Batoulis, K., Weidlich, M., Weske, M.: Extraction, correlation, and abstraction of event data for process mining. Data Min. Knowl. Discov. **10**(3) (2020)
7. Dunzer, S., Stierle, M., Matzner, M., Baier, S.: Conformance checking: a state-of-the-art literature review. In: S-BPM ONE 2019, pp. 1–10. ACM (2019)
8. Esparza, J., Nielsen, M.: Decidability issues for petri nets. BRICS Rep. Ser. **1**(8) (1994)
9. Fettke, P., Reisig, W.: Systems Mining with Heraklit: the Next Step (2022). arXiv:2202.01289 [cs]
10. Gaaloul, W., Baïna, K., Godart, C.: Log-based mining techniques applied to Web service composition reengineering. Serv. Oriented Comp. Appl. **2**(2), 93–110 (2008)
11. Gutnik, G., Kaminka, G.: A scalable petri net representation of interaction protocols for overhearing. In: Agent Communication, pp. 50–64. Springer (2005)
12. Hernandez-Resendiz, et al.: Merging event logs for inter-organizational process mining. In: New Perspectives on Enterprise Decision-Making Applying Artificial Intelligence Techniques, pp. 3–26. Springer (2021)
13. Jablonski, S., Bussler, C.: Workflow management: modeling concepts, architecture and implementation. ITP New Media (1996)
14. Kwantes, P., Kleijn, J.: Distributed synthesis of asynchronously communicating distributed process models. In: ToPNoC, pp. 49–72. Springer (2022)

15. Liu, C., Li, H., Zhang, S., Cheng, L., et al.: Cross-department collaborative healthcare process model discovery from event logs. IEEE Trans. Autom. Sci. Eng. **20**(3), 2115–2125 (2023)
16. Liu, C., et al.: Cross-organization emergency response process mining: an approach based on petri nets. Math. Probl. Eng. **2020**, e8836007 (2020)
17. Murata, T.: Petri nets: properties, analysis and applications. Proc. IEEE **77**(4), 541–580 (1989)
18. Nesterov, R., Bernardinello, L., Lomazova, I., Pomello, L.: Discovering architecture-aware and sound process models of multi-agent systems: a compositional approach. SoSyM **1**, 351–375 (2023)
19. Nooijen, E.H.J., van Dongen, B.F., Fahland, D.: Automatic discovery of data-centric and artifact-centric processes. In: BPM Workshops, pp. 316–327 (2013)
20. Peña, L., Andrade, D., Delgado, A., Calegari, D.: An approach for discovering inter-organizational collaborative business processes in BPMN 2.0. In: Process Mining Workshops. ICPM 2023, pp. 487–498 (2024)
21. Popova, V., Fahland, D., Dumas, M.: Artifact lifecycle discovery. Int. J. Coop. Inf. Syst. **24**(01), 1550001 (2015)
22. Rafiei, M., Van Der Aalst, W.M.P.: An abstraction-based approach for privacy-aware federated process mining. IEEE Access **11**, 33697–33714 (2023)
23. Stroiński, A., Dwornikowski, D., Brzeziński, J.: A distributed discovery of communicating resource systems models. Trans. Serv. Comput. **12**(2), 172–185 (2019)
24. Tour, A., Polyvyanyy, A., Kalenkova, A., Senderovich, A.: Agent miner: an algorithm for discovering agent systems from event data. In: BPM, pp. 284–302 (2023)
25. Van Glabbeek, R.J., Weijland, W.P.: Branching time and abstraction in bisimulation semantics. J. ACM **43**(3), 555–600 (1996)
26. Zeng, Q., Duan, H., Liu, C.: Top-down process mining from multi-source running logs based on refinement of petri nets. IEEE Access **8**, 61355–61369 (2020)
27. Zeng, Q., Sun, S., Duan, H., Liu, C., Wang, H.: Cross-organizational collaborative workflow mining from a multi-source log. Decis. Support Syst. **54**, 1280–1301 (2013)

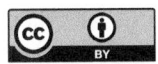

Revealing One-to-Many Event Relationships in Event Knowledge Graphs

Alessio Giacché[1], Sara Pettinari[2]($^{\boxtimes}$) (iD), and Lorenzo Rossi[1] (iD)

[1] School of Science and Technology, University of Camerino, Camerino, Italy
`alessio.giacche@studenti.unicam.it`, `lorenzo.rossi@unicam.it`
[2] Gran Sasso Science Institute, L'Aquila, Italy
`sara.pettinari@gssi.it`

Abstract. Object-centric process mining is recognized to overcome the limitations of traditional process mining by offering approaches for the analysis of processes with multiple case notions such as collaborations. Event knowledge graphs are an effective tool for gathering, manipulating, and visualizing event and entity relations. Current approaches focus on inferring correlations between events and objects and directly-follows relationships between events correlated to the same object. However, object-to-object relations may hide one-to-many relations between events essential for understanding the actual flow among processes. We propose an approach to reveal these one-to-many causal relationships in an event knowledge graph. By defining when two events are causally related and extending the standard approach of event knowledge graphs construction to reveal them. We assess the approach using two case studies.

Keywords: Collaborations · Object-Centric Process Mining · Event Knowledge Graph · One-to-Many Relationships

1 Introduction

Process mining collects well-established techniques for analyzing event logs produced during the execution of processes [2]. By its nature, process mining techniques target the analysis of event logs from the perspective of a single case, i.e., an identifier shared by the events that belong to the same process instance. However, many real-life event logs contain different case notions since the events and the associated activities are shared by more than one process [1]. For instance, in an order handling process, a single order can trigger as many pick-up processes as there are items in the order. Therefore, some of the events in the log could be related to a unique order identifier as a case notion, while others could also refer to an item identifier. This creates a one-to-many relationship between orders and items, which must be considered in analyzing the processes.

In recent years, Object-Centric Process Mining (OCPM) has emerged from traditional process mining to address convergence and divergence issues in real-life process analysis [1]. OCPM has been proposed to connect processes not based on the same case notion but to explore and filter the behavior recorded

A. Delgado and T. Slaats (Eds.): ICPM 2024 Workshops, LNBIP 533, pp. 184–196, 2025.
https://doi.org/10.1007/978-3-031-82225-4_14

in the logs considering different classes of objects and their interaction [4]. So far, most of the work has been done in providing process models capable of capturing event-to-object and object-to-object interactions, whereas less work also investigated the representation of event-to-event relationships [5].

In this context, an Event Knowledge Graph (EKG) is a flexible and expressive event data model to capture different aspects of the system behavior [11]. It enables the representation of the correlation between events and objects, and the relations between objects [18], while inferring the directly-follows relationships of events correlated with the same object. This approach establishes directly-follows relationships between events by considering each object individually. However, when multiple objects are involved, their interrelations can affect the event relationships. These relationships can vary in nature, ranging from one event triggering many others to multiple events impacting a single event.

This paper discusses causal event relationships and presents an approach to reveal them on EKGs. The approach leverages domain knowledge to identify the object types impacting event relationships. Using this information, the approach constructs the EKG which reveals the causal relation between events correlated to the identified objects. Finally, the nodes and relationships in the resulting EKG can be aggregated to discover a multi-entity Directly-Follows Graph (DFG) [12] representing the underlying system.

The rest of the paper is organized as follows. Section 2 introduces the main EKGs' concepts. Section 3 motivates the necessity of revealing causal event relationships through two case studies and the current state of the art. Section 4 presents the approach for revealing the causal relationships on EKGs. Section 5 discusses and applies the proposed approach in the two case studies. Finally, Sect. 6 concludes the paper by discussing the results, and touches upon future directions.

2 Background

An EKG is built on the concepts of events, entities (i.e., objects), and relations, which are interconnected to represent the analyzed system [12]. It is a labeled property graph with a limited set of node and relationship labels. In an EKG, event nodes store at least the *activity* name and its *timestamp*, and entities store at least a property defining its *type*. Event-to-event relations are defined via the directly-follows relationship, while, event-to-entity relations are defined via the correlation relationship. Formally, given the set Λ of labels, and the set *Attr* of property names over a value domain Val, an EKG is defined as follows.

Definition 1 (EKG). *An EKG is a graph $G = (N, R, \lambda, \#)$ where N is a set of nodes, $R \subseteq N \times N$ is a set of relationships, $\lambda : N \cup R \to \Lambda$ is a function assigning a label to nodes and relationships, and $\# : (N \cup R) \times Attr \nrightarrow Val$ is a partial function assigning properties (attribute-value pairs) to nodes and relationships.*

We adopt the notation $n.a$ as shorthand for $\#(n, a)$. Given an EKG, we distinguish two node sets, $N = N^{Event} \cup N^{Ent}$ where N^{Event} and N^{Ent} are

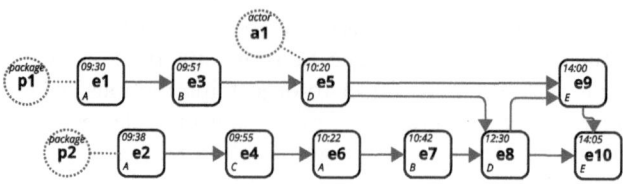

Fig. 1. EKG example

respectively the set of event and entity nodes. Similarly, we distinguish two sets of relations, $R \subseteq R^{corr} \cup R^{df}$, where $R^{corr} = \{r : \lambda(r) = corr\} \subseteq N^{Event} \times N^{Ent}$ is the set of correlations between events and entities, and $R^{df} = \{r : \lambda(r) = df\} \subseteq N^{Event} \times N^{Event}$ is the set of directly-follows relationships. For the sake of simplicity, we say that $r = (e, a) \in R^{corr}$ if $a \in e.\mathcal{A}$; $(e, A) \in R^{corr}$ to mean that $(e, a') \in R^{corr}$, $\forall a' \in A$ with $a'.type = \mathcal{A}$; and $r = (e_i, e_j) \in R^{df}$ with respect to a (we write $r \in R_a^{df} \subseteq R^{df}$ for convenience) if $(e_i, a), (e_j, a) \in R^{corr} \land e_i.time < e_j.time \land (\nexists e : (e, a) \in R^{corr} \land e_i.time < e.time < e_j.time)$.

Figure 1 shows an EKG example. Events are represented with rectangles; entities as circles; and correlation and directly-follows relationships as dashed and solid edges. For convention, the correlations are depicted only between an entity and the first event in time correlated to it, and directly-follows relationships over a specific entity are colored uniquely. For example, the relations in R_{a1}^{df} form the trace of events $\langle e_5, e_8, e_9, e_{10} \rangle$. EKGs allow for their manipulation and navigation through queries, facilitating the extraction of desired insights. Among the other manipulations, *aggregation* enables grouping multiple nodes and relations sharing common properties [11]. This produces a summarized view of event data therefore resulting essential to construct a multi-entity DFG, that stores in each directly-follows relationship the corresponding entity type.

3   Motivation

This section presents two case studies exhibiting collaborative patterns [16], showing the need to represent causal event relationships. Following this, current research relevant to this topic is reviewed.

3.1   Case Studies

The first collaborative scenario represents an order-handling process. It has been synthetically generated and keeps track of the ordering procedures in which each order can be composed of several items. The system receives an order, breaks it down into individual items, and prepares them for packing and shipping. Therefore, each order hierarchically involves several sub-processes for each item. An excerpt of the event log of the order-handling system is depicted in Fig. 2. Here the log stores as entity type the order identifier, i.e., *order*, and the item identifier, i.e., *item*, composing an order. Constructing an EKG from this log would enable

(a)

e_id	activity	time	order	item
e1	receive order	21:32:23	O1	⊥
e2	start order	21:42:23	O1	⊥
e3	picking item	21:47:34	O1	i1
e4	picking item	21:47:45	O1	i2
e5	picking item	21:47:49	O1	i3
e6	out-of-stock	21:49:49	O1	i3
e7	item available	21:57:34	O1	i1
e8	item available	21:57:45	O1	i2
e9	picking completed	22:01:18	O1	i1
e10	picking completed	22:01:50	O1	i2
e11	item available	13:02:00	O1	i3
e12	picking item	13:05:04	O1	i3
e13	item available	13:09:28	O1	i3
e14	picking completed	13:14:51	O1	i3
e15	create pack	13:25:31	O1	⊥
e16	ship order	13:32:31	O1	⊥

(b)

e_id	activity	time	msg	robot
e1	takeoff	15:33:22	⊥	drone
e2	explore	15:33:25	⊥	drone
e3	weed_found	15:34:45	⊥	drone
e4	weed_position!	15:34:50	wp_1	drone
e5	weed_position?	15:35:06	wp_1	tractor_1
e6	weed_position?	15:35:07	wp_1	tractor_2
e7	tractor_position!	15:35:31	tp_2	tractor_1
e8	tractor_position?	15:35:32	tp_2	drone

Fig. 2. Excerpt of order-handling (a) and robotic system (b) event logs

the visualization of distinct processes for each order and item. Focusing on the *order* entity type, inferring the directly-follows relationships only based on order identifier and the time would create a trace like $\langle e_1, e_2, e_3, e_4, e_5, \ldots, e_{15}, e_{16} \rangle$. This implies that the activities of $O1$, but correlated to different items, would be related via a directly-follow relationship, as in the case of e_3 and e_4. However, since each item follows a unique process, the order process flow should depict a partial ordering of events. Therefore, the actual order process should start by initializing the order with $\langle e_1, e_2 \rangle$, then it triggers the item flows, for instance for item $i1$ it performs $\langle e_3, e_7, e_9 \rangle$, and concludes the order shipment with $\langle e_{15}, e_{16} \rangle$. Notably, this scenario also serves as a running example throughout this paper.

The second collaborative scenario is from the robotic domain [7]. The scenario consists of one drone and two tractors cooperating to identify and remove weed grass in farmland. The system workflow relies on the direct interaction among the robots via messages-exchange. Specifically, the drone identifies weed grass areas and broadcasts their location to the tractors. Tractors share their positions back, and the drone notifies the nearest one to cut the weed grass. An excerpt of the event log of the robotic system is depicted in Fig. 2. Here the log stores as entity types the robot identifier, i.e., *robot*, and the message identifier, i.e., *msg*, generated during robots' interaction. Constructing an EKG from this log would enable the visualization of distinct processes for each robot and each message flow. Focusing on the *msg* entity type, inferring the directly-follows relationships solely based on the message identifier and the time would lead to a trace like $\langle e_4, e_5, e_6 \rangle$. This implies that the message-sending event of the *drone* directly-follows the message-receiving event of *tractor_ 1*, which in turn directly-follows the message-receiving event of *tractor_ 2*. However, this sequence does not accurately reflect the actual system behavior. Since the drone sends a broadcast message, the trace of the entity wp_1 should reflect the partial order among events where the message-sending event of the *drone* directly-follows both message-receiving events, i.e., $\langle e_4, e_5 \rangle$ and $\langle e_4, e_6 \rangle$.

3.2 State of the Art

To discover the causal relationship between two events, i.e., when one event occurs as a result of another [10], it is important to consider the concept of partial ordering. This concept implies that when two events are causally unrelated, their chronological order can be disregarded, and a partial ordering can be used instead [1]. The partial order concept has been investigated with traditional process mining techniques to depict causal relationships between events [15]. With the advent of OCPM, a partial order of events has been obtained by inferring directly-follow relationships based on the object shared between two sequential events [3]. Thus, for each object, the corresponding trace represents a total order of events [12]. However, depending on the requirements and characteristics of different scenarios, these approaches may lead to incorrect and misleading connections. Differently from these approaches and in line with the idea of depicting one-to-many and many-to-one relationships among events, causal event models based on object types that can trigger different object types have been investigated in [20,21]. The authors introduce and define the Causal Event Graph (CEG) data structure. This structure, along with its aggregated version, represents event causalities through many-to-many relationships tied to the corresponding objects. However, the CEG data structure only models events and excludes objects and their relationships.

Instead, considering the characteristics of the case studies, the literature proposes traditional process mining techniques to handle the hierarchical dependency between processes and message interactions. One can refer to approaches for discovering multiple instance subprocesses [6,22], or for the discovery of collaborative systems [8,17], as well as agent system mining approaches [19]. However, these approaches are purpose-specific and not suited for object-centric event logs. To address this limitation, we propose the use of EKGs to reveal causal event relationships in terms of causality, and related object types.

4   Approach

This section presents an approach for creating an EKG that reveals the causal relationship between events related to multiple interrelated objects. Specifically, we define when two events are in a causal relationship over two entities. Moreover, we extend EKG creation guidelines presented in [12] to infer the causal relationship and avoid the wrongly inferred directly-follows relationships. Finally, we applied existing aggregation operations to retrieve causal activity relationships.

4.1   Defining Causal Event Relationship

To reveal causal relationships between events, we start from an EKG with two entity types in a one-to-many relation, we call *trigger* the entity with cardinality 1 and *target* the entity with cardinality N. In a nutshell, two events in an EKG are in a causal relationship if they are correlated to the same entity of the trigger type and to different entities of the target type. Moreover, there must not exist a third event that happens in between the first two events, and that either is correlated to the same entities of one of them.

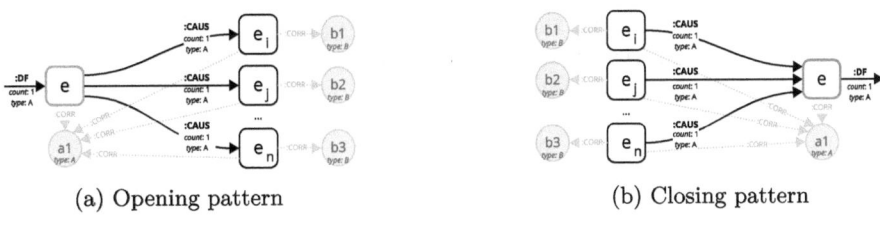

(a) Opening pattern   (b) Closing pattern

Fig. 3. Causal Event Relationships

Definition 2 (Causal relationship). *Let $G = (N, R, \lambda, \#)$ be an EKG, $\mathcal{A}$ and $\mathcal{B}$ two entity types in a one-to-many relation, e and e_i two events, a and b two entities respectively of type $\mathcal{A}$ and $\mathcal{B}$. We say that $r = (e, e_i)$ with $\lambda(r) =$ "causal" is a causal relation over a, b if the following hold:*

- *$(e, a), (e_i, a) \in R^{corr} \wedge (e_i, b) \in R^{corr}$; and*
- *$(e, B') \in R^{corr}$ with $(b \in B' \wedge B' \neq \{b\}) \vee B' = \emptyset$; and*
- *$\nexists\ e_j : (e_j, a), (e_j, b) \in R^{corr} \wedge (e.time < e_j.time < e_i.time \vee e_i.time < e_j.time < e.time)$.*

We call $R_{a,B'}^{caus}$ the set of all causal relationships over an entity a of type $\mathcal{A}$ and the set B' of entities of type $\mathcal{B}$. This set of causal relationships creates two kinds of patterns, namely *opening* and *closing* patterns. An **opening pattern** consists of a node, named *opening*, with outgoing causal relationships (Fig. 3a); a **closing pattern** consists of a node, named *closing* with incoming causal relationships (Fig. 3b). Following, we provide a formal definition of opening and closing nodes.

Definition 3 (Opening and closing nodes). *Let $G = (N, R, \lambda, \#)$ be an EKG, $e \in N^{Event}$ an event node and a and entity node of type $\mathcal{A}$ such that $(e, a) \in R^{corr}$, B' a set of entities of type $\mathcal{B}$, and $R_{a,B'}^{caus}$ the set of all causal relationships over a and B', we call e:*

- *an opening node if either $\exists\ e_i, e_j \in N^{Event} : (e, e_i) \in R_{a,B'}^{caus} \wedge (e, e_j) \in R_{a,B'}^{caus}$ or $(\exists\ e_i \in N^{Event} : (e, e_i) \in R_{a,B'}^{caus}) \wedge (\nexists\ e_k \in N^{Event} : (e_k, e_i) \in R_{a,B'}^{caus})$*
- *a closing node if either $\exists\ e_i, e_j \in N^{Event} : (e_i, e) \in R_{a,B'}^{caus} \wedge (e_j, e) \in R_{a,B'}^{caus}$ or $(\exists\ e_i \in N^{Event} : (e_i, e) \in R_{a,B'}^{caus}) \wedge (\nexists\ e_k \in N^{Event} : (e_i, e_k) \in R_{a,B'}^{caus})$*

Moreover, opening and closing nodes are identified by property rel i.e., $e.rel =$ "opening" and $e.rel =$ "closing" respectively.

4.2 Constructing the EKG

Following, we present the approach for revealing causal relationships in an EKG. Let $G = (N, R, \lambda, \#)$ be an EKG, a be a trigger entity of $\mathcal{A}$ type, and $\mathcal{B}$ a target entity type. The approach consists of applying the following steps for each trigger entity of type $\mathcal{A}$. First, we *combine traces* of events correlated to trigger and target entities. Then, we *reveal opening and closing patterns*. Finally, we *infer directly-follows relationships*.

Combine Traces. To identify the opening and closing patterns for a trigger entity a, we need to retrieve from the graph the set of traces by looking at events correlated with both a and the set of target entities. The function in Algorithm 1 represents the proposed step. It defines an empty dictionary E_a for containing the traces; the set E' of events correlated to a; and the set B' of values for the property $e.\mathcal{B}$ (lines 2 to 4). Then, the function cycles the elements of E' and B' to populate the dictionary E_a that will match each entity of B' with the set of events of E' correlated to that entity (lines 5 to 11).

Algorithm 1. Combine Traces

```
1:  function COMBINE(a)
2:      E_a ← [][]
3:      E' ← {e : (e, a) ∈ R^corr}
4:      B' ← {e.B : e ∈ E'}
5:      for e ∈ E' do
6:          for b ∈ B' do
7:              if e.B = b then
8:                  E_a[b] ← E_a[b] ∪ {e}
9:              end if
10:         end for
11:     end for
12:     return E_a
13: end function
```

Algorithm 2. Reveal opening and closing Patterns

```
1:  Input: E_a
2:  first = head(E_a)
3:  remaining = E_a \ {first}
4:  for rel ∈ {"opening", "closing"} do
5:      first' = FILTER(first, remaining, rel)
6:      e_c = IDENTIFY(first', rel)
7:      REVEAL(e_c, rel)
8:  end for
9:  function FILTER(tr, remaining, relation)
10:     if relation = "opening" then
11:         tr' ← {e ∈ tr : ∄ e_r ∈ remaining s.t. e.time < e_r.time}
12:     else if relation = "closing" then
13:         tr' ← {e ∈ tr : ∄ e_r ∈ remaining s.t. e.time > e_r.time}
14:     end if
15:     return tr'
16: end function
17: function IDENTIFY(tr, relation)
18:     e_c ← null
19:     if relation = "opening" then
20:         e_c ← e ∈ tr : ∄ e'' ∈ tr s.t. e''.time > e.time
21:     else if relation = "closing" then
22:         e_c ← e ∈ tr : ∄ e'' ∈ tr s.t. e''.time < e.time
23:     end if
24:     e_c.rel = relation
25:     return e_c
26: end function
27: function REVEAL(e_c, remaining, relation)
28:     r ← null
29:     if relation = "opening" then
30:         for tr ∈ remaining do
31:             e_r ← e ∈ tr : ∄ e'' ∈ tr s.t. e''.time < e.time
32:             r ← (e_c, e_r)
33:         end for
34:     else if relation = "closing" then
35:         for tr ∈ remaining do
36:             e_r ← e ∈ tr : ∄ e'' ∈ tr s.t. e''.time > e.time
37:             r ← (e_r, e_c)
38:         end for
39:     end if
40:     R_{a,B'}^{caus} ← R_{a,B'}^{caus} ∪ {r}
41: end function
```

Reveal Opening and Closing Patterns. To reveal opening and closing patterns, we use the set of combined traces E_a for the a entity. We consider the *relation* variable that indicates whether we are looking for an *opening* or a *closing*. We extract $first = head(E_a)$ where function $head()$ returns the trace with the event occurring for first in all events of E_a, and the set $remaining = tail(E_a)$ as the set of other traces except for the first one. The opening and closing pattern identification follows a similar path composed of three main steps: (*i*) filter, (*ii*) identify, and (*iii*) reveal. Algorithm 2 depicts the functions to reveal opening and closing patterns. Starting from the FILTER function, it retrieves events from the *first* trace where their timestamps are lower than those in the events of the *remaining* traces (if looking for an opening pattern) or higher than those in remaining events (if looking for a closing pattern) (lines 10 to 14). This function results in the $first'$ set of events, used to identify the opening or closing nodes.

The IDENTIFY function retrieves the node e_c from $first'$ as the one with a higher timestamp (opening) (line 20) or the one with a lower timestamp (closing) (line 22). Finally, it marks the identified node with the corresponding relation (line 24). Finally, the REVEAL function uses the identified node e_c and the set *remaining* to create a causal relationship. For each trace in *remaining*, it gets the event with a lower timestamp (opening) (line 31) or the event with a higher timestamp (closing) (line 36) and creates a causal relationship (lines 32 and 37), via r such that it stores in the rel property, the *causal* value. The revealed causal relation is then added to $R_{a,B'}^{caus}$ to include in the relations of the EKG (line 40).

Infer Directly-Follows Relationship. Once the opening and closing patterns are identified and the causal relationships revealed, the last step is inferring the remaining directly-follows relations. Algorithm 3 describes the final step.

For the a entity and each

Algorithm 3. Infer R^{df}

1: **Input:** a, B'
2: **function** INFER(a, B')
3: $\quad R^{df} \leftarrow R_a^{df} \cup \{R_b^{df}, \forall \, b \in B'\}$
4: $\quad e_{op} \leftarrow e : (e, a) \in R^{corr} \wedge e.rel = \text{``opening''}$
5: $\quad e_{cl} \leftarrow e : (e, a) \in R^{corr} \wedge e.rel = \text{``closing''}$
6: $\quad R^{df} \leftarrow R^{df} \setminus \{(e_{op}, e_{cl})\}$
7: **end function**

---

entity of $\mathcal{B}$ type, a directly-follows relationship of the respective type is inferred following the formalization prescribed by [12] (line 3). Additionally, for the a entity a directly-follows relationship is not inferred between the opening and the closing node (lines 4 to 6). Notably, for each trigger entity, an opening pattern generates as many causal relationships as the number of unique occurrences with the target entity. A closing pattern collects as many causal relationships as the number of unique occurrences with the target entity.

4.3 Revealing Causal Activity Relations

Let $G = (N, R, \lambda, \#)$ be a graph constructed considering causal event relations. To reveal causal activity relations we performed node and relation aggregation as prescribed by the current state-of-the-art [11]. The aggregation operation relies on a generic aggregation function $Agg(class, G) = G^c$ to produce a multi-entity

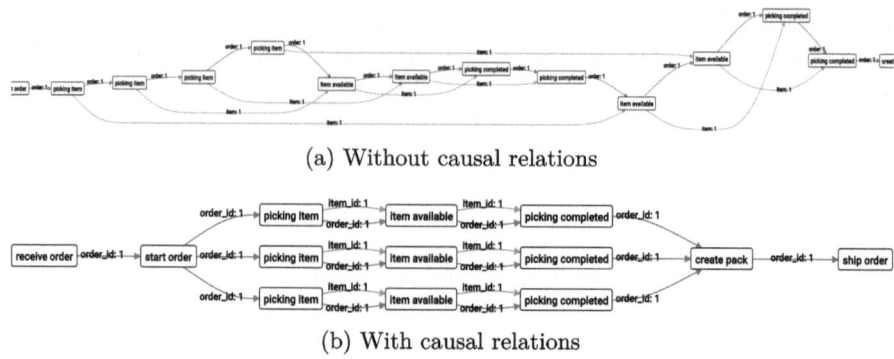

(a) Without causal relations

(b) With causal relations

Fig. 4. EKGs excerpt of the order-handling case study

DFG, following the node aggregation property *class* to create *Class* nodes. Usually, the aggregation property refers to the events *activity* name, but it can also be a combination of properties, such as aggregating event nodes with the same *activity* and *order*. Moreover, the event-to-event relationships are aggregated to derive class-to-class relationships. The *type* of the class-to-class relationship is set based on the event-to-event relationship type, and the node causal *rel* information, i.e., opening or closing, is kept. Additionally, the occurrences of each observed event pair are stored as a relationship property *count*. Therefore, after EKG aggregation, the resulting multi-entity DFG shows class nodes and the relations among them, keeping track of the causal activity relations.

5   Proof of Concept

In this section, we show the proposed approach compared to the standard EKG creation of [12]. The approach has been applied to the case studies presented in Sect. 3 by implementing it as a collection of queries[1] in the *Cypher* language [13], enriched with the trigger and target information selected by the domain expert.

Order-Handling. This case study is characterized by a hierarchical behavior where each order is split into several item lines composing it. Thus, an event produced by an order triggers multiple flows for item preparation. Therefore, the approach has been assessed considering the *order* entity type as the trigger and the *item* as the target entity type. Figure 4 shows an excerpt of the EKGs generated without considering causal relationships (Fig. 4a) and with causal relationships (Fig. 4b). As illustrated in Fig. 4a, the flow of an order entity based on temporal order incorrectly links different *picking item* activities, even if they belong to different items. Additionally, it links an *item available* activity to a *picking completed* activity across different items, as shown by looking both at the *order* and the *item* flow. Differently, Fig. 4b reveals the causal relationships

---

[1] https://bitbucket.org/proslabteam/soup/wiki/CausalRelationships.

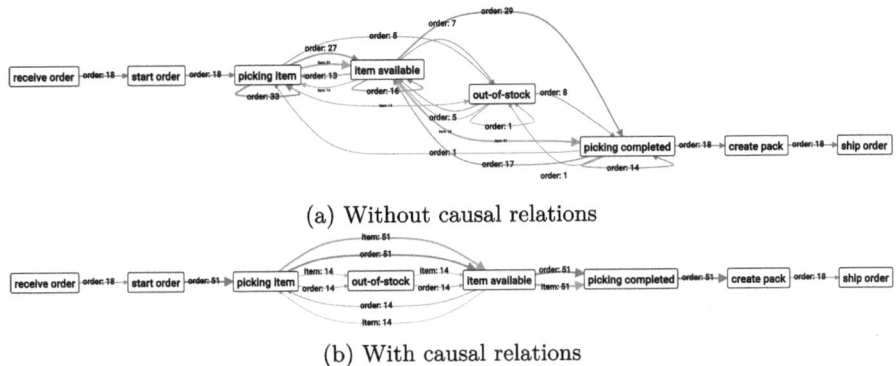

(a) Without causal relations

(b) With causal relations

Fig. 5. Multi-entity DFG of the order-handling case study

between an order and the items composing it. It shows that the start order activity splits its flow into three item lines, each of which independently executes its process. After a *picking completed* items' flows collide into the order *create pack* activity. Performing the aggregation operation for the *activity* property results in Fig. 5. Specifically, Fig. 5a shows the aggregation of the EKG without considering the causal relationships between events correlated to orders and items. As a result, the order flow only reflects the sequence of activities performed on the orders over time. In contrast, Fig. 5b depicts the multi-entity DFG, which incorporates causal relationships. This view captures the entire process: 18 orders are received and started, generating 51 items. Of these, 14 were initially out-of-stock but were later prepared to assemble an order pack and ship the order.

Robotic System. This case study involves direct communication among robots. In a collaborative system with broadcast communication, a single event that generates a message can trigger multiple message-catching events by different participants. Therefore, the *msg* entity type has been identified as the trigger entity, and the *robot* entity type has been identified as the target entity affected by events correlated with a message. Figure 6 shows an excerpt of the EKG constructed using the current state-of-the-art method (Fig. 6a) and the proposed approach (Fig. 6b). This excerpt focuses on the interaction between events from the message and robot perspectives. In Fig. 6a, the *msg* flow is constructed by following the temporal order of events correlated to the same message, leading to a one-to-one relationship between events, where two message-receive events, belonging to different robots, are connected. In contrast, Fig. 6b splits the message flow, creating a one-to-many relationship between a message-sending event and two message-receiving events. The structure of the EKG influences its aggregated version, which is used for system analysis. In this case study, events are aggregated following the activity name and the robot identifier to retrieve the collaboration between robots. However, for the sake of presentation, the result of EKG aggregation is in the online documentation.

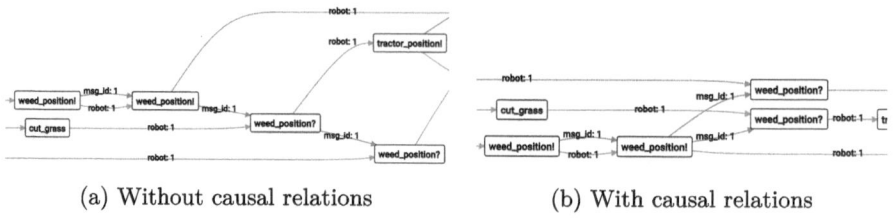

(a) Without causal relations   (b) With causal relations

Fig. 6. EKG excerpt of the robotic case study

Summing up, the generated EKGs demonstrate the potential of the proposed approach through two case studies with different characteristics but exhibiting collaboration patterns. Specifically, the comparison between the EKGs generated with causal relations and those generated with existing approaches highlights the necessity of considering not only one-to-one event relations but also one-to-many relations between events.

6   Concluding Remarks

We presented an approach for revealing causal relationships between events correlated to objects in one-to-many relations. The approach has been assessed on two case studies, showing its effectiveness in revealing causal relationships over an EKG. The approach highlights the limitation of constructing event-to-event relations solely based on the shared entity and the temporal occurrence, emphasizing the necessity of representing the partial order of events from an object-centric perspective. Although it has been applied only to pairs of entity types, the approach can be extended to multiple entity pairs. For instance, an order can be in a one-to-many relation with items in a many-to-one relation with packages, which could be related in a many-to-one fashion to an order.

With this work, we aim to focus on the importance of causal relationships between events when dealing with object-centric event logs in which objects are related among them. We acknowledge that the proposed approach may be limited by the need for domain knowledge to identify which objects are causally related and to determine which entities are the triggers and which are the targets. Nevertheless, domain knowledge is crucial for guiding process mining analysis [9], especially in OCPM, where multiple processes are interrelated [14]. In future work, we intend to deepen the study of causal relationships by including additional case studies where more entities are causally related to each other.

Acknowledgments. This work has been funded by the European Union - NextGenerationEU under the Italian Ministry of University and Research (MUR) National Innovation Ecosystem grant ECS00000041 - VITALITY - CUP J13C22000430001

References

1. Aalst, W.M.P.: Object-centric process mining: dealing with divergence and convergence in event data. In: Ölveczky, P.C., Salaün, G. (eds.) SEFM 2019. LNCS, vol. 11724, pp. 3–25. Springer, Cham (2019). https://doi.org/10.1007/978-3-030-30446-1_1
2. van der Aalst, W.M.P., Carmona, J.: Process Mining Handbook. Springer, Cham (2022)
3. Berti, A., van der Aalst, W.M.P.: Extracting multiple viewpoint models from relational databases. In: Data-Driven Process Discovery and Analysis. LNBIP, vol. 379, pp. 24–51. Springer (2019)
4. Berti, A., van der Aalst, W.M.P.: OC-PM: analyzing object-centric event logs and process models. Int. J. Softw. Tools Technol. Transfer **25**(1), 1–17 (2023)
5. Berti, A., Montali, M., van der Aalst, W.M.P.: Advancements and challenges in object-centric process mining: a systematic literature review. CoRR **abs/2311.08795** (2023)
6. Conforti, R., Dumas, M., García-Bañuelos, L., Rosa, M.L.: BPMN miner: automated discovery of BPMN process models with hierarchical structure. Inf. Syst. **56**, 284–303 (2016)
7. Corradini, F., Pettinari, S., Re, B., Rossi, L., Tiezzi, F.: A methodology for the analysis of robotic systems via process mining. In: Enterprise Design, Operations, and Computing. LNCS, vol. 14367, pp. 117–133. Springer (2023)
8. Corradini, F., Pettinari, S., Re, B., Rossi, L., Tiezzi, F.: A technique for discovering BPMN collaboration diagrams. Softw. Syst. Model. 1–21 (2024)
9. Dixit, P.M., Buijs, J.C.A.M., van der Aalst, W.M.P., Hompes, B.F.A., Buurman, J.: Using domain knowledge to enhance process mining results. In: Data-Driven Process Discovery and Analysis, pp. 76–104. Springer (2017)
10. van Dongen, B.F., Van der Aalst, W.M.: Multi-phase process mining: aggregating instance graphs into EPCS and petri nets. In: PNCWB Workshop, pp. 35–58 (2005)
11. Esser, S., Fahland, D.: Multi-dimensional event data in graph databases. J. Data Semantics **10**(1–2), 109–141 (2021)
12. Fahland, D.: Process mining over multiple behavioral dimensions with event knowledge graphs. In: Process Mining Handbook, vol. 448, pp. 274–319. Springer (2022)
13. Francis, N., et al.: Cypher: an evolving query language for property graphs. In: Management of Data, pp. 1433–1445. ACM (2018)
14. Goossens, A., De Smedt, J., Vanthienen, J., van der Aalst, W.M.P.: Enhancing data-awareness of object-centric event logs. In: Process Mining Workshops, pp. 18–30. Springer (2023)
15. Leemans, S.J.J., van Zelst, S.J., Lu, X.: Partial-order-based process mining: a survey and outlook. Knowl. Inf. Syst. **65**(1), 1–29 (2023)
16. Lonchamp, J.: Process model patterns for collaborative work. In: World Computer Congress-Telecooperation 1998, p. 12 (1998)
17. Peña, L., Andrade, D., Delgado, A., Calegari, D.: An approach for discovering inter-organizational collaborative business processes in BPMN 2.0. In: Process Mining Workshops. LNBIP, vol. 503, pp. 487–498. Springer (2023)
18. Swevels, A., Fahland, D., Montali, M.: Implementing object-centric event data models in event knowledge graphs. In: Process Mining Workshops, LNBIP, vol. 513, pp. 431–443. Springer (2024)
19. Tour, A., Polyvyanyy, A., Kalenkova, A.A., Senderovich, A.: Agent miner: an algorithm for discovering agent systems from event data. In: Business Process Management. LNCS, vol. 14159, pp. 284–302. Springer (2023)

20. Waibel, P., Novak, C., Bala, S., Revoredo, K., Mendling, J.: Analysis of business process batching using causal event models. In: Process Mining Workshops. LNBIP, vol. 406, pp. 17–29. Springer (2020)
21. Waibel, P., Pfahlsberger, L., Revoredo, K., Mendling, J.: Causal process mining from relational databases with domain knowledge. arXiv:2202.08314 (2022)
22. Weber, I., Farshchi, M., Mendling, J., Schneider, J.: Mining processes with multi-instantiation. In: Symposium on Applied Computing, pp. 1231–1237. ACM (2015)

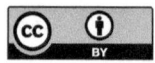

5th International Workshop on Leveraging Machine Learning in Process Mining (ML4PM 2024)

Preface

5th International Workshop on Leveraging Machine Learning in Process Mining (ML4PM 2024)

The integration of Machine Learning (ML) and Process Mining (PM) can allow organizations to anticipate problems, delays or deviations and proactively intervene to improve the efficiency and quality of their processes. Recent academic studies and cutting-edge industrial developments have increasingly underscored the importance of integrating ML techniques to boost the effectiveness of PM methods. By bringing together practitioners and researchers from both fields, the 5th International Workshop on Leveraging Machine Learning in Process Mining aimed to explore recent research advances at the intersection of ML and PM. The broad call for papers invited submissions in various areas, including process modeling, predictive process mining, deep learning techniques and online process mining.

The workshop received nineteen submissions, which underwent a thorough review process involving three to four members of the program committee. Finally, eight papers were accepted for presentation and inclusion in the post-proceedings. A summary of these papers is given below.

The paper by Comuzzi M. et al. addresses the problem of data quality by examining the impact of errors in event log data, particularly problems involving task labels. Specifically, the authors focus on the prediction of the next activity, outcome and completion time.

The paper by Roider J. et al. introduces a method to handle previously unseen categorical values during the training phase of predictive process mining models. The authors explore some enterprise-wide strategies, such as temporary stops or manual intervention, and introduce five technical variants of one-hot encoding designed to handle unseen values without interrupting predictions.

The paper by Wuyts B. et al. addresses the problem of the case-length bias in deep learning models trained for predictive process mining tasks. Longer cases are overrepresented by distorting model training and evaluation. To overcome this problem, the authors introduce a framework to align training and evaluation to real case-length distributions.

The paper by Ueck H. introduces a privacy-preserving framework for publishing event logs that ensure differential privacy for both control flow and case attributes. This addresses a limitation of traditional methods that focus on control flow only.

The paper by [Yuan J. et al.] proposes a novel approach to enhancing predictive process mining approaches by leveraging semantic information extracted from event logs. The authors focus on business object statuses associated with process instances. They adopt large language models to extract this semantic information and apply it to outcome-oriented and next activity prediction tasks.

The paper by Hennig M. C. proposes a novel transformer-based architecture for predictive process mining in IT service management to improve the accuracy of service process performance predictions.

The paper by Yu Y. et al. proposes a novel approach using multivariate time series models to predict direct-follows relationships. Through extensive benchmarking on real-world event logs, the authors find that the model performance varies significantly across processes, emphasizing the importance of selecting a suitable model for accurate forecasting.

The paper by Xian Z. et al. introduces a counterfactual-based method designed to enhance process efficiency by identifying activity transitions that most impact overall trace durations. This approach provides actionable insights for optimizing process flow by enabling targeted interventions.

In addition to these papers, the workshop program included a keynote talk titled "Predictive Process Monitoring: the story so far and trends for the future" by Chiara Ghidini and Massimiliano Ronzani, as well as a technical talk "Process Mining the Scikit-Learn Way: Introducing SkPM" by Sylvio Barbon Junior.

We would like to thank all the authors who submitted papers for publication in this book. We are also grateful to the members of the Program Committee and the external reviewers for their excellent work in reviewing the submitted and revised papers with expertise and patience.

November 2024

Paolo Ceravolo
Sylvio Barbon Junior
Vincenzo Pasquadibisceglie

Organization

Workshop Chairs

Paolo Ceravolo   Università degli Studi di Milano, Italy
Sylvio Barbon Junior   Università degli Studi di Trieste, Italy
Vincenzo Pasquadibisceglie   Università degli Studi di Bari, Italy

Program Committee

Rafael Accorsi   Accenture, Switzerland
Mario Luca Bernardi   University of Sannio, Italy
Marco Comuzzi   Ulsan National Institute of Science and
                                 Technology, South Korea
Carl Corea   University of Koblenz, Germany
Jochen De Weerdt   KU Leuven, Belgium
Shridhar Devamane   Global Academy of Technology, India
Gabriel Marques Tavares   LMU Munich, Germany
Luigi Pontieri   ICAR, National Research Council of Italy
                                 (CNR), Italy
Domenico Potena   Università Politecnica delle Marche, Italy
Rafael Seidi Oyamada   University of Milan, Italy
Emerson Paraiso   Pontificia Universidade Católica do Paraná,
                                 Brazil
Flavia Santoro   UERJ, Brazil
Tijs Slaats   University of Copenhagen, Denmark
Fang Wang   Khalifa University, UAE
Bruno Zarpelao   State University of Londrina, Brazil
Rabia Maqsood   National University of Computer and
                                 Emerging Sciences, Pakistan

On the Impact of Low-Quality Activity Labels in Predictive Process Monitoring

Marco Comuzzi[1(✉)], Sungkyu Kim[1], Jonghyeon Ko[2], Musa Salamov[3], Cinzia Cappiello[3], and Barbara Pernici[3]

[1] Ulsan National Institute of Science and Technology, Ulsan, Korea
{mcomuzzi,kimkangf3}@unist.ac.kr
[2] Jeonju University, Jeonju, Korea
whd1gus2@jj.ac.kr
[3] Politecnico di Milano, Milan, Italy
{musa.salamov,cinzia.cappiello,barbara.pernici}@polimi.it

Abstract. While event log data quality is recognized as a crucial concern in process mining, the impact of event log errors on different types of process mining tasks has remained largely unexplored. This paper aims to fill such a gap by analyzing how various errors affect analysis results. In particular, we aim to assess whether and to what extent different types of errors that impact the quality of activity labels affect the performance of predictive process monitoring models, considering the three main tasks of next activity, outcome, and remaining time prediction, using publicly available and simulated event logs. The results of the experiments are used to extract preliminary insights into the design of data preparation pipelines for predictive process monitoring.

Keywords: data quality · data science pipeline · classification

1 Introduction

Process mining aims to extract insights on business processes using the data in so-called event logs [19]. Event logs collect digital traces of events, capturing the occurrence of process steps. Events may be logged by human actors or information systems used in the execution of the process. For each event, an event log must contain at least an ID of the process execution to which the event belongs, a.k.a. case ID, a label indicating the activity that the event has recorded, and a timestamp. As a (process) data science and analytics discipline, process mining is subject to the tenet of *garbage in, garbage out*: the lower the quality of the

This work has been supported by the PRIN 2022 Project "Discount quality for responsible data science: Human-in-the-Loop for quality data", by the PNRR-PE-AI "FAIR" project funded by the NextGenerationEU program, and by the NRF Korea, Grant Number 2022R1F1A1072843. We thank Federico Toschi from Politecnico di Milano for his support in data profiling and the Apromore Process Mining Academic Alliance for providing log analysis tools.

A. Delgado and T. Slaats (Eds.): ICPM 2024 Workshops, LNBIP 533, pp. 201–213, 2025.
https://doi.org/10.1007/978-3-031-82225-4_15

input event logs, the lower the quality and reliability of the insights that we can extract using process mining [17].

Understanding the effect of errors on the quality of the data analysis results is crucial for designing and improving data science pipelines [3,8]. On the one hand, it can inform the design and configuration of the data-gathering landscape. For instance, information systems and sensors could be configured to avoid practices more likely to lead to high-impact errors during data gathering. On the other hand, it helps designers to prioritize cleaning actions in the input data preparation phase. Data cleaning has a cost, at least in terms of computational time and effort. As such, a trade-off between input data cleaning actions and the expected impact on the data analytics output quality must be found when designing a data science pipeline.

While several research contributions focus on characterizing event log data quality [3,17], the issue of how low-quality logs impact the quality of process mining results has remained largely unexplored. This paper aims to start a research journey to close this gap. Specifically, as far as errors are concerned, we restrict our attention to the ones affecting the activity labels. This is a fundamental attribute of an event log that is crucial for all process mining tasks. As a process mining task, we focus on Predictive Process Monitoring (PPM) [4], a task falling within our realm of expertise that has seen exponentially growing interest from the process mining research community during the past ten years. Thus, our research question is: "How do errors on event log activity labels affect the performance of PPM models?".

To answer the research question, we present and discuss in this paper the results of a comprehensive experiment. To model the errors, we consider the event log imperfection patterns in [17] that target activity labels, i.e., distorted, polluted, homonym, and synonym labels. We consider the established tasks of the next event, outcome, and remaining time prediction as PPM tasks, using state-of-the-art long short-term memory (LSTM) recurring neural networks. As expected, erroneous labels impact the performance of the PPM model. However, the type of errors and some data characteristics may also have an important influence, thus possibly driving the choice of which cleaning operations to prioritize.

The paper is structured as follows. The next section discusses the related work. Section 3 illustrates a general data pipeline design framework. The detailed design of the experiment and the results obtained are presented in Sect. 4 and 5, respectively. Conclusions are drawn in Sect. 6.

2   Related Work

The design of an effective data preparation pipeline for data-centric AI systems mainly consists of techniques for detecting and repairing errors in the input data. Several approaches proposed in the literature aim to support the early stages of the data analysis pipeline, such as data exploration, profiling, and data quality (DQ) assessment [5]. Other approaches also consider the DQ improvement of input data, e.g., exploiting reinforcement learning [1] or leveraging the knowledge of data preparation pipelines performed in the past [11].

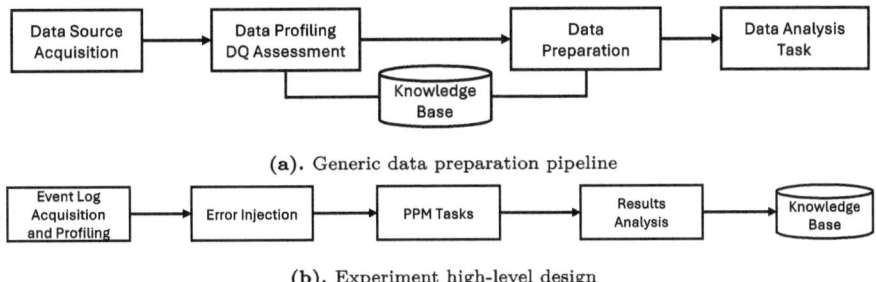

(a). Generic data preparation pipeline

(b). Experiment high-level design

Fig. 1. High-level framework.

Along the direction of the approach presented in this paper, other approaches focus on assessing the effect of DQ errors and DQ improvement techniques, e.g., data cleaning, on the performance of ML applications [6,15]. All these papers conclude that the impact of errors depends on the characteristics of the dataset and the ML model used.

The process mining manifesto [19] assumes that high-quality event logs are the ones that record all the relevant events and in which all the events are well-defined. Bose et al. [2] have further defined the source of low data quality of event logs as missing, incorrect, imprecise, and irrelevant data, which can affect different types of information recorded in an event log. Suriadi et al. [17] have instead developed a bottom-up, pattern-based approach to characterizing the sources of poor event log data quality, proposing 11 imperfection patterns based on the insights of industrial case studies. The methods to identify data quality issues in event logs and address them focus on specific patterns, such as synonymous or polluted labels [14], or more artificial problems on timestamp accuracy and event ordering [16]. While the event log preparation phase is usually included in process mining methodologies and deemed crucial to obtain high-quality results [20], systematic approaches to this phase are missing and, in our humble view, under-investigated in the literature.

3   High-Level Framework

A typical data preparation pipeline for data analytics is shown in Fig. 1a. After having acquired the data and before the data analysis task is performed, the DQ of the data is assessed and possibly improved in the data preparation phase. Both central phases rely on a Knowledge Base recording knowledge about the type of errors that are found, or could potentially be found, in the data and possible ways to fix them.

The experiment that we present in this paper (see Fig. 1b) focuses on extracting insights for such a knowledge base, considering PPM as the Data Analysis Task. As a first step, we acquired five different data sources (event logs) and performed some general data profiling. Then, for each of the sources, we systematically introduced imperfections in the activity labels, creating new datasets

Table 1. Event logs used in the experiment.

Log	Events	Act. Labels	Traces	Avg. case durat.
BPIC11	29004	186	1026	8.64 m
BPIC15	33574	281	696	3.16 m
Credit	63980	12	5000	2.05 h
Pub	66524	12	5000	1.47 w
Justice	669693	1141	24465	18.9 m

to be analyzed. For each of these datasets, we created predictors for the three PPM tasks and tested them using a test set based on clean data (traces from the original dataset). The goal of this phase is to gather evidence on how much building a model with data containing imperfections impacts future predictions on cleaned data. In other words, we follow the principle that it is important to obtain predictive models that are accurate on the correct reality of process execution, as captured by the clean traces. The results obtained are analyzed to obtain preliminary insights regarding the design of data preparation pipelines for the PPM task in process mining.

4   Experiment Design

4.1   Event Log Acquisition and Error Injection

Table 1 lists the event logs considered in the experiments. The BPIC11 and BPIC15 are sets of event logs made available by the Business Process Intelligence Challenge (BPIC) in 2011 and 2015, respectively (the reduced logs from [18] have been considered in the analyses). For each set of logs, we use the one labeled as number one. These logs have been chosen because they are widely used in the literature and have outcome labels. We also consider two synthetic logs (Pub and Credit) used in previous research [10] and for which we can control the error injection of homonymous and synonymous labels. Note that no outcome labels are defined for these synthetic logs. Finally, we acquired an event log about judicial cases execution in an Italian court (dataset "Justice" in Table 1), which has both cleaned labels (standardized event codes) and polluted labels (event codes polluted by case-level attributes and resource information) [13]. This log allows comparing the impact on the PPM performance of training with cleaned and polluted labels (without the need to inject artificial errors).

We model the errors that can affect the activity labels based on the event log imperfection patterns defined by Suriadi et al. [17]. Note that the error injection process is supported by the scripts implementing the FLAWD language publicly available.[1] Among the 11 imperfection patterns, we consider the four ones that directly affect categorical labels in an event log:

---

[1] https://github.com/jonghyeonk/FLAWD.

Distorted Labels (DIST). This pattern refers to the existence of two or more values of an activity label that, while not an exact match, have strong similarities syntactically and semantically. In the experiments, we distort activity labels by randomly introducing one of five possible types of typos.[2]

Polluted Labels. This pattern refers to a situation where the values assumed by an attribute are structurally the same, yet they are distinct due to differences in the values that further qualify the meaning of the value. We distinguish two types of polluted labels: a) *non-random* (POL-NORND), when pollution is performed systematically by attaching to the activity label the resource label of the same event and b) *random* (POL-RND) when, additionally, a randomly generated string is attached to the combination of the activity and the resource label.

Homonymous Labels (HOM). This pattern describes a situation where an activity is repeated multiple times in a log to refer to two or more distinct process steps. Given the domain-specific nature of this error, we consider it only for the synthetic datasets. In both the Pub and Credit datasets, we created four homonym labels, each of which can be used to substitute two or three activity labels in the original dataset.

Synonymous Labels (SYN). This pattern refers to a situation where a group of activity labels are syntactically different but semantically equivalent. Like HOM, we consider this error type only for the synthetic datasets. For each activity label, we created from one up to three synonym labels.

Table 2. Number of distinct activity labels for each dataset per error type (avg. of 8 training datasets, rounded to the unit) for $X \in \{0.1, 0.2, 0.3, 0.4, 0.5\}$.

Log	Error Type	0.1	0.2	0.3	0.4	0.5
BPIC11	DIST	1894	3214	4387	5416	6372
	POL-RND	2571	4958	7344	9730	12115
	POL-NORND	392	443	469	484	495
BPIC15	DIST	2344	4080	5624	7027	8318
	POL-RND	2948	5626	8304	10981	13659
	POL-NORND	906	1114	1251	1352	1441
Credit	DIST	1854	2874	3696	4369	4962
	POL-RND	5144	10277	15410	20543	25676
	POL-NORND	59	59	59	59	59
	HOM	16	16	16	16	16
	SYN	33	33	33	33	33
Pub	DIST	1844	2814	3594	4231	4781
	POL-RND	5326	10640	15954	21268	26582
	POL-NORND	52	52	52	52	52
	HOM	15	15	15	15	15
	SYN	33	33	33	33	33

---

[2] deleting a character, inserting a random character, swapping two characters randomly chosen, substituting a character with one randomly chosen from the ones close to it on a keyboard, changing a lowercase character to uppercase or vice versa.

Each pattern is injected randomly in an event log until a given ratio X of events (rows) in it have been affected by an error, with $X \in \{0.1, 0.2, 0.3, 0.4, 0.5\}$ (that is, we consider an error rate of the events in a log varying from 10% to 50%). For instance, for the HOM and SYN error types, $X = 0.1$ means that in 10% of the events of a log, one activity label is substituted by its homonym and one of its synonyms, respectively. To be able to assess the impact of individual patterns, logs are injected with one individual pattern at a time.

As a result of the error injection process, new activity labels appear in an event log. Table 2 shows the total number of activity labels (that is, the original ones, plus the ones generated by the error injection process) in the logs for different values of the error ratio X. Note that, because the injection process involves randomness, we generated 8 different datasets per error type-ratio combination. The results shown in Sect. 5 refer to averages obtained across these 8 randomly generated datasets for a given error type and error ratio. It must also be noted that the number of new labels introduced by the error injection process strongly depends on the type of injected error and it does not follow directly the error ratio X. For errors characterized by randomness (DIST, POL-NORND), the number of activity labels increases with the error rate, whereas the other types of errors introduce only a fixed number of new activity labels. The DIST error type introduces fewer new activity labels than POL-RND because (i) the classifiers are not case sensitive, so changing the case of characters in a label (i.e. one of the possible typos) does not introduce new labels, and (ii) some of the other simulated typos may yield the same erroneous activity label, e.g., when by chance the same character is deleted in more than one occurrence of the same activity label.

In the experiments, we considered both a *random* and a *temporal* train/test set split. In the random split, we randomly split the traces in the original dataset into train/test sets with 80%/20% ratio. In temporal split, the earliest 80% of the traces in a log constitute the train set and the remaining 20% the test set. We anticipate here that, unless specified, the results obtained with these two types of splits do not differ significantly.

The experiment for the dataset for the Justice datasets incorporates some specific adjustments tailored to the unique characteristics of the dataset. First, the stakeholders who provided the dataset wanted us to focus on the case remaining time prediction PPM task. The log contains 24,465 finished cases starting from January 2017 to March 2023. Several incomplete cases start earlier than 2017, but they are kept in the training and test sets to maintain authenticity. The dataset is split based on the cut-off date of January 1, 2020. The test dataset includes only cases active after this date, while the remaining cases are used for the training set. This results in an approximate split of 80% for training and 20% for testing. As far as the error rate is concerned, the number of unique activity labels for which there is also a polluted value is 68 out of 1,141 activity labels.

4.2   Predictive Models

To keep the focus on the event log errors impact, we consider relatively simple LSTM learning models, which have proved effective in PPM tasks [12], with reasonable hyperparameter values. For all PPM tasks, we used a LSTM model with two layers of 128 nodes, trained using the ADAM optimizer with learning rate 0.001 and 300 epochs with 20% of the training set used for validation, and early stopping when, after 100 epochs, the loss function does not decrease for 10 straight epochs. Note that the activity label vocabulary is built using both the training and the validation set. For the classification problems, we consider a batch size of 16 and use the cross-entropy loss for the next activity task and the binary cross-entropy loss combined with sigmoid layer for the outcome prediction task. The F1-score is considered as evaluation metric (note that AUC could not be used in this case because of unseen labels in the test sets). For the remaining time prediction, we consider a batch size of 32, the mean square error (MSE) loss function with early stopping, and the mean absolute error (MAE) serves as the evaluation metric. The predictive models and the error-injected datasets (excluding the private Justice dataset) used in the experiments are publicly available.[3]

As far as feature engineering and encoding are concerned, we generated features using the (categorical) activity and resource attributes, and two features derived from the event timestamp: time since the start of the case (TSSC) and time since the previous event (TSP). The activity labels are encoded into a 32-dimensional feature vector using an embedding layer with the stochastic gradient descent. The resource attribute is one-hot encoded and time features are standardized to handle categorical data effectively. For sequence encoding, we used prefixes padded as necessary to handle varying sequence lengths [12].

5   Results and Discussion

5.1   Experimental Results

For brevity, we only present a set of representative results for each PPM task. The next activity prediction PPM task is the one that is affected the most by the errors, which could have been expected since the errors modify the errors of the classification task.

Figure 2a and 2b show the value of the F1-score of the next activity prediction task in the real-world datasets BPIC11 and BPIC15, respectively. The performance of the next activity appears to degrade linearly with the ratio of errors injected. At an error ratio of 30%, the performance is at least 30% of the one achieved using the clean training set. The performance degradation also depends on the type of errors that are introduced. The performance degradation associated with the POL-NORND errors is less than the one introduced by the DIST errors, which is less than the one introduced by the POL-RND. This can be explained by considering the number of new activity labels introduced by each type of error (see Table 2): the higher the number of new activity labels introduced by errors, the higher the performance degradation. This result is aligned with the literature on open set recognition in multi-class classification [7], which

---

[3] https://github.com/brucks1217/Imperfection-pattern.

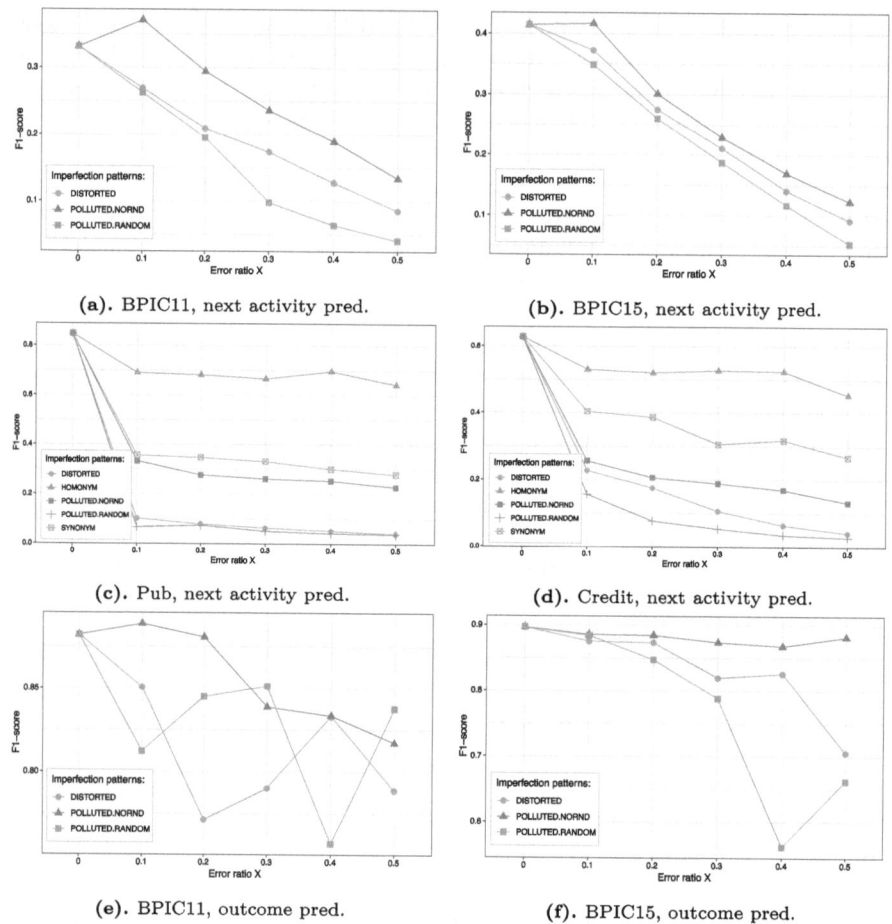

Fig. 2. Next activity and outcome prediction performance (F1-score) for different error ratios X.

has recognized that random noise on labels can dramatically decrease the classifier performance. Note that the results shown in Fig. 2 consider a random training/test split. When using the temporal split for next activity prediction, the performance obtained on the full dataset is about one order of magnitude lower. This is due to the fact that, towards the end of the timeline, both datasets contain several cases that remain incomplete. Using the temporal split, we obtained a performance similar to the random split when deleting 30% of the cases starting last in the original logs.

The results on the synthetic datasets Pub and Credit, shown respectively in Fig. 2c and 2d, confirm the results obtained on the real-world datasets for the POL-NORND, DIST and POL-RND types of errors, and they allow us to discuss the effect on the performance of the HOM and SYN errors. The performance degradation associated with the HOM errors is limited. The SYN errors are associated with higher performance degradation, albeit lower than the label polluting/distorting errors discussed earlier. Again, this result can be explained by referring to the number of activity labels introduced (see Table 2). The HOM type of error type introduces only a few new activity labels, while the SYN error type introduces about half the number of new labels introduced by the POL-NORND type of error.

The classification performance (F1-score) of outcome predictors is shown in Fig. 2e and 2f. We draw two insights from the results shown in the figure: (i) while errors induce a performance degradation, this remains limited compared to the next activity prediction task, and (ii) while it appears like the non-random errors (POL-NORND) are associated with lower performance degradation, the performance degradation patterns associated with different error types are not clearly discernible as in the next activity prediction task. Both insights can be explained by the nature of the outcome prediction PPM task, whereby the importance of the activity labels in the classifier learning process may be limited due to several factors, such as the outcome labels depending on factors not captured in the event log or other features derived from case-level attributes being highly correlated with the outcome label values. Similar considerations on the limited importance of features derived from event-level attributes in outcome prediction have been drawn by [9] studying the impact of features derived from event resource labels.

Figure 3 shows, as a representative example, the results obtained for the BPIC11 dataset for remaining time predictions. In Fig. 3a, we see the case durations in this log have a significant variability, as captured by a median of 1.84 months with some cases spanning even the whole event log timeframe (3.13 yrs). We can notice that differences in the MAE with different types of imperfections remain limited (within 10% of the MAE for the clean training set). A possible explanation is that the activity labels for remaining time predictions are less important than the event time series in the prediction model. In general, as shown in Fig. 3b, there is a relatively low variability in the errors. When labels are distorted (DIST), the remaining time predictions are slightly worse than the baseline (around 5% in the worst case). For the POL-NORND error type, the impact of the errors is negligible, which may also be justified by the low number of new labels introduced (cfr. Table 1). For the POL-RND error type, the MAE even slightly improves compared to the baselines. This could be due to the fact that a high number of randomly inserted values changes the world of which the predictor tries to learn a model.

The results for the Justice dataset—not shown in Fig. 2—highlight a clear impact of the errors, with a MAE[4] of 212 days obtained with a clean training set, i.e., using the standardized event codes, and 269 days with the polluted labels. This performance difference between the predictions is remarkable, particularly considering that the unique labels appearing both in the clean and the polluted

---

[4] Note that trials can span several years, so an MAE of a few months may still be acceptable in many decision-making scenarios.

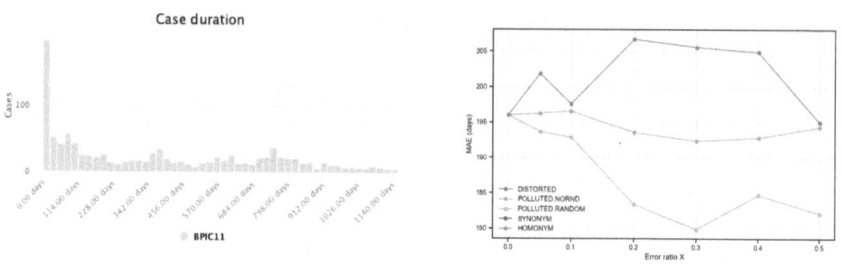

(a). BPIC11 case duration distribution   **(b).** MAE for different values of error ratio X

Fig. 3. BPIC11 log trace durations and test MAE.

datasets are only 68 out of 1,141. It could be explained by considering that, in a long-lived process like trial scheduling and execution, the order of activity labels may still play a key role (as compared to the timestamps series) in the remaining time predictor learning process. Further testing would be needed to understand the learning dynamics with this dataset.

5.2 Discussion

The development of the experiments presented in this paper was driven primarily by the aim of understanding how to design data preparation pipelines for the PPM process mining task. Although the experiment design is subject to limitations (discussed in the next section), based on the results presented in this paper, we argue that the following insights should be considered when designing a data preparation pipeline for activity labels of input datasets for PPM tasks:
(i) Activity label cleaning must be prioritized for next activity prediction, since the impact on the model performance of low-quality activity labels in this task is massive even at low error rates.
(ii) Activity label cleaning is less important for the outcome and remaining time PPM prediction tasks, where the model performance may depend strongly on other contextual factors, such as the nature of outcome labels in the case of outcome prediction or the distribution of timestamps in the remaining time prediction.
(iii) Among the considered imperfection patterns, the POL-RND and DIST bear the highest impact on the performance of PPM models, because they introduce a higher number of activity labels that do not appear in the *clean* event log. Homonym and synonym labels appear to be a less critical quality issue, even in the next activity prediction task.
(iv) Fixing the errors that introduce a higher number of new distinct activity labels in a log should be prioritized over other types of errors that introduce a lower number of new activity labels. Hence, perhaps counter-intuitively, fixing the sources of random errors (e.g., using automated scripts to fix random typos) should be prioritized over fixing the sources of systematic, non-random

errors (e.g., setting up a panel of domain experts to understand how homonymous/synonymous labels could be substituted by their correct values).

5.3   Limitations

The experiments presented in this paper suffer from several limitations. First, while the event logs considered are diverse in terms of the number of variants and activities, we considered a limited set of logs, which could hamper the external validity of the results. While the LSTM model is widely adopted for PPM, we consider only one type of encoding and fixed hyperparameter settings. Note, however, that the objective of the experiments is to compare the impact on the performance of different types of errors, not to optimize the predictive performance of the PPM models. Moreover, injecting errors increases the variability of activity label values, which in turn increases the chance of having activity labels in the (clean) test sets unseen in the training sets. To handle this issue, a common solution that we also applied in this work is to map all the unseen labels to a default value. Other choices would have been possible. For example, in the case of polluted labels, a more refined encoding could try to extract the activity label information from the polluted label. However, we think that such approaches would already require the definition of event log quality improvement methods, which is not the focus of this paper. Finally, as discussed in [21], the train-test split of traces may introduce different types of bias when executed either randomly or accounting for temporal relations. As discussed earlier, we found such a bias in the next activity prediction results for the real-world datasets when using the temporal split.

6   Concluding Remarks

The impact of imperfections in training datasets in PPM has been evaluated in this paper through a set of experiments injecting systematically four types of errors in the logs: distortions, pollutions, synonyms, and homonyms of activity labels. The experiments have been performed on five datasets presenting different characteristics, considering the three main tasks of PPM: next activity, outcome, and remaining time prediction. The results of the experiments show that impacts are diverse and depend on the type of imperfection and the intended prediction. As discussed in the last section, these results open the way to further investigations in the direction of building effective and efficient data preparation pipelines for preparing datasets for high-performing predictive process models.

References

1. Berti-Équille, L.: Active reinforcement learning for data preparation: Learn2Clean with Human-In-The-Loop. In: CIDR 2020 Proceedings (2020). www.cidrdb.org
2. Bose, J.C., Mans, R.S., van der Aalst, W.M.P.: Wanna improve process mining results? It's high time we consider data quality issues seriously. In: IEEE Symposium on Computational Intelligence and Data Mining, pp. 127–134 (2013)

3. Cappiello, C., Comuzzi, M., Plebani, P., Fim, M.: Assessing and improving measurability of process performance indicators based on quality of logs. Inf. Syst. **103**, 101874 (2022)
4. Di Francescomarino, C., Ghidini, C.: Predictive process monitoring. In: Process Mining Handbook, pp. 320–346. Springer, Cham (2022)
5. Ehrlinger, L., Wöß, W.: A survey of data quality measurement and monitoring tools. Front. Big Data **5**, 850611 (2022)
6. Foroni, D., Lissandrini, M., Velegrakis, Y.: Estimating the extent of the effects of data quality through observations. In: ICDE 2021, pp. 1913–1918. IEEE (2021)
7. Geng, C., Huang, S.J., Chen, S.: Recent advances in open set recognition: a survey. IEEE Trans. Pattern Anal. Mach. Intell. **43**(10), 3614–3631 (2020)
8. Ilyas, I.F., Rekatsinas, T.: Machine learning and data cleaning: which serves the other? ACM J. Data Inf. Qual. (JDIQ) **14**(3), 1–11 (2022)
9. Kim, J., Comuzzi, M., Dumas, M., Maggi, F.M., Teinemaa, I.: Encoding resource experience for predictive process monitoring. Decis. Support Syst. **153**, 113669 (2022)
10. Ko, J., Comuzzi, M.: Keeping our rivers clean: information-theoretic online anomaly detection for streaming business process events. Inf. Syst. **104**, 101894 (2022)
11. Mahdavi, M., Abedjan, Z.: Semi-supervised data cleaning with Raha and Baran. In: 11th Conference on Innovative Data Systems Research, CIDR 2021 (2021). www.cidrdb.org
12. Navarin, N., Vincenzi, B., Polato, M., Sperduti, A.: LSTM networks for data-aware remaining time prediction of business process instances. In: 2017 IEEE Symposium Series on Computational Intelligence (SSCI), pp. 1–7. IEEE (2017)
13. Pernici, B., Bono, C.A., Piro, L., Del Treste, M., Vecchi, G.: Improving the analysis of the judiciary performance - the use of data mining techniques to assess the timeliness of civil trials. Int. J. Public Sect. Manag. **37**(1), 59–76 (2024)
14. Sadeghianasl, S., ter Hofstede, A.H., Wynn, M.T., Suriadi, S.: A contextual approach to detecting synonymous and polluted activity labels in process event logs. In: Proc. Intl. Conf. Cooperative Information Systems. pp. 76–94 (2019)
15. Sancricca, C., Cappiello, C.: Supporting the design of data preparation pipelines. In: Proc. SEBD 2022. CEUR Workshop Proceedings, vol. 3194, pp. 149–158. CEUR-WS.org (2022)
16. Schmid, S.J., Moder, L., Hofmann, P., Röglinger, M.: Everything at the proper time: Repairing identical timestamp errors in event logs with generative adversarial networks. Inf. Syst. **118**, 102246 (2023)
17. Suriadi, S., Andrews, R., ter Hofstede, A.H., Wynn, M.T.: Event log imperfection patterns for process mining: towards a systematic approach to cleaning event logs. Inf. Syst. **64**, 132–150 (2017)
18. Teinemaa, I., Dumas, M., Rosa, M.L., Maggi, F.M.: Outcome-oriented predictive process monitoring: review and benchmark. ACM Trans. Knowl. Discov. Data (TKDD) **13**(2), 1–57 (2019)
19. van Der Aalst, W., et al.: Process mining manifesto. In: Business Process Management Workshops: BPM 2011 Workshops, pp. 169–194. Springer (2012)
20. Van Eck, M.L., Lu, X., Leemans, S.J., van der Aalst, W.M.: PM^2: a process mining project methodology. In: Proceedings of CAiSE, pp. 297–313. Springer (2015)
21. Weytjens, H., De Weerdt, J.: Creating unbiased public benchmark datasets with data leakage prevention for predictive process monitoring. In: International Conference on Business Process Management, pp. 18–29. Springer (2021)

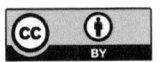

Towards Accurate Predictions in ITSM: A Study on Transformer-Based Predictive Process Monitoring

Marc C. Hennig$^{(\boxtimes)}$ (iD)

University of Applied Sciences Munich, Lothstr. 64, 80335 Munich, Germany
mhennig@hm.edu

Abstract. The accurate prediction of service process performance, particularly in IT service management (ITSM), is critical for adhering to service-level agreements and avoiding associated penalties. However, existing predictive process monitoring solutions, predominantly based on recurrent neural networks, have been found to be inadequate in handling ITSM processes. Notably, the heterogeneity in process artifacts and environments impairs process predictions. This research proposes a novel transformer-based architecture to effectively handle IT service process event logs. By integrating advanced positional encoding techniques and distinguishing between static and dynamic attributes, a novel transformer architecture is evaluated using multiple publicly available ITSM event logs. This architecture demonstrates its potential to deliver more accurate predictions than LSTM models in terms of remaining time predictions. This work provides experimental results into the application of transformer architectures for predictive process monitoring, paving the way for enhanced efficiency in ITSM.

Keywords: predictive process monitoring · remaining time prediction · transformer · GLU · ITSM · SLA

1 Introduction

In today's economy, the success of a service provider is increasingly tied to an organization's ability to provide its processes in time [1]. Ensuring an efficient execution of the underlying service processes is particularly relevant in this regard, as providers are bound by contractual service-level agreements (SLA) [1]. SLAs usually involve severe penalties in case of time or quality-related deviations, and adherence to them is an important performance indicator.

In this setting, service process instances benefit greatly from predictive insights of the expected remaining time to facilitate decision-making and avoid time-related SLA violations. Predictive process monitoring (PPM) has emerged as a tool for forecasting the future states of ongoing process instances [2]. However, IT service management (ITSM) processes, in particular, exhibit an inherent complexity due to heterogeneity in artifacts [3] and process environments [4]. Additionally, their ad-hoc nature and reliance

© The Author(s) 2025
A. Delgado and T. Slaats (Eds.): ICPM 2024 Workshops, LNBIP 533, pp. 214–226, 2025.
https://doi.org/10.1007/978-3-031-82225-4_16

on individual expertise complicate the accurate forecast of process instance runtimes and outcomes, often leading to results that are too inaccurate for practical use [4]. This underscores the need for innovative solutions in this area.

These challenges in ITSM processes have hindered the widespread adoption of PPM. Although many predictive process monitoring architectures have been created [2], only a few have been successfully applied to ITSM event logs. Given this limited application of predictive process monitoring in ITSM, there is a clear need for innovative approaches. This research addresses this need by designing a transformer architecture [5] that can effectively handle complex IT service process event logs. The transformer architecture [5] has replaced commonly used recurrent neural networks (RNN) and their derivatives for many sequence-related tasks [6]. Still, it has yet to gain significant traction in PPM compared to other domains [2]. It is therefore assessed in this work, attempting to answer the following research question: *How can a predictive process monitoring transformer architecture be designed to accommodate the intricacies of IT service processes?*

As part of a research project investigating how PPM can transform ITSM operations, this work's approach consists of three main parts. First, the literature regarding transformers in PPM in terms of their architecture and the different approaches taken is analyzed. Second, a transformer architecture is designed and implemented based on these insights. Finally, the model is applied to event logs from ITSM's incident management, and the results are quantitatively evaluated to assess how techniques new to PPM can be used therein, potentially outperforming other solutions. Due to its relevance for highly operational incident management [4], the focus lies on the remaining time prediction, contributing to a better understanding of transformers in PPM.

2   Research Method

In this work, design science research is applied, as described by [7], as the central framework with the steps outlined in Fig. 1. The research problem is analyzed by reviewing the ongoing research on transformers in PPM and innovations from other domains using transformers that might be transferable to PPM. A transformer architecture is then designed and developed based on the insights from the literature research, the special requirements, and the unique properties of ITSM processes outlined in the previous section. During the architecture development, the focus is explicitly laid on the input preparation and positional encoding in addition to providing a ground-up explanation of the different model components.

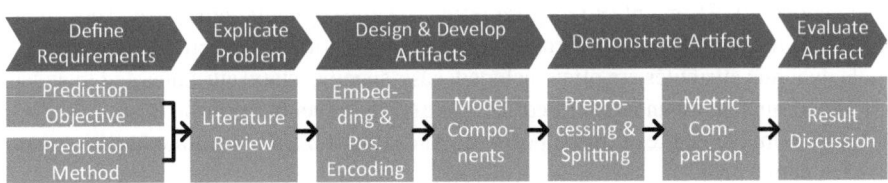

Fig. 1. Design science research framework following [7]

The results are subsequently demonstrated and experimentally evaluated using multiple publicly available event logs from ITSM, focusing specifically on applying a reproducible preprocessing setup using strict temporal splitting [8] to ensure comparable results. The models are trained on the prepared event logs, and their performance is measured using regression metrics appropriate for the remaining time prediction. Finally, the results are compared with baseline solutions to allow an interpretation of the findings and the developed transformer architecture.

3 Research Background

PPM has traditionally depended extensively on RNNs, particularly Long-Short-Term Memory (LSTM) networks, which are commonly used for their capacity to handle sequential data effectively [2, 9]. However, other architectures and use cases have continuously evolved. This study focuses on the usage of transformers in PPM, which is motivated by both theoretical and practical benefits [5]. To achieve this, the existing literature on the application of transformers in PPM is first collected and analyzed. Transferable architectural features from other domains are then identified and contextualized within the findings of prior studies to identify possible research gaps.

3.1 Transformer in Predictive Process Monitoring

Most earlier works in PPM use simpler transformer architectures consisting primarily of single transformer encoders [10, 11] close to the original implementation [5]. The *ProcessTransformer* [10] is particularly notable as it is an often-used baseline model consisting of a transformer encoder and minimal preprocessing. Transformers have diversified in newer research, resorting to more specialized solutions. However, transformer encoders are still popular, while decoders remain a niche choice. Despite their popularity in natural language processing, models like BERT [12] and GPT-2 [13] are not widely used, possibly due to their low performance compared to later solutions [10].

The strategies for attaining improved prediction performances vary widely. Hierarchical architectures, either as a hybrid of RNNs with the transformer's central attention mechanism [15, 16] or stacked attention over different granularities [6], outperformed several earlier solutions. This might be due to their improved ability to capture local process structures and long-range dependencies, which is hypothesized to improve model performance [21]. Additionally, the integration of further attributes might contribute to the performance [22]. While not hierarchical, other approaches have adopted multiple encoders [17], mainly to capture event-specific, dynamic attributes. Thus, these attributes are integrated as concurrent sequences in addition to the activity. Interestingly, while dynamic attributes are often included, case-specific, static attributes and their separate handling remain underexplored. They are often sequentialized and treated similarly to the dynamic attributes despite positive indications for their separate handling from other domains [23].

The next activity (*NA*) classification is the most popular choice regarding the prediction targets with transformers, as seen in Table 1. In contrast, regression problems like the remaining time (*RT*) and next timestamp (*NT*) prediction are far less commonly

Table 1. Overview of the work on PPM and transformers oriented on [2]

Ref	Network Type	Seq. Encoding	Attr. Handling	Pos. Encoding	Target
[14]	Hybrid	BiLSTM + Attention	Dynamic	–	OUT
[11]	Transformer	Decoder	–	Fixed	NA
[15]	Hybrid	LSTM + Attention	–	–	NA, SEQ
[10]	Transformer	Encoder	–	Learned	NA, NT, RT
[13]	Transformer	Decoder (GPT2)	Dynamic	Learned	NA
[12]	Transformer	Encoder (BERT)	–	Learned	NA, OUT
[16]	Hybrid	BiLSTM + Attention	Dynamic	–	NA
[17]	Transformer	Encoder	Dynamic	Fixed	NA, ATTR
[18]	Hybrid	LSTM + Attention	Dynamic	–	NA
[19]	Transformer	Encoder	–	Custom	NA
[6]	Transformer	Encoder	Dynamic	Fixed, Learned	NA, RT
[20]	Transformer	Encoder	Dynamic	Learned	NA, NT, RT

approached. Predicting specific process instance outcomes (*OUT*) or other attributes (*ATTR*) is also less often performed, similar to sequence-to-sequence (*SEQ*) predictions [2]. Various transformer architectures have been developed, with a trend toward multiple attentions for dynamic attributes. This suggests a gap in the current research on investigating the benefits of distinctly integrating static attributes to enhance the prediction performance of PPM models.

3.2 Architectural Features in Transformer Models

Transformers are widely used in other domains, leading to several improvements that could benefit PPM. One key innovation is in positional encodings, where supplementary information beyond the absolute position of an element in a sequence enriches the data. While encoding static context information through additional domain knowledge has been described [19] in PPM, most works use fixed or learned positional encodings, as shown in Table 1. From outside PPM, timestamp encoding seems especially relevant and has succeeded in transformer-based time series predictions [24]. Also, it is currently suspected that relative encodings might outperform commonly used absolute encodings, leading to the development of combinations [25] to mitigate disadvantages.

Another essential aspect is converting transformer layer outputs from two-dimensional matrices into single vectors suitable for downstream prediction tasks. Standard techniques in PPM include average pooling layers [10, 20], weighted summation of outputs [16], and flattening [6]. In natural language processing, hidden states are often extracted based on a special token or the last position [12], but techniques vary widely.

Additionally, the enhanced performance of transformers using gated linear units (GLU) and gated residual networks (GRN) is notable. The *Temporal Fusion Transformer* [23], which employs these techniques to incorporate static attributes and enhance self-regularization, is a well-known example. In other studies, GLUs have also been shown to benefit transformers [26], suggesting their utility for PPM. None of these approaches have been applied to PPM, indicating an actionable research gap.

4   Model Development

Based on the analysis of the related research, it was identified that integration methods for static attributes are missing, especially, and that the use of GLUs and alternative positional embedding methods is under-researched. A transformer-based architecture is developed using these insights, focusing on incorporating static attributes separately from dynamic ones. Static and dynamic attributes can be distinguished with scarce detailed knowledge of the event logs, and this distinction is commonly made in PPM [22]. First, some general design decisions are clarified, and then the implementation of further model parts is detailed. Figure 2 provides a general overview of the architecture.

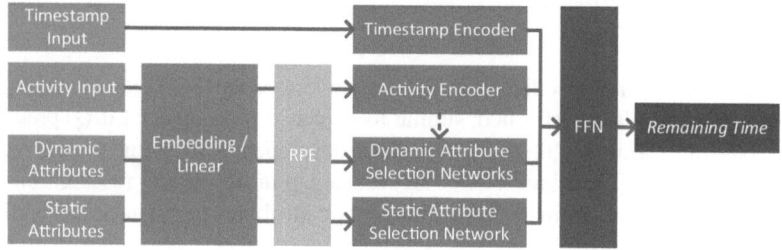

Fig. 2. Overview of the architecture of the developed transformer

4.1   Embedding and Positional Encoding

The input for the transformer varies for the different types of attributes in the datasets and follows a general approach depending on the type, as described below.

Categorical Attributes. Nominal categorical attributes are encoded using learnable embeddings, as is usual with transformers. This balances expressiveness and dimensionality and increases the model's capacity. A single embedding length is used to facilitate handling vector and matrix dimensions throughout the model.

Numerical Attributes. Min-max scaling is applied to all numerical attributes; thus, attributes are scaled linearly using the minimum and maximum derived from the training set. The same approach is used for ordinal categorical attributes, numbered according to their natural order in advance. As numerical attributes cannot be embedded without discretization, a linear projection is applied to the scaled attributes instead to maintain identical dimensions for numerical and categorical attributes across the model.

Unlike RNNs, transformers do not impose positional information on their inputs, so positional encodings are added [5]. This work uses rotary position encoding (RPE), which combines relative and absolute position information and reportedly outperforms other encodings [25].

4.2 Activity and Timestamp Encoder

Activity and timestamps are special event log attributes, as both are central elements of an event log and are handled separately from other event log attributes. A transformer encoder is used to encode both sequences for each of these attributes separately. The activity is embedded and positionally encoded beforehand, while the time features are handled as numerical attributes and concatenated.

Central to the transformer is the attention mechanism which is applied to the input sequences $X = \langle x_1, x_2, \ldots, x_n \rangle$ with x_i commonly being a vector representation of a sequence elements. In this case, X is an embedded sequence of activities. The input to the attention consists of queries in a matrix Q, keys of dimension d_k in a matrix K, and values in a matrix V [5]. In case identical sequences are used as input to the attention, so that $Q = XW_Q$, $K = XW_K$, and $V = XW_V$ with W denoting learned weight matrices, this is known as self-attention. Instances with different query and key matrices are commonly called cross-attention [6]. Multiple attentions are usually applied to the inputs separately and concatenated, leading to multi-head attention [5].

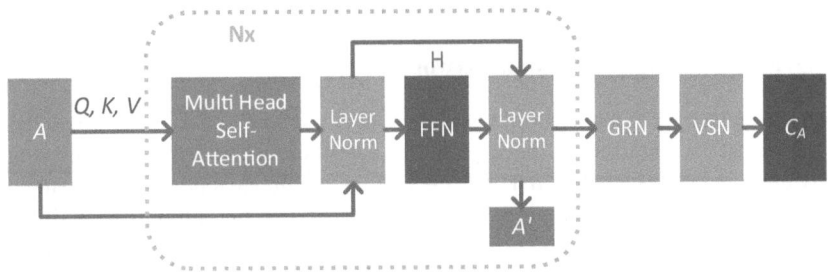

Fig. 3. Activity and timestamp encoder

The outputs of the multi-head attention are subsequently subjected to layer normalization and a position-wise feed-forward network. In addition, residual connections are added so that the encoded sequence X' as a result of self-attention on X with an activation function ϕ, which also describes a transformer encoder block, is given as:

$$H = \text{LayerNorm}(\text{MultiHeadAttention}(Q, K, V) + X)$$
$$X' = \text{LayerNorm}(\text{FFN}(H) + H)$$
$$\text{FFN}(a) = \phi(W_1 a + b_1)W_2 + b_2$$
$$\phi(x) = \text{Mish}(x) = \tanh(\text{softplus}(x))x$$

The *Mish* [27] activation function, which has self-regularizing properties and is well-suited for deep networks, is used throughout the model. Multiple encoders are stacked four times, leading to a deeper model. The encoded activity and timestamp matrices are denoted as A' and T', respectively. The matrices are then flattened using a variable selection network [23], as shown in Fig. 3, similar to the dynamic attribute sequences.

4.3 Static Attribute Selection Network

A variable selection network (VSN) [23] is used to include the static attributes and handle them separately from the dynamic ones. VSNs are based on GRNs and provide a weighting of input attributes. Given several static attributes $S = [s_1, s_2, \ldots, s_m]$ with s_i being a preprocessed vector of an encoded attribute, a VSN weighs inputs by applying a GRN followed by a softmax function, resulting in a weight vector v_i and again feeding each variable in its own GRN and summarizing the outputs. The final static context vector C_S is derived as follows:

$$C_S = \text{VSN}(S) = \sum_{i=1}^{m} v_i \tilde{s}_i$$
$$v = \text{softmax}(\text{GRN}(S))$$
$$\tilde{s}_i = \text{GRN}_{s_i}(s_i)$$

The GLU and GRN are defined using the following equations and extensively use residual connections, with W indicating a trained weight matrix and a bias b. Please note that weights and biases are not shared between individual GLUs and GRNs.

$$\text{GRN}(a) = \text{LayerNorm}(a + \text{GLU}(W_1\phi(W_2a + b_2) + b_1))$$
$$\text{GLU}(a) = \phi(W_1a + b_1) \circ (W_2a + b_2)$$

4.4 Dynamic Attribute Selection Network

Given a sequence of dynamic attribute values, $D_k = \langle d_1^k, d_2^k, \ldots, d_n^k \rangle$ of the dynamic attribute k that is concurrent to the sequence of activities, each attribute is encoded separately applying self-attention first. The encoded dynamic attributes are then subjected to cross-attention using the previously encoded activities. This setup is quite similar to the original transformer decoder [5]. However, no causal masking is applied. Please note that k is omitted in the following equation to improve clarity:

$$H_D = \text{LayerNorm}(\text{MultiHeadAttention}(Q_D, K_D, V_D) + D)$$
$$H_{D'} = \text{LayerNorm}(\text{MultiHeadAttention}(Q_{D'}, K_{A'}, V_{A'}) + H_D)$$
$$D' = \text{LayerNorm}(\text{FFN}(H_{D'}) + H_{D'})$$
$$C_D = \text{VSN}(D')$$
$$Q_D = DW_Q^D, K_D = DW_K^D, V_D = DW_V^D \text{ and } Q_{D'} = D_{k'}W_Q^{D'}, K_{A'} = A'W_K^{A'}, V_{A'} = A'W_V^{A'}$$

This is done to extract importances from the attribute sequence itself and then exploit the relationship between the activities and further attributes, similar to [6]. After that, the encoded dynamic attribute sequence is flattened using a VSN to weigh the importance of the individual time steps, resulting in the attribute's dynamic context vector C_{Dk}, as shown in Fig. 4. While many solutions in PPM use simpler desequentialization mechanisms, such as global average pooling [10, 20] layers or simple flattening [6], we suspect that targeted feature selection might improve the model's prediction quality.

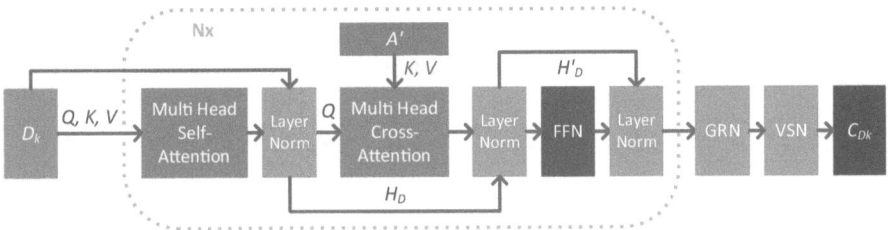

Fig. 4. Dynamic attribute selection network

5   Experimental Evaluation

Five datasets from different industries in ITSM's incident management are used to evaluate the developed architecture. These datasets show various event and case counts and event log attributes, ensuring a broad coverage and validity of the findings. The models are trained using early stopping up to a maximum of one hundred epochs on these logs.

- The "enriched event log of an incident management process" [28] derived from an IT company's ServiceNow platform and is referred to as "ServiceNow".
- The "Dataset belonging to the help desk log of an Italian Company" [29] originating in an Italian software company referred to as "Italian Company".
- The "Helpdesk" event log [30] from a software company without extra attributes.
- The BPIC 2014 [31] event log, created by Rabobank's IT organization.
- The BPIC 2013 [32] incident log from the car producer Volvo's IT organization.

5.1   Event Log Filtering and Splitting

The data undergoes unified preprocessing to prepare it for the training. This involves removing duplicates and highly correlated attributes (≥ 0.9 or ≤ -0.9). All parts are combined using the provided identifiers for event logs with multiple files. The event logs are then split into 80/20 partitions using strict temporal splitting [8] to create unbiased and reproducible splits. Chronological outliers at the beginning and end of the BPIC 2014, BPIC 2013, and ServiceNow datasets are filtered, while the top 5% of cases by event count are filtered out in all event logs following the recommendation by [8].

The strict temporal splitting approach performs well, covering over 85% of events of the original, unfiltered logs, as shown in Table 2. Applying this method to the BPIC 2013 event log results in many invalid events between the train and test set splits, rendering it unsuitable for strict temporal splitting [8]. Consequently, it was opted for a temporal split of the cases without debiasing for this event log, leading to a high coverage of 89.55% of the unfiltered event log, with 17.81% of events in the test set.

Table 2. Split distribution and coverage analysis after filtering and strict temporal splitting [8]

	Train		Test		Total	
	Abs	Rel	Abs	Rel	Abs	Rel
Helpdesk	11,029	81.45%	2,512	18.55%	13,541	98.77%
Italian Company	15,391	72.09%	4,477	20.97%	19,868	93.07%
ServiceNow	96,350	77.69%	27,670	22.31%	124,020	87.52%
BPIC 2013	8,653	31.15%	19,124	68.85%	27,777	42.39%
BPIC 2014	318,228	80.13%	78,901	19.67%	397,129	85.09%

5.2 Evaluation Results

Predicting the remaining time is a regression task requiring metrics to determine the deviation between the label and the predicted values. Although the mean absolute error (MAE) shows some sensitivity to outliers, it is less than other metrics and offers intuitive interpretability [33]. The mean squared error (MSE) complements this metric with a stronger penalization for larger errors and potential outliers [33]. To assess whether the models have learned adequately, a naïve model, which predicts the train set's median for the remaining time, is added for reference. A baseline model is also implemented using an LSTM approach as described in [9], with the identical handling of numerical and categorical attributes as the transformer without positional encoding.

The evaluation results are shown in Table 3 and indicate that most models have learned better predictions than the naïve models. An exception to this is the Italian company event log, where the LSTM performs worse. This may indicate potential instability of the model that might be alleviated by using more attributes or different preprocessing in this model, especially using embeddings might not be suitable. Additional model fine-tuning might also be beneficial in the case of the LSTM.

Table 3. Results of the evaluation on the test set with the MAE and MSE in days

Event Log	Naïve		LSTM		Transformer		Mean	
	MAE	MSE	MAE	MSE	MAE	MSE	MAE	MSE
Helpdesk	5.05	109.50	4.94	107.29	**3.55**	**68.71**	4.51	95.17
Italian Company	15.58	147.98	21.61	699.71	**7.81**	**113.97**	15.00	320.55
ServiceNow	3.26	31.68	2.29	**20.49**	1.95	22.66	2.50	24.94
BPIC 2013	4.26	28.88	2.95	14.21	**2.46**	**11.35**	3.22	18.15
BPIC 2014	1.93	14.37	1.79	**11.51**	**1.71**	13.22	1.81	13.03

The transformer model generally outperforms the LSTM and naïve models regarding MAE and MSE across most datasets. This suggests that it is a more accurate prediction model for the event logs used in this work, measured by MAE. Interestingly, despite the transformer model's significantly better MAE, the LSTM slightly outperforms the transformer in terms of MSE in some instances, suggesting a better handling of outliers.

Regarding the training, it must be stated that the deep transformer model exhibited significant overfitting in the first tries, while the LSTM was unproblematic in this regard. This necessitated a low learning rate and the extensive use of dropout, L2 regularization, and weight decay in the model. During training, linear warm-up epochs were incorporated at the start, and a linear decay rate was added for the later epochs. This was done to help the used adaptive *AdamW* optimizer learn accurate gradient statistics first and later decrease the magnitude of weight updates as the training progresses. This increased the epochs required to converge, again adding to the training time.

6 Discussion and Limitations

The empirical results in this work underscore the transformer's performance and feasibility in the novel architecture presented for the domain of ITSM. The developed architecture shows promise in handling ITSM processes' complexities and outperforms naïve baselines and LSTMs on several event logs. Notably, the utility of several architectural features new to PPM is shown, such as advanced positional encoding techniques [25] and the distinguishing between static and dynamic attributes [22], which enable the model to effectively capture the inherent contextual and temporal dynamics of ITSM processes. As a novel approach, this complements earlier work that eschewed this distinction [6] or omitted additional attributes [10], offering insights into the design of transformer architectures. Integrating GLUs and GRNs also contributes to a more refined handling of these attributes, replicating findings outside of PPM [23], showing their transferability, and improving the model's performance. Additionally, several insights into training transformer models could be gained, specifically regarding the mitigation of overfitting, which was found to be pivotal in such deep models.

Nonetheless, this study has some limitations. First, further ablation studies of the model might be necessary to assess the independent impact of each component, such as the VSNs and positional encoding. Also, as this work focused on a newly developed architecture, a comprehensive tuning of the hyperparameters was omitted. The evaluation results might be more favorable if separate tuning is applied for each event log. This should also be combined with a further comparison of more event logs and additional benchmark models to assess the architecture on a broader scale.

7 Conclusion and Future Research

This study introduced a novel transformer-based architecture for predictive process monitoring in IT Service Management (ITSM), addressing the challenges posed by the complexity and heterogeneity of ITSM processes. The proposed model incorporates advanced techniques such as rotary position encoding, GLUs, and separate handling of static and dynamic attributes, which have not been widely explored in predictive process monitoring. Generally, the transformer model demonstrates a robust capability to generalize across different datasets, as evidenced by its performance metrics attained in this work. The enhanced prediction capabilities of transformers in ITSM can drive operational effectiveness by facilitating decision-making and proactive SLA management. However, this work shows that deep transformers tended to overfit, necessitating careful regularization techniques during training. Addressing these challenges of overfitting and optimizing the training process will be crucial for advancing the application of these models in future works. Overall, the results validate the hypothesis that transformers can meet the complex demands of ITSM predictive process monitoring with appropriate modifications, potentially leading to more operational efficiency and service-level adherence. To ensure optimal models are selected, future work on this architecture should include more extensive studies on separate model components of the transformer to assess their impact on prediction performance. This should be supplemented with an extended evaluation containing additional event logs and prediction targets, such as the next activity and timestamp.

Many relevant data sources in ITSM, such as configuration management databases and organizational and technical structures, form multi-layered network structures. In this regard, the work with non-tabular network data and geometric deep learning remains interesting for future analyses.

References

1. Bardhan, I.R., Demirkan, H., Kannan, P.K., Kauffman, R.J., Sougstad, R.: An interdisciplinary perspective on it services management and service science. JMIS. **26**, 13–64 (2010). https://doi.org/10.2753/mis0742-1222260402
2. Rama-Maneiro, E., Vidal, J., Lama, M.: Deep learning for predictive business process monitoring: review and benchmark. IEEE Trans. Serv. Comput. **16**, 739–756 (2022). https://doi.org/10.1109/tsc.2021.3139807
3. Loewenstern, D., Shwartz, L.: IT Service management of using heterogeneous, dynamically alterable configuration item lifecycles. In: Cordeiro, J. and Filipe, J. (eds.) 10th International Conference on Enterprise Information Systems, pp. 155–160. Barcelona, (2008)
4. Mao, H., Zhang, T., Tang, Q.: Research framework for determining how artificial intelligence enables information technology service management for business model resilience. Sustainability. **13**, 11496 (2021). https://doi.org/10.3390/su132011496
5. Vaswani, A., et al.: Attention is all you need. In: Guyon, I., Luxburg, U. von, Bengio, S., Wallach, H.M., Fergus, R., Vishwanathan, S.V.N., and Garnett, R. (eds.) Advances in Neural Information Processing Systems, pp. 5998–6008. NeurIPS, Long Beach, CA, USA (2017)
6. Ni, W., Zhao, G., Liu, T., Zeng, Q., Xu, X.: Predictive business process monitoring approach based on hierarchical transformer. Electronics **12**, 1273 (2023). https://doi.org/10.3390/electronics12061273
7. Johannesson, P., Perjons, E.: An Introduction to Design Science. Springer, Cham, Switzerland (2021). https://doi.org/10.1007/978-3-030-78132-3
8. Weytjens, H., De Weerdt, J.: Creating unbiased public benchmark datasets with data leakage prevention for predictive process monitoring. In: Marrella, A. and Weber, B. (eds.) Business Process Management Workshops. pp. 18–29. Springer, Cham (2022). https://doi.org/10.1007/978-3-030-94343-1_2
9. Tax, N., Verenich, I., La Rosa, M., Dumas, M.: Predictive business process monitoring with LSTM Neural Networks. In: Dubois, E. and Pohl, K. (eds.) Advanced Information Systems Engineering, pp. 477–492. Springer, Essen, Germany (2017). https://doi.org/10.1007/978-3-319-59536-8_30

10. Bukhsh, Z.A., Saeed, A., Dijkman, R.M.: ProcessTransformer: Predictive Business Process Monitoring with Transformer Network (2021). http://arxiv.org/abs/2104.00721

11. Philipp, P., Jacob, R., Robert, S., Beyerer, J.: Predictive analysis of business processes using neural networks with attention mechanism. In: 2020 International Conference on Artificial Intelligence in Information and Communication, pp. 225–230. IEEE, Fukuoka, Japan (2020). https://doi.org/10.1109/icaiic48513.2020.9065057

12. Chen, H., Fang, X., Fang, H.: Multi-task prediction method of business process based on BERT and Transfer Learning. Knowl. Based Syst. **254**, 109603 (2022). https://doi.org/10.1016/j.knosys.2022.109603

13. Moon, J., Park, G., Jeong, J.: POP-ON: prediction of process using one-way language model based on NLP approach. Appl. Sci. **11**, 864 (2021). https://doi.org/10.3390/app11020864

14. Wang, J., Yu, D., Liu, C., Sun, X.: Outcome-oriented predictive process monitoring with attention-based bidirectional LSTM neural networks. In: 13th International Conference on Web Services. pp. 360–367. IEEE, Milan (2019). https://doi.org/10.1109/icws.2019.00065

15. Jalayer, A., Kahani, M., Beheshti, A., Pourmasoumi, A., Motahari-Nezhad, H.R.: Attention mechanism in predictive business process monitoring. In: 24th International Enterprise Distributed Object Computing Conference, pp. 181–186. IEEE, Eindhoven, Netherlands (2020). https://doi.org/10.1109/edoc49727.2020.00030

16. Jalayer, A., Kahani, M., Pourmasoumi, A., Beheshti, A.: HAM-Net: predictive business process monitoring with a hierarchical attention mechanism. Knowl. Based Syst. **236**, 107722 (2022). https://doi.org/10.1016/j.knosys.2021.107722

17. Rivera-Lazo, G., Ñanculef, R.: Multi-attribute transformers for sequence prediction in business process management. In: Pascal, P. and Ienco, D. (eds.) Discovery Science. pp. 184–194. Springer, Montpellier (2022). https://doi.org/10.1007/978-3-031-18840-4_14

18. Wickramanayake, B., He, Z., Ouyang, C., Moreira, C., Xu, Y., Sindhgatta, R.: Building interpretable models for business process prediction using shared and specialised attention mechanisms. Knowl. Based Syst. **248**, 108773 (2022). https://doi.org/10.1016/j.knosys.2022.108773

19. Irwin, C., Dossena, M., Leonardi, G., Montani, S.: Structural positional encoding for knowledge integration in transformer-based medical process monitoring. In: Calimeri, F., Dragoni, M., and Stella, F. (eds.) 2nd AIxIA Workshop on Artificial Intelligence for Healthcare, pp. 18–30. CEUR, Rome, Italy (2023)

20. Wang, J., Huang, J., Ma, X., Li, Z., Wang, Y., Yu, D.: MTLFormer: multi-task learning guided transformer network for business process prediction. IEEE Access **11**, 76722–76738 (2023). https://doi.org/10.1109/access.2023.3298305

21. Amiri Elyasi, K., van der Aa, H., Stuckenschmidt, H.: PGTNet: a process graph transformer network for remaining time prediction of business process instances. In: Guizzardi, G., Santoro, F., Mouratidis, H., and Soffer, P. (eds.) Advanced Information Systems Engineering, pp. 124–140. Springer, Cham (2024). https://doi.org/10.1007/978-3-031-61057-8_8

22. Brunk, J.: Structuring business process context information for process monitoring and prediction. In: 22nd Conference on Business Informatics, pp. 39–48. IEEE, Antwerp, Belgium (2020). https://doi.org/10.1109/cbi49978.2020.00012

23. Lim, B., Arik, S.O., Loeff, N., Pfister, T.: Temporal fusion transformers for interpretable multi-horizon time series forecasting (2020). http://arxiv.org/abs/1912.09363

24. Wen, Q., et al.: Transformers in time series: a survey. In: Elkind, E. (ed.) 32nd International Joint Conference on Artificial Intelligence, pp. 6778–6786. Macao, PRC (2023). https://doi.org/10.24963/ijcai.2023/759

25. Su, J., Ahmed, M., Lu, Y., Pan, S., Bo, W., Liu, Y.: RoFormer: enhanced transformer with rotary Position Embedding. Neurocomputing **568**, 127063 (2024). https://doi.org/10.1016/j.neucom.2023.127063

26. Shazeer, N.: GLU Variants Improve Transformer (2020). http://arxiv.org/abs/2002.05202
27. Misra, D.: Mish: a self regularized non-monotonic activation function. In: 31st British Machine Vision Virtual Conference. Virtual (2020)
28. Amaral, C., Fantinato, M., Peres, S.: Incident management process enriched event log, (2018). https://doi.org/10.24432/c57s4h
29. Polato, M.: Dataset belonging to the help desk log of an Italian Company (2017).https://doi.org/10.4121/uuid:0c60edf1-6f83-4e75-9367-4c63b3e9d5bb
30. Verenich, I.: Helpdesk (2016). https://doi.org/10.17632/39bp3vv62t.1
31. van Dongen, B.F.: BPI Challenge 2014 (2014). https://doi.org/10.4121/uuid:c3e5d162-0cfd-4bb0-bd82-af5268819c35
32. Steeman, W.: BPI Challenge 2013 (2013). https://doi.org/10.4121/uuid:a7ce5c55-03a7-4583-b855-98b86e1a2b07
33. Jadon, A., Patil, A., Jadon, S.: A comprehensive survey of regression based loss functions for time series forecasting (2022). http://arxiv.org/abs/2211.02989

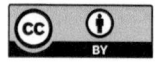

Predictions in Predictive Process Monitoring with Previously Unseen Categorical Values

Johannes Roider[1(✉)], Weixin Wang[2], Dario Zanca[1], Martin Matzner[2], and Bjoern M. Eskofier[1]

[1] Machine Learning and Data Analytics (MaD) Lab, Friedrich-Alexander Universität Erlangen-Nürnberg, Erlangen, Germany
`johannes.roider@fau.de`
[2] Chair of Digital Industrial Service Systems, Friedrich-Alexander Universität Erlangen-Nürnberg, Nürnberg, Germany

Abstract. Predictive process monitoring (PPM) methods provide users with real-time predictions about ongoing process instances. Machine learning models used for such tasks do not account for data variability, such as the occurrence of previously unseen categorical feature values. Concept drift adaptation solutions are suggested in such scenarios. However, adapting to new feature values requires time and a sample size large enough to train a well-generalizing model. Still, users expect seamless communication during the timeframe between the first occurrence of a new value and the availability of an updated model. Dedicated solutions are needed since encoding techniques like one hot encoding cannot handle previously unseen values by default. In this work, we first introduce and discuss possible solutions from a business perspective, ranging from temporary shutdowns to dedicated manual and technical solutions for an uninterrupted continuation of predictive services. Next, we present five variants for one hot encoding to handle previously unseen categorical values. This is followed by a case study using six real-world event logs and two machine learning models, XGBoost and LSTM, to identify the variants that produce the most reliable remaining time predictions. The study also includes the evaluation of two baseline models as an alternative to the machine learning models. The results show that previously unseen categorical values can be handled on a technical level without severely affecting the remaining time prediction quality. However, future research is required to provide more practical recommendations.

Keywords: Predictive Process Monitoring · Remaining Time · Machine Learning

1 Introduction

Predicting the remaining time of business processes is a major task in predictive process monitoring (PPM), next to outcome and next activity prediction. To

A. Delgado and T. Slaats (Eds.): ICPM 2024 Workshops, LNBIP 533, pp. 227–239, 2025.
https://doi.org/10.1007/978-3-031-82225-4_17

provide remaining time prediction services, machine learning models are first trained on historical data (offline phase) and then deployed and applied to real-time streaming data (online phase) [2].

Users of predictive services expect an uninterrupted, consistent prediction quality. However, business process data is subject to change over time. Examples include the occurrence of new activities, customers, or products over time. These are examples of data variability on the level of categorical values [7]. One solution to such concept drifts discussed in previous work is to (re)train machine learning models with the new data [6,10]. However, there are two practical challenges:

1. When a previously unseen categorical value is encountered, there are no ground truth labels available to (re)train a model. Still, predictions are expected by end users.
2. Machine learning models need a sample size large enough in order not to overfit to the training data. Even if a small sample size with ground truth labels is available for new categorical values, there is a risk that a (re)trained model overfits and produces low-quality predictions. Collecting a certain amount of data before (re)training a model is required.

In both scenarios there is a gap in time where new categorical values occur but a machine learning model that incorporates them is not available. Predictive service providers are challenged to bridge this time interval without negatively impacting user satisfaction. Therefore, we list and discuss possible solution strategies from a business perspective in Sect. 4.

Challenges with previously unseen categorical values also arise on a technical level. Many machine learning models require specifying the number of distinct values for categorical features in advance. However, it is not foreseeable whether and how many new values will occur in the future. If a new value occurs during the online phase that has not been considered in the offline phase, it can lead to service disruptions.

For these reasons, our evaluations focus on previously unseen categorical values occurring over time and its handling with one hot encoding. This encoding technique is commonly used to encode categorical features. In Sect. 5, we discuss one-hot encoding and the reasons of technical failures with new categorical values in detail. Furthermore, we present five specific ways to encode previously unseen categorical values with one-hot encoding. This is followed by a benchmark study in the context of remaining time prediction. We evaluate the proposed solutions with two variants of XGBoost and a Long Short-Term Memory (LSTM) model on six real-world datasets and compare them to the performance of two simple baselines presented in prior literature.

The remainder of this work is structured as follows: In Sect. 2 we discuss related work, followed by general concepts relevant to this work in Sect. 3. New concepts are introduced in Sect. 4 by discussing possible solution strategies from a business perspective, and in Sect. 5 by presenting one-hot encoding schemes for previously unseen categorical values. In Sect. 6 we outline our experiments which are discussed in Sect. 7. In Sect. 8 we conclude our work.

2   Related Work

Predicting the remaining time has been studied in several works. It has been analyzed with structured reviews and benchmarking methods. Verenich et al. [13] conducted a review and benchmark study where they compared process-aware methods, variants of XGBoost, and a neural network based method. They found that DA-LSTM, introduced by Navarin et al. [8], outperforms process-aware and classical machine learning methods. Rama-Maneiro et al. [11] focused on deep learning in their benchmark study. They compare four methods for remaining time prediction and also determined DA-LSTM as the best method. Recently, classical methods were investigated again due to their lower computational needs. Aalikhani et al. [1] compare four different methods in their regression-based and classification-based counterparts. The latter methods require a discretization of labels, but they often outperform regression-based models. Oyamada et al. [9] compare three models with a focus on time-related feature engineering. They find that LSTM outperforms the classical methods, but classical methods can be improved with a careful choice of time-related features.

Few works in PPM have motivated the problem of new categorical values during the online phase. Mangat and Rinderle-Ma [7] propose two solution strategies for one-hot feature encoding (void encoding and reserving additional capacities). However, they only consider void encoding and not different variants during their evaluation for predicting the next activity. Pasquadibisceglie et al. [10] use word2vec from the Gensim package[1] since it provides automatic handling of new categorical values. However, the original implementation of Word2vec does not support new values, and the Gensim package provides one specific implementation. There might be a variety of possible solutions available. The same applies to one-hot encoding, for which we will discuss several variations.

Other domains also encounter the challenge of handling previously unseen categorical values. Dedicated work exists in the field of recommendation systems. An overview of encoding strategies is given by Shiao et al. [12]. Some of the proposed solutions overlap with the work by Mangat et al. [7], for example both papers propose zero encoding. Shiao et al. [12] propose further solutions like mean embedding and random embeddings, some of which we consider in Sect. 5.

3   Prerequisites

Data. The data used in predictive process monitoring are *event logs*. Event logs are sets of sequences, also called *cases* or *traces*. Each trace is a sequence of *events*. Events are standardized data structures which have specific attributes assigned. Common attributes are *case identifiers*, *activities*, and *timestamps*, which identify to which trace an event belongs, the task that is being performed, and when it has been performed, respectively. Further optional attributes, called *context attributes*, can be assigned. Examples include resources or costs.

---

[1] https://radimrehurek.com/gensim/.

Training samples called *prefixes* are generated from each trace to train a machine-learning model. For each event in the trace one prefix is created by including the whole history of the trace up to this specific event. The corresponding remaining time label is represented by the difference in time from the last event of the trace to the specific event at hand.

Prefixes are preprocessed to reflect a data format which can be utilized by machine learning algorithms. The specific representation depends on the algorithm used. We differentiate between numerical and categorical features. Numerical features take on continuous values. Categorical features are discrete. While numerical features can be directly utilized, optionally with a predefined normalization beforehand, categorical features often require specific encoding.

Encoding of Categorical Features. The encoding of categorical values depends on the machine learning model employed. Tree-based models like random forests or XGBoost process categorical features by determining splits in individual trees directly on the discrete feature values. Another approach for XGBoost is to transform categorical features first into a numerical representation like one-hot encoding. In one-hot encoding, a feature vector is created whose length corresponds to the number of categories observed in the dataset at hand (see Sect. 5). The type of encoding for tree-based methods depends heavily on the implementation. For example, XGBoost[2] up to version 1.6 did not support direct categorical encodings but required a numerical representation like one-hot encoding. Scikit-learn[3], a commonly used library for tree-based methods like random forests, requires numerical representation and direct categorical splits are not supported as of the latest version 1.5.

Neural networks require a numerical encoding and one-hot encoding is often chosen. Since one-hot encoding is applicable with both, XGBoost and neural networks, and since it was also used in prior literature (see Verenich et al. [13]), we conducted our experiments with one-hot encoding.

4 Handling Previously Unseen Categorical Values from a Business Perspective

We motivated in Sect. 1 the problem of previously unseen categorical values. From a business perspective this should be handled without negative impact on the satisfaction levels of end users. Service providers need to be aware of possible solutions and cope with the challenge based on their individual end users' needs. We have identified four different solutions strategies:

1. Disable the service (partially): To avoid inaccurate predictions, the service is disabled for samples where previously unseen values are encountered. A more rigid approach is to deactivate the service completely. The service is resumed

---

[2] https://xgboost.ai.

[3] https://scikit-learn.org.

after a large enough sample size for the new value is collected, a new model is trained, evaluated and deployed.

2. Escalate predictions: Traces containing new values are escalated to human experts. These take over the task and provide a prediction based on their domain knowledge. While the service can be continued, extra resources are required to uphold it. Furthermore, human interventions take more time to finish, and dedicated user interfaces are needed to support the manual work.

3. Exclude features with previously unseen values: A backup model is used which does not use the affected feature. This can be a model using all other available features or a simple baseline solution predicting a standard value. This ensures that the service is continued fully automated, but there is a high risk that the quality of predictions drops. Furthermore, backup models need to be maintained to be immediately available.

4. Encode feature value as "new value": Use the deployed model, but provide an input signal that there is a previously unseen categorical value encountered. There are different possibilities for such an encoding which we discuss in Sect. 5. Advantages are that the service is not interrupted and there is only one model to be maintained. However, such a strategy can lead to a reduced prediction accuracy.

Table 1. Solution strategies to handle previously unseen categorical values

Mitigation Strategy	Advantages	Disadvantages
1. Disable service (partially)	No risk of low quality predictions;	Service interruptions can affect customer satisfaction;
2. Escalate predictions	High quality predictions;	Time consuming due to manual work; Risk of inconsistent predictions (different experts make different predictions); Escalation procedure and additional user interfaces needed;
3. Exclude categorical feature	Fast response times;	Risk of reduced prediction quality; Additional model(s) to be maintained;
4. Encode "new value"	Fast response times; Only one model to be maintained;	Risk of reduced prediction quality;

The derived advantages and disadvantages are summarized in Table 1. The right strategy to be chosen depends on individual business requirements. If high-quality predictions are paramount, strategies 1. and 2. might be preferred. If fast response times and no interruptions are required while reduced accuracy can be tolerated, strategies 3. and 4. may offer the better choice.

In our case study, we will compare strategies 3. and 4. We investigate whether models receiving the input signal of a "new value" can outperform simple baseline models or if they fail to produce reliable predictions. This will give practitioners insights on whether technical solutions are feasible.

5   Encoding of Previously Unseen Categorical Values

Let's assume a categorical feature for which n distinct values occur in the training set, i.e. the set of distinct values is defined as $C_{train} = \{c_1, c_2, ..., c_n\}$. Next, we define a bijective function f that maps a value c_j to a unique integer i_j, i.e. $f : C_{train} \to I$ where $I = \{0, 1, ..., n - 1\}$. In other words, each categorical value can be mapped uniquely to exactly one integer value, and vice versa.

For one-hot encoding, we create a feature vector V with length n and set all values to 0 (zero), i.e. $V = [v_0, v_1, ..., v_{n-1}]$ where $\forall v_m \in V : v_m = 0$. Given attribute value c_j, we obtain i_j by applying $f : c_j \to i_j$ and set $\forall v_m \in V : v_m = 1$, if $m = i_j$. As an example, let's assume $C_{train} = \{A, B, C, D\}$. Function f gives the following mappings: $A \to 0, B \to 1, C \to 2, D \to 3$. The one-hot encoded feature vector for event C is given by $V = [0, 0, 1, 0]$.

Let's now assume a test set c_{test} such that $C_{test} \setminus C_{train} \neq \emptyset$. That means a new feature value c_k occurs in the test set which is not present in the training set. A mapping by f for c_k is not defined. In technical implementations such an approach can lead to execution errors. Therefore, a contingency method needs to be established on how to encode previously unseen values to avoid such errors and ensure the continuation of a service.

We present solutions to situations where $c_k \notin C_{train} \land c_k \in C_{test}$ and c_k needs to be one-hot encoded. The corresponding example assumes that $C_{train} = \{A, B, C, D\}$ and $C_{test} = \{A, B, C, D, E\}$ where value E represents c_k. *Zero encoding* and *Dummy encoding* were previously mentioned by Mangat and Rinderle-Ma [7] and denoted as *Void encoding* and *Additional Capacity*, respectively.

Zero Encoding. If there is no mapping defined by f for c_k, the one-hot encoding for c_k is defined as a zero vector, i.e. $V = [v_0, v_1, ..., v_{n-1}]$ where $\forall v_j \in V : v_j = 0$. Encoding value E corresponds to the following vector: $V = [0, 0, 0, 0]$.

Dummy Encoding. With this encoding we reserve an additional position in the one-hot encoded vector, such that $V = [v_0, v_1, ..., v_n]$. During training, v_n will always be 0. On an algorithmic level, we then set $v_n = 1$ in case f is not defined for c_k. In our example, value E is therefore defined as $V = [0, 0, 0, 0, 1]$. Please note that this encoding is used for any new categorical value. If another value F occurs, the encoding is also $V = [0, 0, 0, 0, 1]$.

One-over-n Encoding. The idea for one-over-n encoding is to provide an uninformative input to a model, similar to zero encoding, but to keep the sum of all elements of the input vector to 1, i.e. $\sum_{j=0}^{n-1} v_j = 1$, where $v_j \in V$. Instead of 0, we assign to each $v_j \in V$ a value of $\frac{1}{n}$, i.e. $V = [v_0, v_1, ..., v_{n-1}]$ where

$\forall v_j \in V : v_j = \frac{1}{n}$. Categorical value E in our example would therefore be encoded as $V = [0.25, 0.25, 0.25, 0.25]$ since $n = 4$.

Distribution-Based Encoding. In distribution-based encoding we provide for each element in the one-hot encoded vector the relative frequency of the corresponding feature value. In order to do so, we define a function $\text{count}(c_j)$ that counts for each value $c_j \in C_{\text{train}}$ the number of occurrences in the training set, i.e. $\text{count} : C \to \mathbb{N}_0$. The sum of all events is defined as $M = \sum_{j=1}^{n} \text{count}(c_j)$ where $c_j \in C_{\text{train}}$. For any $v_j \in V$ we retrieve the distribution-based encoding with $v_j = \frac{\text{count}(f^{-1}:i_j \to c_j)}{M}$ where $i_j \in I$ and f^{-1} is the inverse of f such that we retrieve the original categorical value given an index of the one-hot encoding. In other words, we count for each categorical value how often it occurs and then divide it by the total number of events in the training set.

Let's assume that $\text{count}(C_{train})$ defines the following mappings: $A \to 100, B \to 200, C \to 400, D \to 300$. Encoding previously unseen value E gives the following one-hot encoded vector: $V = [0.1, 0.2, 0.4, 0.3]$. This encoding has the same property as one-over-n encoding such that $\sum_{j=0}^{n-1} v_j = 1$.

Random Encoding. To benchmark the other encoding techniques, we define random encoding which we assume to produce less accurate results. The one-hot encoding is defined as $V = [v_0, v_1, ..., v_{n-1}]$ where we sample uniformly and independently any $v_j \in V$ in the value range of $[0, 1)$ where $v_j \in \mathbb{R}$.

6   Experimental Setting

In our experiments we use XGBoost and LSTM's, representing state-of-the-art classical and deep learning methods, as outlined in Sect. 2. XGBoost has the advantage of fast computations with competitive performance. LSTM neural networks are computationally demanding, but show high prediction quality.

We trained the models with two features: Activities and a time-related feature. Activities represent the categorical feature in our study due to its consistent presence in all event logs. The time related feature is numerical and indicates for an event the time that has passed since the process has started.

We use six publicly available event logs[4] which show an occurrence of new activities over time. We preprocessed them such that they only contain completed cases and split them temporally into training, validation and test sets. 64% of the oldest cases, determined by the timestamp of the first event, are used for training, the next 16% represent the validation set and the last 20% of cases are used for testing. This is close to a real-life situation in which new activities occur over time. The datasets as well as statistics on the test sets relevant to our study are listed in Table 2.

To encode the activity feature we use one-hot encoding. We determine the number of activities for one-hot encoding on the training set solely. If a new

---

[4] Available at https://data.4tu.nl/.

activity occurs in the validation set we encode it as "unknown". We have not considered additional values from the validation set for one-hot encoding during training since this would effectively lead to dummy encoding for these activities. To avoid this danger of mixing different encoding techniques, we defined "known" activities strictly on the training set. Since we apply this approach consistently to all models, it allows for a fair comparison.

Table 2. Test Set Statistics. First row: Total number of prefixes in the test set. Second row: Number of prefixes for which at least one new activity is present. These are the samples which are considered in our experimental evaluation. Third row: Average proportion of events which are previously unseen in the affected prefixes.

Dataset	2015_1	2015_2	2015_3	2015_4	2015_5	helpdesk
Num. Prefixes	5,827	8,526	11,526	4,699	10,896	3,415
Num. Affected Prefixes	5,104	3,640	4,777	1,516	5,730	207
Avg. Percentage of New Activities per Affected Prefix	16.41	4.75	4.01	5.10	5.67	29.04

We trained two variants of XGBoost models. One with aggregation encoding and one with last-state encoding. Aggregation encoding embeds the relative frequency of how often an activity is present in the prefix and the mean of the time-related feature over all events in the prefix. For last state encoding we applied one-hot encoding to the last activity and appended its associated time-related feature. We used the parameters of the standard implementation of the XGBoost package. The only exception is the loss function, for which we used the mean absolute loss instead of a square error loss.

For the LSTM model, we defined a fixed setting with three LSTM layers with a hidden size of 100 neurons each. As optimizer we use NAdam with a learning rate of 0.001. The hyperparameters are determined based on the insights from prior studies [8,13]. The input is provided as tensor-encoded vector [13] and we use the mean absolute error (MAE) as optimization metric. For the implementation we built on a generic codebase by Liessmann et al. [5][5].

We evaluated all results with the mean absolute error (MAE). Furthermore, we trained each model variant five times and calculated the average MAE achieved over the five runs. We repeated training because random factors like the order of the data can influence a model's convergence during training. To average out random effects we train and evaluate each model five times.

We evaluated two baseline models to cover Solution 3. as presented in Sect. 4. The first baseline by van der Aalst et al. [3] simply predicts half of the average runtime of traces in the training set. The second baseline by Ceci et al. [4] uses the time-related feature and predicts the difference between the average runtime of traces in the training set and the time that has passed for the last event of a prefix. We denote the approaches as *baseline1* and *baseline2*, respectively.

---

[5] https://github.com/fau-is/ECIS24-TL4PM.

Since previous work has shown that machine learning models outperform simple baselines, we focused our analysis only on prefixes of the test set where a previously unseen activity is encountered for any event. In this way we avoid that good predictions for prefixes without new activities average out potentially bad predictions when calculating the MAE.

7   Results and Discussion

The results of our case study are displayed in Table 3. The values show the mean MAE across the five runs. Bold numbers indicate the overall best model for a dataset. For the baselines, no encoding techniques are applied, therefore only one number is reported.

Table 3. Results of benchmark study. Abbreviations: Dst: Distribution; Dm: Dummy; N: One-over-n; Rnd: Randomg; Zro: Zero; b1: baseline1; b2: baseline2.

bpic2015_1						bpic2015_2				
	LSTM	XGB Agg	XGB Last	b1	b2		LSTM	XGB Agg	XGB Last	b1	b2
Dst	36.75	41.15	35.03			Dst	65.35	65.02	**31.02**		
Dm	35.30	41.48	34.72			Dm	72.55	68.82	31.05		
N	**33.03**	39.80	34.59	38.99	41.03	N	64.10	64.37	31.14	48.89	68.40
Rnd	40.81	134.33	35.13			Rnd	44.90	441.05	31.05		
Zro	34.82	41.53	35.17			Zro	68.3	65.18	31.23		

bpic2015_3						bpic2015_4				
	LSTM	XGB Agg	XGB Last	b1	b2		LSTM	XGB Agg	XGB Last	b1	b2
Dst	6.85	7.72	7.42			Dst	49.18	46.08	44.12		
Dm	**5.45**	8.61	7.41			Dm	44.00	46.25	44.08		
N	5.61	7.35	7.41	29.11	22.91	N	47.07	46.29	43.95	44.85	58.41
Rnd	5.88	92.68	7.39			Rnd	**37.58**	60.46	44.40		
Zro	5.64	10.69	7.46			Zro	48.53	46.20	44.79		

bpic2015_5						helpdesk				
	LSTM	XGB Agg	XGB Last	b1	b2		LSTM	XGB Agg	XGB Last	b1	b2
Dst	41.55	36.50	34.68			Dst	**3.70**	5.06	3.98		
Dm	35.58	36.43	34.69			Dm	3.97	4.76	3.98		
N	**34.51**	36.94	34.78	40.80	42.11	N	3.85	4.76	3.98	8.72	7.30
Rnd	37.82	244.45	34.81			Rnd	5.01	7.42	3.98		
Zro	34.86	36.81	34.72			Zro	3.88	4.76	3.98		

Comparing Machine Learning Methods to Baseline Methods. The overall best model for a given dataset outperforms the two baseline models each time. A variant of the LSTM model is the overall best model for the datasets helpdesk, bpic2015_1, bpic2015_3, bpic2015_4, and bpic2015_5, however, with changing one-hot encodings. For bpic2015_2, XGBoost (Last) performs best, whereas most variants of LSTM and XGBoost (Agg) are outperformed by baseline1. This shows that machine learning models are generally capable of handling previously unseen categorical values efficiently, compared to simple baseline models. However, further research is required to determine the best suited model type for a given dataset. We have not found any insights based on specific dataset characteristics which explain the best methods for a given dataset.

Robustness of Machine Learning Models to Encoding Techniques. The least deviation in MAE across different encoding techniques is shown by XGBoost (Last). The numbers in Table 3 are close to each other for each dataset. XGBoost (Agg) produces the worst results with random one-hot encoding. One-over-n encoding is the best approach for XGBoost (Agg) on 4 datasets and close to the best-performing approach for bpic2015_3 and bpic2015_4. For LSTM the results are less clear. Random encoding is the worst approach for the datasets helpdesk and bpic2015_1. In Table 2 we show the average percentage of new activities present in prefixes of the test set for which at least one new activity is occurs. It shows the highest numbers for the datasets helpdesk and bpic2015_1 and it is a result of previously unseen activities being mainly present at the end of traces. Therefore, we conclude that random encoding has a negative effect in prefixes with many new activities. However, random encoding also produces the best results with considerable distance for the datasets bpic2015_2 and bpic2015_4. We could not not identify any unique dataset characteristic for these datasets which differentiates them from others. Leaving random encoding aside we found one-over-n encoding delivering stable results for LSTM. A future challenge is to investigate the results obtained with random encoding further to allow more specific recommendations to practitioners.

Comparison of Encodings over All Machine Learning Methods. There is no single approach that is clearly the best. Across all datasets, regardless of the machine learning method, each encoding produces once the best result, except for one-over-n encoding, which is best on two datasets (bpic2015_1, bpic2015_5). However, we observed that one-over-n encoding produces for each model consistently results which are competitive to the best performing one. The only exception is given for LSTM when random encoding is best.

Discussion. To minimize the overall risk of low performance with new categorical values, we recommend using one-over-n encoding. However, the type of selected machine learning model is difficult to determine in advance. There are scenarios in which one-over-n encoding can lead to low performance if the right machine learning model is not chosen. The relatively good performance of last state encoding indicates that the time-related features as well knowledge of the last event are the most important features for accurate predictions, whereas knowledge about all events of a prefix adds additional minor information for predicting the remaining time. Providing complete traces could even lead to overfitting, which is a possible reason for the good performance of the random encoding for LSTM on datasets bpic2015_2 and bpic2015_4. For bpic2015_4 overfitting might even apply to the last activity where the performance of all methods is close to the baseline models. This suggests that mainly the time-related feature is informative in this case. For future studies we recommend ablation studies to understand the importance of individual features such that the effect of new categorical values can be isolated in more detail.

Besides these challenges, we have found that machine learning models can handle newly occurring categorical feature values and outperform simple baseline models. Therefore, it is a viable alternative for practitioners to avoid additional maintenance and escalation overhead. One-over-n encoding showed stable results. Still, open questions remain to provide fully informed recommendations.

8   Conclusion and Outlook

In this work, we motivated the need for solutions when concept drifts, represented by previously unseen categorical values, occur over time. However, (re)trained models are not immediately available for predictions. We have discussed four solution strategies from a business perspective that can help practitioners decide on a strategy based on the needs of their end users. Next, we focused on technical solutions to maintain predictive services. We have presented five different one-hot encoding strategies and compared them in a benchmark study in combination with LSTM models and two variants of XGBoost with two simple baseline solutions. The results show that one-over-n encoding provides the most promising results.

However, this study only represents a first investigation of the topic; further research is required in the future to provide more practical insights. This includes tackling limitations of our study. For example, only a small number of event logs is available where new activities occur over time and most of them, namely the bpic 2015 datasets, relate to the same underlying process execution. Also, we focused our study only on two features, activity and a time-related feature, but the complex interplay of several categorical features where new values occur over time, but also numerical features, needs to be evaluated, especially in light of recent suggestions of extending contextual data sources even further, for example by using data from complete enterprise process networks instead of isolated processes, as motivated by Weinzierl et al. [14]. Furthermore, our statistical approach of training five versions of each model and calculating the average MAE on the test set of these five models does not allow for statistically significant tests. We highlight that our approach is more reliable than just training one model variant which is mostly done in related literature. However, more runs will give statistically more significant insights. Besides these limitations, further aspects can be investigated in future research. Different encoding techniques such as word2vec might be evaluated. Also, other model types and additional tasks for PPM, like next activity prediction or outcome prediction, can be assessed.

Overall, we have motivated the need for handling previously unseen categorical values during runtime. Practitioners need to decide if services are continued and in which form. Technical solutions exist, but have not been compared with each other previously. Our study suggests that these technical solutions can provide reliable performance which are better than simple baseline solutions. However, clear recommendations are hard to give at this point. To close this gap, more research is required in the future.

Acknowledgments. This study was supported by Deutsche Forschungsgemeinschaft (DFG, German Research Foundation) (grant number 456415646).

Disclosure of Interests. The authors have no competing interests to declare that are relevant to the content of this article.

References

1. Aalikhani, R., Fathian, M., Rasouli, M.R.: Comparative analysis of classification-based and regression-based predictive process monitoring models for accurate and time-efficient remaining time prediction. IEEE Access (2024)
2. van der Aalst, W.M., Carmona, J.: Process Mining Handbook. Springer (2022)
3. van der Aalst, W.M., Schonenberg, M.H., Song, M.: Time prediction based on process mining. Inf. Syst. **36**(2), 450–475 (2011)
4. Ceci, M., Lanotte, P.F., Fumarola, F., Cavallo, D.P., Malerba, D.: Completion time and next activity prediction of processes using sequential pattern mining. In: Džeroski, S., Panov, P., Kocev, D., Todorovski, L. (eds.) DS 2014. LNCS (LNAI), vol. 8777, pp. 49–61. Springer, Cham (2014). https://doi.org/10.1007/978-3-319-11812-3_5
5. Liessmann, A., Wang, W., Weinzierl, S., Zilker, S., Matzner, M.: Transfer learning for predictive process monitoring. In: ECIS 2024 Proceedings, vol. 4 (2024)
6. Maisenbacher, M., Weidlich, M.: Handling concept drift in predictive process monitoring. In: 2017 IEEE International Conference on Services Computing (SCC), pp. 1–8. IEEE (2017)
7. Mangat, A.S., Rinderle-Ma, S.: Next-activity prediction for non-stationary processes with unseen data variability. In: International Conference on Enterprise Design, Operations, and Computing, pp. 145–161. Springer (2022)
8. Navarin, N., Vincenzi, B., Polato, M., Sperduti, A.: LSTM networks for data-aware remaining time prediction of business process instances. In: 2017 IEEE Symposium Series on Computational Intelligence (SSCI), pp. 1–7. IEEE (2017)
9. Oyamada, R.S., Tavares, G.M., Junior, S.B., Ceravolo, P.: Enhancing predictive process monitoring with time-related feature engineering. In: International Conference on Advanced Information Systems Engineering, pp. 71–86. Springer (2024)
10. Pasquadibisceglie, V., Appice, A., Castellano, G., Malerba, D.: DARWIN: an online deep learning approach to handle concept drifts in predictive process monitoring. Eng. Appl. Artif. Intell. **123**, 106461 (2023)

11. Rama-Maneiro, E., Vidal, J.C., Lama, M.: Deep learning for predictive business process monitoring: review and benchmark. IEEE Trans. Serv. Comput. **16**(1), 739–756 (2021)
12. Shiao, W., et al.: Improving out-of-vocabulary handling in recommendation systems. arXiv preprint arXiv:2403.18280 (2024)
13. Verenich, I., Dumas, M., Rosa, M.L., Maggi, F.M., Teinemaa, I.: Survey and cross-benchmark comparison of remaining time prediction methods in business process monitoring. ACM Trans. Intell. Syst. Technol. (TIST) **10**(4), 1–34 (2019)
14. Weinzierl, S., Zilker, S., Dunzer, S., Matzner, M.: Machine learning in business process management: a systematic literature review. Exp. Syst. Appl. **253** (2024)

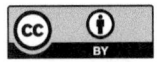

Differentially Private Event Logs with Case Attributes

Hannes Ueck[1]([✉]), Robert Andrews[2], Moe T. Wynn[2],
and Sander J. J. Leemans[1,3]

[1] RWTH Aachen, Aachen, Germany
hannes.ueck@rwth-aachen.de, s.leemans@bpm.rwth-aachen.de
[2] Queensland University of Technology, Brisbane, Australia
[3] Fraunhofer FIT, Sankt Augustin, Germany

Abstract. Event logs capture the execution of processes, record activities and additional information. A trace represents a single instance of a process and includes a sequence of activity records and case attributes with additional information. Event logs may contain sensitive personal information that could harm an individual's privacy if it is published without pre-processing. Differential privacy (DP) limits the disclosure of new information about any individual when publishing an event log beyond the publicly available background knowledge. Many privacy-preserving approaches to event log publishing ensure DP. Traditional methods focus on preserving the control flow but omit case attributes, limiting comprehensive process analysis based on these attributes. This work addresses this limitation by proposing a novel privacy-preserving event log publishing framework. Our approach ensures privacy for the control flow and case attributes, utilising synthetic tabular data generation approaches based on machine learning that guarantee DP. The framework allows for the use of various tabular data generation approaches. Experimental results with real-world event data demonstrate the framework's feasibility and highlight the trade-off between data utility and the guaranteed levels of privacy.

Keywords: Differential Privacy · Process Mining · Event Logs · Machine Learning

1 Introduction

Modern information systems are designed to record the activities executed in processes across different domains such as businesses or healthcare [1]. This information is consolidated into event logs, which are collections of the executed activities. Each activity is part of a sequence of activities that comprise a case and additional attributes on the case level might be recorded.

Process mining aims to generate insights from event logs [1]. This could include discovering a process's control flow, optimising it, detecting deviations from the expected behaviour, or predicting future activities. Combined with case

A. Delgado and T. Slaats (Eds.): ICPM 2024 Workshops, LNBIP 533, pp. 240–252, 2025.
https://doi.org/10.1007/978-3-031-82225-4_18

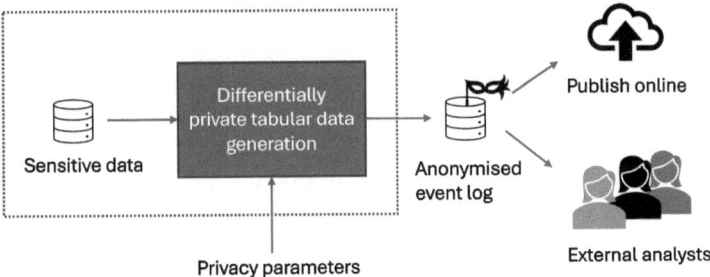

Fig. 1. Conceptual overview

attributes more detailed analyses are possible, e.g. predictive monitoring of processes [19] or identifying differing process behaviour for cohorts of patients [15].

Event logs contain personal data about the individuals involved in the process. Legislation enforces the protection of personal data, the General Data Protection Regulation (GDPR) in the European Union (*Regulation 2016/679, European Parliament*) or the Privacy Act in Australia (*Privacy act 1988, Commonwealth of Australia*). Personal data is considered sensitive and thus needs additional protection when it reveals, for instance, health-related information, ethnic origin or political opinions of individuals. Event logs contain possibly sensitive information in the recorded activities or information included in the additionally collected attributes. For a hospital process, this might be a patient's treatment, the time when the treatment is executed, or the patient's treatment outcome. An adversary might be able to link an individual to a case and re-identify the individual. To protect the privacy of the individuals, it is necessary to apply transformations to the data before publishing it [6,17].

After applying the transformations, the data should still be useful for subsequent analysis [12]. It has been shown that simple removal of names and unique identifiers from the data might lead to re-identification [25]. Differential privacy (DP) provides mathematically proven privacy that limits the impact of any single individual on a dataset [3]. Consequently, publishing a differentially private dataset offers only negligible additional information to adversaries beyond general background knowledge. Unlike group-based techniques where records are generalised or suppressed to create groups of similar records [26], DP also prevents predicate singling out attacks, to which group-based techniques are vulnerable [2].

Most existing methods to guarantee DP for event logs focus on the control flow by omitting other information contained in the event log [8,9,17]. [10] proposed a method to include contextual information, timestamps and case attributes in the anonymised event log. However, this method assumes that the case attributes are independent, which is unrealistic for most common event logs. To the best of our knowledge, no other approaches support the privatisation of an event log with case attributes while guaranteeing DP.

Methods to guarantee DP for purely tabular data have been the focus of research [18,27,31]. These tabular data generation algorithms (TDG) reproduce a dataset by estimating the underlying distribution of the data [31]. Since this does not inherently ensure DP, noise is added to the estimation process to achieve it. We argue that because of the similarities between tabular data and event log data, applying those proven approaches to event log data is possible. However, we argue that additional measures are required to ensure that the characteristics of event logs are accounted for.

In this paper, we propose a framework to apply synthetic tabular data generation methods to event logs while guaranteeing DP for the generated event log. Our contribution is threefold: (1) We propose a framework (DP-ELCA) to anonymise event logs with case attributes while guaranteeing DP. (2) We discuss the privacy implications when applying tabular data generation techniques to event logs. (3) We benchmark our framework using different TDGs on multiple real-life event logs and assess the similarity of the anonymised event log to the original data.

The remainder of this paper is structured as follows. Section 2 introduces the necessary background information. In Sect. 3 we present our approach. We evaluate our approach in Sect. 4. In Sect. 5 we discuss related work and conclude in Sect. 6.

2   Preliminaries

2.1   Event Logs

An event log L is composed of traces, where each trace consists of a sequence of activities. The traces represent the executions of cases in the process and next to the sequence of activities each trace can have case attributes that provide additional information about the case. We consider only the control flow information and the case attributes in this approach.

Definition 1 (Event log). *An event log L with case attributes is defined as a set of tuples, where each tuple consists of a trace and a set of case attributes: $L = \{(\sigma_1, \mathbf{ca_1}), (\sigma_2, \mathbf{ca_2}), \ldots, (\sigma_n, \mathbf{ca_n})\}$. Each trace σ is a sequence of activities $\sigma_i = \langle a_1, a_2, \ldots, a_l \rangle$, where a_j is the j-th activity in the trace and l its varying length. The set of case attributes $\mathbf{ca_i} = \{att_i^1, att_i^2, \ldots, att_i^p\}$, where p is the number of case attributes, provides additional information about the case.*

2.2   Differential Privacy

Differential privacy (DP) is a probabilistic privacy guarantee given on the output of a data processing mechanism $\mathcal{M}$ given an input in form of a dataset $\mathbf{X}$ [3]. It states that anyone examining the output draws the same conclusions about an individual's private information regardless of whether that individual's data was part of the input to the mechanism or not. We apply the definition of DP in [3] to event logs.

Definition 2 (ε,δ-DP for event logs). *Let L_1 and L_2 be two event logs differing in at most one trace σ. Further, let $\varepsilon > 0$ and $\delta \in [0, 1]$ be privacy parameters. Then a randomised mechanism $\mathcal{M}$ provides (ε, δ)-DP if for all subsets S of the output space of $\mathcal{M}$,*

$$\frac{\Pr[\mathcal{M}(L_1) \in S]}{\Pr[\mathcal{M}(L_2) \in S]} \leq e^{\varepsilon} + \delta \tag{1}$$

where the probability $\Pr$ is taken over the randomness introduced by the mechanism $\mathcal{M}$.

Intuitively, ε represents the privacy loss incurred when including an individual's data in the dataset. δ is the probability for a deviation from this guarantee.

Proven theorems give bounds for the privacy budget when applying multiple differentially private mechanisms to the same dataset. The k-fold adaptive composition theorem allows chained heterogeneous mechanisms to access the outputs of the previous mechanisms:

Theorem 1 (k-fold adaptive composition [13]). *Let $\mathcal{M}_1, \mathcal{M}_2, \ldots, \mathcal{M}_k$ be $(\varepsilon_i, \delta_i)$-differentially private mechanism for $i \in [k]$, $\varepsilon_i > 0$, $\delta_i \in [0, 1]$ and $\tilde{\delta} \in [0, 1]$. Then the combined mechanism using k-fold adaptive composition of $\mathcal{M}_i$ provides $(\tilde{\varepsilon}_{\tilde{\delta}}, 1 - (1 - \tilde{\delta}) \prod_{i=1}^{k} (1 - \delta_i))$-DP with $\tilde{\varepsilon}_{\tilde{\delta}} =$*

$$\min \left\{ \sum_{i=1}^{k} \varepsilon_i, \sum_{i=1}^{k} \frac{(e^{\varepsilon_i} - 1)\varepsilon_i}{e^{\varepsilon_i} + 1} + \sqrt{\sum_{i=1}^{k} 2\varepsilon_i^2 \log \left(e + \frac{\sqrt{\sum_{i=1}^{k} \varepsilon_i^2}}{\tilde{\delta}} \right)}, \right.$$
$$\left. \sum_{i=1}^{k} \frac{(e^{\varepsilon_i} - 1)\varepsilon_i}{e^{\varepsilon_i} + 1} + \sqrt{\sum_{i=1}^{k} 2\varepsilon_i^2 \log \left(\frac{1}{\tilde{\delta}} \right)} \right\} \tag{2}$$

2.3 TraVaS: Differentially Private Trace Variant Selection

TraVaS is a framework that allows for releasing the distribution of trace variants based on a private partition selection algorithm with a privacy budget of (ε, δ). It utilises a k-Truncated Symmetric Geometric Distribution (k-TSGD) to add noise to the frequencies of the trace variants. Based on the privacy budget noise values are drawn from the k-TSGD and added to each trace variant count. The output then only contains trace variants where the perturbed count is above a threshold that is calculated using the privacy budget. This ensures DP for the resulting trace variant distribution [23].

2.4 Tabular Data Generation

Tabular data generation aims to generate synthetic data that closely resembles the statistical properties of the original data [30]. It can be used to provide data for analysis without revealing sensitive information about the individuals in the dataset. While the original data is not disclosed, the synthetic data should keep the statistical properties of the original data, such as the distribution of the data points and the correlations between the columns.

Methods Based on Graphical Models. The methods based on graphical models first measure the conditional distributions in the dataset [18,31]. Noise is introduced into the measurements to achieve DP, where the scale of the noise is computed based on the provided privacy parameters. Then, the parameters of a probabilistic graphical model are estimated based on the noisy measures. Finally, the estimated model is sampled to generate an anonymised dataset. This ensures the privacy of individuals in the dataset while allowing the synthetic data to retain the properties of the original data.

Methods Based on Generative Neural Networks. Generative neural networks are used to generate data that resembles the features of the original data [29]. Differentially private stochastic gradient descent (DP-SGD) is used to train the models to achieve DP. This includes adding noise to the gradients and clipping them to ensure that the model does not learn exact copies of data points in the original dataset.

3   Approach: DP-ELCA

DP-ELCA, as shown in Fig. 2, guarantees (ϵ, δ)-DP for the control flow and the case attributes, while ensuring the utility of the anonymised event log by keeping the statistical properties of the original event log.

3.1   Transforming the Event Log to Tabular Data

The event log is transformed into a tabular data format by aggregating the event log on the case level. Each case in the event log corresponds to a row in the tabular data and each row contains a list of activities, i.e. the variant, and the case attributes.

Definition 3 (Aggregated event log). *Let L be an event log and $\mathbf{X}$ the tabular dataset constructed from L. For each tuple $(\sigma_i, \mathbf{ca_i}) \in L$, a datapoint $\mathbf{x_i} \in \mathbf{X}$ is created. A datapoint is the concatenation of the numerical representation of the trace variant $c_i^v = f(\sigma_i)$ with k case attributes in $\mathbf{ca_i}$. Thus, $\mathbf{x_i} = c_i^v \circ c_i^{att^1} \circ c_i^{att^2} \circ \cdots \circ c_i^{att^k}$.*

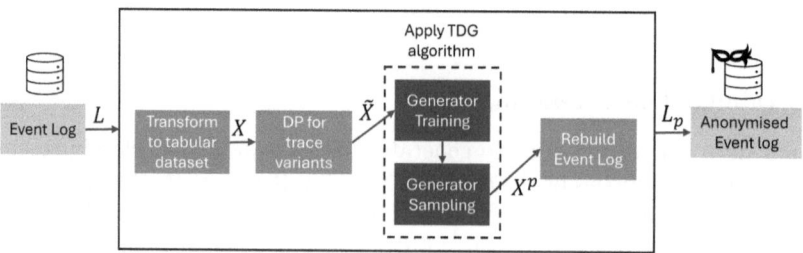

Fig. 2. Overview of the DP-ELCA.

3.2   Privacy Implications of Trace Variants for Private Tabular Data Generation

In traditional tabular data generation settings, it is assumed that the domains of the columns of the dataset are public knowledge, meaning that for a dataset $\mathbf{X}$ with l columns and n rows, $dom(c_j)$ for $j \in [l]$ are publicly known. The algorithms are applied to datasets where the usual range of values or categories within the columns are known and do not depend on the dataset, e.g., the range of blood pressure measurements or categories of diseases. For a categorical column $dom(c_c)$, it is assumed that there are many more rows of data than the number of categories ($|dom(c_c)| << n$).

Given these assumptions, differentially private TDG algorithms reproduce the exact domains of the original dataset in the generated data ($dom(c_j) = dom(c_j^p), j \in [l]$). For datasets that are derived from event logs as defined in Definition 3, this assumption of independence holds for the columns $c^{att^k}, i \in [k]$ that contain data taken directly from the case attributes. However, for c_v, which contains the categories of the trace variants, this assumption does not hold. The domain of the trace variants $dom(c_v)$ is dependent on the traces contained in the event log.

Consider a scenario where an attacker knows the trace variant related to an individual and knows that only this individual could produce this trace variant. Then there are two ways how the attacker could infer information:

(1) If the individual is in the event log, the anonymised event log would contain cases with such a trace variant. In that case, the attacker could infer that the individual is included in the event log.
(2) If the individual is not in the event log, the anonymised event log would not include cases with such a trace variant. In that case, the attacker could infer that the individual was not part of the event log.

This scenario illustrates that information about an individual could be leaked if the algorithm does not change the domain of the attributes in the output ($dom(c_v) = dom(c_v^p)$). The same problem holds for infrequent trace variants where the existence of a group of individuals in the dataset could be leaked. Therefore, filtering infrequent trace variants is needed to ensure privacy. Note that the information leakage is independent of the privacy budget (ϵ, δ) because it has no influence on the domain produced by the TDG. We showed that after filtering out infrequent traces the attacker cannot single out an individual or a group of individuals as described above.

We conclude that directly applying traditional tabular data generation approaches is possible but needs a filtering step beforehand. For this reason our approach applies a DP trace selection algorithm [23] before applying the TDG.

3.3   DP-ELCA

The framework $\mathcal{F}$ receives an event log L as input and generates a differentially private event log L_p as output. Figure 2 shows the four steps of the framework. First, for each case, the sequence of activities and the case attributes are extracted from L. Next, infrequent sequences of activities are filtered out, using [23], and a table is created. Second, a TDG is trained to estimate the statistical properties of the tabular data. Third, synthetic tabular data is sampled from the estimated model. The generated tabular data is then transformed into an event log containing the sequences of activities and case attributes. Next, we introduce each of the steps in more detail.

Transform Event Log to Tabular Data. This step involves the transformation of the event log L to a tabular dataset $\mathbf{X}$. According to Definition 3, the tabular dataset is constructed by aggregating the event log by case identifier. We build a look-up table to convert the trace variants into their numerical representation. Further, we let the user choose which case attributes to include in the tabular dataset $\mathbf{X}$. Any directly identifying information, such as case IDs or patient IDs, is omitted during the aggregation process.

Apply Differential Privacy to Trace Variants. After constructing the tabular dataset $\mathbf{X}$ from the previous step, we limit the trace variants c_v to a (ε, δ)-differentially private selection of trace variants. This ensures that no information leakage occurs, as discussed in Sect. 3.2. We use the *TraVaS* algorithm proposed by [23] to obtain a set $\tilde{c}_v$ of (ε, δ)-differentially private trace variants. By removing all rows where the trace variant is not in the set $\tilde{c}_v$ from the tabular dataset $\mathbf{X}$, we obtain a new tabular dataset $\tilde{\mathbf{X}}$.

Apply Tabular Data Generation Algorithm. This step takes the tabular data set $\tilde{\mathbf{X}}$, applies a TDG $\mathcal{A}$ and returns the anonymised tabular dataset $\mathbf{X}^{\mathbf{P}}$. As defined in Sect. 2.4, we denote the application of the TDG by $\mathbf{X}^{\mathbf{P}} = \mathcal{A}(\tilde{\mathbf{X}})$. After this step, $\mathbf{X}^{\mathbf{P}}$ satisfies (ε, δ)-DP, given that $\mathcal{A}$ guarantees (ε, δ)-DP. Note that any tabular data generation method that guarantees (ε, δ)-DP can be interchangeably used. Some methods additionally require the user to specify types for the columns in the dataset. This is abstracted in the framework and must be specified once in the beginning for each case attribute in the event log.

Rebuild Event Log. The generated tabular data can be transformed back into an event log format by creating a case for each row in the generated tabular dataset $\mathbf{X}^{\mathbf{P}}$. For each row, a case is created that is annotated with the information from the case attributes and corresponding activity from the variant information. Based on the post-processing theorem of DP [4], the privacy guarantee of the anonymised dataset is preserved under any data transformation that does not involve additional queries to the original data. This means that any derived event log from L_p remains differentially private. Thus, improving the data utility after generation, e.g. by removing impossible combinations of case attributes, does not violate the privacy guarantee.

Calculating the Final Privacy Budget. The framework takes as input two privacy budgets $(\varepsilon_{\text{TraVaS}}, \delta_{\text{TraVaS}})$ and $(\varepsilon_{\mathcal{A}}, \delta_{\mathcal{A}})$. Both budgets are used to ensure (ε, δ)-DP for the final event log. The output from the first mechanism, *TraVaS*, is used as input for the TDG. Therefore, instead of using the sequential composition

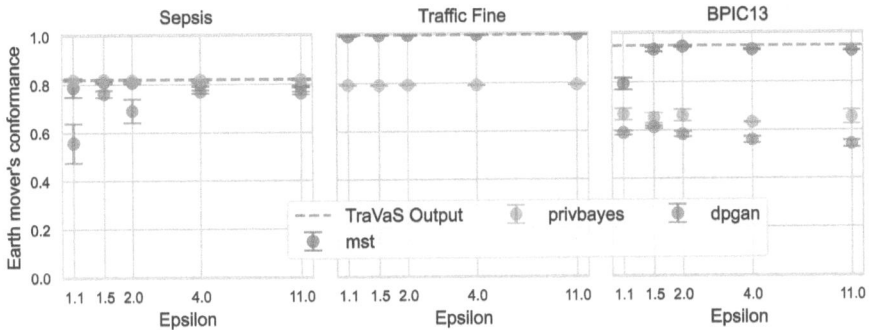

Fig. 3. Earth mover's conformance for values of ε.

theorem, the resulting composed privacy budget (ε, δ) needs to be calculated using the k-fold adaptive composition theorem as in Theorem 1.

4   Evaluation

This section evaluates the results of DP-ELCA when applying it to three real-life event logs using three different TDGs. The resulting anonymised event logs are evaluated regarding the similarity of the stochastic process behaviour, case attributes and the relationships within the event log to the original event logs. Further, each combination of tabular data generation is evaluated for different privacy budgets ($\varepsilon \in \{1.1, 2, 2.5, 4, 11\}$, $\delta = 0.75$. We set $(\varepsilon_{\text{TraVaS}}, \delta_{\text{TraVaS}}) = (0.1, 0.5)$ and $\tilde{\delta} = 0.0001$. Each combination of event log, TDG and privacy budget is run five times to account for the non-determinism of the TDG.

We choose *PrivBayes* [31], *MST* [18] and *DPGAN* [29] as TDGs, based on the availability of the implementation of each algorithm and the results in the literature [27]. For *PrivBayes* and *DPGAN* we use the implementation in the framework Synthcity [21]. *MST* is implemented in the framework Smartnoise-sdk github.com/opendp/smartnoise-sdk.

Stochastic Process Behaviour. We use the earth mover's conformance (EMC) [16] to measure the similarity of the stochastic process behaviour between the original and anonymised event log. This metric quantifies how closely the distribution of trace variants in the anonymised log matches the original distribution, using a value $d \in [0, 1]$. Figure 3 shows the results we obtained where an earth mover's conformance of 1 signifies perfect conformance. We observe a high conformance of the anonymised process behaviour to the original process behaviour. Further, *MST* produces better results for the traffic fine event log and the BPIC13 event log. The output from *TraVaS* is part of the input for the TDG algorithm in our framework. When comparing its EMC to the EMC of the TDG algorithms, we see only a slight decrease in conformance for the best TDG algorithms. Additional results for precision and fitness values are shown in [28].

Table 1. Means and standard deviations for different ε for Sepsis.

MST

ε	μ_{age}	$\mu_{infectionsuspected}$	$\mu_{hypotensie}$	$\mu_{infusion}$	$\mu_{oligurie}$	$\mu_{hypoxie}$
orig	70.08 ± (17.36)	0.81 ± (0.39)	0.05 ± (0.22)	0.76 ± (0.43)	0.02 ± (0.15)	0.02 ± (0.14)
11.0	66.77 ± (19.34)	0.67 ± (0.47)	0.03 ± (0.18)	0.62 ± (0.49)	0.02 ± (0.14)	0.02 ± (0.14)
4.0	65.25 ± (20.26)	0.67 ± (0.47)	0.03 ± (0.18)	0.61 ± (0.49)	0.04 ± (0.19)	0.02 ± (0.15)
2.0	55.64 ± (21.86)	0.67 ± (0.47)	0.05 ± (0.21)	0.62 ± (0.48)	0.04 ± (0.19)	0.04 ± (0.17)
1.5	55.66 ± (21.63)	0.70 ± (0.45)	0.05 ± (0.19)	0.62 ± (0.48)	0.05 ± (0.15)	0.02 ± (0.08)
1.1	55.27 ± (21.55)	0.51 ± (0.50)	0.50 ± (0.50)	0.50 ± (0.50)	0.51 ± (0.50)	0.40 ± (0.40)

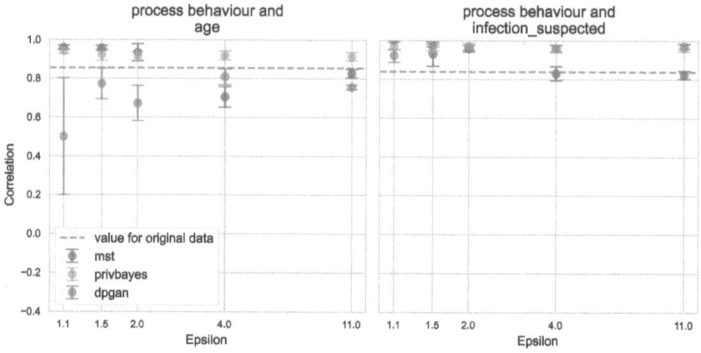

Fig. 4. Process behaviours' correlation with case attributes for Sepsis.

Descriptive Statistics of Case Attributes. Table 1 shows the statistical properties for the Sepsis event log for *MST*. We observe that for stricter privacy budgets the means and variances of the case attributes deviate more from the values of the original event log. *PrivBayes* and *DPGAN* do not show such a clear trend with the values, as shown in [28]. We find that the results for the different TDG algorithms do not differ significantly. However, in some cases, *DPGAN* fails to reproduce the distribution of binary case attributes.

Correlation Process Behaviour - Case Attributes. To test how our approach influences the relation between process behaviour and case attributes, we measure this correlation using [14] for several values of ϵ. Figure 4 shows the results for the Sepsis event logs, the other results are shown in [28]. We see that all TDG algorithms reproduce the existing correlations in the original event log. However, *MST* and *PrivBayes* produce more stable results than *DPGAN*, which deviates in some cases from the original values, especially for lower privacy budgets. Further, we see a higher variance in the results of *MST* for the lowest privacy budget.

Correlation Between Case Attributes. We compare the Pearson correlation coefficient of the numerical case attributes between the original and anonymised event logs. Figure 5 shows the correlations between the case attributes of the traffic

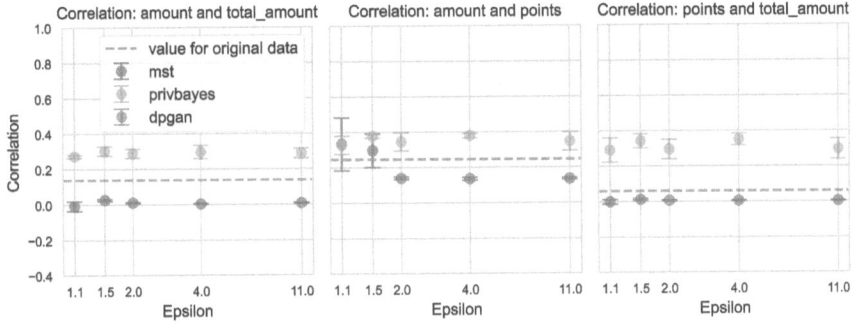

Fig. 5. Correlation measures: case attributes for Traffic fine.

fine event log. We find that the *MST* algorithm underestimates the correlations, while the *PrivBayes* algorithm overestimates them. *DPGAN* is missing due its long run times for large event logs and computational limitations. The traffic fine event log is the only one of the chosen event logs containing multiple numerical case attributes.

5   Related Work

Several papers argue for privacy in process mining by highlighting the importance of protecting individuals' data [1,6]. A direction of research is to develop algorithms to provide group-based privacy guarantees, e.g. k-anonymity [26], for event logs [11,20,22]. These methods differ to our approach in the privacy guarantee given for the anonymised event log.

DP has been applied to anonymise event logs in process mining. Prefix-based methods utilise a noisy prefix tree to anonymise the trace variants [17]. This potentially introduces new, non-original trace variants. To limit this, the construction of the prefix tree can be guided using a score function that is derived from the usefulness of the possible trace variants [9]. Similarly, methods based on Deterministic Acyclic Finite State Automata (DAFSA) add noise to the transition frequencies [7]. This reduces the spent privacy budget while maintaining a high utility, which is achieved by combining the results of applying the algorithms to subsamples of the event log [5]. A method for trace variant anonymisation using a generative adversarial network has been proposed [24]. However, this approach does not filter out infrequent trace variants or modify them, thus posing re-identification risks, see Sect. 3.2. More recently, *TraVaS*, the adoption of a differentially private partition selection algorithm for trace variants, was proposed that enables the publication of unmodified trace variants where the noisy counts are above a certain threshold [23]. All of the before mentioned approaches to guarantee DP to event logs only include control flow information and no additional information in the anonymised event logs. Finally, Fahrenkrog-Petersen et al. [10] propose a two-step approach that anonymises control flow and adds contextual information. This method assumes the independence of case attributes, limiting its applicability to real-world logs. Our framework builds on the *TraVaS* approach, further enhancing the utility by using TDG to anonymise dependent case attributes.

6   Conclusion

This work proposed DP-ELCA, a differentially private framework, to anonymise event logs with case attributes ensuring (ε, δ)-DP while ensuring data quality. We make use of TDG algorithms that provide differential privacy for tabular data. Further we discuss privacy implications when using TDG algorithms on event logs and propose to filter the event log based on a differentially private set of trace variants obtained by using *TraVaS*. This allows for the release of the anonymised event logs with dependent case attributes. The k-fold adaptive composition theorem is used to compute the resulting privacy budget.

The evaluation of three real-life event logs shows that of the chosen TDG algorithms, the MST algorithm yields the best results in terms of the similarity of the anonymised event log to the original event log. In some cases, however, a trade-off between privacy and utility can be noticed. A lower privacy budget, i.e. a stronger privacy guarantee, decreases the similarity of the original and anonymised event log.

The framework's flexibility in the choice of the TDG algorithm ensures that future advancements in the field can be leveraged. Further evaluation with other TDG algorithms and systematic evaluation of hyperparameters could improve the framework's performance. Additionally, evaluation with other real-life event logs or controlled synthetic event logs could reveal further strengths and weaknesses. An avenue for future work lies in extending the framework to include additional dimensions, such as timestamps or more granular event attributes. Additionally, the task of choosing the right epsilon value balancing the trade off between privacy and utility could be investigated and methods to detect suitable privacy budgets developed.

References

1. van der Aalst, W., et al.: Process mining manifesto. In: Business Process Management Workshops, pp. 169–194. Springer, Cham (2012)
2. Cohen, A., Nissim, K.: Towards formalizing the GDPR's notion of singling out. Proc. Natl. Acad. Sci. **117**(15), 8344–8352 (2020)
3. Dwork, C.: Differential privacy. In: Automata, Languages and Programming. Lecture Notes in Computer Science, pp. 1–12. Springer, Cham (2006)
4. Dwork, C., Roth, A., et al.: The algorithmic foundations of differential privacy. Found. Trends Theor. Comput. Sci. **9**(3–4), 211–407 (2014)
5. Elkoumy, G., Dumas, M.: Libra: high-utility anonymization of event logs for process mining via subsampling. In: ICPM, pp. 144–151 (2022)
6. Elkoumy, G., et al.: Privacy and confidentiality in process mining. ACM Trans. Manag. Inf. Syst. **13**(1), 1–17 (2022)

7. Elkoumy, G., Pankova, A., Dumas, M.: Mine me but don't single me out: differentially private event logs for process mining. In: ICPM, pp. 80–87 (2021)
8. Elkoumy, G., Pankova, A., Dumas, M.: Differentially private release of event logs for process mining. Inf. Syst. **115**, 102161 (2023)
9. Fahrenkog-Petersen, et al.: Sacofa: semantics-aware control-flow anonymization for process mining. In: 2021 ICPM, pp. 72–79 (2021)
10. Fahrenkrog-Petersen, S.A., van der Aa, H., Weidlich, M.: PRIPEL: privacy-preserving event log publishing including contextual information. In: Fahland, D., Ghidini, C., Becker, J., Dumas, M. (eds.) BPM 2020. LNCS, vol. 12168, pp. 111–128. Springer, Cham (2020). https://doi.org/10.1007/978-3-030-58666-9_7
11. Fahrenkrog-Petersen, S.A., et al.: Optimal event log sanitization for privacy-preserving process mining. Data Knowl. Eng. **145**, 102175 (2023)
12. Fung, B.C.M., Wang, K., Chen, R., Yu, P.S.: Privacy-preserving data publishing: a survey of recent developments. ACM Comput. Surv. **42**(4) (2010)
13. Kairouz, P., Oh, S., Viswanath, P.: The composition theorem for differential privacy. In: ICML, pp. 1376–1385 (2015)
14. Leemans, S.J.J., McGree, J.M., Polyvyanyy, A., ter Hofstede, A.H.: Statistical tests and association measures for business processes. IEEE Trans. Knowl. Data Eng. **35**(7), 7497–7511 (2023)
15. Leemans, S.J.J., Shabaninejad, S., Goel, K., Khosravi, H., Sadiq, S., Wynn, M.T.: Identifying cohorts. In: Conceptual Modeling, pp. 92–102 (2020)
16. Leemans, S.J.J., et al.: Stochastic process mining: earth movers' stochastic conformance. IS **102**, 101724 (2021)
17. Mannhardt, F., et al.: Privacy-preserving process mining: differential privacy for event logs. Bus. Inf. Syst. Eng. **61**, 595–614 (2019)
18. Mckenna, R., Sheldon, D., Miklau, G.: Graphical-model based estimation and inference for differential privacy. In: ICML, vol. 97, pp. 4435–4444 (2019)
19. Márquez-Chamorro, A.E., Resinas, M., Ruiz-Cortés, A.: Predictive monitoring of business processes: a survey. IEEE Trans. Serv. Comput. **11**(6), 962–977 (2018)
20. Pika, A., et al.: Privacy-preserving process mining in healthcare. Int. J. Env. Res. Pub. Health **17**(5) (2020)
21. Qian, Z., Cebere, B.C., van der Schaar, M.: Synthcity: facilitating innovative use cases of synthetic data in different data modalities (2023)
22. Rafiei, M., Wagner, M., van der Aalst, W.M.: TLKC-privacy model for process mining. In: International Conference on Research Challenges in Information Science, pp. 398–416 (2020)
23. Rafiei, M., Wangelik, F., van der Aalst, W.M.P.: Travas: differentially private trace variant selection for process mining. In: Process Mining Workshops, pp. 114–126 (2023)
24. Rafiei, M., Wangelik, F., Pourbafrani, M., van der Aalst, W.M.P.: TraVaG: differentially private trace variant generation using GANs. In: Research Challenges in Information Science: Information Science and the Connected World, pp. 415–431 (2023)
25. Sweeney, L.: Simple demographics often identify people uniquely. Health (San Francisco) **671**(2000), 1–34 (2000)
26. Sweeney, L.: k-anonymity: a model for protecting privacy. Int. J. Uncertain. Fuzziness Knowl.-Based Syst. **10**(05), 557–570 (2002)
27. Tao, Y., McKenna, R., Hay, M., Machanavajjhala, A., Miklau, G.: Benchmarking differentially private synthetic data generation algorithms. arXiv (2021)

28. Ueck, H., Andrews, R., Wynn, M.T., Leemans, S.J.J.: Technical report: differentially private event logs with case attributes. https://github.com/hueck/DP-ELCA/blob/6cf7f578d3ee18f9cad2405fb25f0be0c43dd63b/technical_report.pdf

29. Xie, L., Lin, K., Wang, S., Wang, F., Zhou, J.: Differentially private generative adversarial network (2018)

30. Yale, A., et al.: Generation and evaluation of privacy preserving synthetic health data. Neurocomputing **416**, 244–255 (2020)

31. Zhang, J., Cormode, G., Procopiuc, C.M., Srivastava, D., Xiao, X.: PrivBayes: private data release via Bayesian networks. ACM Trans. Datab. Syst. **42**(4) (2017)

CaLenDiR: Mitigating Case-Length Distortion in Deep-Learning-Based Predictive Process Monitoring

Brecht Wuyts[1]([✉]) [iD], Seppe Vanden Broucke[1,2] [iD], and Jochen De Weerdt[1] [iD]

[1] LIRIS, Faculty of Economics and Business, KU Leuven, Leuven, Belgium
brecht.wuyts@kuleuven.be
[2] Department of Business Informatics and Operations Management, Ghent University, Ghent, Belgium

Abstract. Predictive Process Monitoring (PPM) in Process Mining (PM) focuses on forecasting future aspects of ongoing business processes. Recent Deep Learning (DL) models excel at these tasks but suffer from *case-length distortion*, where longer cases dominate training and skew evaluation metrics. We propose the *CaLenDiR* (Case Length Distribution-Reflective) framework to address this, aligning DL training and evaluation with true case length distributions. *CaLenDiR* incorporates *Uniform Case-Based Sampling (UCBS)* and *suffix-length-normalized loss functions* for balanced training, along *case-based metrics* for evaluation. Our experiments show that *CaLenDiR* enhances model robustness and provides new insights into the interaction between log characteristics and model behavior.

Keywords: Process Mining · Predictive Process Monitoring · Deep Learning · Case-Length Distortion

1 Introduction

Predictive Process Monitoring (PPM) aims to predict aspects like remaining runtime, outcomes, next events, and even entire suffixes of business processes (e.g., [1,9,13]). While deep learning (DL) techniques have proven effective across these tasks [6,15], an issue we term *case-length distortion* emerges due to instance creation practices that over-represent longer cases. This distortion impacts training by reducing model generalization over true case distributions and skews evaluation metrics, potentially leading to misleading performance assessments. For suffix prediction, non-normalized loss functions further intensify this distortion.

To address case-length distortion, we introduce the *CaLenDiR* (Case Length Distribution-Reflective) PPM framework for DL-based models. CaLenDiR consists of two components: (1) *CaLenDiR training*, which applies *Uniform Case-Based Sampling (UCBS)* across PPM tasks to ensure balanced case representation in training and employs *Suffix-Length-Normalized Loss Functions* for suffix prediction; and (2) *Case-Based (CB) metrics* for evaluation, offering a more accurate alternative to traditional, skewed Instance-Based (IB) metrics.

© The Author(s) 2025
A. Delgado and T. Slaats (Eds.): ICPM 2024 Workshops, LNBIP 533, pp. 253–266, 2025.
https://doi.org/10.1007/978-3-031-82225-4_19

Extensive suffix prediction experiments demonstrate *CaLenDiR*'s ability to improve DL models' generalization and robustness, while also revealing insights into how event log characteristics and model features impact performance, enhancing our understanding of effective suffix prediction.

2   Background and Related Work

2.1   DL-Based PPM and Event Log Data

DL-Based PPM. Most DL-based PPM approaches utilize Long Short-Term Memory (LSTM) networks. Hinkka et al. [4] were early adopters of Recurrent Neural Networks (RNN) for outcome prediction, exploring LSTM variants. Weytjens et al. [14] demonstrated that Convolutional Neural Networks (CNNs) could serve as a fast, competitive alternative to LSTMs for outcome prediction. For runtime prediction, Navarin et al. [7] introduced an LSTM model to directly estimate remaining time, while Tax et al. [9] and Camargo et al. [1] employed LSTM networks for multi-task next-event prediction, targeting activity labels and timestamps, with [1] also predicting roles. Suffix and remaining time predictions were subsequently derived from these models using feedback loops. More recently, Philipp et al. [8] introduced Transformer components for next-event prediction, marking a shift toward advanced architectures. Numerous DL-based techniques for suffix prediction have also emerged, relevant to our *CaLenDiR* framework, detailed further in Sect. 2.2.

PPM neural networks, despite architectural differences, share a common training method. Data is processed in small *batches*, with predictions compared to actual targets via a *loss function*. Model parameters are iteratively adjusted to minimize this error across all batches within an *epoch*. Multiple epochs enable refinement of predictions, improving accuracy as the dataset is repeatedly processed.

Event Log Data. An *event log* $L = \{\sigma_i | 1 \leq i \leq |L|\}$ records cases σ_i that represent a sequence of chronologically ordered events $\langle e_{i,1}, \ldots, e_{i,n_i} \rangle$, with n_i being the number of events executed for that particular case. For notational simplicity, unless explicitly needed, the subscript i referring to the case is omitted. An *event* is a tuple $e = (a, c, t, f_1, \ldots, f_m)$ with a the activity label, c the case ID, t the timestamp, and $f_1, \ldots, f_m$ (with $m \geq 0$) the potential case and event features. All elements comprising the event tuple e can be accessed individually, and are denoted by means of the subscript of the event. E.g., the activity label of the j-th event e_j ($j \in \{1, ..., n\}$) is denoted by a_j, while the timestamp of that same event is denoted by t_j.

Moreover, to enable algorithms to interpret (and predict) timestamps, it is necessary to convert them into a numerical proxy. As such, they are converted into the numerical feature *time elapsed since the previous event* $t_j^p = t_j - t_{j-1}$ ($\forall j = 2, ..., n$), capturing the absolute amount of time elapsed since the previous event. For the first event e_1, $t_1^p = 0$.

PPM techniques are trained and evaluated on historical data. To do so, event log L is subdivided into a training log L_{train} ($\subset L$) and test log L_{test} ($\subset L$). Afterwards, for both L_{train} and L_{test}, each case σ_i is parsed into n_i prefix-target pairs or instances $\{(\sigma_{i,k}^p, y_{i,k})|1 \leq k \leq n_i\}$ (e.g. $[1,3,7,12–15]$)[1] ultimately resulting in the training and test set of instances, N_{train} & N_{test}. The prefix $\sigma_{i,k}^p = \langle e_{i,1}, \ldots, e_{i,k} \rangle$ contains the first k events, mimicking a real-life unfinished case, serving as the input, while the target $y_{i,k}$ encapsulates the ground-truth prediction target(s), the form of which depends on the specific prediction task at hand.

For instance, in remaining time prediction, the target $y_k = r_k$ represents the total remaining runtime from the last observed prefix event e_k until the case completion e_n, calculated as $r_k = t_n - t_k$. For next event prediction, the target $y_k = a_{k+1}$ is the activity label of the event that directly follows the last observed prefix event e_k (e.g. [2]). Alternatively, other next event prediction approaches (e.g., [1,9,10]) opt for the multi-task target $y_k = (a_{k+1}, t_{k+1}^p)$, simultaneously predicting the next event's activity label and its timestamp (proxy). In (binary) outcome prediction, the target $y_k = o$ with $o \in \{0,1\}$ represents a binary label indicating a particular outcome of the process. Note that the subscript k is omitted since true label o does not depend on event index k. Lastly, in suffix prediction, a commonly used (multi-task) target y_k is the sequence $\langle (a_{k+1}, t_{k+1}^p), \ldots, (a_n, t_n^p), (EOS) \rangle$, which includes the remaining activity labels and their corresponding timestamps, i.e. the activity and timestamp suffix, with an *End Of Sequence* (EOS) token added during preprocessing to denote the end of a case. Additionally, many suffix prediction techniques produce an additional scalar remaining runtime prediction $\hat{r}_k$, either directly (e.g. [3,15]), or indirectly (e.g. [1,5,9,11]).

2.2   Suffix Prediction

The majority of (DL-based) suffix prediction techniques are developed to jointly predict the activity suffix $\langle a_{k+1}, \ldots, a_n, EOS \rangle$, timestamp suffix $\langle t_{k+1}^p, \ldots, t_n^p \rangle$ and remaining runtime r_k, when being presented with a prefix σ_k^p. As such, the multi-task target y_k comprises two sequences and one scalar target.

All suffix prediction networks are trained using a multi-task loss function for joint optimization. Most use an additive loss function, summing the individual loss functions for each target. Commonly used loss functions for these targets include:

1. **Activity Suffix Prediction - Categorical Cross Entropy**: Let $\hat{a}_{j,t}$ be the predicted probability for the t-th activity label in the suffix of the j-th instance, and $a_{j,t}$ be the true activity label. The cross-entropy loss for the activity suffix is given by:

$$\mathcal{L}_{\text{activity}} = -\frac{1}{\sum_{j=1}^{B} N_j} \sum_{j=1}^{B} \sum_{t=1}^{N_j} \sum_{c=1}^{C} a_{j,t,c} \log(\hat{a}_{j,t,c}) \tag{1}$$

---

[1] Other approaches (e.g. [5,9,11]) slightly deviate, and construct $n_i - 1$ instances, with $2 \leq k \leq n_i$.

where B is the batch size, N_j is the number of events in the (ground-truth) suffix of the j-th instance, and C is the number of possible activity labels.

2. **Timestamp Suffix Prediction - Mean Absolute Error (MAE):** Let $\hat{t}^p_{j,t}$ be the predicted timestamp for the t-th event in the suffix of the j-th instance, and $t^p_{j,t}$ be the true timestamp. The MAE loss for the timestamp suffix is given by:

$$\mathcal{L}_{\text{timestamp}} = \frac{1}{\sum_{j=1}^{B} N_j} \sum_{j=1}^{B} \sum_{t=1}^{N_j} |\hat{t}^p_{j,t} - t^p_{j,t}| \tag{2}$$

3. **Remaining Runtime Prediction - Mean Absolute Error (MAE):** Let $\hat{r}_j$ be the predicted remaining runtime for the j-th instance, and r_j be the true remaining runtime. The MAE loss for the remaining runtime is given by:

$$\mathcal{L}_{\text{runtime}} = \frac{1}{B} \sum_{j=1}^{B} |\hat{r}_j - r_j| \tag{3}$$

However, the way in which different techniques are trained to ultimately deliver these predictions, differs. Most recently, Wuyts et al. [15] proposed a Data-Aware (DA) encoder-decoder Transformer-based network, the only technique explicitly trained for jointly predicting all three targets, using the following composite loss function $\mathcal{L}_{\text{batch}} = \mathcal{L}_{\text{activity}} + \mathcal{L}_{\text{timestamp}} + \mathcal{L}_{\text{runtime}}$. Taymouri et al. [11] introduced a Non-Data-Aware (NDA) encoder-decoder LSTM network trained to generate activity and timestamp suffixes, with the remaining runtime implicitly derived by computing the sum over the predicted timestamp (proxy) suffix, i.e., $\hat{r}_k = \sum \hat{t}^p_{k+i}$. They furthermore complement supervised training with adversarial learning, resulting in performance gains for the largest beam widths. They used the following supervised loss function: $\mathcal{L}_{\text{batch}} = \mathcal{L}'_{\text{activity}} + \mathcal{L}'_{\text{timestamp}}$, with $\mathcal{L}'_{\text{activity}} = \sum_{i=1}^{B} \sum_{t=1}^{N_i} \sum_{c=1}^{C} a_{i,t,c} \log(\hat{a}_{i,t,c})$, which is highly similar to Eq. 1, except for the omission of averaging, and with $\mathcal{L}'_{\text{timestamp}} = \sum_{i=1}^{B} \left((\sum \hat{t}^p_{k+i}) - \sum t^p_{k+i} \right)^2$. Ketykó et al. [5] compared various NDA suffix prediction models, including encoder-decoder LSTM and Transformer architectures. These seq2seq models were trained for activity and timestamp suffix prediction, with remaining runtime derived during inference ($\hat{r}_k = \sum \hat{t}^p_{k+i}$), using a weighted sum of categorical cross-entropy and Mean Squared Error (MSE) losses. The MSE loss is akin to the MAE loss (Eq. 2), but with $(\hat{t}_{i,t} - t_{i,t})^2$ replacing $|\hat{t}_{i,t} - t_{i,t}|$. The DA LSTM-based technique by Gunnarsson et al. [3] is explicitly trained to predict the activity and remaining time suffix $\langle r_k, \ldots, r_{n-1} \rangle$, deviating from the common timestamp suffix approach. During inference, timestamp suffix predictions can be derived by subtracting consecutive timestamp predictions ($\hat{t}^p_{k+i} = \hat{r}_{k+i-1} - \hat{r}_{k+i}$), while only the first element of the predicted remaining time suffix ($\hat{r}_k$) is used for remaining time estimation. They used the following loss function: $\mathcal{L}_{\text{batch}} = \mathcal{L}_{\text{activity}} + \mathcal{L}'_{\text{runtime}}$. It should be noted that the latter component ($\mathcal{L}'_{\text{runtime}}$) is the MAE as defined in Eq. 2, except that it is computed over the predicted remaining time suffixes instead of the timestamp suffixes.

Moreover, earlier DL suffix prediction techniques, referred to as *Single-Event Prediction (SEP)* techniques, are explicitly trained for next event (instead of suffix) prediction, i.e. the joint prediction of the next event's activity and timestamp proxy (a_{k+1}, t^p_{k+1}). Only upon inference, they are leveraged for suffix generation by means of an iterative feedback loop, updating event prefixes after every consecutive prediction, with remaining time derived as in [5,11]. Examples are the techniques proposed by [1,9] (as discussed in Sect. 2.1), with [9] utilizing the unweighted sum of $\mathcal{L}^1_{\text{activity}}$ and $\mathcal{L}^1_{\text{timestamp}}$, which are similar to their suffix counterparts, Eq. 1 and 2 respectively, but with $N_j = 1$, and [1] adding a third component to the loss: the cross entropy loss $\mathcal{L}^1_{\text{role}}$ for predicting the next 'role' as well.

2.3   Case-Length Distortion

Without further domain knowledge or specific attention to a specific set of cases, one would prefer PPM techniques to generalize well over the underlying distribution of cases and their case lengths. However, the common practice of *instance creation* (Sect. 2.1) and, in the case of suffix prediction, the prevalent use of *non-normalized loss functions* in seq2seq DL architectures (Sect. 2.2, 4.1), introduces case-length distortions, hindering this ideal generalization and skewing evaluation metrics.

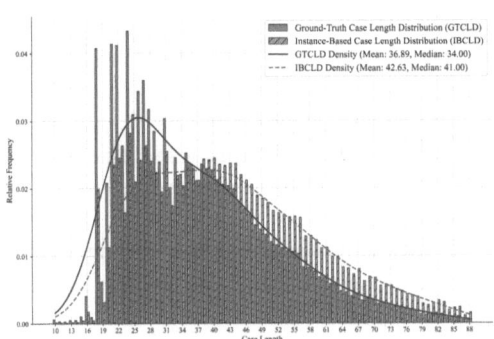

Fig. 1. Ground-Truth and Instance-Based Case Length Distributions for BPIC17 (post-preprocessing), highlighting the overrepresentation of longer cases in the instance-based distribution.

Instance Creation. Creating instances by parsing each original case σ_i into n_i prefix-target pairs (Sect. 2.1) leads to an overrepresentation of longer cases among the derived instances in both the training N_{train} and test N_{test} sets, compared to their original distribution of case lengths. This artificially induced bias towards longer cases in N_{train} skews the models' learning process and negatively influences the degree to which the models generalize across the underlying case length distribution. Similarly, by default, evaluation metrics should measure models' true performance across all test log cases $\sigma_i \in L_{test}$, with each case weighted equally, regardless of its length and resulting instances in N_{test}. However, evaluation metrics are typically computed by averaging over all instances in the test set N_{test}, unintentionally amplifying the influence of longer cases (Sect. 3.3).

Figure 1 illustrates case-length distortion in the BPIC17[2] event log postpreprocessing. It compares the original case length distribution (GTCLD) with that after instance parsing (IBCLD). Note that the IBCLD represents the distribution of case lengths among the created instances, where each instance is labeled with the length of the original case it was derived from. The comparison shows a clear shift towards longer cases in the IBCLD, where they are overrepresented at the expense of cases pertaining to more representative lengths, as also reflected in the means and medians.

Additionally, event logs' case length distributions generally exhibit a pronounced right-skew, with outliers often containing significantly more events than the median. Further investigation revealed these extended cases to be frequently characterized by multiple repetitions of the same activity or group of activities, often executed in quick succession, which raises important considerations regarding their representativeness in modeling and whether models should be designed to accommodate or mitigate the influence of such disproportionately represented cases.

Non-normalized Loss Functions. In suffix prediction, instances originating from longer cases inherently possess longer ground-truth suffixes on average. Standard sequential loss functions, such as $\mathcal{L}_{activity}$ (Eq. 1) and $\mathcal{L}_{timestamp}$ (Eq. 2), average across all time steps within these suffixes for every instance in the batch, resulting in a greater number of terms in the loss calculation for instances from longer cases, disproportionately amplifying their influence on the overall loss. Consequently, these longer cases exert a stronger effect on the gradient updates during training, further skewing the models' learning process towards them.

3   Case Length Distribution-Reflective (*CaLenDiR*) PPM

In this section, we introduce the three core components of the *CaLenDiR* PPM framework designed to address case-length distortion: Uniform Case-Based Sampling (UCBS) (Sect. 3.1), Suffix-Length-Normalized Loss Functions for suffix prediction (Sect. 3.2), and Case-Based Evaluation Metrics (Sect. 3.3).

---

[2] https://doi.org/10.4121/uuid:5f3067df-f10b-45da-b98b-86ae4c7a310b.

3.1   Uniform Case-Based Sampling (*UCBS*)

UCBS counteracts case-length distortion by equalizing the contribution of each case to the training set. At the start of each epoch, it samples a uniform number of instances from each case σ_i in training log L_{train}, regardless of its original length. Let $N_{\sigma_i} = \{(\sigma^p_{i,k}, y_{i,k}) | 1 \leq k \leq n_i\}$ be the set of instances (i.e., prefix-target pairs) derived from case σ_i. The training set $N_{train} = \bigcup_{\sigma_i \in L_{train}} N_{\sigma_i}$ encompasses all instances derived from all cases $\sigma_i \in L_{train}$, with $\tilde{n}_{train} = \text{median}(\{n_i \mid \sigma_i \in L_{train}\})$ as the median case length. The *UCBS* procedure, detailed in Algorithm 1, begins by setting a random seed equal to the epoch number, ensuring slightly different sampled sets $N^{(e)}_{train}$ each epoch e, which aids regularization and maintains reproducibility.

The procedure iterates over each case in L_{train}, sampling $\tilde{n}_{train}$ instances from N_{σ_i}. If the number of instances for a case is less than $\tilde{n}_{train}$, sampling is done with replacement; otherwise, without replacement[3]. This design balances uniform instance contribution with diversity, reducing the risk of overfitting and improving training stability. The sampled instances are then aggregated to form the training set for epoch e: $N^{(e)}_{train}$.

Algorithm 1. Uniform Case-Based Sampling (UCBS) Procedure

1: **Input:** Training log L_{train}, training set N_{train}, median case length $\tilde{n}_{train}$, epoch number e
2: **Output:** Sampled training set $N^{(e)}_{train}$
3: **Set random seed** $s = e$
4: $N^{(e)}_{train} \leftarrow \emptyset$
5: **for all** $\sigma_i \in L_{train}$ **do**
6:     $N_{\sigma_i} \leftarrow \{(\sigma^p_{i,k}, y_{i,k}) \in N_{train} \mid 1 \leq k \leq n_i\}$
7:     **if** $|N_{\sigma_i}| < \tilde{n}_{train}$ **then**
8:         $N^{(e)}_{\sigma_i} \leftarrow$ sample $\tilde{n}_{train}$ instances from N_{σ_i} with replacement
9:     **else**
10:         $N^{(e)}_{\sigma_i} \leftarrow$ sample $\tilde{n}_{train}$ instances from N_{σ_i} without replacement
11:     **end if**
12:     $N^{(e)}_{train} \leftarrow N^{(e)}_{train} \cup N^{(e)}_{\sigma_i}$
13: **end for**
14: **return** $N^{(e)}_{train}$

3.2   Suffix-Length-Normalized Loss Functions

CaLenDiR's *Suffix-Length-Normalized Loss Functions* provide an alternative to the standard loss functions commonly used in seq2seq neural networks (e.g.,

---

[3] In the commonly applied instance creation approach, as described in Sect. 2.1, $|N_{\sigma_i}| = n_i$. We use the generic $|N_{\sigma_i}|$ to ensure UCBS is applicable to methods where this may not hold, such as those creating only $n_i - 1$ instances (i.e., $N_{\sigma_i} = \{(\sigma^p_{i,k}, y_{i,k}) \mid 2 \leq k \leq n_i\}$).

[3,5,11,15]), which exacerbate case-length distortion. These functions normalize each instance's contribution by its suffix length N_j, rather than summing over all suffix elements in a batch, ensuring equal weighting of all instances and preventing overemphasis on longer cases. The normalized versions of Eq. 1 and 2 are provided in Eq. 4 and 5, respectively. This normalization can also be applied to other timestamp loss functions, such as Mean Squared Error (MSE) used in, e.g., [5]. For SEP techniques (e.g., [1,2,9]), suffix-length normalization is unnecessary, as they predict only the next event, with a single error per instance contributing to the loss.

$$\widetilde{\mathcal{L}}_{\text{activity}} = -\frac{1}{B} \sum_{j=1}^{B} \left(\frac{1}{N_j} \sum_{t=1}^{N_j} \sum_{c=1}^{C} a_{j,t,c} \log(\hat{a}_{j,t,c}) \right) \tag{4}$$

$$\widetilde{\mathcal{L}}_{\text{timestamp}} = \frac{1}{B} \sum_{j=1}^{B} \left(\frac{1}{N_j} \sum_{t=1}^{N_j} |\hat{t}^p_{j,t} - t^p_{j,t}| \right) \tag{5}$$

3.3   Case-Based Evaluation Metrics

The test log $\boldsymbol{L}_{test}$ is transformed into a test set $\boldsymbol{N}_{test} = \bigcup_{\sigma_i \in \boldsymbol{L}_{test}} \boldsymbol{N}_{\sigma_i}$ (Sect. 2.1, 3.1). In multi-task settings, the target $\boldsymbol{y}_{i,k}$ comprises multiple prediction tasks. Let $\boldsymbol{y}^x_{i,k} \in \boldsymbol{y}_{i,k}$ denote the ground truth for prediction task x and prefix $\boldsymbol{\sigma}^p_{i,k}$, and let $\widehat{\boldsymbol{y}}^x_{i,k}$ be the corresponding model prediction. The evaluation function $m_x : (\boldsymbol{y}^x_{i,k}, \widehat{\boldsymbol{y}}^x_{i,k}) \mapsto \mathbb{R}$ rates the prediction $\widehat{\boldsymbol{y}}^x_{i,k}$ against the ground truth $\boldsymbol{y}^x_{i,k}$. Finally, let $\alpha_{i,k}$ denote the pair $(\boldsymbol{\sigma}^p_{i,k}, \boldsymbol{y}_{i,k})$. The standard instance-based (IB) evaluation metric for prediction task x, averaging over all instances $\alpha_{i,k} \in \boldsymbol{N}_{test}$, is then defined as:

$$\overline{M}_{IB} = \frac{1}{|\boldsymbol{N}_{test}|} \sum_{i=1}^{|\boldsymbol{L}_{test}|} \sum_{\alpha_{i,k} \in \boldsymbol{N}_{\sigma_i}} m_x(\boldsymbol{y}^x_{i,k}, \widehat{\boldsymbol{y}}^x_{i,k}) \tag{6}$$

In this approach, longer cases disproportionately influence the results due to their higher instance count. To mitigate this, we propose case-based (CB) evaluation metrics, where each test case $\boldsymbol{\sigma}_i$ is weighted equally, regardless of length. This is done by first averaging the score per case and then averaging across all cases in the test set, as shown in Eq. 7. This method provides a more balanced evaluation, accurately reflecting the model's performance across all cases in the test log $\boldsymbol{L}_{test}$.

$$\overline{M}_{CB} = \frac{1}{|\boldsymbol{L}_{test}|} \sum_{i=1}^{|\boldsymbol{L}_{test}|} \frac{1}{|\boldsymbol{N}_{\sigma_i}|} \left(\sum_{\alpha_{i,k} \in \boldsymbol{N}_{\sigma_i}} m_x(\boldsymbol{y}^x_{i,k}, \widehat{\boldsymbol{y}}^x_{i,k}) \right) \tag{7}$$

4   Experimental Setup

In our previous work [15], we introduced a Transformer-based seq2seq architecture for suffix prediction and re-implemented five existing architectures, applying consistent data preprocessing and scaling. All models were trained and evaluated on four real-life event logs using the standard approach. In this study, we replicate the experimental setup from [15] to evaluate *CaLenDiR* training for suffix prediction. The same models are retrained on the same event logs with identical hyperparameters, except for *(1)* the use of *UCBS* instead of processing the entire training set N_{train} each epoch (Sect. 3.1), and *(2)* suffix-length normalization of the loss functions (Sect. 3.2).

While [15] primarily reported conventional Instance-Based (IB) metrics, this paper expands the analysis by including Case-Based (CB) metrics (Sect. 3.3, 4.2) for both *CaLenDiR*-trained models and those trained using the standard approach in [15]. To provide a comprehensive perspective, we also report IB metrics for both training approaches. This dual reporting offers a more nuanced understanding of case-length distortion and the impact of *CaLenDiR* training on model performance and generalization.

By directly comparing the evaluation metrics of *CaLenDiR*-trained models with those trained using the standard approach, we isolate the impact of the training methodology, clearly measuring the improvements facilitated by *CaLenDiR*.

4.1 Data and Models

The four real-life event logs are: BPIC17 (see Footnote 2), BPIC17-DR, BPIC19[4], and BAC. Table 1 summarizes their main properties, including the average and standard deviation of the case length (event count) and case duration. BPIC17-DR is a variant of BPIC17 with subsequent repetitions of the same activity removed to enhance data quality. The BAC log, sourced from a major European airport's luggage handling system, is not publicly available. Adopting a chronological 75–25% out-of-time train-test split, each event log L is subdivided into a training and test log (L_{train} & L_{test}). The former was further divided into final training and validation logs (L_{train} & L_{val}) by assigning the last 20% of cases to L_{val}. The final train, validation and test sets (N_{train}, N_{val} & N_{test}) are derived from L_{train}, L_{val} and L_{test} as discussed in Sect. 2.1. Please refer to [15] for further details regarding the preprocessing pipeline.

Table 1 summarizes the six implementations, re-trained using the *CaLenDiR* framework. The *'DA'* column indicates whether the architecture is *Data-Aware*,

Table 1. Overview of the models (left) and event logs (right) included in the experimental comparison [15].

Benchmark	seq2seqDA	Explicit RT prediction	Explicit timestamp prediction	Default loss	CaLenDiR loss
SEP-LSTM	✗	✗	✗	✓	$\mathcal{L}_{activity}^1 + \mathcal{L}_{timestamp}^1$	$\mathcal{L}_{activity}^1 + \mathcal{L}_{timestamp}^1$
CRTP-LSTM (NDA)	✓	✗	✓	✗	$\mathcal{L}_{activity} + \mathcal{L}_{runtime}^*$	$\mathcal{L}_{activity} + \mathcal{L}_{runtime}$
CRTP-LSTM	✓	✓	✓	✗	$\mathcal{L}_{activity} + \mathcal{L}_{runtime}^*$	$\mathcal{L}_{activity} + \mathcal{L}_{runtime}$
ED-LSTM	✓	✗	✗	✓	$\mathcal{L}_{activity} + \mathcal{L}_{timestamp}$	$\mathcal{L}_{activity} + \mathcal{L}_{timestamp}$
SuTraN (NDA)	✓	✗	✓	✓	$\mathcal{L}_{activity} + \mathcal{L}_{timestamp} + \mathcal{L}_{runtime}$	$\mathcal{L}_{activity} + \mathcal{L}_{timestamp} + \mathcal{L}_{runtime}$
SuTraN	✓	✓	✓	✓	$\mathcal{L}_{activity} + \mathcal{L}_{timestamp} + \mathcal{L}_{runtime}$	$\mathcal{L}_{activity} + \mathcal{L}_{timestamp} + \mathcal{L}_{runtime}$

Log	Cases · Events	Variants	avg. - SD Length	avg. - SD Duration
BPIC17	30,078 – 1,109,665	14,745	36.90 – 14.55	20.52 – 10.81 (days)
BPIC17-DR	30,078 – 704,202	3,592	23.42 – 6.85	20.52 – 10.81 (days)
BPIC19	181,395 – 986,077	5,767	5.44 – 1.78	71.76 – 36.78 (days)
BAC	362,563 – 1,767,186	13,496	4.87 – 2.49	732 – 912.24 (sec.)

---

[4] https://doi.org/10.4121/uuid:d06aff4b-79f0-45e6-8ec8-e19730c248f1.

leveraging (all) available payload data beyond just the timestamp and activity information of the prefix events. *SEP-LSTM* is a re-implementation of [9], trained solely for next event prediction, only generating suffixes during inference using an external feedback loop (Sect. 2). *CRTP-LSTM* re-implements the DA architecture from [3], while *ED-LSTM*, an encoder-decoder LSTM, is based on NDA techniques from [5,11]. *SuTraN* is the encoder-decoder Transformer network from [15]. *SuTraN* and *CRTP-LSTM* are the only DA models, with NDA versions (*SuTraN (NDA)* and *CRTP-LSTM (NDA)*) also implemented.

During inference, all implementations generate an activity suffix, timestamp suffix, and remaining runtime prediction, though the specific targets trained for, differ (Sect. 2.2). Each implementation uses a simple additive loss function, summing the losses for its explicit prediction targets. The individual loss components (Table 1) are standardized across implementations to ensure a level playing field. For *CaLenDiR* training, seq2seq models use Suffix-Length-Normalized Cross Entropy (Eq. 4) for activity suffix prediction and Normalized MAE (Eq. 5) for timestamp suffix prediction. In *CRTP-LSTM*, the MAE is applied to remaining time suffixes instead of timestamp suffixes. *SuTraN*, which predicts all three targets, adds a third loss function (Eq. 3) for remaining time prediction, but no normalization is needed since it outputs a scalar instead of a sequence. *SEP-LSTM*, trained only for next event prediction, uses non-sequential cross-entropy $\mathcal{L}^1_{activity}$ and MAE $\mathcal{L}^1_{timestamp}$ for next activity and timestamp prediction (Sect. 2.2), respectively, which do not require normalization. Aside from these training specifics, all other hyperparameters and inference settings, were kept consistent with those in [15].

4.2 Evaluation - Uniform Case-Based vs. Instance-Based

We evaluate the three prediction tasks using (normalized) Damerau-Levenshtein Similarity (DLS) for activity suffix prediction and mean absolute error (MAE) for both timestamp suffix and remaining time prediction. DLS measures sequence similarity on a scale from 0 (completely different) to 1 (identical) and is calculated as $DLS(X, Y) = 1 - \frac{DL(X,Y)}{\max(|X|,|Y|)}$, where $DL(X, Y)$ is the Damerau-Levenshtein distance between sequences X and Y, and $\max(|X|, |Y|)$ the length of the longer sequence. For activity suffix prediction, DLS is computed for each instance $\alpha_{i,k} = (\sigma^p_{i,k}, y_{i,k})$ in N_{test} as $DLS(y^{activity}_{i,k}, \widehat{y}^{activity}_{i,k})$, where $y^{activity}_{i,k}$ is the ground-truth activity suffix and $\widehat{y}^{activity}_{i,k}$ the predicted suffix. The IB and CB metrics ($\overline{DLS}_{IB}$ & $\overline{DLS}_{CB}$) are derived by setting $m_x(y^x_{i,k}, \widehat{y}^x_{i,k})$ to $DLS(y^{activity}_{i,k}, \widehat{y}^{activity}_{i,k})$ in Eqs. 6 and 7 respectively. The IB and CB metrics for remaining time ($\overline{MAE}^{runtime}_{IB}$ & $\overline{MAE}^{runtime}_{CB}$) are calculated by setting $m_x(y^x_{i,k}, \widehat{y}^x_{i,k})$ to $|\widehat{r}_{i,k} - r_{i,k}|$.

In contrast, the MAE for timestamp suffix prediction is computed across the $N_{i,k}$ predicted timestamps in the suffix. Let $\widehat{t}^p_{i,k;t}$ and $t^p_{i,k;t}$ represent the predicted and true timestamps, respectively. The IB MAE is given by:

$$\overline{MAE}_{IB}^{timestamp} = \frac{1}{|N_{test}|} \sum_{i=1}^{|L_{test}|} \sum_{\alpha_{i,k}\in N_{\sigma_i}} \sum_{t=1}^{N_{i,k}} |\widehat{t}_{i,k;t}^{\,p} - t_{i,k;t}^{p}|$$

To counter the resulting additional distortions (cf. Sect. 2.3 and 3.2), the CB MAE includes both case-based weighting and suffix-length normalization:

$$\overline{MAE}_{CB}^{timestamp} = \frac{1}{|L_{test}|} \sum_{i=1}^{|L_{test}|} \frac{1}{|N_{\sigma_i}|} \left(\sum_{\alpha_{i,k}\in N_{\sigma_i}} \frac{1}{N_{i,k}} \sum_{t=1}^{N_{i,k}} |\widehat{t}_{i,k;t}^{\,p} - t_{i,k;t}^{p}| \right)$$

5 Results

Tables 2a and 2b present IB and CB performance metrics for models trained using both standard and *CaLenDiR* methods. The best results are bolded and underlined, with second-best in bold. Table 2c shows percentage changes in these metrics, comparing *CaLenDiR* to standard training. Our analysis focuses on the less distorted CB metrics unless noted otherwise.

Overall, *CaLenDiR* training improves CB metrics across all prediction tasks, as shown in the *Average Change* row in Table 2c. Minor exceptions include slight declines in CB DLS, MAE_{suffix}, and $MAE_{runtime}$ for BPIC19 by approximately 1.99%, 2.35%, and 1.18%, respectively. These findings indicate that *CaLenDiR* improves generalization and robustness. IB metrics often decrease with *CaLenDiR*, as anticipated, with a significant 16.31% IB DLS improvement on BPIC17 as an exception.

Table 2. Performance comparison across different techniques and datasets

(a) Standard Training

Model	DLS BPIC17-DR IB	CB	DLS BPIC17 IB	CB	DLS BPIC19 IB	CB	DLS BAC IB	CB	MAE$_{suffix}$ BPIC17-DR IB	CB	BPIC17 IB	CB	BPIC19 IB	CB	BAC (sec.) IB	CB	MAE$_{runtime}$ BPIC17-DR IB	CB	BPIC17 IB	CB	BPIC19 IB	CB	BAC (sec.) IB	CB
SEP-LSTM	0.6733	0.6902	0.2160	0.2823	0.8425	0.8183	0.7206	0.7488	1178	1219	762	1048	16604	13930	113	64	10139	9699	11823	11683	30572	33645	420	262
CRTP-LSTM (NDA)	0.6525	0.6734	0.3357	0.3692	0.8435	0.8188	0.7320	0.7640	1391	1313	1009	1248	17182	14511	113	66	8931	8520	8906	8788	29323	33400	318	204
CRTP-LSTM	0.6741	0.7149	0.4095	0.4660	0.8522	0.8427	0.8374	0.8647	1556	1414	996	1184	15708	13572	112	61	8000	7287	8685	8059	21345	24360	301	191
ED-LSTM	0.6737	0.6902	0.3239	0.3623	0.8477	0.8201	0.7424	0.7663	1200	1224	739	993	16485	13810	108	61	9705	9298	12160	11889	31000	33914	338	217
SuTraN (NDA)	0.6723	0.6895	0.2669	0.3161	0.8435	0.8193	0.7355	0.7645	1201	1224	745	1008	16621	13897	109	61	8896	8452	8860	8754	29209	33387	308	200
SuTraN	0.7274	0.7621	0.3843	0.4621	0.8699	0.8601	0.8461	0.8698	1157	977	749	882	14542	12446	106	58	7727	6945	7913	7260	20182	23462	290	183

(b) CaLenDiR Training

Model	DLS BPIC17-DR IB	CB	DLS BPIC17 IB	CB	DLS BPIC19 IB	CB	DLS BAC IB	CB	MAE$_{suffix}$ BPIC17-DR IB	CB	BPIC17 IB	CB	BPIC19 IB	CB	BAC (sec.) IB	CB	MAE$_{runtime}$ BPIC17-DR IB	CB	BPIC17 IB	CB	BPIC19 IB	CB	BAC (sec.) IB	CB
SEP-LSTM	0.6738	0.6931	0.2132	0.2818	0.8425	0.8217	0.7421	0.7764	1190	1218	759	1001	16909	14139	112	60	9821	9405	11940	11590	30134	33324	382	234
CRTP-LSTM (NDA)	0.6268	0.7014	0.4285	0.5207	0.7851	0.7784	0.7077	0.7421	1655	1298	1160	1136	18005	15046	122	72	9878	8775	10252	9157	33173	33730	331	201
CRTP-LSTM	0.6868	0.7551	0.4700	0.5523	0.8498	0.8451	0.8338	0.8665	1525	1318	1088	1209	16207	14105	109	54	8035	7072	8503	7513	22509	24938	301	177
ED-LSTM	0.6485	0.7141	0.3862	0.4809	0.7931	0.7883	0.7127	0.7564	1265	1181	804	948	17268	14061	115	62	9231	8795	10817	10078	36490	36624	385	252
SuTraN (NDA)	0.6521	0.7137	0.3704	0.4669	0.7907	0.7870	0.7097	0.7535	1288	1153	909	930	17260	14455	115	62	8943	8422	9015	8657	29716	32734	313	195
SuTraN	0.7278	0.7848	0.3795	0.4780	0.8656	0.8612	0.8386	0.8708	1187	943	765	833	14620	12341	107	52	7770	6939	7859	7092	20076	23146	285	169

(c) Percentage Change Comparison

Model	DLS BPIC17-DR IB	CB	DLS BPIC17 IB	CB	DLS BPIC19 IB	CB	DLS BAC IB	CB	MAE$_{suffix}$ BPIC17-DR IB	CB	BPIC17 IB	CB	BPIC19 IB	CB	BAC (sec.) IB	CB	MAE$_{runtime}$ BPIC17-DR IB	CB	BPIC17 IB	CB	BPIC19 IB	CB	BAC (sec.) IB	CB
SEP-LSTM	+0.07	+0.42	-1.30	-0.18	+0.00	+0.42	+2.98	+3.69	+1.02	-0.08	-0.39	-4.48	+1.84	+1.50	-0.88	-6.25	-3.14	-3.03	+0.99	-0.80	-1.43	-0.95	-9.05	-10.69
CRTP-LSTM (NDA)	-3.94	+4.16	+27.64	+41.03	-6.92	-4.93	-3.32	-1.48	+18.98	-1.14	+14.97	-8.97	+4.79	+3.69	+7.96	+9.09	+10.60	+2.99	+15.11	+4.20	+13.13	+0.99	+4.09	-1.47
CRTP-LSTM	+1.88	+5.62	+14.77	+18.52	-0.28	+0.28	-0.43	+0.21	-1.99	-6.79	+9.24	+2.11	+3.18	+3.93	-2.68	-11.48	+0.44	-2.25	-2.10	-6.78	+5.45	+2.37	+0.00	-7.3
ED-LSTM	-3.74	+3.46	+19.23	+32.74	-6.44	-3.88	-4.00	-1.29	+5.42	-3.51	+20.97	-4.53	+1.60	+1.82	+6.48	+1.64	-4.88	-5.41	-11.04	-15.23	+17.71	+7.99	+13.91	+16.13
SuTraN (NDA)	-3.00	+3.51	+38.78	+47.71	-6.26	-3.94	-3.51	-1.44	+7.24	-5.80	+22.01	-7.74	+3.84	+4.02	+5.50	+1.64	+0.53	-0.35	+1.75	-1.11	+1.71	-1.96	+1.62	-2.50
SuTraN	+0.05	+2.98	-1.25	+3.44	-0.49	+0.13	-0.89	+0.11	+2.59	-3.48	+2.14	-5.56	+0.54	-0.84	+0.94	-10.34	+0.56	-0.09	-0.68	-2.31	-0.53	-1.35	-1.72	-7.65
Average Change	-1.45	+3.36	+16.31	+23.88	-3.49	-1.99	-1.53	-0.03	+5.54	-3.47	+11.49	-4.86	+2.63	+2.35	+2.89	-2.62	+0.68	-1.47	+0.67	-3.67	+6.01	+1.18	+1.47	-2.25

Eliminating case-length distortion has implications for model evaluation and benchmarking. *CaLenDiR*-trained models see shifts in CB rankings across logs, especially for activity and timestamp suffix predictions, and in three of four logs for remaining time predictions, indicating that model susceptibility to distortion varies with log characteristics. Similar shifts in IB rankings for all logs further support this.

Distortion's impact increases with right-skewness in case length distribution, as shown in BPIC17, which exhibits highly repetitive events in longer cases. Results confirm that such cases contribute more noise than predictive value. Here, *CaLenDiR* training improves CB DLS by 23.88%, reduces $MAE_{suffix}$by 4.86%, and decreases $MAE_{runtime}$by 3.67%, reflecting better predictions on moderate-length cases. The IB DLS metric, still influenced by long cases, shows a notable 16.31% improvement, suggesting that *CaLenDiR*'s effect on representative cases outweighs any negative impact on IB metrics.

BPIC19 has the least skewed distribution, suggesting lower case-length distortion. Despite preprocessing to mitigate drift, minor changes persist, particularly with slightly longer test cases and short two-event cases in training. *CaLenDiR* training reduces the disproportionate impact of longer cases while balancing the influence of short outliers, contributing to the generally divergent BPIC19 results. Interestingly, data-aware (DA) models like CRTP-LSTM and SuTraN are not negatively affected and even show a slight increase in CB DLS, suggesting resilience to activity suffix prediction under moderate drift conditions.

SEP-LSTM, the only model trained for next-event prediction, shows mild DLS and $MAE_{runtime}$ improvements with *CaLenDiR* on BPIC19. This indicates that *CaLenDiR* helps SEP-LSTM focus on short-case patterns typical of BPIC19. Similar results are observed in BAC, where SEP-LSTM shows notable improvements in DLS (+3.69%) and $MAE_{runtime}$ (−10.69%), moving it from the lowest to third-best performing model. However, SEP-LSTM struggles with longer cases, as seen in BPIC17-DR and BPIC17, where it uniquely shows a slight decrease in DLS (−0.18%), contrasting with other models. This highlights SEP-LSTM's sensitivity to case length and its reliance on reduced noise from atypical long cases.

DA models also consistently improve on the BAC log, unlike their non-data-aware (NDA) counterparts, which experience slight DLS and MAE_{suffix}declines. This indicates that irregular long cases disrupt the predictive signal for models using additional data.

6   Conclusion

This study presented the *CaLenDiR* PPM framework to address case-length distortion in DL-based PPM, enhancing model generalization, performance, and robustness. Central to *CaLenDiR* is the *Uniform Case-Based Sampling (UCBS)* technique, which mitigates distortion from traditional instance creation. For suffix prediction, *CaLenDiR* also integrates *Suffix-Length-Normalized Loss Functions* to reduce distortion in model training. To ensure unbiased evaluation,

CaLenDiR proposes *Case-Based (CB) metrics* over the commonly used Instance-Based (IB) metrics.

Our experiments, conducted with real-life event logs and six DL-based suffix prediction models, reveal that *CaLenDiR* significantly improves model performance and robustness. Results show that addressing case-length distortion affects model rankings and highlights dependencies between log characteristics and model susceptibility to distortion. Findings suggest that right-skewed case length distributions intensify distortion, making *CaLenDiR* especially impactful in such cases. This analysis deepens our understanding of factors essential for effective suffix prediction and their complex relationship with model performance.

Future research could examine *CaLenDiR*'s applicability to other PPM prediction tasks. To support further research, the code and implementation of *CaLenDiR* components are publicly available at https://github.com/BrechtWts/CaLenDiR-PPM.

References

1. Camargo, M., Dumas, M., González-Rojas, O.: Learning accurate LSTM models of business processes. In: Hildebrandt, T., van Dongen, B.F., Röglinger, M., Mendling, J. (eds.) Business Process Management, pp. 286–302. Springer, Cham (2019)
2. Evermann, J., Rehse, J.R., Fettke, P.: Predicting process behaviour using deep learning. Decis. Support Syst. **100**, 129–140 (2017). https://doi.org/10.1016/j.dss.2017.04.003. Smart Business Process Management
3. Gunnarsson, B.R., vanden Broucke, S., De Weerdt, J.: A direct data aware LSTM neural network architecture for complete remaining trace and runtime prediction. IEEE Trans. Serv. Comput. **16**(4), 2330–2342 (2023). https://doi.org/10.1109/TSC.2023.3245726
4. Hinkka, M., Lehto, T., Heljanko, K., Jung, A.: Classifying process instances using recurrent neural networks. In: Daniel, F., Sheng, Q.Z., Motahari, H. (eds.) Business Process Management Workshops, pp. 313–324. Springer, Cham (2019)
5. Ketykó, I., Mannhardt, F., Hassani, M., van Dongen, B.F.: What averages do not tell: predicting real life processes with sequential deep learning. In: Proceedings of the 37th ACM/SIGAPP Symposium on Applied Computing, SAC 2022, pp. 1128–1131. Association for Computing Machinery, New York (2022). https://doi.org/10.1145/3477314.3507179
6. Kratsch, W., Manderscheid, J., Röglinger, M., Seyfried, J.: Machine learning in business process monitoring: a comparison of deep learning and classical approaches used for outcome prediction. Bus. Inf. Syst. Eng. **63**(3), 261–276 (2021). https://doi.org/10.1007/s12599-020-00645-0
7. Navarin, N., Vincenzi, B., Polato, M., Sperduti, A.: LSTM networks for data-aware remaining time prediction of business process instances. In: 2017 IEEE Symposium Series on Computational Intelligence (SSCI), pp. 1–7 (2017). https://doi.org/10.1109/SSCI.2017.8285184
8. Philipp, P., Jacob, R., Robert, S., Beyerer, J.: Predictive analysis of business processes using neural networks with attention mechanism. In: 2020 International Conference on Artificial Intelligence in Information and Communication (ICAIIC), pp. 225–230 (2020). https://doi.org/10.1109/ICAIIC48513.2020.9065057

9. Tax, N., Verenich, I., La Rosa, M., Dumas, M.: Predictive business process monitoring with LSTM neural networks. In: Proceedings of the 29th International Conference on Advanced Information Systems Engineering, pp. 477–492. Springer, Cham (2017)

10. Taymouri, F., Rosa, M.L., Erfani, S., Bozorgi, Z.D., Verenich, I.: Predictive business process monitoring via generative adversarial nets: the case of next event prediction. In: Fahland, D., Ghidini, C., Becker, J., Dumas, M. (eds.) Business Process Management, pp. 237–256. Springer, Cham (2020)

11. Taymouri, F., Rosa, M.L., Erfani, S.M.: A deep adversarial model for suffix and remaining time prediction of event sequences. In: Demeniconi, C., Davidson, I. (eds.) Proceedings of the 2021 SIAM International Conference on Data Mining, SDM 2021, Virtual Event, 29 April–1 May 2021, pp. 522–530. SIAM (2021). https://doi.org/10.1137/1.9781611976700.59

12. Teinemaa, I., Dumas, M., Rosa, M.L., Maggi, F.M.: Outcome-oriented predictive process monitoring: review and benchmark. ACM Trans. Knowl. Discov. Data (TKDD) **13**(2), 1–57 (2019)

13. Verenich, I., Dumas, M., Rosa, M.L., Maggi, F.M., Teinemaa, I.: Survey and cross-benchmark comparison of remaining time prediction methods in business process monitoring. ACM Trans. Intell. Syst. Technol. **10**(4) (2019). https://doi.org/10.1145/3331449

14. Weytjens, H., De Weerdt, J.: Process outcome prediction: CNN vs. LSTM (with attention). In: Del Río Ortega, A., Leopold, H., Santoro, F.M. (eds.) Business Process Management Workshops, pp. 321–333. Springer, Cham (2020)

15. Wuyts, B., Vanden Broucke, S., De Weerdt, J.: SuTraN: an encoder-decoder transformer for full-context-aware suffix prediction of business processes. In: 2024 6th International Conference on Process Mining (ICPM), pp. 17–24 (2024). https://doi.org/10.1109/ICPM63005.2024.10680671

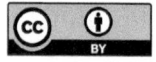

CC-HIT: Creating Counterfactuals from High-Impact Transitions

Zhicong Xian[1,2(✉)], Ludwig Zellner[1,2], Gabriel Marques Tavares[1,2], and Thomas Seidl[1,2]

[1] Database Systems and Data Mining, LMU Munich, Munich, Germany
{xian,zellner,tavares,seidl}@dbs.ifi.lmu.de
[2] Munich Center for Machine Learning, Munich, Germany

Abstract. Smooth process execution relies on high-quality insights extracted from event data. For instance, trace durations heavily affect performance and increase resource consumption. While many predictive systems aim to identify these inefficiencies, they often focus on individual process instances, missing the global perspective. It is essential to detect where delays occur globally and pinpoint specific activity transitions causing them. To address this, we propose CC-HIT (Creating Counterfactuals from High-Impact Transitions), which identifies temporal activity dependencies across the process. CC-HIT uses a modified game theoretic approach and counterfactual information to generate reference event logs to estimate the consequences of activity transitions. It highlights key activity transitions impacting process performance, offering actionable insights for optimization. Validation on the BPIC 2020 dataset demonstrates its effectiveness over baseline methods.

Keywords: Local Explanation · Impact Ranking · Shapley Value · Counterfactuals

1 Introduction

Improving processes to exploit their full potential is critical to survive in a competitive market. When processes are optimized, they may use fewer resources, improve their output, and decrease their duration, leading to better overall performance [3]. This way, identifying performance issues is important for smooth executions. Current solutions focus their explanations and recommendations on a trace-level scope, which causes them to miss the overall view of processes [2,16,18].

When we take temporal optimization of processes as an example we might ask ourselves the following questions: *Which process paths entail the highest delays and lags? Which activities are involved? Are there specific activity transitions that are to blame?* The order of these questions reveals an important aspect: although it is essential to identify objectively slow traces, pinpointing interdependent activities, i.e., specific activity transitions, is much more beneficial. A

© The Author(s) 2025
A. Delgado and T. Slaats (Eds.): ICPM 2024 Workshops, LNBIP 533, pp. 267–278, 2025.
https://doi.org/10.1007/978-3-031-82225-4_20

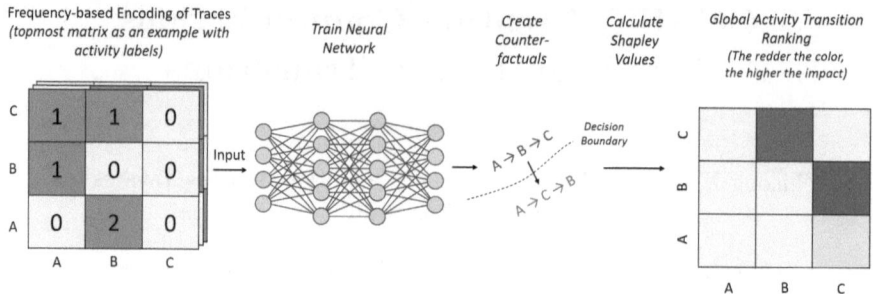

Fig. 1. Main idea of CC-HIT: After training the neural network on the transition matrices of each trace, counterfactuals are generated. Using these counterfactuals, Shapley values are computed for each transition between activity pairs, leading to a global ranking of activity transitions.

reason for that, on the one hand, is the multiple occurrences of these activity combinations in different process paths influencing multiple traces. On the other hand, a transition can manifest itself differently in various traces leading to different impacts. From the second reason follows that pinpointing and explaining transitions locally is imperative to understand the source of inefficiency. However, the key point involves maintaining a global view, as these insights are drawn from it.

Key performance indicators (KPIs), which can be based on factors like time or cost, are used to measure the success of specific entities in relation to these attributes. Using CC-HIT, we analyze processes based on a chosen KPI, giving full control of the analysis to the process owner. With this, we manage to derive the impact of activity transitions for a trace regarding the specified KPI, i.e., we handle the event log as input and produce a ranking of transitions, showing how each one impacts the trace. Additionally, CC-HIT provides alternative insights in the event log by incorporating counterfactuals [13, p. 262]. Hence, we explore how changing certain factors would affect outcomes and use these insights to provide a global activity transition ranking. Figure 1 demonstrates the steps of our approach. We start by training a model using the activity transition data from all traces in the event log. This helps the model learn patterns and relationships between different activities. Next, we create hypothetical scenarios, i.e. counterfactuals, to explore how changing certain factors might affect the results. We then use these counterfactuals to calculate Shapley values, which measure the impact of each activity transition on KPIs. This procedure precisely identifies activity transitions that are high-impacting on KPIs providing deeper insights than typical shallow analysis.

In this paper, we first review related work to contextualize our research and identify existing gaps (Sect. 2). We then present our preliminary section (Sect. 3), which covers the theoretical foundations and definitions pertinent to our study. Our methodology section details the research design and analysis techniques employed (Sect. 4). Following this, we describe our experiments, present and analyze the results, and evaluate our findings (Sect. 5). Finally, we conclude with a summary of our key findings and suggest directions for future research (Sect. 6).

2 Related Work

Explainable AI (XAI) techniques have been extensively applied in event data. Special focus is observed in predictive and prescriptive tasks aiming to forecast future outcomes (e.g., remaining time, next-activity) [4] and to recommend actions [14]. For instance, Pauwels and Calders [16] take advantage of Bayesian Networks to provide reasoning behind predictions. Galanti et al. [7] combined a machine learning KPI predictor with Shapley values to leverage explanations. Similarly, a post-hoc explanation is obtained by the application of Local Interpretable Model-Agnostic Explanations (LIME) in [18]. As performance in predictive tasks is improved with deep learning models, Mehdiyev and Fettke [12] tailored a method for local post-hoc analysis for deep neural networks. Concerned with cross-assessment, El-khawaga et al. [6] introduced a framework for comparison of local and global XAI methods for predictive tasks with a focus on empirical evaluation. Additionally, [19] proposed a blockchain-based auditing system that utilizes maximum-likelihood evidential reasoning to attribute the impact of legal facts in legal documents to a final decision. However, its applicability to process mining must be investigated, as legal documents and event data have different intrinsic characteristics, such as logical reasoning based on closed-world assumptions.

In the realm of prescriptive process monitoring, Bozorgi et al. [2] applied Shapley values on top of a causal effect approach. For that, the authors fix the prefix vector representation to assess feature importances and provide an analysis of causalities. Stevens et al. [21] investigated the trade-off between interpretable models versus model-agnostic XAI techniques and introduced a notion of explainability that allows comparisons of methods from different families.

Although XAI has been extensively used in event data, its application is limited to predictive tasks for providing explanations that support model decisions, i.e., to justify model choices. Moreover, these approaches work on trace prefixes since the task is to predict forthcoming steps [8,15]. Contrarily, our approach aims at looking at historical event data to uncover hidden patterns that influence on KPI performance. Thus, supporting more informed decision-making within organizations.

3 Preliminaries

This section covers the definitions regarding process mining and Shapley value applications.

Definition 1 (Activity, Event). *An event contains the information about an activity occurring at a specific time in a specific context. Additionally, it can provide further data attributes. Here, we refer to the realm of activities by $\mathcal{A}$. An* *event is defined as a tuple $e = (c, a, t) \in (\mathbb{N}, \mathcal{A}, \mathbb{N})$ consisting of a case identifier c, an activity a, a timestamp t. The universe of all possible events is denoted by $\mathcal{U}_e$.*

An ordered, finite sequence of events constitutes a case, whereas an event log contains multiple cases.

Definition 2 (KPI). *We assign a key performance indicator (KPI) $\mathcal{K}$ to each case. This numerical value can represent any case attribute, such as time, money, or other measurable attributes.*

Definition 3 (Activity Transition). *Given our set of activities $\mathcal{A}$ and a transition relation $\mathcal{T}$ being a subset of $\mathcal{A} \times \mathcal{A}$. We define a transition from a_1 to a_2 iff $(a_1, a_2) \in \mathcal{T}$.*

In our work, we calculate Shapley values [20] by treating each activity transition as a player.

Definition 4 (Contribution, Coalition). *A subset of players is called a coalition S where the set of possible coalitions corresponds to the powerset of players $\mathcal{P}(\mathcal{N})$. A contribution function v maps a subset of players to the real numbers $v : 2^{\mathcal{N}} \to \mathbb{R}$, with $v(\emptyset) = 0$, where $\emptyset$ denotes the empty set. Hence, given v the calculation of $v(S)$ yields the contribution of the coalition S.*

We utilize a transition matrix where each cell represents the transition value of each pair in $(a_i, a_j) \in \mathcal{M}$. This matrix helps us capture and analyze the transition value between consecutive events regarding its respective attribute $\mathcal{K}$. For instance, if we assign time as $\mathcal{K}$, we derive the value for an event transition as the time difference between two consecutive events $\Delta_t(e^i, e^{i+1}) = t_{e^{i+1}} - t_{e^i}$.

Definition 5 (Shapley Value [20]). *The Shapley value is defined by the following equation:*

$$\phi_j(v) = \sum_{S \subseteq \mathcal{A} \setminus \{a_j\}} \frac{|S|!(|\mathcal{A}| - |S| - 1)!}{|\mathcal{A}|!} (v(S \cup \{a_j\}) - v(S))$$

Hence, $\forall a_j \in \{a_k\}_{k=1}^{|\mathcal{A}|}$ we calculate the average marginal contribution to every possible coalition which eventually yields the impact for each activity transition regarding $\mathcal{K}$.

The exact relationship between activity transitions and the final case KPI in cases is often unknown and usually surrogate models are used to approximate it. One such possibility is to use machine learning prediction models.

Definition 6 (Prediction models for activity transitions). *The oracle function $\Phi : \mathcal{E} \to \mathcal{K}$ maps a case containing activity transitions to its KPI. For a case, σ with activity sequences, we can derive a list of activity transitions $\sigma' = \langle (a_1, a_2), (a_2, a_3), \cdots, (a_{|\sigma'|-1}, a_{|\sigma'|}) \rangle$. A prediction model $f : \mathcal{E}' \to \mathcal{K}$ maps activity transitions in a case to its KPI. It is an approximation of the oracle function Φ, i.e., $f \approx \Phi$.*

4   Methodology

We assume the activities happen instantaneously (atomic event assumption) and apply the Markov assumption, which states that the probability of the next activity occurring, given the current and past activities, depends only on the current activity [10]. In the scope of this paper, we mainly focus on the types of activities and their inter-relationships that can contribute to the case KPI $\mathcal{K}$.

4.1   Activity Transition Matrix

In process mining, representing the sequential orders of activities is crucial for understanding how processes flow and identifying inefficiencies or deviations. We propose using transition matrices to represent the interaction among activities. Given a total number of activities $|\mathcal{A}|$ as N, we construct a matrix M of size $N \times N$ with preceding activities represented in the rows and succeeding activities represented in the columns. Furthermore, each entry $M_{i,j}$ is defined as follows:

$$M_{i,j} = \begin{cases} n, & \text{if there are transitions from activity } i \text{ to activity } j \text{ in one case} \\ & \text{then the number of these transitions} \\ 0, & \text{otherwise} \end{cases}$$

(1)

Multiple occurrences of the same activity within a single case are possible in an event log. As a result, there may be different subsequent activities for a single activity, leading to several entries in the same column of the transition matrix. Additionally, by representing the temporal sequencing of activities as a transition matrix, we can easily observe self-loops on the diagonal matrix, indicating instances where activities transition to themselves. Another benefit of this representation is that it encodes the temporal relationships among activities. It allows us to identify infeasible transitions as zero entries in the transition matrix across the entire event log. This matrix representation resembles an image, facilitating the use of machine learning models for predicting case KPIs.

Consequently, we treat the transition matrices as two-dimensional images and apply deep neural networks to predict the final case KPI. We then derive estimations for coalition functions from the trained model to compute Shapley values.

4.2   The Shapley Additive Explanation Framework (SHAP)

As described in Definition 5, the computation of Shapley values requires estimating coalition values $v(S)$. When using machine learning models to approximate the relationship between case activity transitions and their KPIs, it is important to address the issue of missing activity transitions that only appear in some cases within the event log. Lundberg et al. [11] addresses this challenge by proposing the SHapley Additive exPlanation framework (SHAP).

In this framework, the coalition values for player subsets are computed as the conditional expectation of the outcome given these player subsets marginalizing over all the other missing players, i.e., $v(S) = \mathbb{E}[f(x)|x_S]$. x are the input features to our prediction model f, equal to the activity transitions $(a_i, a_j) \in \mathbf{M}$ in event logs with x_S denoting the activity transitions defined in the player subset S. Since trace activity transitions resemble 2D images, and we aim to extract both local features, such as adjacent activity transitions, and global features, such as distant influences, we employ a residual neural network (ResNet) [9] to obtain the prediction function $f(x)$.

A common practice in SHAP for estimating coalition values for player subsets is to predict the outcomes for these subsets while replacing missing players with mean values from background datasets. The resulting Shapley values then explain the input predictions relative to these background datasets [1]. The background datasets are selected by uniformly sampling from the given datasets. However, in process mining, our focus extends beyond identifying which activity transitions increase overall case throughput time on average; we are also interested in actionable insights for improving process KPIs. Assume a dataset with two features, x_1 and x_2. To estimate x_1's contribution to the predicted outcome, we compare samples with actual x_1 values to those with dummy x_1 values, often set as the average x_1. However, this may be unrealistic since x_1 could depend on x_2, and different x_2 values may restrict the range of x_1. Albini et al. [1] proposed using counterfactual Shapley values to improve the predicted outcomes. We will adapt this approach for process mining in the next section.

4.3   The Generation of Counterfactuals

While standard Shapley value computations assign importance scores to activity transitions based on an average case—such as one with average frequencies of all occurring activity transitions—in the given event logs, this average case may not be viable in the real world. A case may not necessarily experience all feasible activity transitions, as some are mutually exclusive. Standard Shapley values do not capture this limitation. To address this, we propose using counterfactuals—minimal feasible changes in the sequence of activities that can lead to significant deviations in case KPIs—as reference cases. This section focuses on generating counterfactuals for process mining. Consider a loan approval process with the following sequence of activities: "Application Submitted High/Medium/Low Loan" (A) → "Automated/Manual Document Verification" (B) → "Initial Automated/Manual Credit Check Performed" (C) → "Loan Officer Detailed Risk Assessment" (D) → "Loan Offer Generated" (E) → "Loan Decision (Approved/Declined)" (F) → "Customer Notification" (G), and we aim to generate counterfactuals to accelerate the loan application process. Before introducing our algorithm to generate counterfactuals, we must first examine the properties that qualify as good counterfactuals in process mining:

- *Plausibility.* Some activity transitions are mandatory, and certain steps must occur in a specific order. In the previous loan application example, having C occuring B before does not make sense because credit checks should only be performed on verified documents.

- *Proximity.* The generated counterfactual must be similar to the sample of interest. In the loan approval process, a minimal change in the activity sequence, such as swapping C and D, can lead to a significant deviation in the runtime. If the D occurs before C, manual effort is wasted as the officer reviews the application without the necessary credit information. Reordering these two activities can substantially impact the process runtime, making this change a valuable counterfactual.
- *Feasibility.* Some transition changes are only possible depending on previous workflows. In the previous loan approval application, a "Pre-Approved Loan Offer" can be generated if B is completed, no discrepancies are found, and activity C identifies the application as low-risk. If any documents are missing or incorrect or the loan amount is large, the process moves to a manual review, and pre-approval is not possible.

To satisfy the aforementioned properties, we propose generating counterfactuals by projecting onto decision boundaries based on constraints and along directions derived from the principal components of the nearby neighborhood. We describe this method in the following steps and apply it to the loan application process introduced at the beginning of this section to enhance understanding:

Step 1: Definition of the counterfactual outcome: If the prediction outcome is continuous, we categorize it into discrete labels such as desired and undesired. For instance, if the loan application considers throughput time as its KPI $\mathcal{K}$, it could be categorized as fast-tracked or delayed. If the queried samples are delayed, we define counterfactual outcomes as fast-tracked or on time.

Step 2: Obtaining immutable constraints: Creates a binary mask matrix for activity transitions, with zeros for infeasible transitions and ones for feasible ones. Since the steps of the loan application process are causal, we can mask reverse orderings of steps with zeros for infeasible changes.

Step 3: Initial generation of counterfactual samples: Randomly sample data and use prediction models to select candidates that match the counterfactual outcomes. We randomly draw samples and resample for the loan application process until we have enough instances with no delays.

Step 4: Finding K-nearest neighbors: To determine feasible directions for altering samples to their counterfactuals, we first identify the nearest neighbors for the queried samples. For example, clustering delayed samples may reveal that they all have "Application Submitted HIGH Loan". In contrast, other samples that follow similar steps, such as "Automated/Manual Document Verification" $\rightarrow$ "Initial Credit Check Performed", have a lower overall run-time due to a smaller loan amount.

Step 5: Calculation of principal axes of the clusters: We derive feasible changes in the activity transitions by analyzing their correlations. Mathematically, this involves performing Principal Component Analysis (PCA) on the clustered data near the query points to capture correlations among activity transitions. For instance, the previous step shows a strong correlation between the requested loan amount and final throughput time. Thus, one feasible change is to decrease the requested loan amount.

Step 6: Projection of the counterfactual candidates onto decision boundary along the principal axes of the clusters: Iteratively project the difference between the query data points and counterfactual candidates onto the principal components, gradually pulling the counterfactual candidates closer to the query sample points until they are near the decision boundary. In the loan application process, this means successively reducing the loan amount to align with cases with a faster approval track.

5   Evaluation

In this section, we focus on the impact of activity transitions on the throughput time as the KPI. For our experiments, we use the permit log from the BPIC Challenge 2020 event log [5], focusing on throughput time as the key KPI. We aim to identify potential activity transitions for improvement.

5.1   Dataset Description

The travel permit log documents the billing process at the Eindhoven University of Technology from 2017 to 2018. The event log contains 7,065 cases, some of which are also included in the international declaration event log. This overlap occurs because international trips require supervisor permission, obtained by filing a travel permit. This permit must be approved before any travel arrangements are made. Statistical analysis reveals an average throughput time of 87.4 days compared to a median of 71.73 days. The maximum and minimum throughput times are 1190 and 0.53 days, respectively. This indicates that the case duration is slightly skewed across the entire event log, with some cases experiencing significant delays.

A standard process workflow typically proceeds as follows: employees submit travel requests, which are then forwarded to budget owners, supervisors, directors, and finally, administrative departments for approval. Once travel is granted, employees can begin their trips. After the trip ends, employees must submit travel declarations detailing their expenses, followed by a request for payment to cover these expenses. The approval procedures for travel declarations and payment requests follow similar steps to those for travel approval. Pufahl et al. [17] find out that the event log conforms to the standard procedure in most cases.

5.2   Experiment Results

Most methods discussed in Sect. 2 focus on trace-level assessments using case or activity attributes while we uniquely study the impact of activity transitions. To evaluate and compare different methods for analyzing activity transitions, we visualize various plots that rank the importance of these transitions. Additionally, we discuss the additional insights our approach provides by directly incorporating throughput time into the analysis.

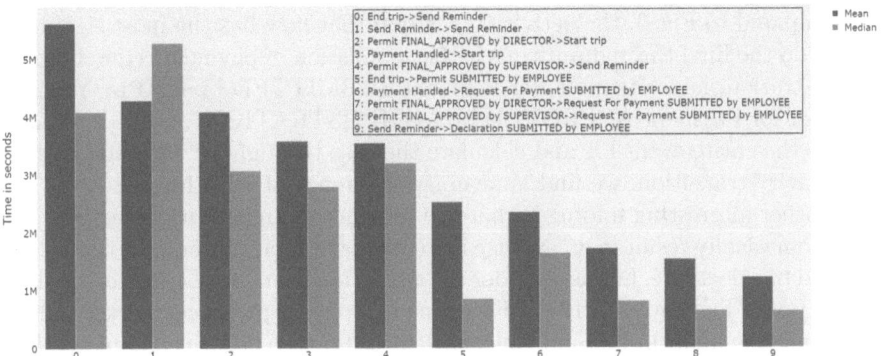

Fig. 2. Ranking of the activity transitions based on mean and median duration.

Baseline. The classical approach to analyzing the importance of activity transitions on the final throughput time involves calculating the mean and median for each possible activity transition across the event log. The event log contains 51 unique activities, resulting in 51×51 possible activity transitions. We then filter out the infrequent transitions to reduce the number of transitions to consider. Next, we rank the remaining activity transitions according to their *median* duration and select the top 10 for visualization. As shown in Fig. 2, the activity transition "Send Reminder" $\rightarrow$ "Send Reminder" consumes the most time, with the transition "End trip" $\rightarrow$ "Send Reminder" in the second place. We observe that transitions involving the "Send Reminder" activity significantly impact the throughput, which makes sense because a reminder will only be sent when the expected next activity is pending. Other activities, such as "Start trip" and "End trip", are also associated with high-duration transitions. However, from Fig. 2, we cannot determine the expected next activity to prevent the system from sending a reminder, even when examining transitions with minimal duration.

CC-HIT. Unlike traditional analysis, which only considers the absolute activity transition time in the event log, our approach encodes the activity transitions to predict the final throughput time and uses the prediction model to assess the impact of these transitions compared to what-if scenarios. We then quantify these impacts using Shapley values. If changing the state of an activity transition from absence to presence (or vice versa) reduces throughput time, that activity transition will have a higher Shapley value. Since the original SHAP framework provides instance-wise interpretation, and we are focused on the overall Shapley values in the event log, we average these values across the entire event log and rank the activity transitions based on the mean of their Shapley values. This allows us to generate a bee swarm plot, as shown in Fig. 3. As depicted in Fig. 3, the activity transitions are shown on the x-axis. At the same time, each point represents the Shapley value for a specific activity transition, plotted along the y-axis. The color of the points in the figure represents the original transition encoding, with zero values indicating absence and positive values indicating presence.

Compared to Fig. 2, the activity transition that now has the most significant impact on the final throughput time is the submission of payment requests to the administration, i.e., "Request For Payment SUBMITTED by EMPLOYEE" → "Request for Payment APPROVED by ADMINISTRATION". Indeed, when we analyze the entire event log and calculate the case throughput with and without this activity transition, we find an average difference of 22.9 days.

Another interesting finding is that the presence of an activity transition does not automatically result in an average increase in the final throughput time; it can also lead to a decrease. Let us consider the transition from "End trip" to "Declaration SUBMITTED by EMPLOYEE" as an example. Its presence, marked in blue, can reduce the final throughput time, as depicted by the negative Shapley values. This occurs because employees should submit their declaration immediately after the trip. If they do not, the system will send a reminder, which increases the final throughput. This is illustrated by the activity transition from "End trip" to "Send reminder", which ranks ninth in terms of throughput impact.

Another advantage of our approach is that less frequent activity transitions, which may be time-consuming, do not necessarily have a high impact on changing throughput time. For example, the transition from "Permit FINAL_APPROVED by DIRECTOR" to "Start trip", while present in Fig. 2, does not appear prominently in our analysis. This is because it occurs infrequently in only 362 out of 7,065 cases. Therefore, our approach provides a more robust and insightful view of the impact of activity transitions, shining light on influential transitions and further supporting decision-makers in improving their processes.

However, when we consider the transition from "End trip" to "Permit SUBMITTED by EMPLOYEE" as an example, we see that submitting a permit after the trip can speed up the process. Nonetheless, this may introduce other risks, such as the potential rejection of the reimbursement. Therefore, a reduction in throughput time does not necessarily indicate an optimal outcome, as our prediction model does not account for other risks, such as final activity labels like rejection. Consequently, it remains up to the process owner to determine which transition links can be improved.

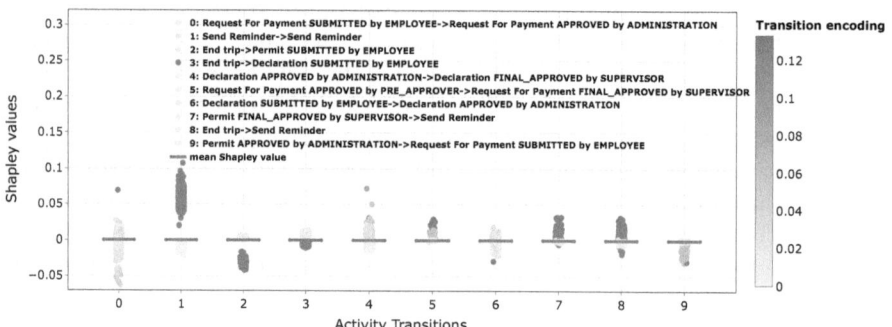

Fig. 3. Ranking of the activity transitions based on Shapley values referencing counterfactual cases.

Nevertheless, our data-driven approach provides valuable insights based on the data, reflecting the practices and outcomes observed.

6   Conclusion

Process performance is often measured by KPIs. However, identifying transitions that influence process outcome is challenging. Standard approaches focus on instance-level analysis or assess impact based on mean throughput time. We propose CC-HIT, a framework for identifying influential activity transitions that stakeholders can further improve once identified. We compared CC-HIT to traditional statistical analysis and demonstrated its advantages. Our approach identifies transitions that differentially impact the final process KPIs and shows how the presence or absence of these transitions can influence the final KPI. Our method is more data-driven and provides deeper insights than traditional statistical approaches. While we aggregate Shapley values by their average to obtain a global assessment of activity transitions, we still retain local information, such as the distribution of Shapley values across instances for each activity transition, as visualized in Fig. 3. A product owner can design additional metrics, such as incorporating the variance of Shapley values, to aggregate individual impacts. Nonetheless, our approach highlights all significant transitions worth noting and offers opportunities for future process optimization. In future work, we aim to use the identified transitions to support stakeholders in making direct decisions, suggesting potential ways to overcome bottlenecks.

References

1. Albini, E., Long, J., Dervovic, D., Magazzeni, D.: Counterfactual shapley additive explanations. In: Proceedings of the 2022 ACM Conference on Fairness, Accountability, and Transparency, FAccT 2022, pp. 1054–1070. Association for Computing Machinery, New York (2022)
2. Dasht Bozorgi, Z., Teinemaa, I., Dumas, M., La Rosa, M., Polyvyanyy, A.: Prescriptive process monitoring based on causal effect estimation. Inf. Syst. **116**, 102198 (2023)
3. Di Cunzolo, M., et al.: Combining process mining and optimization: a scheduling application in healthcare. In: International Conference on Business Process Management, pp. 197–209. Springer, Cham (2022)
4. Di Francescomarino, C., Ghidini, C.: Predictive Process Monitoring, pp. 320–346. Springer, Cham (2022)
5. van Dongen, B.: BPI challenge 2020 (2020). https://doi.org/10.4121/UUID: 52FB97D4-4588-43C9-9D04-3604D4613B51
6. El-khawaga, G., Abu-Elkheir, M., Reichert, M.: XAI in the context of predictive process monitoring: an empirical analysis framework. Algorithms **15**(6) (2022)
7. Galanti, R., Coma-Puig, B., Leoni, M., Carmona, J., Navarin, N.: Explainable predictive process monitoring. In: 2020 2nd International Conference on Process Mining (ICPM), pp. 1–8 (2020)
8. Galanti, R., et al.: An explainable decision support system for predictive process analytics. Eng. Appl. Artif. Intell. **120**(C) (2023)

9. He, K., Zhang, X., Ren, S., Sun, J.: Deep residual learning for image recognition. In: Proceedings of 2016 IEEE Conference on Computer Vision and Pattern Recognition, CVPR 2016, pp. 770–778. IEEE (2016)
10. Helske, J., Helske, S., Saqr, M., López-Pernas, S., Murphy, K.: A Modern Approach to Transition Analysis and Process Mining with Markov Models in Education, pp. 381–427. Springer, Cham (2024)
11. Lundberg, S.M., Lee, S.I.: A unified approach to interpreting model predictions. In: Guyon, I., et al. (eds.) Advances in Neural Information Processing Systems, vol. 30. Curran Associates, Inc. (2017)
12. Mehdiyev, N., Fettke, P.: Explainable Artificial Intelligence for Process Mining: A General Overview and Application of a Novel Local Explanation Approach for Predictive Process Monitoring, pp. 1–28. Springer, Cham (2021)
13. Molnar, C.: Interpretable machine learning. Lulu.com (2020)
14. Padella, A., de Leoni, M., Dogan, O., Galanti, R.: Explainable process prescriptive analytics. In: 2022 4th International Conference on Process Mining (ICPM), pp. 16–23 (2022)
15. Pasquadibisceglie, V., Appice, A., Ieva, G., Malerba, D.: TSUNAMI - an explainable PPM approach for customer churn prediction in evolving retail data environments. J. Intell. Inf. Syst. **62**(3), 705–733 (2024)
16. Pauwels, S., Calders, T.: Bayesian network based predictions of business processes. In: Fahland, D., Ghidini, C., Becker, J., Dumas, M. (eds.) Business Process Management Forum, pp. 159–175. Springer, Cham (2020)
17. Pufahl, L., et al.: Performance variant and conformance analysis of an academic travel reimbursement process. In: BPI Challenge 2020 (2020)
18. Rizzi, W., Di Francescomarino, C., Maggi, F.M.: Explainability in predictive process monitoring: when understanding helps improving. In: Fahland, D., Ghidini, C., Becker, J., Dumas, M. (eds.) Business Process Management Forum, pp. 141–158. Springer, Cham (2020)
19. Sachan, S., Liu, X.: Blockchain-based auditing of legal decisions supported by explainable AI and generative AI tools. Eng. Appl. Artif. Intell. **129**, 107666 (2024)
20. Shapley, L.S., et al.: A value for n-person games (1953)
21. Stevens, A., De Smedt, J., Peeperkorn, J.: Quantifying explainability in outcome-oriented predictive process monitoring. In: Munoz-Gama, J., Lu, X. (eds.) Process Mining Workshops, pp. 194–206. Springer, Cham (2022)

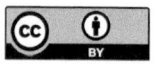

Multivariate Approaches for Process Model Forecasting

Yongbo Yu$^{(\boxtimes)}$, Jari Peeperkorn , Johannes De Smedt ,
and Jochen De Weerdt

Research Center for Information Systems Engineering (LIRIS), KU Leuven,
Leuven, Belgium
{yongbo.yu,jari.peeperkorn,johannes.desmedt,jochen.deweerdt}@kuleuven.be

Abstract. Recently, inspired by predictive process monitoring, the modeling and prediction of the entire process information system has been proposed as process model forecasting. By forecasting individual elements of a directly-follows graph, the future state of the system can be predicted. However, the current state-of-the-art principally employs univariate forecasting of direct-follows relationships (DFs). This univariate approach overlooks the process structure and possible relations between different elements within the process. This paper introduces a comprehensive deployment of multivariate time series models, more specifically a range of different machine- and deep learning approaches, to forecast DFs. These are benchmarked on different event logs collected from real-life event processes. Our extensive experiments reveal that the performance of these forecasting models varies significantly across different processes, highlighting the importance of model selection.

Keywords: Process Model Forecasting · Time Series Forecasting · Deep Learning

1 Introduction

In recent years numerous research advancements in the field of predictive process monitoring (PPM) have been proposed, driven by the rapid development and widespread application of machine learning and deep learning. PPM aims to forecast future elements of ongoing cases in the information system, including the most probable next activities [8], outcomes [26], and remaining runtimes [25]. Notably, the integration of recurrent neural networks (RNNs) into this domain has improved predictive performance significantly.

Recently, a new paradigm known as Process Model Forecasting (PMF) has emerged, focusing on predicting future states of the overall process model over a long-term horizon [6]. The forecasted process model represents the will-be process, enabling the exploration of tactical and strategic questions such as "Are my bottlenecks persistent over time?" and "Will the ratio of granted loan applications change in the next quarter?". The evolution of process behavior can be

A. Delgado and T. Slaats (Eds.): ICPM 2024 Workshops, LNBIP 533, pp. 279–292, 2025.
https://doi.org/10.1007/978-3-031-82225-4_21

captured through the shift in the direct-follows occurrences (DFs) over time. By deconstructing the time dimensions, DFs are predicted by univariate time series techniques and transformed to the directly-follows graphs (DFGs) as the forecasted process model. However, the dependencies and interactions between DFs might influence each other or be influenced by the temporal evolution of the system in general (e.g. drifts), which is not considered by univariate time series forecasting techniques that handle each DF separately. For example, if a DF pair of activity A to B is followed by another DF pair of activity B to C, the growth of the former DF tends to also result in an increase in the occurrence of the latter one. The underlying pattern of DFs could be captured by leveraging the multivariate time series forecasting models.

Inspired by the extensive research of deep learning applications in PPM, we explore the use of current state-of-the-art time series forecasting models based on machine learning (ML) and deep learning (DL) to do multivariate PMF. More specifically, we incorporate the classes of Gradient Boosting Decision Tree (GBDT), Recurrent Neural Networks (RNNs), Convolutional Neural Networks (CNNs), Multilayer Perceptrons (MLPs), and Transformers to capture the dependencies between DFs and tackle the high dimensionality stemming from a high number of DFs interacting over time when making predictions. In a benchmark, we aim to quantify the benefits of using multivariate PMF, and specifically the use of state-of-the-art ML and DL time series techniques.

The rest of this paper is structured as follows. Section 2 discusses related work and introduces several state-of-the-art time series forecasting approaches. Section 3 gives a high-level overview of how PMF works. Section 4 introduces the data used in our benchmark and shows the model selection. The section also explains the benchmark setup and accompanying results. Next, Sect. 5 discusses the implications of these results and some of the limitations. Finally, Sect. 6 summarizes the main findings and provides some suggestions for future work.

2   Background and Related Work

2.1   Background of PMF

There has been a significant surge of interest in the exploration and application of predictive modeling techniques in process analytics. PMF moves from a case-level perspective towards process system-wide predictions. In an event log, directly-follows relations between activities can be calculated as counting functions for activity pairs over traces. Thus, a directly-follows graph can be obtained with the activities as nodes and DF relations as weighted edges. In this sense, the dynamics of a process model are expressed as the evolution of a DF Graph (DFG). By utilizing aggregations, the event log is split into multiple intervals, and the DFGs are constructed from every subset of the log. In PMF, the directly-follows time series over the time intervals are modeled and forecasted to build up a sequence of predicted DFGs, reflecting the long-term system-wide changes. To predict the DFs, [6] leverage Holt Winter's (HW) model, autoregressive model (AR), ARIMA model, GARCH model, and VAR models. Note that the first four models are classical univariate time series models, and VAR is a simple multivariate time series model that does not operate well on high-dimensional time series. The key distinction lies in whether considering the time series as separate single time-dependent variables (univariate) or multiple interrelated time-dependent variables together (multivariate). Thus, the univariate time series forecasting models overlook correlations between different DFs induced by the process structure. As the time series in actual applications become increasingly higher dimensional and complex, the importance of multivariate time series techniques becomes more important to capture the relationships and interactions between the different time series. In addition to VAR, as an extension of the AR model, multivariate time series models based on deep learning such as RNNs attract more attention recently, and are widely used in PPM [23]. Recently, other time series-based approaches to analyze these system-wide aspects of a process system have surfaced, such as [21] proposing a shift towards proactive and future-oriented business process management (BPM). [22] provide a generic approach to create time series abstractions of event logs. [24] present time-based conformance checking. [19] use a transition matrix with probabilities, possibly over time, to detect concept drift. The most similar work is [18], who demonstrate the effectiveness of temporal convolution networks on the prediction of work-in-progress (WiP) distributions in business processes. However, the predicted WiP is calculated as the total of all activities rather than on individual changes, resulting in insufficient granularity in describing and forecasting the process as PMF focuses on the joint prediction of the individual time series.

In the various DF time series selected from the event logs used in the evaluation section visualized in Fig. 1, it can be seen that DF time series are typically not well-behaved and exhibit a variety of particular time series behavior. Sample 1a shows a common white noise serie with a trend and cycle, however, Sample 1b contains intermittency common to process systems such as weekends, resting periods, or activities not used throughout a process in combination with another (e.g. batching is happening, or resources are on holidays). Sample 1c shows similar low and high spikes which are typically hard to model with parametric (univariate) time series like ARIMA. Finally, Sample 1d shows the warm-up period of the system, which requires appropriate trimming of the time series. Given that these patterns can become complex and are often intertwined, e.g., Samples 1c through 1d are from the same system and can have been produced under similar resource schedules, it is necessary to use models that can cope with these irregularities which are not common to, e.g., econometric time series for which many typical time series techniques are tailored to. Below, we cover the most recent machine learning and deep learning approaches to tackle these.

2.2   ML and DL Time Series Forecasting

Forecasting plays a crucial role in anticipating future trends by extrapolating time series data. The communities of data science and operations research have extensively researched time series forecasting by incorporating machine learning

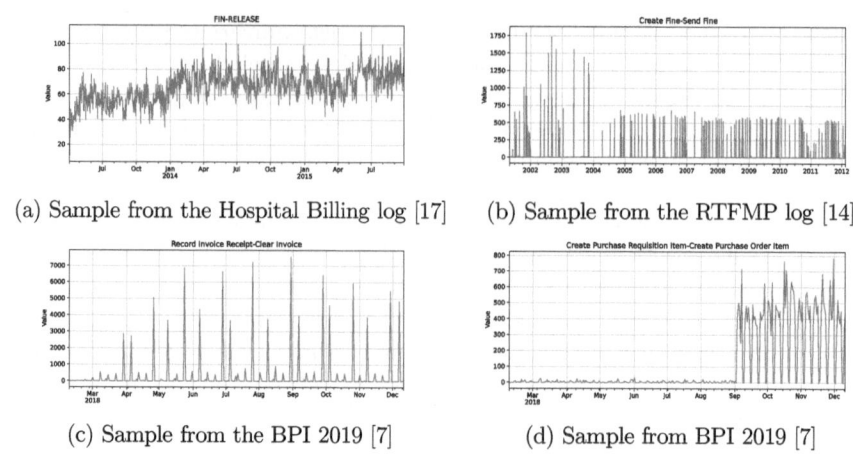

(a) Sample from the Hospital Billing log [17]   (b) Sample from the RTFMP log [14]

(c) Sample from the BPI 2019 [7]   (d) Sample from BPI 2019 [7]

Fig. 1. Sample of DF time series

and deep learning techniques. In comparison to traditional forecasting methods, modern approaches often involve handling large sets of interconnected time series data, all of which require simultaneous forecasting. Gradient Boosting Decision Tree (GBDT) [9] is a widely-used machine learning algorithm due to its accuracy and interpretability, and Extreme Gradient Boosting (XGBoost) [4] and Light Gradient Boosting Machine (LightGBM) [12] were developed to be highly efficient and scalable. XGBoost grows trees level-wise and introduces regularization to prevent overfitting, while LightGBM grows trees leaf-wise, allowing deeper trees and better performance in some cases.

In deep learning, Recurrent Neural Networks (RNNs) are specifically designed to capture and learn patterns in sequential data such as time series. Connecting the hidden layers recurrently back to themselves enables the neural network to build memory. Furthermore, Long Short-Term Memory networks (LSTMs) [10] and a simplified version called Gated Recurrent Units (GRUs) [5] improve the gradient vanishment problem when revealing long-term dependencies. In process mining, LSTMs are widely applied in Predictive Process Monitoring (PPM) [25]. Besides RNNs, Multilayer Perceptrons (MLPs) as a simpler architecture are adopted for time series forecasting to achieve faster training and better generalization. N-BEATS [20] is designed specifically for forecasting tasks, relying on a structure of stacked MLPs. Each MLP block has a backward residual connection to improve the learning of the trend and seasonality components. Furthermore, N-HITS [3] introduces a hierarchical interpolation mechanism for multi-scale modeling of time series data, capturing different scales of information and features along the time axis. Unlike the general-purpose time series forecasting of N-BEATS, N-HITS provides better performance when time series data involves multiple temporal resolutions or significant short-term and long-term variations. Convolutional Neural Networks (CNNs) are tailored to handling input data such as images and time series A variation is dilated casual convolutions which are stacked on top of each other for efficient modeling of long-range dependencies in sequences. [2] propose a simple dilated casual convolution model, Temporal Convolutional Networks (TCNs), and provide empirical evidence showing its outperforming traditional recurrent models in many sequence modeling tasks.

Another recent architecture for time series forecasting is based on the attention mechanism [1] by focusing on specific parts of the input data and dynamically weighting different elements. The Transformers [27] are built entirely on the attention mechanism allowing parallelized training and a large number of parameters. Temporal Fusion Transformers (TFTs) [16] combine RNNs and attention mechanisms to capture both temporal dynamics and feature importance. In addition, the gating components in TFTs allow the model to skip irrelevant parts of the context, increasing flexibility and reducing the risk of overfitting. For long-term time series forecasting, DLinear and NLinear [29] were recently proposed as lightweight MLP model alternatives to Transformers. DLinear decomposes a time series into trend and seasonal components and modeling these components separately using linear models, while NLinear directly applies a linear model to the raw time series data without separating trend and seasonality. [29] demonstrate that these linear models outperform more complex Transformer models for long-term time series forecasting on several benchmarks.

An effective variant of neural networks for prediction tasks is the family of Graph Neural Networks (GNNs), modeling network-based data like traffic networks [11]. GNNs allow to model both spatial and temporal dependency together for time series forecasting. For instance, [28] propose STGCN to tackle the time series prediction problem in the traffic domain with complete convolutional structures.

Given the various modeling capabilities of these multivariate models, a study into whether these multivariate correlations can be captured in DF time series, and how these relate to the characteristics of business processes underpinning various systems. This is done by an extensive benchmark by a wide range of the aforementioned techniques over a set of widely-used event logs.

3   Methodology

This work aims to perform DF forecasting using time series. More concretely, these are built by counting the occurrence of each DF in certain predefined timesteps (e.g. each day), determined by looking at the occurrence of the corresponding activity pairs in a process. Note that, for now, we assume atomic events, i.e., we only have a completion timestamp for each performed activity. In this way, we assume the activities taking a long time to finish and a long time to start are both reflected in a bottleneck in the DF. Figure 2 illustrates the transformation from event logs to DF time series. By dividing the event log into day-based intervals, a sequence of DFG matrices can be extracted from each subset of logs. The DFG matrices are flattened to one-dimensional DF vectors and stacked together in chronological order to obtain tabular time series data. However, a significant amount of DF relations in such a matrix never occur in the event log (as the activity pairs forming the DFs beginning- and end points are not present), so those are filtered out. Thus, the final tabular DF data excludes the empty DF columns and retains the observed DFs coinciding with the number of activity pairs present in the event log (of which there can be many) for prediction. To summarize, our approach takes an event log as input and predicts the DF time series as output. In the end, the predicted DFs support the construction of a DFG to represent the forecasted process model, which is not in the scope of this paper.

4   Experimental Evaluation

In this section, we give an overview of the data, its preprocessing, the models used, and finally we present the results of the benchmark.

4.1   Selected Data and Preprocessing

In the experiment, three publicly available event logs are used: BPI challenge of 2019 [7], a Hospital Billing event log [17], and a Road Traffic Fine Management Process log (RTFMP) [14], covering a diverse set of processes. The BPI challenge of the 2019 event log contains four types of flows, and the used sub-log is the category of "3-way match, invoice before GR", indicated as BPI2019_1. In the current experiments, to more accurately characterize process changes and provide insights for practical applications, we take timesteps of one day.

Table 1 describes three event logs and the preprocessing. Firstly, to only retain process behavior with enough signal in the event log, the infrequent variants are removed, and we retain the variants with a coverage percentage of 99.99% of the number of traces. Secondly, artificial "start" and "end" activities are added to the beginning and end of every case. Finally, the time lengths of the filtered event logs are reduced by trimming the first and last 10% of the time horizon as many systems have warm-up periods in which behavior is different, as illustrated in Fig. 1d. By focusing on the steady-state part of processes, models can be trained on data that better represents typical operations, improving its generalization capabilities and predictive performance. Due to a large number of variants occurring rarely, the preprocessed event logs contain less than half of the variants but keep more than 90% traces. The activities "start" and "end" increase the number of activities and possible DFs after preprocessing.

4.2   Model Selection

As shown in Sect. 2.1, the intricacies of the DF time series such as intermittency, long-distance dependencies and severe multicollinearity motivate the selection of time series forecasting approaches. The BPI2019_1 event log has a narrow time range (so fewer time steps) and may be trackable for ML-based models of XGBoost and LightGBM due to their low training data requirements. The

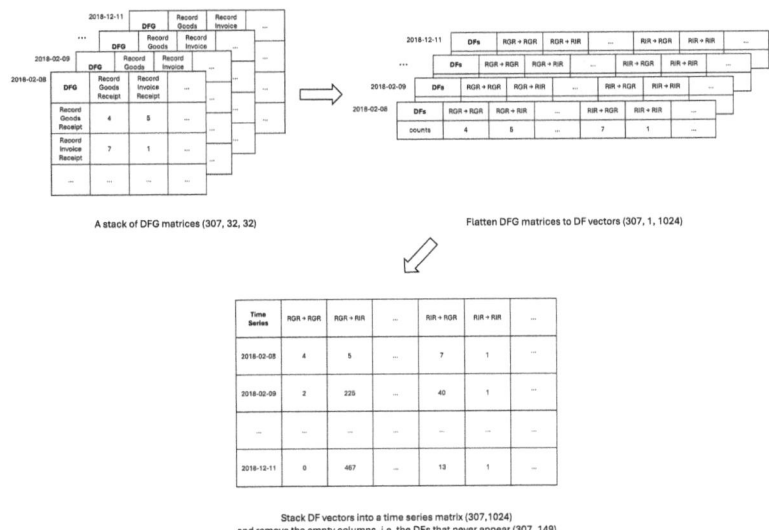

Fig. 2. Data transformation of BPI2019_1 [7] as an example, where "RGR" is short for "Record Goods Receipt" and "RIR" is short for "Record Invoice Receipt". The time step granularity is set at 1 day.

Table 1. Log Preprocessing

	BPI2019_1			Hospital Billing			RTFMP		
	original	preprocessed		original	preprocessed		original	preprocessed	
time range (days)	383	307	80%	1,132	906	80%	4,917	3,938	80%
# variants	7,835	740	9%	1,020	301	30%	231	106	46%
# traces	221,010	198,018	90%	100,000	90,604	91%	150,370	138,260	92%
# activities	39	32	82%	18	17	94%	11	13	118%
# events	1,234,494	1,301,182	105%	451,359	539,658	120%	561,470	720,625	128%
# unique DFs	413	149	36%	143	69	48%	70	39	56%
# DFs	1,013,484	1,103,164	109%	351,359	449,054	128%	411,100	582,365	142%

widely used RNNs and their capabilities of finding autoregressive and potentially longer-distance dependencies (in PPM) encourage us to extend them to PMF, including vanilla RNNs, LSTMs, and GRUs. Given the effectiveness of simple MLP architectures, N-BEATS is utilized for its robustness and N-HITS is included to capture the multi-scale seasonality, such as for the DFs in Fig. 1b and 1c. TCNs have the advantage of forecasting business process changes by [18]. For long-term time series predictions like the RTFMP log, uncovering the dynamic trends involves using Transformers, TFTs, DLinear, and NLinear.

Therefore, the selected models include XGBoost, LightGBM, RNNs, LSTMs, GRUs, N-BEATS, N-HITS, TCNs, Transformers, TFTs, DLinear, and NLinear, compared with baselines of persistence, mean forecast, and linear regression. The persistence forecast, also known as naive forecast, takes the value of the last observed data point as the prediction for the future. The mean forecast predicts future values as the average of all past observations. The RNN, LSTM, and GRU have the same structure, with 2 hidden layers and 64 units in each. The N-BEATS and N-HITS have the same structure of 3 blocks with 4 hidden layers and 256 units on each. All the deep learning models are trained for 100 epochs.

GNN-based approaches, such as DCRNN [15], which would more directly use the process graph structure (e.g. the DFG), were omitted from this benchmark due to preliminary results indicating the data requirements are too strong for this type of problem (without significant architectural changes). Besides, the DFGs have time series on the edges instead of the nodes, which is not typical of GNNs.

4.3   Experimental Setup

First, the event logs are preprocessed by removing infrequent variants, adding "start" and "end" activities, and reducing the time length, as described in Sect. 4.1. Then, the number of occurrences of each DF within the determined time step of one day is extracted as time series. To cover sufficient business days and provide strategic forecasting, which is the main aim of PMF being a system-wide forecasting exercise, we designed the model to learn the historical one-month data for predicting the future half month. For this experiment, different sample time series of 32 time steps (days) were used to forecast over an output horizon consisting of the next 16 days. Time series data is divided into training and test sets by a 4:1 ratio.

To visualize the overall evolution of DFs on three event logs, Fig. 3 illustrates the summed DF time series, where the dotted green line represents the boundary between training and test sets and the red dots indicate the points exceeding the 3-sigma limit, i.e. the points that lie out of an interval 3 standard deviations removed from the mean. The high spikes in Fig. 3a and 3c show the challenges for modeling. Note that BPI2019_1 appears to exhibit periodic patterns while RTFMP contains more intermittency. The majority of red dots in Fig. 3b lie in the test set, posing challenges to learning these from the training data.

We evaluate the forecasted horizon of 16 days in different ways. Firstly, we measure the mean absolute error (MAE) and root mean square error (RMSE) between the forecasted time series and the true values over the whole horizon. However, since forecasting one timestep or multiple (like 16) time steps ahead

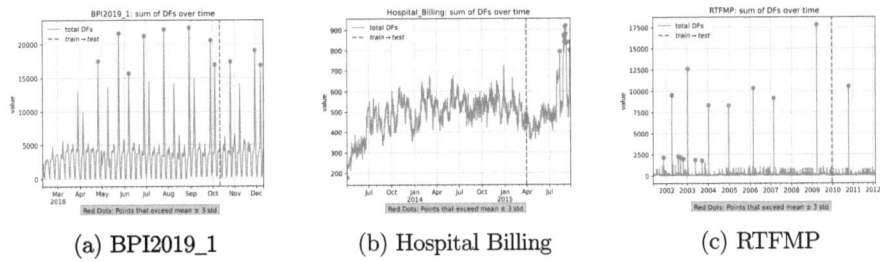

(a) BPI2019_1   (b) Hospital Billing   (c) RTFMP

Fig. 3. Summed DFs Time Series Plots

can be regarded as different problems we also evaluate the MAE and RMSE between forecast and true value for only the last timestep 16 days ahead, as this reflects the most difficult part of the horizon to forecast.

All preprocessing and models are implemented in Python with pm4py[1] and Darts[2] packages separately. The models' hyper-parameters are selected as the default settings in Darts. The code is publicly available[3].

4.4 Results

As mentioned earlier, the predictions are evaluated for all 16 time steps (all predictions of output sequences) as measured in Table 2 and the last time step (the last predictions of output sequences) as measured in Table 3 by mean absolute error (MAE) and root mean square error (RMSE). Note that the MAE and RMSE in Table 2 is the average error over the full horizon (16 days). The bottom lines in Table 2 and 3 show the number of evaluated output sequences and the number of predicted DFs in each sequence. The additional "Rank" columns indicate the prediction performance of different models according to the metrics of MAE or RMSE. The results show that different approaches rank vastly differently for different processes but XGBoost is best-performing in general. The boosting models produce more accurate predictions across all three datasets. However, the models of the RNN class perform poorly overall, especially on the BPI2019_1 log. N-HITS outperforms N-BEATS, potentially due to the capability of multi-scale time series techniques, but both achieve only moderate predictive capabilities. TCN stands out only on the RTFMP but loses the strength on the BPI2019_1. Transformer and TFT models have shown limited forecasting accuracy across the three datasets. DLinear and NLinear models demonstrate poor performance on the Hospital Billing and RTFMP, similar to the poor results of the linear regression.

---

[1] https://pm4py.fit.fraunhofer.de.
[2] https://unit8co.github.io/darts/index.html.
[3] https://github.com/YongboYu/multi_PMF.

Table 2. Evaluation for All 16 Output Predictions of All DFs

Model	BPI2019_1				Hospital Billing				RTFMP			
	MAE	Rank	RMSE	Rank	MAE	Rank	RMSE	Rank	MAE	Rank	RMSE	Rank
Persistence	26.80	5	47.66	10	2.47	2	2.99	2	3.75	3	6.89	3
Mean	25.76	4	41.53	6	**2.09**	1	**2.54**	1	3.48	2	**6.27**	1
LinearRegression	24.13	3	35.43	3	5.13	15	5.80	15	16.95	15	23.14	15
XGBoost	**17.99**	1	35.04	2	2.92	4	3.48	4	**3.22**	1	7.15	4
LightGBM	22.54	2	**33.34**	1	2.89	3	3.39	3	4.72	5	8.67	6
RNN	39.69	12	56.08	11	3.72	11	4.35	10	7.59	9	11.18	8
LSTM	49.22	15	160.99	15	3.54	9	4.19	9	9.04	10	13.94	10
GRU	45.15	14	58.06	12	3.78	12	4.45	12	11.97	12	16.48	12
N-BEATS	31.14	9	45.83	8	3.13	6	3.59	5	10.78	11	14.93	11
N-HiTS	27.87	6	40.75	5	3.12	5	3.59	5	6.87	8	10.56	7
TCN	41.63	13	60.35	14	3.34	7	3.84	7	3.93	4	6.79	2
Transformer	29.81	7	44.52	7	3.45	8	3.94	8	5.28	6	8.37	5
TFT	34.11	10	58.47	13	3.59	10	4.37	11	6.35	7	12.86	9
DLinear	35.84	11	46.97	9	4.56	13	5.16	13	15.64	14	21.02	14
NLinear	30.06	8	40.59	4	4.84	14	5.50	14	15.02	13	20.31	13
(#seq, #DF)	(15, 149)				(134, 69)				(741, 39)			

Table 3. Evaluation for Last One Output Prediction of All DFs

Model	BPI2019_1				Hospital Billing				RTFMP			
	MAE	Rank	RMSE	Rank	MAE	Rank	RMSE	Rank	MAE	Rank	RMSE	Rank
Persistence	33.95	7	161.23	9	2.90	2	9.76	3	3.94	3	15.44	4
Mean	31.28	6	151.23	6	**2.28**	1	**7.54**	1	3.58	2	12.17	2
LinearRegression	28.09	3	140.83	4	5.70	15	18.10	15	17.18	15	56.79	15
XGBoost	**22.11**	1	**105.27**	1	3.01	3	8.93	2	**3.37**	1	12.46	3
LightGBM	24.94	2	120.39	2	3.25	5	10.15	6	4.74	5	16.16	5
RNN	33.96	8	167.09	10	4.11	12	12.50	11	9.10	9	25.74	9
LSTM	53.53	15	272.12	15	3.83	10	11.87	10	9.26	10	28.67	10
GRU	47.77	13	245.05	14	3.83	10	11.13	8	14.77	12	44.70	11
N-BEATS	40.92	12	205.09	12	3.28	6	10.30	7	13.41	11	46.32	12
N-HiTS	28.18	4	134.41	3	3.19	4	9.86	4	6.96	8	22.73	7
TCN	49.07	14	241.16	13	3.40	7	10.10	5	3.94	3	**11.42**	1
Transformer	34.34	11	159.63	8	3.73	9	12.57	12	6.27	6	20.23	6
TFT	34.16	9	172.24	11	3.67	8	11.41	9	6.63	7	24.32	8
DLinear	34.27	10	157.84	7	5.08	13	14.58	13	15.92	14	52.36	14
NLinear	30.60	5	146.63	5	5.25	14	15.55	14	15.30	13	50.23	13
(#seq, #DF)	(15, 149)				(134, 69)				(741, 39)			

5   Discussion

Given the results in Sect. 4.4, it is not possible to definitively confirm whether multivariate approaches are superior. In some cases, even a naive forecast or a mean forecast can lead to only a small prediction error in terms of MAE and RMSE. On the other hand, two traditional ensemble models perform better than deep learning approaches overall, especially on the BPI2019_1 and Hospital Billing, which consist of shorter time lengths and higher dimensions of DF time series. In this section, we discuss the challenges of DF time series prediction in PMF for general forecasting models and multivariate deep learning models specifically.

In general, the evolution in the patterns of DF time series extracted from the event logs are challenging to capture and model. Different information systems tailor the timing of events and uniformly process them based on business content (i.e. batching). Thus, many DF pairs occur intermittently with exceptionally high values and some are present in clusters of a certain period, posing challenges for overall time series forecasting techniques. Concerning the setting up, the DF time series with the step of one day also introduces significant intermittency and fluctuations. A higher time aggregation level is possible to smooth the DF time series and enhance the predictive effect, however, this may again cause even sparser time series levels. In addition, the window size of 32 days might not be large enough to predict the time horizon of 16 days. Large fluctuations and long-term seasonality and trends in DF time series may require a longer window of inputs to learn and fit for more accurate predictions. The above three aspects impact the time series forecasting approaches including univariate and multivariate analysis techniques.

For multivariate deep learning approaches, we can identify several additional reasons for their poor performance in the experiments. First of all, event logs with short time ranges (a limited number of observations) are inadequate for training deep-learning models. Both time series and deep learning models require a large amount of data to fully learn complex multivariate relations and the fluctuations, seasonality, and trends in the time dimension. For example, TCN's performance ranks higher on the event logs with longer time ranges and fewer DFs. On the other hand, training traditional machine learning models is more manageable on small data sets (most commonly used event logs can be considered small). This leads to XGBoost and LightGBM reporting lower error rates in the overall experiments. Secondly, the diverse and widely fluctuating patterns of individual DF time series suggest that the relationships among them are also complex to reveal. The constructed multivariate connections might be insufficient and mislead the information propagated in the neural networks.

6   Conclusion and Future Work

In this paper, we propose data preprocessing for DF time series predictions in PMF. The various intricacies tied to DF time series such as intermittency, long-range dependencies, multi-scale presence, and so on, complicate the (multivariate) forecasting exercise, hence a wide range of techniques of different multivariate forecasting methods from machine learning and deep learning forecasting approaches with diverse architectures were benchmarked over three real-life event logs. XGBoost, as a traditional machine learning technique, performs better than deep learning-based models in general, meaning that the most sophisticated state-of-the-art fails to handle the DF time series' inherent complexity. In line with the several other insights and limitations raised in Sect. 5, several avenues for future work in PMF can be proposed.

For significant intermittency in the DF time series, specialized mechanisms such as [13] can be incorporated to boost the predictive performance. Even though GNNs are not covered in this paper, using the inherent capability to incorporate graph structures of process models would still be worth exploring. In addition to DFs from the control-flow aspect, forecasting process elements along other dimensions such as resource allocation, bottlenecks, and decision points could provide rich insights and enable proactive intervention. To generalize PMF, more event logs and process characters will be investigated.

Acknowledgements. This study was financed by the Research Foundation Flanders under grant number G039923N and Internal Funds KU Leuven under grant number C14/23/031.

References

1. Bahdanau, D., Cho, K., Bengio, Y.: Neural machine translation by jointly learning to align and translate. arXiv preprint arXiv:1409.0473 (2014)
2. Bai, S., Kolter, J.Z., Koltun, V.: An empirical evaluation of generic convolutional and recurrent networks for sequence modeling. arXiv preprint arXiv:1803.01271 (2018)
3. Challu, C., Olivares, K.G., Oreshkin, B.N., Ramirez, F.G., Canseco, M.M., Dubrawski, A.: NHITS: neural hierarchical interpolation for time series forecasting. In: Proceedings of the AAAI Conference on Artificial Intelligence, vol. 37, pp. 6989–6997 (2023)
4. Chen, T., Guestrin, C.: XGBoost: a scalable tree boosting system. In: Proceedings of the 22nd ACM SIGKDD International Conference on Knowledge Discovery and Data Mining, pp. 785–794 (2016)
5. Cho, K., Van Merriënboer, B., Bahdanau, D., Bengio, Y.: On the properties of neural machine translation: encoder-decoder approaches. arXiv preprint arXiv:1409.1259 (2014)
6. De Smedt, J., Yeshchenko, A., Polyvyanyy, A., De Weerdt, J., Mendling, J.: Process model forecasting and change exploration using time series analysis of event sequence data. Data Knowl. Eng. **145**, 102145 (2023)
7. van Dongen, B.: BPI challenge 2019 (2019). https://doi.org/10.4121/uuid: d06aff4b-79f0-45e6-8ec8-e19730c248f1. https://data.4tu.nl/articles/dataset/BPI_Challenge_2019/12715853/1
8. Evermann, J., Rehse, J.R., Fettke, P.: Predicting process behaviour using deep learning. Decis. Support Syst. **100**, 129–140 (2017)

9. Friedman, J.H.: Greedy function approximation: a gradient boosting machine. Ann. Stat. 1189–1232 (2001)
10. Hochreiter, S., Schmidhuber, J.: Long short-term memory. Neural Comput. **9**, 1735–1780 (1997)
11. Jiang, W., Luo, J.: Graph neural network for traffic forecasting: a survey. Expert Syst. Appl. **207**, 117921 (2022)
12. Ke, G., et al.: LightGBM: a highly efficient gradient boosting decision tree. In: Advances in Neural Information Processing Systems, vol. 30 (2017)
13. Kourentzes, N.: Intermittent demand forecasts with neural networks. Int. J. Prod. Econ. **143**(1), 198–206 (2013)
14. de Leoni, M.M., Mannhardt, F.: Road Traffic Fine Management Process (2015). https://doi.org/10.4121/uuid:270fd440-1057-4fb9-89a9-b699b47990f5.   https://data.4tu.nl/articles/dataset/Road_Traffic_Fine_Management_Process/12683249
15. Li, Y., Yu, R., Shahabi, C., Liu, Y.: Diffusion convolutional recurrent neural network: data-driven traffic forecasting. arXiv preprint arXiv:1707.01926 (2017)
16. Lim, B., Arık, S.Ö., Loeff, N., Pfister, T.: Temporal fusion transformers for interpretable multi-horizon time series forecasting. Int. J. Forecast. **37**(4), 1748–1764 (2021)
17. Mannhardt, F.: Hospital Billing - Event Log (2017). https://doi.org/10.4121/uuid:76c46b83-c930-4798-a1c9-4be94dfeb741.   https://data.4tu.nl/articles/dataset/Hospital_Billing_-_Event_Log/12705113
18. Mehrdad Bibalan, Y., Far, B., Eshragh, F., Ghiyasian, B.: Work in progress prediction for business processes using temporal convolutional networks. In: International Conference on Industrial, Engineering and Other Applications of Applied Intelligent Systems, pp. 109–121. Springer, Cham (2024)
19. Meira Neto, A.C., de Sousa, R.G., Fantinato, M., Peres, S.M.: Revisiting the transition matrix-based concept drift approach: improving the detection task reliability through additional experimentation. SN Comput. Sci. **5**, 188 (2024)
20. Oreshkin, B.N., Carpov, D., Chapados, N., Bengio, Y.: N-beats: neural basis expansion analysis for interpretable time series forecasting. arXiv preprint arXiv:1905.10437 (2019)
21. Poll, R., Polyvyanyy, A., Rosemann, M., Röglinger, M., Rupprecht, L.: Process forecasting: towards proactive business process management. In: Weske, M., Montali, M., Weber, I., vom Brocke, J. (eds.) BPM 2018. LNCS, vol. 11080, pp. 496–512. Springer, Cham (2018). https://doi.org/10.1007/978-3-319-98648-7_29
22. Pourbafrani, M., van der Aalst, W.M.: Extracting process features from event logs to learn coarse-grained simulation models. In: International Conference on Advanced Information Systems Engineering, pp. 125–140. Springer, Cham (2021)
23. Rama-Maneiro, E., Vidal, J.C., Lama, M.: Deep learning for predictive business process monitoring: review and benchmark. IEEE Trans. Serv. Comput. **16**(1), 739–756 (2021)
24. Schuster, D., Schade, L., van Zelst, S.J., van der Aalst, W.M.: Temporal performance analysis for block-structured process models in cortado. In: International Conference on Advanced Information Systems Engineering, pp. 110–119. Springer, Cham (2022)
25. Tax, N., Verenich, I., La Rosa, M., Dumas, M.: Predictive business process monitoring with LSTM neural networks. In: Dubois, E., Pohl, K. (eds.) CAiSE 2017. LNCS, vol. 10253, pp. 477–492. Springer, Cham (2017). https://doi.org/10.1007/978-3-319-59536-8_30

26. Teinemaa, I., Dumas, M., Rosa, M.L., Maggi, F.M.: Outcome-oriented predictive process monitoring: review and benchmark. ACM Trans. Knowl. Discov. Data (TKDD) **13**(2), 1–57 (2019)
27. Vaswani, A.: Attention is all you need. arXiv preprint arXiv:1706.03762 (2017)
28. Yu, B., Yin, H., Zhu, Z.: Spatio-temporal graph convolutional networks: a deep learning framework for traffic forecasting. arXiv preprint arXiv:1709.04875 (2017)
29. Zeng, A., Chen, M., Zhang, L., Xu, Q.: Are transformers effective for time series forecasting? In: Proceedings of the AAAI Conference on Artificial Intelligence, vol. 37, pp. 11121–11128 (2023)

Enhancing Predictive Process Monitoring Using Semantic Information

Jiaxin Yuan[1]([✉])(ID), Daniela Grigori[1]([✉])(ID), and Han van der Aa[2]([✉])(ID)

[1] Paris Dauphine University-PSL, Pl. du Maréchal de Lattre de Tassigny,
75016 Paris, France
jiaxin.yuan@dauphine.eu, daniela.grigori@lamsade.dauphine.fr
[2] University of Vienna, Universitätsring 1, 1010 Wien, Austria
han.van.der.aa@univie.ac.at

Abstract. Predictive Process Monitoring (PPM) leverages historical data to forecast information about ongoing business processes. Recent methods have utilized advanced deep learning and classical machine learning models. However, the role of semantic information that can be extracted from event logs has been underexplored, although such information has been demonstrated to have significant advantages for other process mining tasks, such as anomaly detection. Therefore, this paper proposes a novel mechanism that aims to exploit semantic information for PPM, particularly by extracting information regarding the status of business objects associated with process instances from event data. We evaluate this mechanism in outcome-oriented and next activity prediction tasks, using state-of-the-art large language models (LLMs) for semantic extraction. Our results show that integrating semantic information improves prediction performance across these tasks. This work demonstrates that utilizing semantic information in PPM has considerable potential, especially in combination with advanced language models.

Keywords: Process mining · Predictive process monitoring · Semantic information · Large language models

1 Introduction

Predictive process monitoring (PPM) leverages historical data to forecast information about ongoing business process instances, thereby providing organizations with significant competitive advantages [13,18]. To address various tasks within this domain, numerous methods utilizing machine learning and deep learning models have been developed [8]. These methods employ a range of data preprocessing techniques and diverse prediction algorithms to tackle the challenges inherent in PPM [14].

Although few studies have explicitly explored the semantic information embedded within historical data, the potential benefits of incorporating such semantic information into predictive models are evident. For instance, in predicting the outcome of a case, an *application* that is *complete* is more likely to

A. Delgado and T. Slaats (Eds.): ICPM 2024 Workshops, LNBIP 533, pp. 293–305, 2025.
https://doi.org/10.1007/978-3-031-82225-4_22

succeed than an *incomplete* one. Similarly, in scenarios where the goal is to predict the next likely activity, if an *application* has been *rejected*, it is unlikely that it will proceed to *validation* again, thereby narrowing the potential search space. Relevant tasks in process mining such as anomaly detection have demonstrated significant advantages by leveraging semantic information [1,4]. These methods employ natural language processing (NLP) techniques to analyze the semantics of activity labels associated with events, enabling the identification of illogical behaviors. Furthermore, the increasing capabilities of large language models (LLMs) suggest that their integration into process mining is highly promising [2,9].

Therefore, this paper investigates integration of semantic information in PPM. Specifically, we propose a mechanism for PPM that utilizes semantic information by extracting and annotating the statuses of key business objects from event logs, through the use of LLMs. We tested this mechanism on both Outcome-Oriented Prediction (OOP) [13] and Next Activity Prediction (NAP) tasks [22], using real-life logs provided by a benchmark paper [23]. For NAP, we further validate our mechanism on additional logs. Our evaluation demonstrates that adopting our mechanism enhances prediction performance across both tasks. This underscores the potential effectiveness of discovering and leveraging semantic information in prediction tasks, indicating a promising future direction for this field.

The remainder is structured as follows. Section 2 reviews the related works in the field. Section 3 defines essential preliminaries. Section 4 describes the mechanism we introduced, which is further evaluated in Sect. 5. Finally, Sect. 6 concludes the paper by summarizing the findings, discussing their implications, and outlining potential directions for future research in this area.

2   Related Work

Research relevant to our work can be categorized into three areas: traditional methods and textual-aware solutions for PPM, semantic process mining, and the application of LLMs in the process domain.

Our work focuses on OOP and NAP, for which seminal benchmark articles have been published [19,23]. These articles suggest optimal configurations, including encoding, prefix generation, bucketing, and algorithm selection [23]. While extensive research in this area focuses on the discovery of more effective algorithms, ranging from Deep Learning (DL) approaches like transformers and LSTM to Machine Learning (ML) techniques such as SVM and RF [7,12,15,22], textual features remain largely underexplored. However, unstructured text from different process-related sources such as comment fields, emails, or documents is leveraged using traditional vectorization methods like bag of words (BoW) and Latent Dirichlet Allocation (LDA) [17]. More advanced encoding approaches, such as BERT [5], have been employed for textual features, aligning closely with recent studies on next activity prediction using LLMs, particularly from a control-flow perspective [21].

In other process mining tasks like anomaly detection, research has demonstrated significant success in utilizing semantic information, suggesting that integrating such information could enhance PPM tasks. Anomalous process behavior is identified by detecting semantically inconsistent execution patterns, with the benefits clearly demonstrated in real-world scenarios [1]. Combining machine learning methods with NLP techniques has led to significant improvements in precision and recall for semantic anomaly detection [6]. Tasks like the automatic semantic annotation of event data, which identifies specific semantic components from textual attributes, have inspired our approach to extracting business objects and their statuses [20].

Although our focus differs, our work also relates to recent research exploring the integration of LLMs into various aspects of process mining, such as process discovery and conformance checking [10,11]. Some research also delves into causal reasoning and explaining decision points [9]. Emerging benchmarks combining LLMs with process mining, such as those found in [2,3], mainly assess the quality of textual or coding answers provided by LLMs. However, these studies primarily explore how LLMs comprehend process mining artifacts or tasks rather than directly evaluating their performance on downstream tasks. More closely related to our task is a template extraction method performed using LLMs, followed by fine-tuning with a pre-trained language model, though their focus was solely on the next activity prediction task [16].

In our work, we combine these three streams by using LLMs to extract semantic information to be leveraged for different PPM tasks.

3   Preliminaries

In this section, we define preliminaries required for the remainder of the paper.

Event Data. To extract semantic information, our work takes an event log L as input, which is composed of traces. A trace $t = \langle e_1, e_2, \ldots, e_n \rangle \in L$ is a sequence of events associated with the same case. Each event in a trace can be represented as a tuple $(a, c, t, (d_1, v_1), \ldots, (d_m, v_m))$, where a denotes activity label, c is case id, t is the timestamp, and $(d_1, v_1), \ldots, (d_m, v_m)$ represents a number of data attributes and their corresponding values. PPM tasks are conducted over a set of prefixes of an event log. Therefore we define an event prefix of length k, noted as $hd^k(\sigma)$ is $hd^k(\sigma) = \langle e_1, \ldots, e_k \rangle$, where k is between 1 to $n-1$. Beyond these elements, from a broader perspective, the analysis that considers only the sequence of activities is referred to as control-flow analysis.

Classifier. In machine learning, a classifier is an algorithm that categorizes data into predefined classes. It learns from training data to map input features X to target labels y and predicts the class of new data. To be fed into a machine learning model, input features X are typically encoded as vectors, commonly referred to as feature vectors.

Outcome-Oriented Prediction. For OOP, the input X is an event prefix $hd^k(\sigma)$, while y is a finite set of categorical outcomes.

Next Activity Prediction. For NAP, the input X is the same as outcome-oriented tasks. We use a multi-class classifier $f : X \rightarrow \{a_1, a_2, \ldots, a_k\}$, where the label space is the set of unique activity labels $\{a_1, a_2, \ldots, a_k\}$.

4   Mechanism

This section presents our proposed semantic-aware status annotation mechanism for general PPM tasks. As shown in Fig. 1, our mechanism includes two steps specific to our pipeline (in red). *Semantic extraction* creates a static mapping from activity labels to their corresponding business objects and statuses. *Status annotation*, in turn, uses this mapping to annotate a prefix (for training) or an ongoing case (for inference) with information that captures the current status of each of its business objects. The rest of the PPM pipeline is in line with common practice, making our mechanism independent of the choice of a specific machine learning model or other configuration choices.

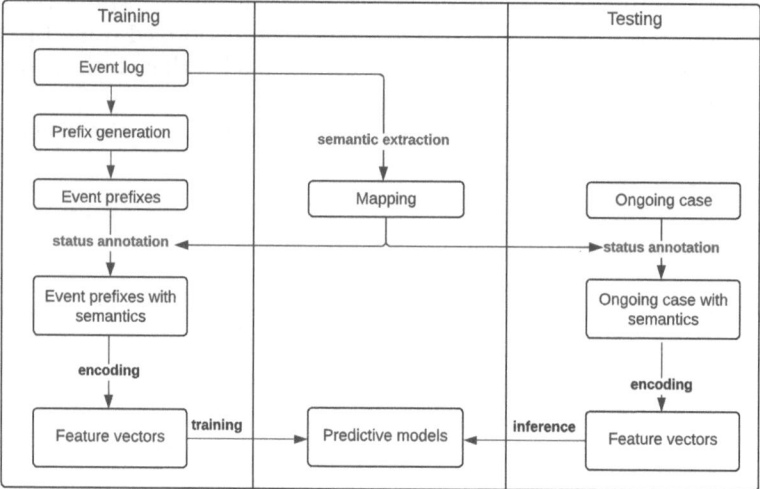

Fig. 1. Overview of our semantic-aware status annotation mechanism. (Color figure online)

4.1   Semantic Extraction

The first step in our mechanism is semantic extraction, which creates a static mapping from each activity label in the label space of an event log to a collection of key-value pairs that identify business objects and their corresponding statuses. This mapping serves as a reference for generating semantic information for each event in the subsequent step. For example, from *Create fine*, we obtain *fine* as the business object and *created* as its status.

Semantic extraction can be conducted using LLMs. By providing a prompt with task-specific instructions, LLMs are able to comprehend the task and return the key-value pairs that identify business objects and their corresponding statuses. Figure 2 illustrates an example of how we extract semantic information using Llama-3[1]. When a verb-substantive combination is present in the activity label, semantic extraction is straightforward. Otherwise, LLMs must rely on learned knowledge to infer meaning. For example, the activity label *Payment* provides no indication of status, but based on its pre-trained knowledge, the LLM assigns status *conducted* to the business object *payment*.

<|begin_of_text|><|start_header_id|>system<|end_header_id|>

You are an expert in process mining. Your task is to extract key business objects and their states from complex activity labels by mapping activity labels to a dictionary in the form of {activity label: {business object: status}}.
A single activity label can contain multiple essential business objects and states.
Business objects must be general and process-related.
Respond strictly in JSON format, providing fields for each activity. Ensure you understand the meaning and don't just extract directly. Output only the dictionary as the answer. Don't forget any of given activity labels.

Example activity labels:

{"Create Fine"}

Example answer:
{"Create Fine": {"fine": "created"}}

<|eot_id|><|start_header_id|>user<|end_header_id|>
{'Create Fine', 'Send Fine', 'Insert Fine Notification', 'Send Appeal to Prefecture',
'Receive Result Appeal from Prefecture', 'Appeal to Judge', 'Add penalty', 'Payment',
'Notify Result Appeal to Offender', 'Insert Date Appeal to Prefecture'}
<|eot_id|><|start_header_id|>expert<|end_header_id|>

Fig. 2. The prompt begins with role *system*, followed by a description of the task and constraints. It then presents examples of extractions, which may include multiple instances. The interaction continues in role *user*, listing activity labels for processing. Finally, the prompt concludes with role *expert*, where introduces the expected results.

4.2   Status Annotation

In this step, we annotate a prefix or ongoing case with information that captures the current status of all business objects, using the mapping derived in the first step. This is done by iteratively processing events that occurred, with each status being updated if a new event occurs that relates to that business object.

---

[1] https://huggingface.co/meta-llama/Meta-Llama-3-8B.

For example, consider an entire trace with a control flow $\langle Create\ Fine,$ $Send\ Fine, Insert\ Fine\ Notification, Add\ Penalty \rangle$, with Case id $A100$. The control flow of event prefix of length 2, denoted as $hd^2(\sigma_{A100})$, is $\langle Create\ Fine, Send\ Fine \rangle$. During status annotation, all business objects extracted from previous step are initialized as *unprocessed*, including *fine* and *penalty*, as well as *payment* from other traces. Then business object *fine* is updated to *created* and subsequently to *sent*, while business objects *penalty* and *payment* remain unaffected and retain its initial status. For the event prefix $hd^2(\sigma_{A100})$, the final statuses of business objects that appear in the trace are recorded as {*fine : sent, penalty : unprocessed, payment : unprocessed*}, as illustrated in Fig. 3. The status annotation process for ongoing cases is similar to that for event prefixes, as both capture the sequence of events that have occurred up to that point.

Case id	Event number	Activity	Resource	Amount	Business objects			Label	
					fine	penalty	payment	NAP	OOP
A100	1	Create Fine	R561	35	created	unprocessed	unprocessed	Send fine	1
A100	2	Send Fine	R561	35	sent	unprocessed	unprocessed	Insert fine notification	1
A100	3	Insert Fine Notification	R561	35	notified	unprocessed	unprocessed	Add penalty	1
A100	4	Add penalty	R1	71	notified	added	unprocessed	End	1
A1	1	Create Fine	R537	36	created	unprocessed	unprocessed	Send fine	0
A1	2	Send Fine	R537	36	sent	unprocessed	unprocessed	Insert Fine Notification	0
A1	3	Insert Fine Notification	R537	36	notified	unprocessed	unprocessed	Add penalty	0
A1	4	Add penalty	R537	74	notified	added	unprocessed	Payment	0
A1	5	Payment	R537	74	notified	added	conducted	End	0

Fig. 3. Snapshot of a collection of an event log with semantics. All unique activities are listed in the column *activity*. The example discussed in the text is highlighted, with the event prefix with semantics of $hd^2(\sigma_{A100})$ in red, and the associated labels for NAP and OOP in green. (Color figure online)

4.3   PPM Pipeline

After obtaining the enriched inputs with semantics, we proceed with a standard process within the PPM pipeline. During the training phase, we utilize the collection of event prefixes and their associated semantics to train predictive models for various PPM tasks. In the testing phase, we use the trained models to make predictions for ongoing cases. Semantic information can be seamlessly integrated into downstream tasks, similar to other categorical features within the inputs, with business objects representing the feature names and their final statuses as the corresponding values.

We particularly apply our mechanism to outcome prediction and next activity prediction tasks from PPM, as these are well-explored in the research and represent distinct concerns—one focusing on immediate prediction ability and the other on cumulative prediction ability. Furthermore, more so than remaining time prediction, these tasks can benefit from the integration of semantic information, as their targets may be closely related to the underlying semantics.

5   Evaluation Experiments

This section reports on the experiments conducted in our study. The objective was to compare prediction results with and without semantic information. The selection of event logs is detailed in Sect. 5.1, and the experimental settings are described in Sect. 5.2. The results of both OOP and NAP task are presented in Sect. 5.3. We discuss the results and limitations of our experiment in Sect. 5.4. The implementation can be found in our repository.[2]

5.1   Log Selection

As OOP requires labeled datasets, we initially limited our selection to the OOP benchmark and generated NAP labels from these datasets [23]. We selected five datasets based on the rule that they must be in English with activity labels having clear linguistic meaning, not cryptic notations. Following this rule, we retained three logs from *BPIC2017*, as well as *production* and *traffic fines* logs. Since generating labels for next activity prediction is straightforward, we further expanded our selection to include additional real-world logs commonly used in research, applying the same rule. This resulted in the inclusion of five logs from *BPIC2020*, *BPIC2019*, and *helpdesk*. All logs are available in our repository.

Data Preprocessing. We filter out traces containing fewer than three events, as they generally provide insufficient information at early stages. On the other hand, training with long prefixes is time-consuming, and the OOP becomes trivial at late stages [23]. Thus, we vary the prefix length from 3 to 20 during both training and testing.

Train-Test Split. Within each log, we use 80% of the traces for training and the remaining 20% for testing. To prevent overfitting, we ensure that the testing traces are completely excluded from the training set.

Characteristics. Table 1 gives a summary of the characteristic of the 12 datasets. Among all the datasets for OOP tasks, the labels are either positive or negative, denoting whether the outcomes deviate from or not to the defined rules [23]. In the table, *Pos rate* indicates the proportion of positive labels.

---

[2] https://github.com/jiaxin-yuan/semantic_status_annotation.

Table 1. Characteristics of the chosen logs.

Dataset	Traces	Trace length		Variants	Events	Activity	OOP
		Avg.	Max			Classes	Pos rate
bpic17_a	31,413	45.45	180	15,846	1,198,366	26	0.41
bpic17_c	31,413	45.45	180	15,846	1,198,366	26	0.47
bpic17_r	31,413	45.45	180	15,846	1,198,366	26	0.12
production	220	20.34	78	203	2,489	26	0.53
traffic	129,615	4.07	20	200	460,556	10	0.46
bpic19	251,734	33.23	990	11,973	1,595,923	42	–
bpic20i	6,449	11.19	27	753	72,151	34	–
bpic20d	10,500	5.37	24	99	56,437	17	–
bpic20permit	7,065	14.80	90	1,478	86,581	51	–
bpic20prepaid	2,099	9.27	21	202	18,246	29	–
bpic20request	6,886	5.74	20	89	36,796	19	–
helpdesk	4,580	4.66	15	226	21,348	14	–

5.2 Experimental Setting

Implementation and Environment. Our implementation comprises two components: semantic extraction with LLMs on 2 Nvidia RTX 2080 Ti GPUs and 32GB RAM, and prediction using XGBoost in Python 3.8 on an Apple M2 CPU with 16GB RAM. The prediction phase was executed using a CPU, as XGBoost shows minimal GPU benefit from acceleration.

Configurations and Baseline. We compare results obtained for three settings:

- *w/o semantics*: This represents a baseline that only captures control-flow information. We specifically use aggregation encoding on the *Activity* attribute. For example, an event prefix of length 2 in the trace $\langle a, b, c, d \rangle$ is encoded as $\{a: 1, b: 1, c: 0, d: 0\}$. The aggregation method was chosen for encoding due to its relatively superior performance, as reported in the OOP benchmark [23].
- *w sem(LLM)*: This configuration adds semantic information as obtained through our mechanism to the feature vector. All other configuration options are the same as for the baseline.
- *w sem(hard)*: This configuration is the same as the previous one, with the exception that we use a manually defined (i.e., hardcoded) mapping as the output for Step 1. This configuration allows us to test if extraction mistakes by the LLM impact the prediction accuracy.

In our LLM-based configuration, we employed in-context learning with LLaMa-3 for extraction. Experimentation with various prompting settings revealed that few-shot prompting with more examples typically yielded more stable and accurate results. Consequently, we used six examples per log in our experiments.

Performance Metrics. For OOP, we adopted the Area Under the Curve (AUC), indicating the likelihood of ranking a positive instance higher than a negative one. For NAP, we employed overall accuracy and Macro-Averaged F1 Score as metrics [19]. Accuracy measures correct classifications, while the F1 Score balances precision and recall. The Macro-Averaged F1 Score averages F1 Scores across classes equally, making it suitable for imbalanced distributions.

5.3   Results

Result of OOP. Table 2 presents the results for the outcome-oriented prediction task, measured by AUC among all testing set. Across almost all datasets, settings that incorporate semantics extracted either through hard coding or LLMs consistently outperform those that do not utilize semantics. Though, an exception is observed in the *production* dataset, where the performance of LLM-extracted semantics is lower compared to non-semantics, whereas semantics extracted manually still perform better than non-semantics. In most cases, manually extracted features perform similarly to those extracted by LLMs.

Table 2. Overall AUC for OOP tasks obtained on the test set, using XGBoost. Bold numbers indicate the best score for that dataset.

method	dataset				
	bpic17_a	bpic17_c	bpic17_r	production	traffic
w/o semantics	0.6624	0.6377	0.5743	0.6440	0.6225
w sem(hard)	**0.6636**	**0.6385**	0.5751	**0.6449**	**0.6228**
w sem(LLMs)	**0.6636**	0.6380	**0.5758**	0.6396	**0.6228**

Result of NAP. Table 3 presents the results for the next activity prediction task, evaluated using overall accuracy and Macro-Averaged F1 Score across the test set. The *BPIC2017* subsets *accepted*, *cancelled*, and *refused* originate from the same process, resulting in identical values. In most datasets (7/10), both metrics consistently show performance improvements with the incorporation of semantics. Inconsistencies between the metrics are observed in datasets with limited samples, such as *Production*, and in those with over 40 activity labels. Only the *traffic* dataset consistently underperforms when semantics are incorporated. In most cases, extraction by LLMs outperforms human extraction for this task.

Table 3. Overall accuracy (first row) and Macro-Averaged F1 Score (second row) for the NAP tasks on the test set, using XGBoost. Bold values represent the highest score for each dataset within the same evaluation metric.

method	dataset				
	bpic17	production	traffic	bpic20d	bpic20i
w/o semantics	0.8680	0.0518	**0.8182**	0.3042	0.7041
	0.7204	0.0289	**0.5506**	0.1191	0.3530
w sem(hard)	0.8959	0.0621	0.8181	0.3045	0.7042
	0.7251	**0.0407**	0.5505	0.1193	0.3540
w sem(LLMs)	**0.8960**	**0.0647**	0.8181	**0.3271**	**0.7098**
	0.7252	0.0397	0.5505	**0.1324**	**0.3759**
	bpic20permit	bpic20prepaid	bpic20request	helpdesk	bpic19
w/o semantics	0.2025	0.6541	0.4937	0.2406	0.0093
	0.2370	0.3913	0.1533	0.1132	**0.0097**
w sem(hard)	**0.2040**	0.6546	0.4941	**0.2427**	**0.0097**
	0.2358	0.3938	0.1556	**0.1146**	0.0093
w sem(LLMs)	0.2034	**0.6610**	**0.5043**	0.2411	**0.0097**
	0.2388	**0.4446**	**0.1702**	0.1143	0.0093

Earliness. For the OOP task, we assess earliness by calculating AUC at each prefix length, as illustrated in Fig. 4. As the three logs from *BPIC2017* exhibit similar trends, only one is presented here. The performance gains from using semantics are more pronounced in the earlier stages, as demonstrated in three datasets from the *BPIC2017* log. The AUC score without semantics is notably poorer compared to two settings with semantics, particularly for prefix lengths between 3 and 5. Despite the performance gains from using semantics in the *traffic fines* figure being less visually apparent, the numerical results show that semantics outperform non-semantics for prefix lengths 5, 6, and 7, with improvements of 0.2%, 0.03%, and 0.009%, respectively, while remaining consistent across other prefix lengths. The *Production* dataset shows no clear pattern, but the inclusion of semantics leads to superior performance for prefix lengths 5 to 10.

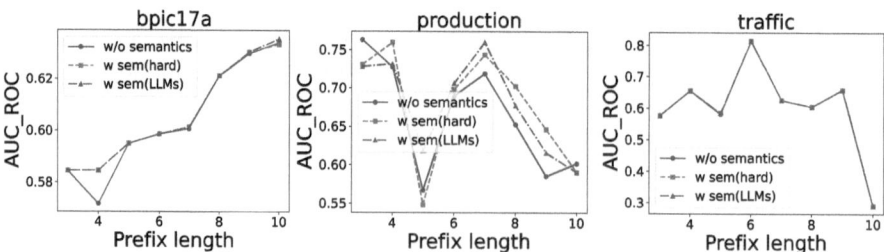

Fig. 4. Earliness of the OOP task across different datasets, limited to prefix lengths below 10.

5.4   Discussion

Overall, we demonstrate that semantics can enhance PPM performance, as indicated by the general performance improvements achieved with our mechanism. However, these improvements vary a lot across datasets and settings. By summarizing the prediction performances from both the OOP and NAP tasks, as well as the earliness of the OOP task, we derive the following key insights.

Task Comparison. Performance gains are generally more evident in NAP than in OOP, indicating that semantics are more beneficial for immediate predictions than for cumulative prediction. On the other hand, performance varies considerably across different datasets, both in terms of overall performance and the magnitude of performance and of performance improvements. This variability suggests that the benefits of our mechanism differ among datasets, which can be attributed to the extent of semantic information contained in the activity labels.

Extraction Method Comparison. Overall, semantic extraction using LLMs outperforms manual extraction in both tasks. Excluding datasets with inconsistent results across both metrics, exceptions are observed in *Helpdesk*. Despite having a limited number of activity labels, similar to *traffic fines* and *BPIC20d*, *Helpdesk* lacks business objects within its activity labels, making it difficult for the LLM to accurately conduct semantic extraction from the context.

Earliness. The consistent performance gains observed in most datasets highlight promising potential in prediction earliness, which is crucial for the OOP task. The oscillations observed in *Production* likely stem from the limited sample size at each prefix length, with the highest number of examples per group being below 40, making the results sensitive to individual samples.

Limitations. Due to the probabilistic nature of LLMs, limitations such as the randomness in optimal extractions are inherent. Additionally, time constraints restricted us from comparing different prefix encoding methods, employing more robust techniques like cross-validation, or exploring the selection of optimal predictive algorithms.

6   Conclusion

This paper addresses the underexplored role of semantic information in PPM. By introducing a novel mechanism for extracting and annotating the statuses of business objects from event logs, we demonstrated that incorporating semantic information can enhance predictive accuracy for outcome-oriented and next activity prediction.

However, our work has some limitations. Currently, our mechanism focuses sorely on statuses associated with individual business objects and does not account for semantic interactions between business objects using linguistic knowledge, such as synonyms, near-synonyms, and antonyms. For example, the status *cancelled* of the business object *booking* may trigger status updates in other related objects, such as changing the status of *bills* from *unpaid* to *cancelled*.

In future work, we plan to explore the role of semantic information in prescriptive process monitoring, incorporating the additional linguistic knowledge mentioned earlier. Building on the foundations of predictive process monitoring, we hope this will help identifying effective intervention actions for different scenarios in advance, thereby offering actionable recommendations for improvement in process monitoring.

Disclosure of Interests. The authors have no competing interests to declare that are relevant to the content of this article.

References

1. van der Aa, H., Rebmann, A., Leopold, H.: Natural language-based detection of semantic execution anomalies in event logs. Inf. Syst. **102**, 101824 (2021)
2. Berti, A., Kourani, H., van der Aalst, W.M.: PM-LLM-benchmark: evaluating large language models on process mining tasks. arXiv preprint arXiv:2407.13244 (2024)
3. Berti, A., Qafari, M.S.: Leveraging large language models (LLMs) for process mining (technical report). arXiv preprint arXiv:2307.12701 (2023)
4. Busch, K., Kampik, T., Leopold, H.: xsemad: explainable semantic anomaly detection in event logs using sequence-to-sequence models. arXiv preprint arXiv:2406.19763 (2024)
5. Cabrera, L., Weinzierl, S., Zilker, S., Matzner, M.: Text-aware predictive process monitoring with contextualized word embeddings. In: International Conference on Business Process Management, pp. 303–314. Springer, Cham (2022)
6. Caspary, J., Rebmann, A., van der Aa, H.: Does this make sense? Machine learning-based detection of semantic anomalies in business processes. In: International Conference on Business Process Management, pp. 163–179. Springer, Cham (2023)
7. Chen, H., Fang, X., Fang, H.: Multi-task prediction method of business process based on BERT and transfer learning. Knowl.-Based Syst. **254**, 109603 (2022)
8. Evermann, J., Rehse, J.R., Fettke, P.: Predicting process behaviour using deep learning. Decis. Support Syst. **100**, 129–140 (2017)
9. Fahland, D., Fournier, F., Limonad, L., Skarbovsky, I., Swevels, A.J.: How well can large language models explain business processes? arXiv preprint arXiv:2401.12846 (2024)
10. Grohs, M., Abb, L., Elsayed, N., Rehse, J.R.: Large language models can accomplish business process management tasks. In: International Conference on Business Process Management, pp. 453–465. Springer, Cham (2023)
11. Kourani, H., Berti, A., Schuster, D., van der Aalst, W.M.: Process modeling with large language models. In: International Conference on Business Process Modeling, Development and Support, pp. 229–244. Springer, Cham (2024)
12. Kratsch, W., Manderscheid, J., Röglinger, M., Seyfried, J.: Machine learning in business process monitoring: a comparison of deep learning and classical approaches used for outcome prediction. Bus. Inf. Syst. Eng. **63**, 261–276 (2021)
13. Maggi, F.M., Di Francescomarino, C., Dumas, M., Ghidini, C.: Predictive monitoring of business processes. In: CAiSE, pp. 457–472 (2014)

14. Neu, D.A., Lahann, J., Fettke, P.: A systematic literature review on state-of-the-art deep learning methods for process prediction. Artif. Intell. Rev. **55**(2), 801–827 (2022)
15. Ni, W., Zhao, G., Liu, T., Zeng, Q., Xu, X.: Predictive business process monitoring approach based on hierarchical transformer. Electronics **12**(6), 1273 (2023)
16. Oved, A., Shlomov, S., Zeltyn, S., Mashkif, N., Yaeli, A.: Snap: semantic stories for next activity prediction. arXiv preprint arXiv:2401.15621 (2024)
17. Pegoraro, M., Uysal, M.S., Georgi, D.B., van der Aalst, W.M.: Text-aware predictive monitoring of business processes. arXiv preprint arXiv:2104.09962 (2021)
18. Philipp, P., Jacob, R., Robert, S., Beyerer, J.: Predictive analysis of business processes using neural networks with attention mechanism. In: 2020 International Conference on Artificial Intelligence in Information and Communication (ICAIIC), pp. 225–230. IEEE (2020)
19. Rama-Maneiro, E., Vidal, J.C., Lama, M.: Deep learning for predictive business process monitoring: review and benchmark. IEEE Trans. Serv. Comput. **16**(1), 739–756 (2021)
20. Rebmann, A., van der Aa, H.: Enabling semantics-aware process mining through the automatic annotation of event logs. Inf. Syst. **110**, 102111 (2022)
21. Rebmann, A., Schmidt, F.D., Glavaš, G., van der Aa, H.: Evaluating the ability of LLMs to solve semantics-aware process mining tasks. arXiv preprint arXiv:2407.02310 (2024)
22. Tax, N., Verenich, I., La Rosa, M., Dumas, M.: Predictive business process monitoring with LSTM neural networks. In: International Conference on Advanced Information Systems Engineering, pp. 477–492. Springer, Cham (2017)
23. Teinemaa, I., Dumas, M., Rosa, M.L., Maggi, F.M.: Outcome-oriented predictive process monitoring: review and benchmark. ACM Trans. Knowl. Discov. Data (TKDD) **13**(2), 1–57 (2019)

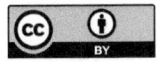

5th International Workshop on Event Data and Behavioral Analytics (EdbA 2024)

Preface

Fifth International Workshop on Event Data and Behavioral Analytics (EdbA 2024)

Over the past decades, capturing, storing, and analyzing event data has gained attention in domains such as process mining, clickstream analytics, IoT analytics, online gaming analytics, website traffic analytics, and preventive maintenance. The interest in event data lies in its analytical potential as it captures the dynamic behavior of people, objects, and systems at a fine-grained level.

Behavior often involves multiple entities, objects, and actors to which events can be correlated in various ways. In these situations, a unique, straightforward process notion does not exist or is unclear, or different processes or dynamics may be recorded in the same data set.

The objective of the Event Data & Behavioral Analytics (EdbA) workshop series is to provide a forum for practitioners and researchers to study a quintessential, minimal notion of events as the common denominator for records of discrete behavior in all its forms. The workshop aims to stimulate the development of new techniques, algorithms, and data structures for recording, storing, managing, processing, analyzing, and visualizing event data in various forms. To this end, different types of submissions are welcome such as original research papers, case study reports, position papers, idea papers, challenge papers, and work-in-progress papers on event data and behavioral analytics.

The fifth edition of the EdbA workshop attracted 27 submissions of which eight were accepted for a full-paper presentation and are included in the proceedings. This year's papers cover a broad spectrum of topics, which can be organized into three main themes: "Extracting Behavioral Insights from Event Data", "Non-traditional Event Data: Sensor, IoT, and Stochastic Event Data", and "Object Centric Event Data".

Throughout the workshop, the topics of IoT/Sensor data as well as Object-Centric Event Data received substantial attention. Both topics were further explored during the final plenary session, where participants engaged in a comprehensive debate. Various outstanding challenges related to these topics were discussed, including: *(i)* to what extent our methods are suitable for the unique challenges of industrial sensor data; *(ii)* the need and importance of a case notion in OCED; *(iii)* the relation between IoT/Sensor data and OCED; and *(iv)* the notion of 'behavior' in Event Data and Behavioral Analytics.

The organizers wish to thank all the people who submitted papers to the Edba 2024 workshop, the many participants who created fruitful discussions and shared insights, and the Edba 2024 Program Committee members for their valuable work in reviewing the submissions. A final word of thanks goes out to the organizers of ICPM 2024 for making this workshop possible.

October 2024

Benoît Depaire
Dirk Fahland
Francesco Leotta
Arik Senderovich

Oragnization

Workshop Chairs

Benoît Depaire   Hasselt University, Belgium
Dirk Fahland   Eindhoven University of Technology,
     the Netherlands
Francesco Leotta   Sapienza University of Rome, Italy
Arik Senderovich   York University, Canada

Program Committee

Simone Agostinelli   Sapienza University of Rome, Italy
Yannis Bertrand   Katholieke Universiteit Leuven, Belgium
Ioannis Chatzigiannakis   Sapienza University of Rome, Italy
Jochen De Weerdt   Katholieke Universiteit Leuven, Belgium
Claudio Di Ciccio   Utrecht University, the Netherlands
Massimiliano de Leoni   University of Padua, Italy
Chiara Di Francescomarino   University of Trento, Italy
Fabrizio Fornari   University of Camerino, Italy
Gert Janssenswillen   Hasselt University, Belgium
Eva Klijn   Eindhoven University of Technology,
     the Netherlands
Felix Mannhardt   Eindhoven University of Technology,
     the Netherlands
Niels Martin   Hasselt University, Belgium
Massimo Mecella   Sapienza University of Rome, Italy
Renata Medeiros de Carvalho   Eindhoven University of Technology,
     the Netherlands
Jan Mendling   Humboldt-Universität zu Berlin, Germany
Barbara Re   University of Camerino, Italy
Stef van den Elzen   Eindhoven University of Technology,
     the Netherlands
Francesca Zerbato   Eindhoven University of Technology,
     the Netherlands

A Classification of Data Quality Issues in Object-Centric Event Data

Maike Basmer[1]([✉])[iD], Martin Kabierski[1,2][iD], Kristina Sahling[1,2][iD],
Agnieszka Patecka[3][iD], Saimir Bala[1][iD], and Jan Mendling[1,2][iD]

[1] Humboldt-Universität zu Berlin, Berlin, Germany
{maike.basmer,martin.kabierski,kristina.sahling,
saimir.bala,jan.mendling}@hu-berlin.de
[2] Weizenbaum Institute, Berlin, Germany
[3] European University Viadrina, Frankfurt (Oder), Germany
patecka@europa-uni.de

Abstract. Process analysis is concerned with analyzing recorded process executions to validate, monitor, or improve the underlying processes according to business goals. In this context, the paradigm of object-centric event data (OCED) has recently emerged, which relates activity executions to multiple objects instead of a single, pre-determined case. Since OCED can integrate various process perspectives simultaneously, it represents real-life activities more accurately than traditional event logs. Being the input of Object-Centric Process Mining (OCPM), the quality of the data recorded in OCED logs directly influences the results of the process analysis. To ensure reliable outcomes, it is imperative to assess potential quality problems manifesting in the data. While frameworks for such an assessment are available for classic event data, equivalent approaches for assessing quality issues in OCED do not yet exist. This paper provides an analysis and classification of data quality issues in OCED, and compares them to the issues in traditional event data. Thus, this study is a first step in the systematic assessment and management of data quality in OCED.

Keywords: event log · data quality · object-centric event data · process mining

1 Introduction

Process mining is a family of techniques that exploits historical data recorded in information systems, with the final goal of understanding, discovering and improving business processes [10]. As with any analysis, the reliability and accuracy of process mining results hinges upon the quality of input data stored in the event logs [5]. Yet, real-life event logs are rarely of perfect quality – in fact, they tend to be imprecise, incomplete and noisy [9]. Not only can low-quality event logs create challenges in converting past data into business value, but also hinder exerting process mining techniques [13]. For that reason, it is important to understand quality issues of event logs and their potential impact on process mining analysis results [16].

© The Author(s) 2025
A. Delgado and T. Slaats (Eds.): ICPM 2024 Workshops, LNBIP 533, pp. 311–323, 2025.
https://doi.org/10.1007/978-3-031-82225-4_23

Recent developments in the storage and analysis of event data, such as the advent of the Object-Centric Event Data (OCED) model [3], require the reconsideration of notions of event log quality. Especially, different data quality (DQ) issues may be identifiable in traditional process mining and Object-Centric Process Mining (OCPM). So far, it is not clear if classifications of DQ issues in case-based event logs can be directly applied to OCPM, or if and where they have to be modified or extended. Moreover, new issues may affect these event logs, such as incorrect information about the relations among objects.

To the best of our knowledge, work on DQ for object-centric event logs has been limited. Numerous authors from the domain have acknowledged the importance of DQ for process mining in general [2,9,19]. These works, however, consider case-based process mining, and therefore do not capture OCPM-specific quality issues. While [12] considers the role of DQ in the discussed context, they almost exclusively focus on storage-related aspects. Given the rising popularity of object-centric event logs and the significance of adequate DQ, it is imperative to propose approaches for assessing the quality of event logs in the object-centric paradigm. To address this problem, we examine an established framework for DQ problems in traditional event data [9], discuss its relevance for OCED, and formulate new quality issues relevant for OCED, based on the proposed OCED base metamodel [22]. While this model is continuously extended, resulting in alternative standards, classifying quality issues on the base model is useful as this identifies quality issues on the essential concepts of object-centricity, which can subsequently be adapted to incorporate changes made by those alternatives.

As a result, we propose a new classification of DQ issues that lifts established DQ issues, and their classification, to OCED.

2   Related Work

We first introduce the developments revolving around OCED in Sect. 2.1 and review existing work on DQ in the context of process mining in Sect. 2.2.

2.1   Object-Centric Event Data

Recently introduced, OCED allows for precise tracking of real-life activities [3]. For example, consider an ordering process. When a customer (e.g., Alice) wants to buy several products in an online shop, she starts by selecting various items (e.g., pen, paper) and placing an order. The items may be available at different points in time. The seller may decide to pack the chosen items together (bundling) or to send them in separate packages, depending on their size or availability. This means that a trace left by this process instance in the information system does not look flat as assumed in traditional event logs. Rather, it can best be represented by considering the various entities and their relations. Figure 1 shows an example of a trace with one Order object and two Item objects, and a sequence of events referring to the objects (based on the exemplary event log in [1]).

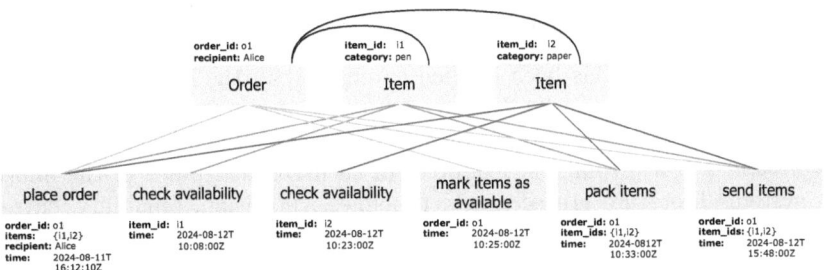

Fig. 1. A simplified example of an object-centric order process.

Besides adapting models and analysis tasks to the object-centric setting [7], several formats have been proposed to store object-centric event logs [12]. In search for a standard format for OCED, a call for reference implementations was put forward by the OCED working group [22]. The call outlines a meta-model, illustrated in Fig. 2, that describes the relation between objects and events. It may be extended to allow for specifying events that operate on object attribute values or object relations. It is divided into three components A, B, and C. Component A captures event-related concepts, namely, events, the corresponding type and attributes together with the notion of time. Similarly, component B encompasses objects along with their attributes and relations between objects. Connecting both worlds, component C represents the relation between objects and events. Alternatively, OCED may be viewed along the *event-to-event (E2E)*, *event-to-object (E2O)*, and *object-to-object (O2O)* relations [7]. Among the implementations answering the call by the OCED working group were the OCEL 2.0 format [7] and an implementation for Event Knowledge Graphs [21].

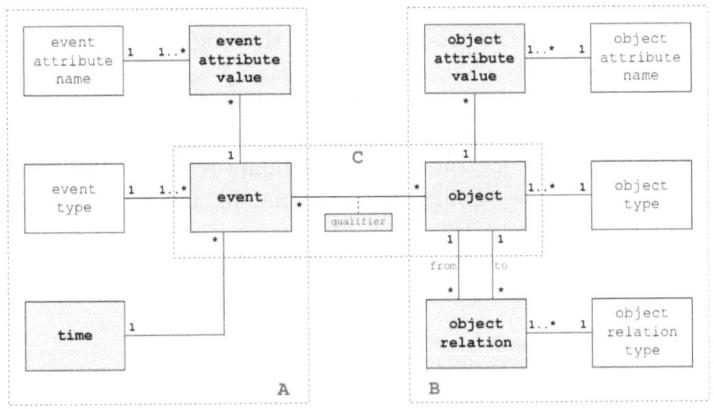

Fig. 2. The OCED base model, taken from [22].

2.2 Data Quality in Process Mining

DQ is a concept that has been studied extensively in the literature across various domains [13] and can be defined as *"data that are fit for use by data consumers"* [23]. It can be described by DQ dimensions, which consist of a set of DQ *attributes* [23]. Prominent examples of such DQ attributes in the information systems literature are accuracy, timeliness, precision, reliability, currency and relevancy [6]. Yet, according to [19], event logs, particularly when considering their temporal dependencies, differ notably from data obtained from usual information systems. Consequently, a typical information systems framework for DQ will not suffice for process mining needs [19].

Various existing DQ taxonomies, DQ assessment frameworks and approaches to data cleaning in process mining are discussed in [17]. Furthermore, the Process Mining Manifesto [2] defines maturity levels describing the quality of event logs on an abstract level and assessment criteria for the quality of event data like trustworthiness, completeness, safety, and well-defined semantics [2]. In [9], DQ issues in event data are classified according to data being missing, incorrect, imprecise or irrelevant. Approaching the definition of DQ issues with observation and experience, [19] suggests the use of imperfection patterns to systematically grasp recurring DQ issues. Similarly, [8] identifies DQ issues specific to sensor data for process mining, while [14] delineates a guideline to cater to quality concerns when extracting event logs from relational databases. In [13], the management of process-data quality is considered as a main driver for the success of process mining initiatives. Based thereon, open challenges are formulated, including the "characterisation of the typical process-data quality problems that may occur in event logs" [13]. In this context, the authors acknowledge that new event formats such as OCED may introduce DQs not yet covered by existing classifications.

Within the context of OCPM, [20] tackles DQ issues in object-centric logs by providing a method to derive missing entity identifiers. On the conceptual side, [12] considers DQ when assessing the state of object-centric event logs, although they mostly focus on storage-related aspects. For example, they emphasize that any value changes should be traceable, which enhances trust and traceability [24]. They further claim that data duplicates should be kept to a minimum, the event log should be maximally scalable, and the format of an object-centric event log should allow for unambiguous identification of each event and object throughout time [12]. Eventually, they define expectations on object-centric event logs, thus pointing to possible DQ issues due to violating these expectations.

3 Deriving Data Quality Issues for OCED

We now turn to the assessment of quality issues in the context of object-centricity, for which we want to provide conceptual groundwork. Section 3.1 outlines our approach, while Sect. 3.2 introduces the framework our work is based on.

3.1   Methodology

To arrive at the classification of DQ problems in OCED, we considered recommendations for systematically building taxonomies based on a conceptual
approach proposed by [15], consisting of six steps. Once we had recognized the
limited research on DQ in OCED as a relevant research gap (step I), we defined
the objectives of our study, that is to arrive at the corresponding classification
(step II). We started our study by assessing potential quality issues in OCED.
During the design and development phase (step III), each author reviewed existing literature on DQ assessment for event data. We then decided to go forward
with the framework for event log quality by [9] due to its simplicity and general applicability. To systematize potential DQ issues for OCED, we took up its
categorization and extended it with object-centric concepts from the proposed
OCED metamodel [22]. Having done the assessment individually, the author
group then discussed the insights and aggregated them into the unified, proposed
quality issue classification (step IV). Subsequently, evaluation of the proposed
classification was conducted, performed through its application to a real-world
event log (see Sect. 5) (step V). Doing so, we arrived at the classification of DQ
for OCED, which will be described in detail in Sect. 4 (step VI).

3.2   Data Quality Issues for Traditional Event Data

In [9], which was the starting point for our work, the authors distinguish two
sources for difficulties faced during the analysis of event data: the process characteristics and the quality of event logs. Concerning the quality of event data, they
identify four categories of problems: missing, incorrect, imprecise, and irrelevant
data. *Missing* refers to required data being absent. *Incorrect* denotes information being logged incorrectly. Data is labeled as *imprecise* when its granularity
is insufficient. Likewise, *irrelevant* data is defined depending on a specific analysis, i.e., the data is irrelevant if the recorded data is not useful for the analysis in
its original form, but may be processed to serve the analysis. According to these
four categories, the authors classify and discuss 27 DQ issues adhering to nine
types of event log items, as shown in Table 1. For instance, if timestamps are

Table 1. Event Data quality issues defined in [9].

	Case	Event	Belongs to	Case Attr.	Position	Activity name	Timestamp	Resource	Event Attr.
Missing Data	I1	I2	I3	I4	I5	I6	I7	I8	I9
Incorrect Data	I10	I11	I12	I13	I14	I15	I16	I17	I18
Imprecise Data	-	-	I19	I20	I21	I22	I23	I24	I25
Irrelevant Data	I26	I27	-	-	-	-	-	-	-

Table 2. Event-level, object-level and relation-level quality issues derived from the OCED base model [22] and [9].

	Events					Objects			Relations	
	Event	Event Type	Time	Event Attr.	Position	Object	Object Type	Object Attr.	O2O	E2O
Missing Data	I2	I6	I7	I9	I5	N1	N2	N3	N4	N5
Incorrect Data	I11	I15	I16	I18	I14	N6	N7	N8	N9	N10
Imprecise Data	-	I22	I23	I25	I21	-	N11	N12	N13	N14
Irrelevant Data	I27	-	-	-	-	N15	-	-	N16	N17

missing, incorrectly logged, or imprecise (i.e., too coarse-granular), the reliability of the analysis is affected significantly, as the ordering of events is determined by timestamps. The authors apply the framework to real-life event logs, observing certain quality issues to prevail. For instance, events are found to be missing or the activity name to be imprecise for four out of five investigated event logs.

This framework applies well to dealing with DQ issues in traditional event data, yet, following our analysis, it is not fully suitable for OCED. Consequently, we suggest a new classification, discussed in detail in the following section.

4   Data Quality Issues for Object-Centric Event Data

As concluded, some of the quality issues identified for classic event data in [9] do not apply to OCED anymore. For instance, issues related to the notion of the case are superfluous. Furthermore, due to the addition of objects and new relation types, emerging quality issues for these concepts have not been categorized yet. Therefore, we propose a new categorization as shown in Table 2 where the dimensions *Events*, *Objects*, and *Relations* for DQ problems are distinguished. The former corresponds to entities relating to events as in the traditional model, whereas the *Objects* dimension is abstracted from entities relating to case and resource, and the *Relations* dimension encompasses both *O2O* and *E2O* relations. Issues beginning with *I* (meaning "Issue") follow the notion introduced in [9] and were directly lifted to OCED, while issues beginning with *N* (meaning "New") had to be newly derived for OCED. In the following, we address the components of each dimension and discuss identified similarities as well as the differences.

4.1   Event-Based Quality Issues

Object-centricity mainly affects the *Objects* as well as the *Relations* dimensions. Similar quality issues as in traditional event logs may be observed for the *Events* dimension. Thus, the proposed classification directly adopts the issues related to the event-dimension as shown in Table 1. However, we conjecture that the $m : n$ relation between events and objects may amplify issues in the *event* dimension, as the occurrence of one flawed event may affect multiple objects. Furthermore, we observe additional implications for *I22* (imprecise activity name) and *I23* (imprecise timestamp). For the former, Bose et al. [9] argue that an activity name is imprecise if the activity name is too coarse-grained and may be interpreted differently depending on the context. In OCED, relations to different objects may now provide the context and hence, reduce the severity of this issue. On the contrary, timestamps also suffer from quality issues if they are too coarse-granular, which may be amplified in object-centric event logs when events for different object types are recorded with varying time granularities and the analysis encompasses the complete process. Furthermore, following the train of thought in [12], deciding whether an event or an object is affected by a quality issue depends on the connection between event attributes and objects. It has to be made clear whether the references in event attributes should be interpreted as simple values (thus, leading to attribute-related issues) or whether they carry meaning for an object (thus inducing object- or *E2O*-level issues).

4.2   Object-Based Quality Issues

The *Objects* dimension lifts issues defined for cases and resources, as these refer to designated object types. Likewise, case attributes are lifted to object attributes, and issues for object types can be defined analogously to issues for event types. However, case issues are not directly applicable, since process instances cannot be easily defined by following one particular object through the process, but rather take relations to other objects into account [4]. Consequently, we obtain the following adapted quality issues. The original issues from [9] are given in square brackets, if applicable.

(N1) Missing Object [I1, I8]: An object from the real world is not represented in the system. This can either mean that there are no events present referring to that object (if it is implicitly represented) or that the object is not present as an entity by itself. Consequently, events cannot refer to the missing object, thus, in such a case a trace is not recorded either. In the example process, this would occur if item i1 (cf. Fig. 1) was missing or if there was a second order, which was not recorded in the log, preventing any relationships from being established.

(N6) Incorrect Object [I10, I17]: An object does not relate to the process in question or may be logged incorrectly, e.g., representing an erroneous duplicate. Assuming there are two orders, with the second order containing the same information as the first one, the second order may represent a duplicate of the first and is thus incorrectly associated with the process.

(N15) Irrelevant Object [I26]: In [9], irrelevant cases refer to cases deemed irrelevant for the analysis. Likewise, irrelevant objects are those objects not considered in a given analysis. Thus, object-centric logs may need to be tailored to an analysis goal as well. However, they allow for more flexible preparation because they do not pre-determine a specific case. For illustration purposes, suppose an analysis is to be conducted on stationary items, such as the number of pens and amount of paper sold in the last month. However, the log may also include data on non-stationary items, which are then irrelevant to the analysis.

(N2) Missing Object Type: In this case, the object type of an object would be unknown, meaning that neither equality nor inequality of objects in terms of type can be established. Not considering objects with missing object types could result in a loss of important information, but introduces difficulties when, e.g., aggregating process behavior based on the object type. In reference to the example in Fig. 1, a missing object type means that, for instance, an object cannot be associated with either Item or Order due to an unknown type.

(N7) Incorrect Object Type: This issue refers to the situation in which an object in the real-world is assigned to the wrong object type in the logging system. In the above example, this issue can occur e.g., if the type Order is mistakenly assigned instead of the type Item, leading to inaccurate analysis outcomes.

(N11) Imprecise Object Type [I24]: If the object type is imprecise, objects may not be distinguishable based on their type. This could lead to blurring process discovery results, e.g., when deriving directly-follows relations based on the entity type. Here, control flows of objects showing distinct behavior may be consolidated and merged due to them sharing the object type, even though they may be distinct sub-types. From the example, we know that the process involves items, but whether there are any differences in the process due to any specific types, such as fragile or luxurious items, remains unknown. With item specifications available, processes could be defined at a more fine-granular level.

(N3) Missing Object Attribute [I4]: This issue refers to two different situations: it either denotes an object missing an attribute entirely or the value for an object attribute not being recorded. In the former case, it is questionable whether the desired analysis can be conducted. In the latter case, objects with missing attribute values may be excluded from the analysis or imputed, possibly distorting the results. Concerning the example process, if the category "pen" is missing, one would only know that the object is of the type Item, without any attributes specifying the particular category. This lack of detail would result in no findings when an analysis specifically for pens is needed.

(N8) Incorrect Object Attribute [I13]: When object attributes are incorrectly logged, the analysis is negatively affected as well. It is then either necessary to exclude objects with incorrect values or clean the data, leading to additional costs, or it results in the unknowing incorporation of wrong attribute values. This issue could be exemplified as follows: Instead of logging the attribute type as "pen" for item id=i1, the attribute type "paper" is recorded.

(N12) Imprecise Object Attribute [I20]: Imprecise object attributes do not offer the granularity levels that are required for the analysis. Assuming that all attribute values have the same granularity for a given attribute name, this issue occurs on the conceptual level. Otherwise, it refers to the granularity of single attribute values. In the example process shown in Fig. 1, suppose the company wants to analyse the inventory of the different types of paper (notepaper, craft paper, copy paper) sold in the last month. However, the log only records the attribute type as "paper" without providing specific details, making it impossible to conduct the precise analysis they require.

We note that the distinction between attributes and attribute values made in issues *N3*, *N8*, and *N12* similarly applies to event attributes.

4.3 Relationship-Based Quality Issues

Lastly, we focus on quality issues in *O2O* and *E2O* relations. *O2O* is newly introduced, whereas *E2O* is lifted from the *belongs to* category in [9]. In contrast to the $1:n$ relation between a case and its events, *E2O* now refers to an $n:m$ relation between events and objects, meaning that an event relates to zero or more objects, and an object relates to zero or more events. Consequently, we obtain the following adapted quality issues, with the issues they are lifted from [9] given in square brackets, if applicable.

(N4) Missing O2O relation: This issue refers to a relation between two objects not being represented in the log, although it exists in the real-world. If cardinality constraints are additionally defined in a data model, these may also be violated by missing *O2O* relations.

(N5) Missing E2O relation [I3]: Likewise, associations between an event and object may be missing. Consequently, the control-flow cannot be correctly reconstructed for that object.

(N9) Incorrect O2O relation: In this case, a relation between two objects is erroneously logged, which implies a correlation that does not exist in the real-world. If a data model additionally imposes cardinality constraints, incorrect *O2O* relations may violate these.

(N10) Incorrect E2O relation [I12]: This issue reflects the situation that a relation between an event and an object is erroneously logged. From the event's point of view, this means it refers to an object that it did not affect in the real world. On the object's side, an event is registered in the log that did not play a role in its actual life-cycle.

(N13) Imprecise O2O relation: This issue refers to coarse-grained relationship types that, e.g., capture a lot of different relations between objects that could be distinguished into more specific types. If relations are only recorded for a general object relation type, it is not possible to differentiate more specific relationships between different objects, thus not allowing for a more detailed analysis.

(N14) Imprecise E2O relation [I19]: In [9], the relationship between events and a case was said to be imprecise if the selected case notion inhibits the correlation of events to other case constructs. This issue should be alleviated in the object-centric world. However, in view of the OCED metamodel [22], qualifiers help to specify the type of relation between object and event. Hence, if a more detailed analysis of the relations between objects and events is required, the use of too general qualifiers may inhibit obtaining the desired insights.

(N16) Irrelevant O2O relation: Irrelevant *O2O* relations refer to relations considered irrelevant for analysis and which should thus be excluded from it. For instance, the items i1 and i2 in Fig. 1 may be related, but for analysing orders, this relation may be inconsequential.

(N17) Irrelevant E2O relation: Similar to *N16*, events may not serve the analysis of designated objects, rendering their relation irrelevant in that context.

5 Evaluating Quality Issues in Object-Centric Event Logs

To explore the applicability and understand the utility of the proposed classification in guiding the identification of quality issues, we applied it to a real-world event log. To do so, we investigated an OCEL 2.0 event log that reflects the development process of the Angular platform via commits in the corresponding GitHub repository [18], as it is one of a few currently publicly available object-centric event logs and provides information about its creation process and intended uses. An event corresponds to one commit in the repository and contains information about the commit, e.g., the author or the timestamp. Two types of objects exist: the Branches a commit is related to as well as the Files that are involved in a commit. A commit is related to at least one branch but is not necessarily linked to a file. Examining the event log in light of the classification in Table 2 revealed several potential issues:

(N4) Missing O2O relation: No *O2O* relations are recorded, although one could assume relations to exist between the object types. If the object relations are approximated based on co-occurrences in the event data, we would likely have to deal with *incorrect O2O relations (N9)*, as commits do not necessarily target only files that are related to each other beyond belonging to the same project.

(N14) Imprecise E2O relation: The *E2O* relation may be underspecified, as a commit is often related to many objects at the same time. Qualifiers indicating the effect of a commit on a file like DELETE, CREATE, or MODIFY would help to distinguish the relation between commits and files, for example.

(I15) Incorrect event type: The extraction of event types relies on labels in commit messages. These labels should adhere to the guidelines defined by the Conventional Commits Initiative[1], which requires a commit message to be preceded by a label indicating the purpose of the commit. Originally, two types of

---

[1] https://www.conventionalcommits.org/en/v1.0.0/.

labels were specified, with the Angular Commit Message Guidelines[2] extending it to 9 types. However, the log reports 67 event types, with event types such as `don't` or `RendererV2` among them. According to [18], some labels had to be corrected manually beforehand, indicating the error-proneness of event types due to e.g. typos.

(I22) Imprecise event type: Related to the previous issue, considering only the official labels for commit messages, many events are assigned to the corresponding event types (given the small number of labels vs. the large number of commits), possibly making it difficult to distinguish more fine-granular activities within the development process.

The proposed framework was effectively leveraged to discover multiple issues in the event log. From the set of identified issues, we conclude that follow-up analysis using this event log may be heavily impaired due to imprecision and missing relations between objects and commits. A precise analysis of the impact of single events on the development process may not be possible. However, the proposed classification only describes which issues may occur. It does not suggest a structured approach to systematically assessing quality issues. Thus, we merely used the classification as guidance here by considering each identified issue type and assessing whether it occurs in the event log, given the available data and knowledge about its creation process. We deem the development of such a structured assessment approach as valuable future work.

6   Discussion

Given the joint development of the proposed classification and its preliminary evaluation on a real-world event log, we believe that the classification is a valuable starting point towards DQ management in OCPM. However, threats to validity consist in the small pool of researchers involved in validating the classification and applying it to only one dataset. We will address this in future work by applying the classification to diverse data sets and involving other researchers and practitioners in the evaluation of the framework. For the former, we intend to examine the BPIC'17 dataset [11]. Beyond that, expecting the event data to comply with the extended OCED metamodel [22] or the OCEL 2.0 metamodel [7] induces other DQ issues, which will have to be investigated in the future. Furthermore, we decided for a high-level view on attributes and relations, which may be further distinguished into attribute names and attribute values as well as object relation and object relation types, respectively.

7   Conclusion

In conclusion, this paper draws from seminal works in the area of DQ in event data for process analysis, to provide a categorization for the recently developed

---

[2] https://github.com/angular/angular/blob/22b96b9/CONTRIBUTING.md#-commit-message-guidelines.

OCED meta-model. This new categorization is intended to help researchers and practitioners to address DQ management, especially when it comes to process mining efforts. In future work, we plan to extensively evaluate our categorization on various object-centric event logs, provide a comprehensive framework for DQ management in OCPM and extend the classification to alternative data models.

Acknowledgement. This research was supported by the Einstein Foundation Berlin under grant EPP-2019-524, by the German Federal Ministry of Education and Research under grant 16DII133, and by Deutsche Forschungsgemeinschaft under grants 496119880 (VisualMine) and 531115272 (ProImpact).

References

1. Aalst, W.M.P.: Object-centric process mining: dealing with divergence and convergence in event data. In: Ölveczky, P.C., Salaün, G. (eds.) SEFM 2019. LNCS, vol. 11724, pp. 3–25. Springer, Cham (2019). https://doi.org/10.1007/978-3-030-30446-1_1
2. van der Aalst, W.M.P., et al.: Process mining manifesto. In: BPM Workshops. Lecture Notes in Business Information Processing, vol. 99, pp. 169–194. Springer, Cham (2011)
3. van der Aalst, W.M.: Object-centric process mining: unraveling the fabric of real processes. Mathematics **11**(12), 2691 (2023)
4. Adams, J.N., Schuster, D., Schmitz, S., Schuh, G., van der Aalst, W.M.P.: Defining cases and variants for object-centric event data. In: Burattin, A., Polyvyanyy, A., Weber, B. (eds.) 4th International Conference on Process Mining, ICPM 2022, Bolzano, Italy, 23–28 October 2022, pp. 128–135. IEEE (2022)
5. Andrews, R., van Dun, C.G.J., Wynn, M.T., Kratsch, W., Röglinger, M., ter Hofstede, A.H.M.: Quality-informed semi-automated event log generation for process mining. Decis. Support Syst. **132**, 113265 (2020)
6. Bailey, J.E., Pearson, S.W.: Development of a tool for measuring and analyzing computer user satisfaction. Manag. Sci. **29**(5), 530–545 (1983)
7. Berti, A., et al.: OCEL 2.0 specification. CoRR abs/2403.01975 (2024)
8. Bertrand, Y., Belle, R.V., Weerdt, J.D., Serral, E.: Defining data quality issues in process mining with IoT data. In: ICPM Workshops. Lecture Notes in Business Information Processing, vol. 468, pp. 422–434. Springer, Cham (2022)
9. Bose, J.C.J.C., Mans, R.S., van der Aalst, W.M.P.: Wanna improve process mining results? In: CIDM, pp. 127–134. IEEE (2013)
10. Dakic, D., Stefanovic, D., Vuckovic, T., Zizakov, M., Stevanov, B.: Event log data quality issues and solutions. Mathematics **11**(13), 2858 (2023)
11. van Dongen, B.: BPI challenge 2017 (2017). https://doi.org/10.4121/UUID: 5F3067DF-F10B-45DA-B98B-86AE4C7A310B
12. Goossens, A., De Smedt, J., Vanthienen, J.: Object-centric event logs: specifications, comparative analysis and refinement. arXiv preprint arXiv:2405.12709 (2024)
13. ter Hofstede, A.H.M., et al.: Process-data quality: the true frontier of process mining. ACM J. Data Inf. Qual. **15**(3), 29:1–29:21 (2023)
14. Jans, M., Soffer, P.: From relational database to event log: decisions with quality impact. In: BPM Workshops. Lecture Notes in Business Information Processing, vol. 308, pp. 588–599. Springer, Cham (2017)

15. Kundisch, D., et al.: An update for taxonomy designers. Bus. Inf. Syst. Eng. **64**(4), 421–439 (2022)
16. Mans, R., van der Aalst, W.M.P., Vanwersch, R.J.B., Moleman, A.J.: Process mining in healthcare: data challenges when answering frequently posed questions. In: ProHealth/KR4HC. Lecture Notes in Computer Science, vol. 7738, pp. 140–153. Springer, Cham (2012)
17. Martin, N.: Data Quality in Process Mining, pp. 53–79. Springer, Cham (2021)
18. Pegoraro, M.: Angular github commits object-centric event log (2023). https://doi.org/10.5281/zenodo.8430332
19. Suriadi, S., Andrews, R., ter Hofstede, A.H.M., Wynn, M.T.: Event log imperfection patterns for process mining: towards a systematic approach to cleaning event logs. Inf. Syst. **64**, 132–150 (2017)
20. Swevels, A., Dijkman, R.M., Fahland, D.: Inferring missing entity identifiers from context using event knowledge graphs. In: BPM. Lecture Notes in Computer Science, vol. 14159, pp. 180–197. Springer, Cham (2023)
21. Swevels, A., Fahland, D., Montali, M.: Implementing object-centric event data models in event knowledge graphs. In: ICPM Workshops. Lecture Notes in Business Information Processing, vol. 503, pp. 431–443. Springer, Cham (2023)
22. TFPM OCED working group: Object-Centric Event Data (OCED) - Call For Action: Reference Implementations. https://www.tf-pm.org/upload/1678694478319.pdf
23. Wang, R.Y., Strong, D.M.: Beyond accuracy: what data quality means to data consumers. J. Manag. Inf. Syst. **12**(4), 5–33 (1996)
24. Wynn, M.T., Sadiq, S.: Responsible process mining - a data quality perspective. In: Hildebrandt, T., van Dongen, B.F., Röglinger, M., Mendling, J. (eds.) BPM 2019. LNCS, vol. 11675, pp. 10–15. Springer, Cham (2019). https://doi.org/10.1007/978-3-030-26619-6_2

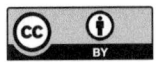

Analyzing the Evolution of Boards in Collaborative Work Management Tools

Alfonso Bravo[1]([✉])[iD], Cristina Cabanillas[1,2][iD], Joaquín Peña[1][iD],
and Manuel Resinas[1,2][iD]

[1] I3US Institute, Universidad de Sevilla, Seville, Spain
{abllanos,cristinacabanillas,joaquinp,resinas}@us.es
[2] SCORE Lab, Universidad de Sevilla, Seville, Spain

Abstract. Board-Based Collaborative Work Management Tools (BBTs) like Trello and Microsoft Planner are widespread today. Their use includes the management of projects, static information, or processes, which is achieved by assigning and moving cards through lists representing specific states, steps, or other classification criteria. BBTs are a flexible solution since boards, lists and cards can be changed by the user to adapt to new situations, e.g., changes in the processes or projects. However, understanding how a board is being used is challenging because what can be seen at a glance is a static snapshot of its current state. BBTs usually produce logs that capture all the activity that has taken place within the boards. In this paper, we leverage that data to mine BBT logs to understand how boards are used and evolve over time. Specifically, we introduce an approach that aims to detect structural changes in the boards, and visualize the evolution of the boards' lists. We have analyzed 63 real-life BBT logs and tested the approach with three case studies.

Keywords: Board-based tools · board mining · board evolution · board use · collaborative work management tools

1 Introduction

The use of Board-Based Collaborative Work Management Tools (BBTs for short) like Trello, Planner, and Asana is widespread today in informal as well as formal contexts. They are built of three main elements: boards, lists and cards. A board contains a set of lists that can be created, updated or closed by the user. Each of these lists contains a set of cards that can also be created, updated and removed or closed. In addition, cards can be moved from one list to another. These three elements represent different concepts of the real world depending

Grants PDC2022-133521-I00 and TED2021-131023B-C22 funded by MCIN/AEI/10.13039/501100011033/ and by the European Union NextGenerationEU/PRTR; and grants PID2021-126227NB-C21 and PID2022-140221NB-I00 funded by MCIN/AEI/10.13039/501100011033/ and by ERDF/EU.

A. Delgado and T. Slaats (Eds.): ICPM 2024 Workshops, LNBIP 533, pp. 324–336, 2025.
https://doi.org/10.1007/978-3-031-82225-4_24

on the context of our problem. For instance, lists usually represent steps of a project, phases of a process, or topics, while cards frequently represent tasks, information or resources related with the project or process represented on the board. The example board of Fig. 1 represents the process of writing research articles, in which each card is a process instance. Thus, cards represent articles (e.g., *Design Patterns for Collaborative Work Management Tools*) which are classified in lists according to their state of publication (e.g., *Inception*). Moving a card from one list to another means a change in the state of the paper.

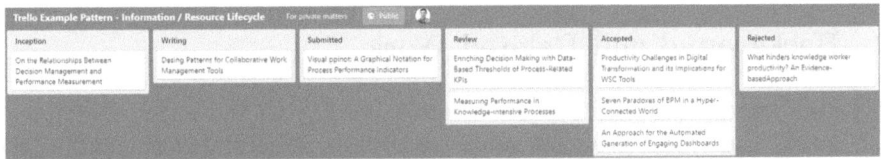

Fig. 1. Screenshot of a Trello board of article production

Organizations adopt these tools to manage their daily work and processes aiming to increase productivity in busy environments [7] given their flexibility and adaptability to manage different projects and processes and to support changes in them. Although they were conceived to manage collaborative work, their actual use expands to other scenarios like sharing knowledge, managing shared processes or representing shared schedules [2,5,6,9,10,14].

When we look at a board at whichever moment, we see a static snapshot of its current state. It is not possible to fully understand how the board has been used without additional information or historical use data. Moreover, as aforementioned, boards may evolve to adapt to new needs or requirements. The changes performed may impact not only the structure of the boards but also how they are used. For instance, the board in Fig. 1 may suffer a structural change to make every list represent a research paper, and the cards within them the tasks to be performed for publication (e.g., write abstract, conduct evaluation, submit paper, etc.). This structural change entails a change in the use of the board.

BBTs usually produce (event) logs that capture all the activity that has taken place within the boards during their design and use. Such log data has been used to analyze how people interact with the boards, usually to identify collaboration patterns or assess participants' performance within educational settings [12,15]. We use the term *board mining* to refer to the extraction of data from BBTs to discover, analyze and optimize boards. In this paper, we apply board mining to investigate and analyze the use and evolution of BBT boards by mining their event logs. Our approach aims to understand how boards are used in real life, analyzing their evolution over time. As a proof of concept, we have analyzed 63 real event logs to show further insights that can be obtained by mining BBT logs. We have also implemented the approach and applied it to three different use cases with publicly available data from Trello to showcase its use to depict the evolution of boards. Other purposes of board mining, such as board discovery and optimization, are out of the scope of this paper, but they entail relevant applications and should be addressed in the future.

The remainder of the paper is structured as follows. Section 2 outlines the BBT concepts relevant in this work and the state of the art on the analysis of boards. Section 3 presents our board mining approach to understand the use of boards. Section 4 describes how we have tested the approach. Section 5 reflects on interesting insights derived from this work and implications for future work. Finally, Sect. 6 summarizes the conclusions drawn and the planned next steps.

2   Background and Related Work

All BBT boards have an implicit design according to the purpose of use of the board. The board design encompasses both its structural elements (i.e., the board itself, its set of lists, and optionally a set of default cards) and the dynamic use of these elements (i.e., the way in which lists and cards are to be created and manipulated). The latter can be implicit to the type of board created (e.g., Kanban boards are used for project management and typically involve moving cards through three lists: "to-do", "doing", and "done" [10]), or explicitly defined elsewhere in natural language.

Considering this, two main phases stand out in the life of a board [11]. The first one is *board design*, which includes all the activities related to the definition of the structure and the dynamic use of the board. Once the board is designed, the *board use* phase begins. This phase involves using the board for the predetermined purpose. Remarkably, the board *evolves* with its use. New lists are created, closed, renamed, or updated. The structural changes that occur while the board evolves may be aligned with its expected dynamic use, or may respond to other organizational needs and imply a redesign that affects the structural elements and/or the dynamic use of the board.

The use of boards has been analyzed so far for different purposes. For instance, BBT logs have been used to analyze aspects related to people involvement and participation in the context of controlled experiments with students. Mora et al. [8] applied gamification to investigate whether personalized learning experiences can better motivate and engage students. They divided the students in groups and subgroups, created Trello boards and used the Trello logs at the end of the gameful experience to perform descriptive analyses on the student involvement. An approach to predict low performance in teams of students was described by Shamshurin and Saltz [15]. They analyzed 80 Kanban projects corresponding to teams' Trello boards on the basis of predefined Kanban metrics [13] as well as on several ad-hoc metrics. Afterward, they used machine learning models to predict risks of low quality results. In [4], Buffardi presented the results of an exploratory analysis of ten software engineering teams of students based on evidence within teams' Git logs and user stories (Kanban boards). The goal was to derive individual assessments from collaborative work results. In this case, BBT log data was not used and the analysis of user stories was done manually by checking the number of cards in a specific list at the end of the experiment. Pisoni et al. [12] identified patterns of collaborative behavior from Trello data obtained from 16 teams collaborating on predefined business cases. Their approach starts with a data preprocessing step to detect sequences of actions that could be separately analysed, followed by the identification of Trello actions, their coding, a data analysis based on these categories and a final clustering to identify similar group activity patterns.

To the best of our knowledge, our work is the first attempt to analyze how BBTs are used in a domain-independent way focusing on understanding how boards evolve over time rather than on analyzing them from a people standpoint.

3   Analysis of Board Evolution

In this section we describe our approach. We first define a BBT log. Then, we discuss about structural updates of a board and how to analyze them.

3.1   Board-Based Event Logs

A BBT log is a collection of the events that occur in a board. Each board has its own event log and we consider the event log of one board to be independent of the others. Conceptually, a BBT log is similar to a business process event log. The main difference is that instead of using the concepts of case and activity, it uses the concepts of lists, cards and actions over them. To formally define a BBT log, we start by defining some universes.

Definition 1 (Universes). *We define the following universes:*

- $\mathcal{U}_{ei}$ *is the universe of event identifiers,*
- $\mathcal{U}_{list}$ *is the universe of lists,*
- $\mathcal{U}_{card}$ *is the universe of cards,*
- $\mathcal{U}_{time}$ *is the universe of timestamps,*
- $\mathcal{U}_{type} = \{c, x, m, d, u, l_c, l_u, l_x\}$ *is the universe of actions that can be performed in a board, namely: create (c), close (x), move (m), delete (d), and update (u) a card; and create (l_c), update (l_u), and close (l_x) a list.*
- $\mathcal{U}_{event} = \mathcal{U}_{ei} \times \mathcal{U}_{time} \times \mathcal{U}_{list} \times (\mathcal{U}_{card} \cup \perp) \times \mathcal{U}_{type} \times (\mathcal{U}_{list} \cup \perp)$ *is the universe of events.*

$e = (ei, time, l, c, type, lt) \in \mathcal{U}_{event}$ is an event with identifier ei, corresponding to the execution of action $type$ on a card c that is in list l. If $type$ is m (moving a card), then lt is the list to which the card is moved. Otherwise, $lt = \perp$. Also, if $type \in \{l_c, l_u, l_x\}$, i.e. it is a list action, then both $c = \perp$ and $lt = \perp$.

Definition 2 (Event Projection). *Given* $e = (ei, time, l, c, type, lto) \in \mathcal{U}_{event}$, $\pi_{ei}(e) = ei$, $\pi_{time}(e) = time$, $\pi_l(e) = l$, $\pi_c(e) = c$, $\pi_{type}(e) = type$, *and* $\pi_{lto}(e) = lto$.

Further attributes could be found in the events of the log, e.g., the name of the lists and cards, due dates, comments, attachments, checklists. We have not included them because they are not used in this paper but they could be added following the same approach that is used to add attributes in process event logs.

A BBT log is a collection of totally ordered events, where event identifiers are unique.

Definition 3 (BBT log). $(E, \prec_E)$ *is a BBT log with* $E \subseteq \mathcal{U}_{event}$ *and* $\prec_E \subseteq E \times E$ *such that:*

- $\prec_E$ *defines a total order,*
- $\forall_{e1,e2 \in E} \pi_{ei}(e1) = \pi_{ei}(e2) \Rightarrow e1 = e2$, *and*
- $e1 \prec e2 \Rightarrow \forall_{e1,e2 \in E} \pi_{time}(e1) < \pi_{time}(e2)$

For convenience, given a BBT log $(E, \prec_E)$, we call e_{first} the first event of the BBT log, and e_{last} the last event.

The set of lists that appear in a BBT log $(E, \prec_E)$ can be defined as the lists that appear in any of the events of the log $L = \{l \in \mathcal{U}_{list} | \exists_{e \in E} \pi_l(e) = l\}$. Each of these lists can only have one creation event that is referred to as $create(l)$. Similarly, each list may have zero or one close events that is referred to as $close(l)$. If there is no close event for the list, then $close(l) = \bot$.

3.2   Analyzing Structural Updates

We define a structural change of a board as any change that affects the lists of the board, e.g., a new list is added (creation), a list changes its name (update), or a list is removed (close). This is signaled in the BBT log by list-related events, i.e., events whose type is l_c (list creation), l_u (list update), and l_x (list close). For a BBT log $(E, \prec_E)$, we call $\phi \subseteq E$ the subset of list-related events of E.

To analyze the structural evolution of a board we define two operations. One involves identifying the timeline of every list in the board, i.e., the moment at which the list is created and the moment at which it is closed, and is specified in Definition 4.

Definition 4 (List timeline). *Let* $(E, \prec_E)$ *be a BBT log, and* L *the set of lists that appear in the log. The timeline of a board list is defined as the function* tl : $L \rightarrow \mathcal{U}_{time} \times \mathcal{U}_{time}$, *such that* $tl(l) = (\pi_{time}(create(l)), \pi_{time}(close(l)))$ *if there is a close event for* l *(i.e.,* $close(l) \neq \bot$) *and* $tl(l) = (\pi_{time}(create(l)), \pi_{time}(e_{last}))$, *otherwise.*

Note that for lists that have not been closed, we take the timestamp of the last event of the board as reference for the last event of the list. It will be the same for all lists of the board that are still open.

The second operation comes from the observation that in many cases, a structural change is not caused by a single list-related event but by a series of several list-related events. For instance, users may reorganize the board by removing one list and adding two new lists. To make the analysis easier and consider all these events together, in this paper we follow a simple heuristic based on time. Specifically, we group together all the structural changes that have occurred within a (small) time interval, e.g., less than 24 h apart from each other.

Definition 5 (Structural change group). *Let $(E, \prec_E)$ be a BBT log, let ϕ be the subset of list-related events of the log, and let θ be a time period (e.g. 24 h), $SG \subseteq \phi$ is a structural change group if for all $e \in SG$:*

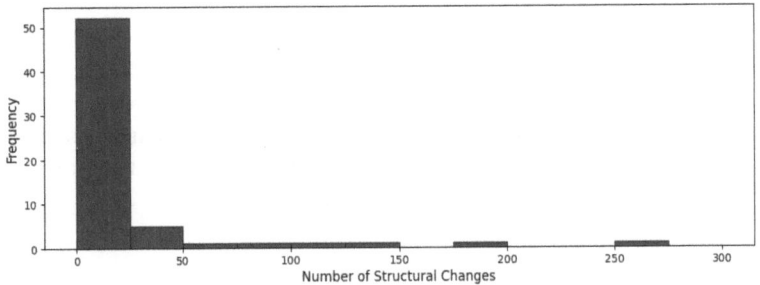

Fig. 2. Number of structural changes in the boards analyzed.

- *there does not exist an $e' \in \phi \setminus SG$ such that $|\pi_{time}(e) - \pi_{time}(e')| < \theta$, and*
- *for all $e'' \in SG \setminus \{e\}$ then $|\pi_{time}(e) - \pi_{time}(e'')| < \theta$ holds.*

Note that a structural change group can contain a single event if no other list-related events occur within the time period θ. For each structural change group, we define its structural change interval as the timestamps of its first and last events.

Together, list timelines and structural change intervals provide a useful tool to analyze the evolution of the structure of a board as discussed in Sect. 4.

4   Empirical Analysis

In February 2022, we scraped the Trello repository[1] obtaining over 600 public boards. We filtered them to keep those with a minimum temporary use (≥ 12 weeks) and a relevant number of events in the log (≥ 2000 events), resulting in a subset of 63 public boards. Boards that are rarely used or have been in use for a short period are not useful for studying their evolution and detecting structural changes, as there has not been enough time for such changes to occur, or they have stopped being used before then. Further information about the scraping,

---
[1] www.trello/b/.

material for replication, the datasets used and produced, and the algorithms implemented are available at https://github.com/isa-group/board-mining. The description of the tool was presented in [3].

Next, we first analyze the 63 public boards together, discussing the joint insights that result from applying our operations, and then we present three real cases of boards selected from among that pool of 63, with which we illustrate our proposal and exemplify the different findings that can be found when applying these operations to BBT event logs.

4.1   Global Analysis

Figure 2 shows the number of structural change groups identified in the boards using the thresholds $\theta = 24$ h. 52 boards went through 1 to 25 of these changes during their lifetime. Most boards with more than 100 structural changes have been used for over three years. Still, delving into their board design and the semantics of the changes would help to determine whether they are due to a regular use of the board or to relevant changes in it.

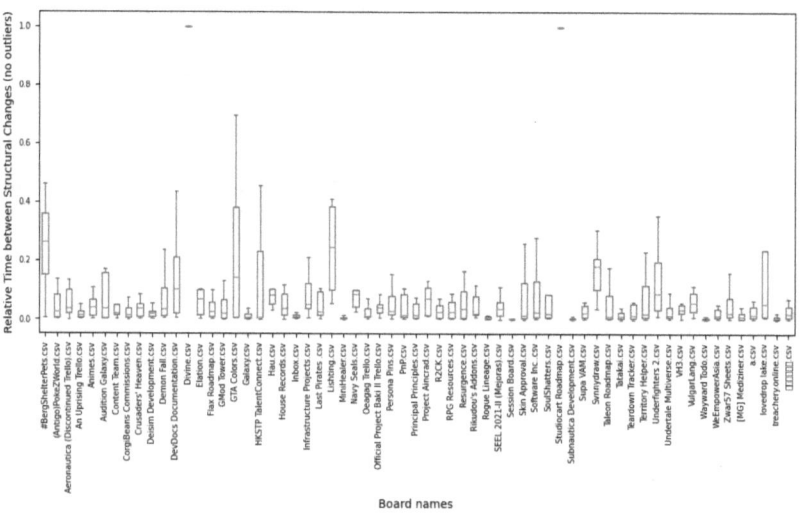

Fig. 3. Relative duration of the periods between structural changes in the boards

Figure 3 depicts the duration of the intervals between structural changes relative to the lifetime of the board. On average, the mean duration of a period between two structural changes is 10% of the life of the board use. We observe that, as expected, the larger number of structural changes a board has, the shorter duration of the intervals between them. For instance, *Subnautica development.csv*, *Wayward Todo.csv*, *Minihealer.csv* and *Session Board.csv* have over 53 structural changes and the average interval duration is below 3% for all of them. On the contrary, for those boards that have suffered only one structural change, the only existing period takes the 100% of the time.

Figure 4 examines the distribution of the structural changes along the lifetime of the boards divided in 10 parts. Regardless of the number of structural changes, the trend is to have the larger number of them in the first half of the use time of a board. The number of structural changes goes down progressively afterwards.

4.2   Case Studies

We have selected three boards from the 63 boards previously analyzed to illustrate the different findings that we can detect with the operations we present. To see graphically the evolution of the boards (cf. Fig. 5, 6 and 7), we represent time on the x-axis, while each row of the y-axis represents a list of the board. The vertical lines represent the structural changes, plotting a line when they start and another line when they finish. These structural changes are computed with the same threshold as before $\theta = 24$ h. Note that for this reason, both lines usually seem to overlap, since the structural change is made in a single day. Lists with very little use (e.g., 3 days) have been filtered, since they tend to be lists that are created and deleted without any action being taken on them in their short lifetime (this way we avoid having horizontal rows without a bar, due to the lack of related list actions).

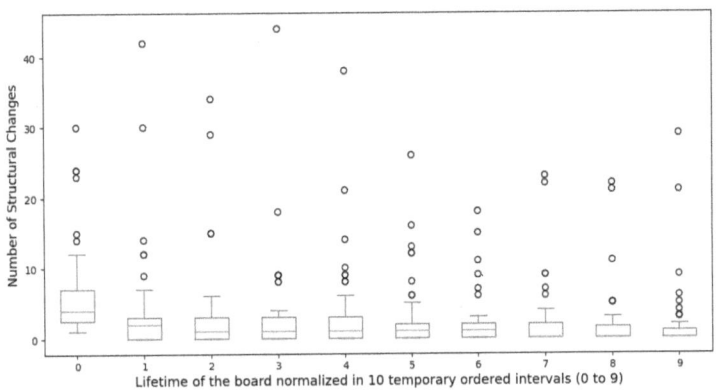

Fig. 4. Structural changes along the lifetime of the boards

Board "ZWar 57 Sheets"[2] is a classification of music by genre. Song titles are represented on the cards, which are classified into the list of their corresponding genre. The board has been used for more than three years, with a total of more than 8,000 actions over the elements of the board. If we open the board at present, we see more than 15 lists corresponding to such different musical genres.

---

[2] https://trello.com/b/5aOH4KDa/zwar57-sheets.

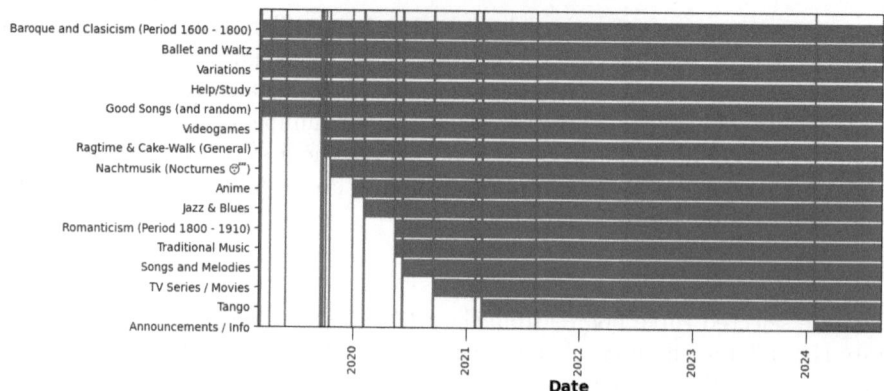

Fig. 5. Evolution of the "Zwar 57 sheets" board noting the structural updates

Within each list, we see all the songs that are classified in that genre. Intuitively, songs should not change their genre (except in case the user makes a mistake when classifying the card), since, for instance, a baroque song does not become a romantic song over time. If we look at the evolution of the board (cf. Fig. 5), we can see how new genres are constantly being added to the board. Although numerous structural changes are noted, most of them are a regular use of the board that do not change its structure or design.

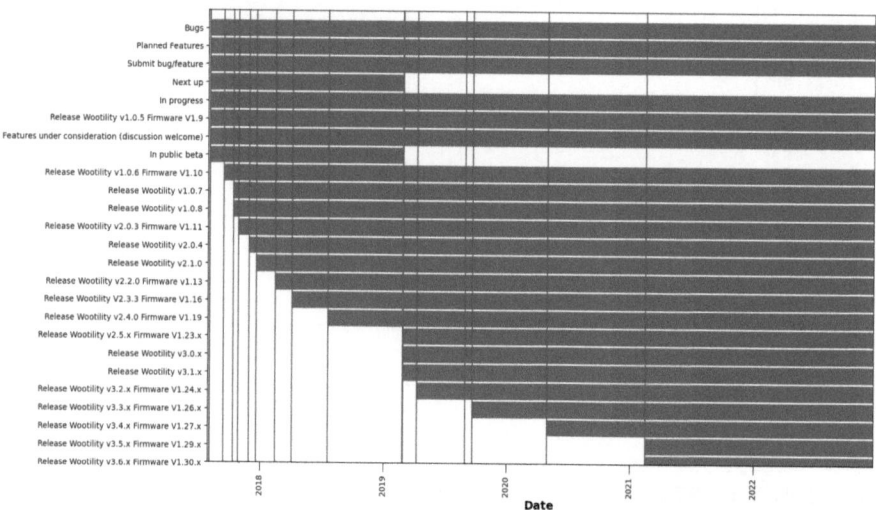

Fig. 6. Evolution of the "Wooting Roadmap" board noting the structural updates

Board "Wooting Roadmap"[3] represents a software development process where the users collect the features to be developed on the cards and classify them by their status, which is indicated on the lists (e.g. "In progress" or "Planned features"). It has been used for more than four years, with more than 2,000 actions during this time.

Figure 6 depicts the list timeline and the structural updates from mid 2017 to mid 2022. The chart shows how the users are continuously creating new lists: one per each new release of their development project. This is an example of structural change that represents a regular use of the board, since the way the board was used before and after adding that new list is the same. Nevertheless, the figure also shows a structural change that happened around February 2019 that did involve a board redesign. In particular, lists *In public beta* and *Next up* were removed, meaning that board users simplified their workflow (or at least the parts managed with the BBT), changing the way in which the board was used or its purpose.

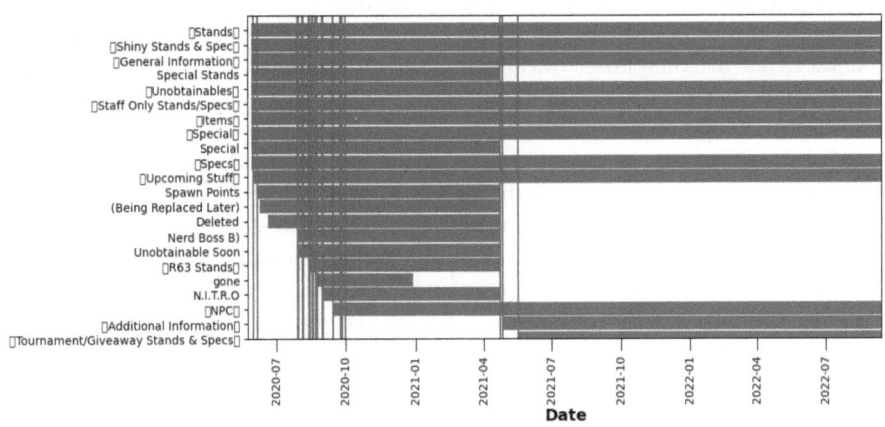

Fig. 7. Evolution of the "Oeagag" board noting its structural updates

Board "Oegag"[4] current snapshot classifies the elements of a video-game (e.g., characters, weapons, levels, or rewards) according to their type. It has been used for about two years, with a total of more than 2,500 actions. However, looking at the output graphs of the algorithms, we could see that it was not always used for the aforementioned purpose. In fact, initially users used this board indicating the features that were being developed in each release and which one of them were included in each version of the video-game. If we look at Fig. 7, we can see how they have been using 14 lists to develop the game, from "R63 Stands" to "gone". After finishing the development, in May 2021,

---

[3] https://trello.com/b/NpKEdAgB/wooting-roadmap.

[4] https://trello.com/b/my8N75db/oeagag-trello.

they put all the information related to the game into the first lists (i.e. from "Stands" to "NPC"). For this reason, we could separate the log of this board into two different fragments, corresponding to the two different uses observed over time: a first phase to develop the video-game, and a second phase to classify the information of the elements of the game statically (current board snapshot).

5 Discussion

This work is a first attempt towards understanding how BBT boards are used in reality. The analysis of BBT logs can tell relevant information about the evolution of the structure and dynamic use of the boards.

The scope of our approach is still limited. On the one hand, the operations presented in this paper focus on actions performed on the lists of the board. These operations could be extended to consider other board elements (e.g. cards, labels, or dates) as well as to pay special attention to its users. On the other hand, the logs analyzed are from public Trello boards. Replicating this analysis using logs from private enterprises could yield new or differing findings and conclusions. The operations presented and their visualizations (cf. Fig. 5, 6, 7) serve to detect that at some point during the use of the boards something happened. The changes occurred have different degrees of importance and implications. Sometimes the pointed structural changes are part of the regular use of the board. For instance, a new list is created for each week, each month and each release containing cards with information or actions related to the list topic (e.g., a to-do list for a new release). In other occasions, the structural update is the result of a major *board redesign* that may completely change the way in which the board represents the problem, as exemplified with the "Oeagag" board. However, the reasons that have led users to undertake such actions on the board and its elements can only be known by including the human in the loop (users in this case). With the information resulting from our operations and graphs, we can intuit reasons for certain actions or behaviors, but to assert them we need the testimony of the board's users, for which private boards would be required.

Regarding the techniques we used to analyze logs, note that advanced process mining approaches such as Object-Centric Process Mining (OCPM) [1] could also align with our proposal. Unlike traditional process mining, OCPM captures one-to-many and many-to-many relationships between multiple objects what aligns with BBT logs since each action is performed on a single element but it may impact other elements of the board. For instance, moving a card from one list to another is an action on the card itself, but it also affects two lists: one that loses a card and another that gains a new one. In this paper, we did not delve into the impact of an event on related objects. However, we plan to explore this approach for future extensions, considering the relationships of board events with other objects affected as a whole instead of analyzing each board element separately, as done with lists in this paper.

Finally, as in process mining, board mining involves applications other than those related to board analysis. *Board discovery* extracts data from boards' history to model the underlying board. A metamodel to represent the structure of a board and its dynamic use based on three aspects, namely, the type of cards, the semantic precedence and the card flow, was introduced in [11]. Eight board design patterns were defined that characterize usual ways of using a board. Further delving into *board analysis* can lead to more applications. For instance, performing conformance checking against the expected board use can reveal deviations in a specific time period. Compliance checking against business rules that shall affect board elements (e.g., the participation of specific people in tasks represented by cards) can also provide useful insights. Board history analysis is also convenient to detect if and why a board has abruptly stopped being used. For example, a reason why people may stop using a board is that its quality has decreased over time due to a large number of structural changes, and consequently, using it has become cumbersome and confusing. The results of the analyses could shed light for possible *board optimizations*. For instance, aligning the structure and dynamic use of the boards to the aforementioned design patterns could be an optimization strategy.

6   Conclusions and Future Work

In this paper, we have devised operations to analyze BBT logs to extract information about the evolution of lists and structural changes. We have also analyzed 63 public Trello boards to further understand how boards are really used, and we have used three boards as use cases to illustrate different possible findings when applying the presented operations.

As next steps, we plan to extend the analyses to include other sources of BBT logs as well as further features of the boards (e.g., cards, people, labels and due dates). Applying advanced process mining techniques could also be of considerable interest, as it would offer a more comprehensive understanding of the board as an entire entity rather than as isolated elements, potentially leading to new insights. Board discovery and optimization should also be addressed in the future to complement board analysis.

References

1. van der Aalst, W.M.: Object-centric process mining: dealing with divergence and convergence in event data. In: SEFM, pp. 3–25 (2019)
2. Ault, A., Krogmeier, J., Buckmaster, D.: Mobile, cloud-based farm management: a case study with Trello on my farm. In: ASABE (2013)
3. Bravo, A., Cabanillas, C., Peña, J., Resinas, M.: Board miner: a tool to analyze the use of board-based collaborative work management tools. In: ICSOC Demos, pp. 345–349 (2022)
4. Buffardi, K.: Assessing individual contributions to software engineering projects with git logs and user stories. In: SIGCSE, pp. 650–656 (2020)
5. Fic, P.: Moved to published: using Trello in content management. Dianoia 15–23 (2019)
6. Gould, E.M.: Workflow management tools for electronic resources management. Ser. Rev. **44**(1), 71–74 (2018)

7. Khoury, A., Bucknor, A., King, I., Kerstein, R., Nduka, C.: Use of Trello as a project management tool for collaborative surgical research and audit. Br. J. Surg. **109** (2022)
8. Mora, A., Tondello, G.F., Nacke, L.E., Arnedo-Moreno, J.: Effect of personalized gameful design on student engagement. In: EDUCON, pp. 1925–1933 (2018)
9. Naik, N., Jenkins, P.: A web based method for managing PRINCE2 projects using Trello. In: IEEE ISSE, pp. 1–3 (2019)
10. Ostergaard, K.: Applying Kanban principles to electronic resource acquisitions with Trello. J. Electron. Resour. Librariansh. **28**(1), 48–52 (2016)
11. Peña, J., Bravo, A., del Río-Ortega, A., Resinas, M., Ruiz-Cortés, A.: Design patterns for board-based collaborative work management tools. In: CAiSE, pp. 177–192 (2021)
12. Pisoni, G., Gijlers, H., Chen, H., Nguyen, T.H.: Collaboration patterns in students' teams working on business cases. In: WSDM Workshops (L2D), vol. 2876, pp. 14–27 (2021)
13. Power, K.: Metrics for understanding flow. In: Agile Conference (2014)
14. Ray, N.: Prioritize, plan, and maintain motivation with Trello. J. Agric. Educ. **88**(6) (2016)
15. Shamshurin, I., Saltz, J.: A predictive model to identify Kanban teams at risk. Model. Assist. Stat. Appl. **14**, 321–335 (2019)

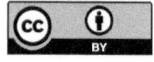

Extending Process Intelligence
with Quantity-Related Process Mining

Nina Graves$^{(\boxtimes)}$ ⒾⒹ, Tobias Brockhoff ⒾⒹ, István Koren ⒾⒹ, and Wil M. P. van
der Aalst ⒾⒹ

Chair of Process and Data Science (PADS), RWTH Aachen University,
Aachen, Germany
{graves,brockhoff,koren,wvdaalst}@pads.rwth-aachen.de

Abstract. Process mining uses data logged during the execution of processes to understand, analyse, and improve processes. Logistics process
management and optimisation are highly relevant for the industry, as
they are crucial to the business' operations but not intrinsically value-
adding. Despite the advantages of applying process mining to logistics
processes, its full potential can not yet be leveraged. Current process
mining techniques assume that an event's execution solely depends on
its associated identifiable objects, their attributes, relationships, and previously executed events. However, in logistics processes, *counts* of items,
which may not be uniquely identifiable, play a crucial role. For instance,
a replenishment order is triggered when the stock level falls below a
threshold, or a second shipment is dispatched if not all ordered items
are available during the first shipment. This work proposes a framework that integrates the concept of a *quantity state* based on properties
derived from common logistics processes. We introduce extensions to
object-centric event logs and object-centric Petri nets that include such
counts of items. We show the feasibility of detecting the quantity state
from the proposed event log class and demonstrate its capability to convey quantity dependencies using a Python-based implementation.

Keywords: object-centric process mining · logistics · event log

1 Introduction

Recently, the need for increasing transparency in supply chains has become more
pronounced, and process mining (PM) is considered a strong contester to provide
it [7]. However, PM is not well established in the domain of logistics [5] as not
all relevant data can be added into the event log format explicitly [8] and techniques do not support a process notion beyond independent workflows [15,16].
Due to their high industrial relevance, inventory management processes (IMPs)
are widely studied and classified in the fields of logistics and supply chains [3].
In several of the common strategies for their handling, the execution of an event
depends on a particular *count* of items, e.g., products in a warehouse or unre-
served products in a planning system. Such counts can be affected by the execution of the workflow of specific objects but are not tied to their lifecycles –

© The Author(s) 2025
A. Delgado and T. Slaats (Eds.): ICPM 2024 Workshops, LNBIP 533, pp. 337–349, 2025.
https://doi.org/10.1007/978-3-031-82225-4_25

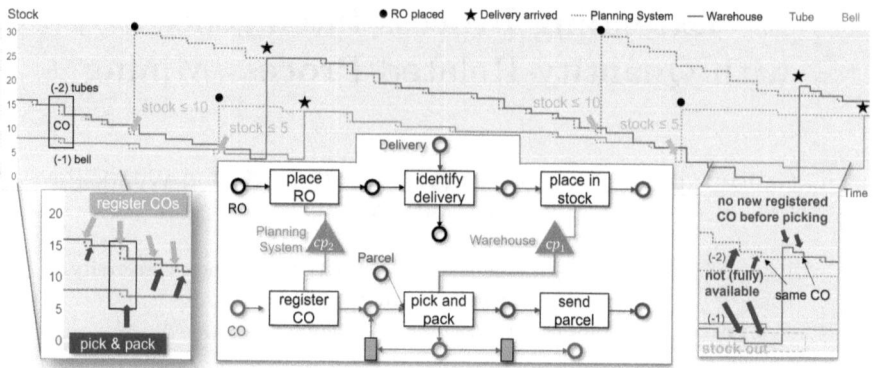

Fig. 1. Example IMP with two products, tubes and bells, and two different counts, cp_1 and cp_2, included in the extended object-centric Petri net (centre). The chart (top) shows the development of the stock levels in the warehouse (solid) and the planning system (dotted) over time. Dotted decreases occur when COs are registered, and solid decreases when products are removed (left). ROs are placed when ten or fewer tubes or five or fewer bells are available in the planning system. If COs arrive that cannot be fulfilled, all available products are removed from the warehouse, and the removal is repeated after the delivery arrives (right).

individual process executions are not independent. Consider, for example, the IMP depicted in Fig. 1, in which a replenishment order (RO) is placed when the number of products in the company's planning system (cp_2) falls to ten tubes or five bells or below. After the order is placed, the in-transit products are registered in the planning system, and when the delivery arrives, the products are placed into the company warehouse (cp_1). Whenever a customer order (CO) arrives, the number of ordered products is removed from the planning system when the order is registered. All available and demanded products are then picked from the warehouse and sent to the customer. If the full CO cannot be fulfilled because the ordered products are not available in the warehouse, a second parcel with the missing products is sent. Current PM techniques implicitly assume that (1) the control flow only depends on the current state of identifiable objects, i.e., object attributes and previously executed activities [1], and (2) activities and object types are the only relevant entities which are represented by uniquely identifiable events and objects in the event log [14]. These assumptions do not hold for IMPs, as the execution of an event can also depend on counts of products without unique identifiers (not every pen or cup has an ID).

This work introduces a basic framework for quantity-related process mining (QRPM) by extending object-centric process mining (OCPM) to allow for the additional consideration of a *quantity state* referring to such counts of items. Motivated by IMPs, we derive generic properties for quantity-related processes to extend object-centric event logs, derive the quantity state from such a log, and include the concept of item counts into process models and discovery. Based

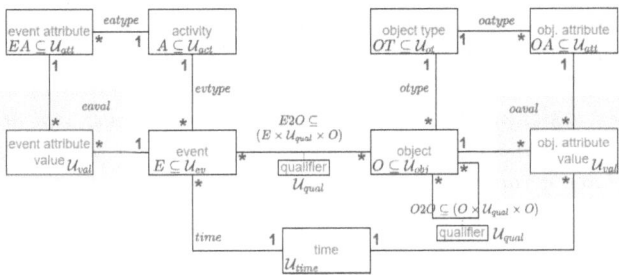

Fig. 2. Meta Model of the Object-Centric Event Log Standard OCEL 2.0 [1].

on the demonstration and discussion of a use case, we conclude the framework's capability of conveying quantity-related behaviour and its suitability as a baseline for further research for PM techniques supporting logistics processes. The remainder of this work is structured as follows: Sect. 2 presents the preliminaries before the framework is introduced in Sect. 3. Section 4 describes the implementation and case study. In Sect. 5, we give an overview of related work before concluding this work in Sect. 6.

2   Preliminaries

A partial function from a set X to a set Y is denoted $f : X \nrightarrow Y$ where $dom(f) \subseteq X$ refers to the function's domain and $rng(f) \subseteq Y$ its range. We denote a total function as $g : X \rightarrow Y$ where $dom(f) = X$. We assume the set-theoretic definition of functions being a relation over tuples, e.g. $g = \{(x_1, f(x_1)), ..., (x_n, f(x_n))\}$ For any finite set A, $|A|$ denotes the number of elements in the set, $\mathcal{P}(A)$ its powerset, and $\mathcal{B}(A)$ the set of all multisets over A. A multiset $b : A \rightarrow \mathbb{N}$ assigns a natural number to every element of a set, $b_1 = [\,]$, $b_2 = [x, y^2, z^3]$, and $b_3 = [y, z^2]$ with $b_1, b_2, b_3 \in \mathcal{B}(A)$ are examples for multisets over a set $A = \{x, y, z\}$. The standard set operators are extended to multisets; $x \in b_2$; $x \notin b_3, b_1$; $b_2 \uplus b_3 = [x, y^3, z^5]$; and $b_2 \cap b_3 = b_3$.

We introduce the following universes and define an Object-Centric Event Log (OCEL) according to the current OCEL 2.0 standard [1]: $\mathcal{U}_{act}$ for activities (i.e., event types), $\mathcal{U}_{ev}$ for events, $\mathcal{U}_{ot}$ for object types, $\mathcal{U}_{obj}$ for objects, $\mathcal{U}_{att}$ for attributes, $\mathcal{U}_{val}$ for attribute values, $\mathcal{U}_{qual}$ for qualifiers, and $\mathcal{U}_{time}$ with $\{0, \infty\} \subseteq \mathcal{U}_{time}$ for time.

Definition 1 (OCEL). *An object-centric event log is a tuple $L_{oc} = (E, O, EA, OA, act, otype, eatype, oatype, eaval, oaval, time, E2O, O2O)$ where $E \subseteq \mathcal{U}_{ev}$ is a set of events, $O \subseteq \mathcal{U}_{obj}$ is a set of objects, $EA, OA \subseteq \mathcal{U}_{att}$ are the sets of event and object attributes, $act : E \rightarrow \mathcal{U}_{act}$ and $otype : O \rightarrow \mathcal{U}_{ot}$ map objects and events to types, $eatype : EA \rightarrow \mathcal{U}_{act}$ and $oatype : OA \rightarrow \mathcal{U}_{ot}$ map attributes to types, $eaval : (E \times EA) \nrightarrow \mathcal{U}_{val}$ and $oaval : (O \times OA \times \mathcal{U}_{time}) \nrightarrow \mathcal{U}_{val}$ partially assign values to event and object attributes, $time : E \rightarrow \mathcal{U}_{time}$*

assign timestamps to events, $E2O \subseteq (E \times \mathcal{U}_{qual} \times O)$ are qualified event-to-object relations, and $O2O \subseteq (O \times \mathcal{U}_{qual} \times O)$ are qualified object-to-object relations, such that $dom(eaval) \subseteq \{(E, ea) \in E \times EA \mid act(e) = eatype(ea)\}$ only attributes assigned to an event's activity have values, and $dom(oaval) \subseteq \{(o, oa, tm) \in O \times EA \times \mathcal{U}_{time} \mid otype(o) = oatype(oa)\}$ only attributes of the object's type have a value.

Figure 2 shows the meta model and the mentioned functions for the current OCEL 2.0 standard. Object-Centric Petri Nets (OCPNs) model the joint workflows of multiple object types, based on labelled Petri nets, $N = (P, T, F, l)$, defined in the usual way. As introduced in [14], they are defined as a labelled Petri net, a mapping of object types to places, and a set of variable arcs. Whereas normal arcs indicate the consumption/production of a single token, variable arcs merely indicate that the number of tokens is not always necessarily one.

Definition 2 (Object-Centric Petri net). *An object-centric Petri net is a tuple $OCPN = (N, pt, F_{var})$ with $N = (P, T, F, l)$ a labelled Petri net, $pt : P \to OT$ maps places to object types, and $F_{var} \subseteq F$ is the subset of variable arcs.*

An OCPN's marking is a multiset of tokens, $m_o \in M_o = \mathcal{B}(P \times O)$; a token being the combination of a place and an object. An *execution binding* (t, b_o) refers to a transition and an object binding function specifying the consumed and produced tokens. An execution binding is only enabled if the current marking includes all to-be-consumed tokens.

3   Quantity-Related Process Mining

This work offers a methodological foundation for PM in processes where the control flow depends on the number of (unidentifiable) entities and the state of objects. As IMPs are a well-defined processes in which this dependency is very explicit, we base our initial framework on an abstraction of IMPs. An *item* is an entity of a particular *item type*, and two items of the same type are considered interchangeable; the process merely depends on their count, not their identities, e.g., tubes and bells in the example process. Similar to [6], we define *counters*, which associate a signed integer with item types, e.g., to denote additions or removals of items from warehouses.

Definition 3 (Counter, Item quantity). *Let $I \subseteq \mathcal{U}_{it}$ be a finite subset of item types from the universe of item types. A counter $c : I \to \mathbb{Z}$ is a function that maps each item type $it \in I$ to an item quantity. The set of all possible counters over I is denoted $\mathcal{I}(I) = I \to \mathbb{Z}$. For counters $c_1, c_2 \in \mathcal{I}(I)$, their composition $c_1 \oplus c_2$ is defined element-wise with $(c_1 \oplus c_2)(it) = c_1(it) + c_2(it)$.*

We write $c_1 = [\![\,]\!]$, $c_2 = [\![x, y^{-1}, y^{-1}, z, z, z]\!] = [\![x, y^{-2}, z^3]\!]$, and $c_3 = [\![x^2, y]\!]$ as examples for counters over a set of item types $I = \{x, y, z\}$. We denote the set of all *active* item types in a counter as $set(c) = \{it \in dom(c) \mid c(it) \neq 0\}$. The composition of a multiset of counters $Q \subseteq \mathcal{B}(\mathcal{I}(I))$ is denoted $c = \bigoplus Q$.

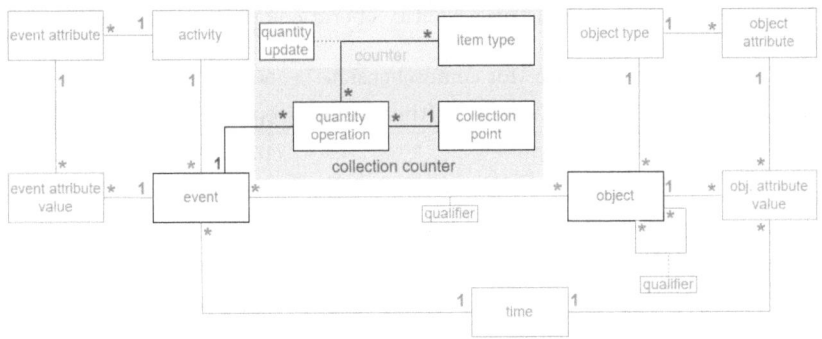

Fig. 3. Meta Model for Quantity Event Logs (QELs).

Collection points (cps) are entities that refer to a particular count of items, e.g., a warehouse. The counts of different item types associated with a cp describe its *item level*, e.g., the item level of the warehouse at the beginning of the example process $[\![tube^{16}, bell^8]\!]$. A collection counter maps every cp in a set to a counter.

Definition 4 (Collection Counter). *Let $CP \subseteq \mathcal{U}_{cp}$ be a finite subset of the universe of cps and $I \subseteq \mathcal{U}_{it}$ a finite set of item types. A collection counter is a function $cc : CP \rightarrow \mathcal{I}(I)$, and $\mathcal{C}(CP, I) = CP \rightarrow \mathcal{I}(I)$ the set of all collection counters over CP and I. The composition of collection counters is $cc_3 = cc_1 \oplus cc_2$ with $cc_3(cp) = cc_1(cp) \oplus cc_2(cp)$ for all $cp \in CP$ for any two collection counters $cc_1, cc_2 \in \mathcal{C}(CP, I)$.*

An example for a collection counter over a set of cps $CP = \{cp_1, cp_2\}$ for the item types $I = \{x, y, z\}$ is $cc_1 = \{(cp_1, [\![x^{-1}, y^{-2}, z^2]\!]), (cp_2, [\![x, y]\!])\}$. Composing cc_1 and $cc_2 = \{(cp_1, [\![x, y, z]\!]), (cp_2, [\![x, y^{-2}, z^{-2}]\!])\}$ leads to $cc_1 \oplus cc_2 = \{(cp_1, [\![y^{-1}, z^3]\!]), (cp_2, [\![x^2, y^{-1}, z^{-2}]\!])\}$. Any $cc \in \mathcal{C}(CP, I)$ is considered *active* if the joint set of active item types is non-empty, i.e., $|\bigcup_{c \in rng(cc)} set(c)| > 0$.

Based on the typology of IMPs presented in [3], we derive three properties characterising quantity-related processes: **(P1) Quantity changes**: An event can change item levels of one or more cps. The affected item levels and the number of items added/removed can differ among events of the same activity. For example, every execution of "place in stock" adds all delivered items to the warehouse, but not all deliveries include the same (number of) items. **(P2) Quantity-dependency for executions**: The execution of an event can depend on the item levels of one or more cps; e.g., tubes are only reordered if the stock level is 5 or below. **(P3) Quantity-dependency for operations**: The number of items added to or removed from a cp in an event can depend on current item levels, e.g., we cannot pick all ordered items if they are not available, so we pick fewer. These three principles highlight the need for PM techniques to explicitly consider a *quantity state*, i.e., the item levels of cps. In logistics, the integration of relevant data into the event log format is a known problem [5,8]: As item types do not require an identifier and the "lifecycle" of a cp cannot be described

Table 1. Data describing active quantity operations for the example process.

event data (for comprehension)			active qops		
eid	activity	timestamp	cp	tube	bell
init	initial item level		cp2	11	7
init	initial item level		cp1	12	7
21	pick and pack	12.10.2019 12:21	cp1	−1	
22	send parcel	12.10.2019 13:16			
23	register CO	12.10.2019 13:56	cp2	−2	−1
24	place RO	12.10.2019 14:01	cp2	21	
25	pick and pack	12.10.2019 14:11	cp1	−2	−1
26	send parcel	12.10.2019 15:19			

by a workflow, their representation as objects is unsuitable. As attributes, they would not be distinct, i.e., automated analyses are impossible. To encompass the inclusion of known collection points and item types, we introduce *quantity event logs* (QELs), which extend OCELs (see Fig. 3). In a QEL, events are connected to *quantity operations*, which describe a change to a cp's item level with *quantity updates* as the number of items added/removed of a specific item type. Consider the example depicted in Fig. 1: when the second CO is registered (black box on the left), the quantity operation to the planning system is $[tubes^{-2}, bell^{-1}]$ – the "steps" in each line represent the quantity updates. To accurately and definitively derive the quantity state from a QEL, we require an entry providing the initial item levels of every cp and a strict total order among the events.

Definition 5 (Quantity Event Log). *A quantity event log is a tuple $QEL = (L_{oc}, I, CP, eqty, \prec_e)$, with $L_{oc} = (E, O, EA, OA, act, otype, eatype, oatype, eval, oval, time, E2O, O2O)$ an OCEL, $I \subseteq \mathcal{U}_{it}$ a set of item types, $CP \subseteq \mathcal{U}_{cp}$ a set of collection points, $eqty : (E \cup \{\blacktriangleright\}) \to \mathcal{C}(CP, I)$ a mapping of events to quantity operations for all collection points, and $\prec_e \subseteq (E \times E)$ the strict total order among the events, such that $\blacktriangleright \notin E$.*

We consider an event $e \in E$ to be active if the corresponding collection counter is active, i.e., $rng(eqty(e)) \neq \{[\![]\!]\}$. Table 1 shows example data containing the active quantity operations associated with events to be added to an event log. The column's activity and timestamp are included to ease comprehension. Assuming all relevant quantity operations are logged in the QEL, the quantity state before every event can be determined by composing all prior quantity operations and the initial item level.

Definition 6 (Quantity State). *Let $QEL = (L_{oc}, I, CP, eqty, \prec_e)$ be a quantity event log referring to the set of events $E \subseteq \mathcal{U}_{ev}$. The function $qstate : E \to \mathcal{C}(CP, I)$ describes the quantity state at the execution of $e \in E$:*

$$qstate(e) = \bigoplus [eqty(\blacktriangleright)] \uplus [eqty(e') \mid e' \prec_e e]$$

Equivalently, the quantity state after an event's execution can be determined by adding the event's quantity operation, $post(qstate(e)) = qstate(e) \oplus eqty(e)$. Figure 1 depicts the quantity state of two collection points (types of lines) of the events in QEL describing the example process ordered by time (x-axis).

To model quantity-related processes, we introduce *Quantity Nets* (q-nets), which convey an activity's ability to impact the system's quantity state. In addition to places whose markings describe the net's object state, q-nets include a set of cps, the marking of which describes the quantity state. Cps are connected to transitions with undirected arcs – firing a transition connected to one or more cps can change each connected cp's item level. The process model in the centre of Fig. 1 shows a fully defined q-net.

Definition 7 (Quantity Net). *A quantity net is a tripartite graph $QN = (OCPN, CP, QA)$, where $OCPN = (N, pt, F_{var})$ is an object-centric Petri net with $N = (P, T, F, l)$, CP is a set of collection points, and $QA \subseteq (T \times CP)$ a set of undirected quantity arcs.*

The q-nets defined here differ from those in [6] where the arcs are directed. Despite making the visualisation less expressive, this increases the model's language and removes the strong requirements for their discovery.

For any transition $t \in T$, the set $CP^t \subseteq CP$ describes the cps it is connected to. The overall state of a q-net is a combination of an object state (marking of places) and a quantity state (marking of collection points), i.e., $M = (m_o, m_q) \in M_o \times \mathcal{C}(CP, I)$. An execution binding $b = (t, b_o, b_q)$ of a q-net refers to an object binding and a valid quantity binding $b_q \in \mathcal{C}(CP^t, I)$. A transition is enabled in a marking $M = (m_o, m_q)$ if the underlying $OCPN$ is enabled in m_o. If a binding is executed, the new marking $m' = (m'_o, m'_q)$ consists of the new object state $m_o \xrightarrow{(t, b_o)} m'_o$ and the new quantity state $m'_q = m_q \oplus b_q$. A q-net can be discovered by identifying the active quantity operations and adding the corresponding cps and arcs to an $OCPN$ mined from the L_{oc}.

Definition 8 (Discovered Q-net). *Let $QEL = (L_{oc}, I, CP, eqty, \prec_e)$ be a QEL. The discovered q-net $QN = (OCPN, CP, QA)$ is a tuple where $OCPN$ is mined from L_{oc} using any discovery algorithm, $CP \subseteq \mathcal{U}_{cp}$ is the set of cps in the QEL, and $QA = \{(t, cp) \in T \times CP \mid (a, cp) \in QR \wedge l(t) = a\}$ the set of quantity arcs with $QR = \{(act(e), cp) \mid eqty_e^{cp} \neq [\![\,]\!]\}$ the set of quantity relations.*

The definitions of q-nets and QELs clearly show that the proposed frameworks are extensions to OCELs and OCPNs, thereby not at all limiting their capabilities but merely adding information. Hence, existing methods, techniques and guarantees remain applicable to the QRPM framework, and all behaviour replayable on the OCPN remains replayable on the q-net.

4   Process Intelligence Using QELs

As suggested in [15], we evaluate the feasibility of our framework for the analysis of non-workflow processes by illustrating its capabilities with an example. With

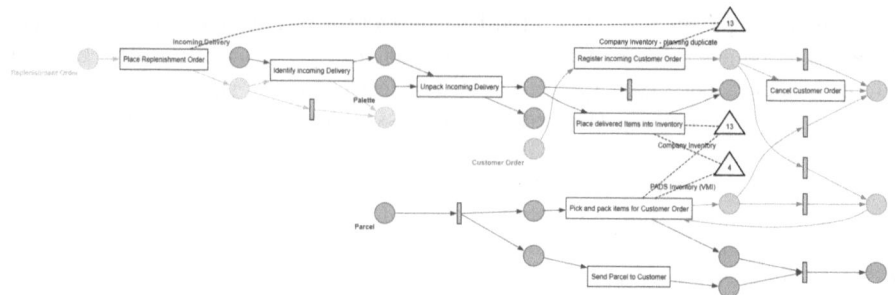

Fig. 4. Q-net discovered from the QEL (only five object types displayed).

a prototypical QEL and implementation of the described framework[1], we demonstrate and discuss its capabilities for the inclusion, detection, and representation of the properties of quantity-related processes.

The Python-based tool *QRPM* (Quantity-related Process Mining) used for this demonstration takes a QEL as an input, which is an OCEL 2.0 in SQLite-format with an additional table *quantity_operations* (like Table 1 without the two columns, "activity" and "timestamp"). Every row refers to an event identifier (*ocel_id*) or the initial item level (*init*), a cp (*ocel_cpid*), as well as one quantity update per item type (columns). The quantity operation table is not required to be complete – active quantity operations are sufficient. QRPM discovers a q-net from an uploaded QEL[2] and detects and visualises the quantity state of every event. It also offers the possibility to perform basic data operations (projections and aggregations) on the quantity operations and quantity state of (selected) events and export this data. For a user-guided analysis, the tool provides descriptive statistics and visualisations on both types of quantity data.

The QEL describing the simulated IMP containing common strategies contains 3622 events of eight activities, with 4097 active quantity operations referring to three collection points and 17 item types. The events are associated with 3441 objects of seven object types; 768 customer orders and 95 replenishment orders. Figure 4 shows the discovered q-net from a sublog only referring to five object types (the two types of employees were removed for easier readability). The numbers in the cps inform of the number of active item types associated with at least one active entry in the quantity operation table. While the underlying OCPN shows two disconnected sub-processes, the discovered q-net can depict a quantity-based connection between them. Furthermore, all quantity operations of the QEL can be represented with the discovered q-net (P1). However, it is unclear what item types the cp refers to and how the execution of an activity impacts its item level in terms of directedness (adding/removing/mixed), involved item types and quantities. This information can be obtained from the QEL and is displayed in QRPM, but it is not part of the model and cannot be incorporated easily, as they may differ among item types. For the discov-

---

[1] Dataset and implementation: https://github.com/rwth-pads/qrpm.git.

[2] The OCPN is discovered with PM4PY [2] which uses the standard Inductive Miner.

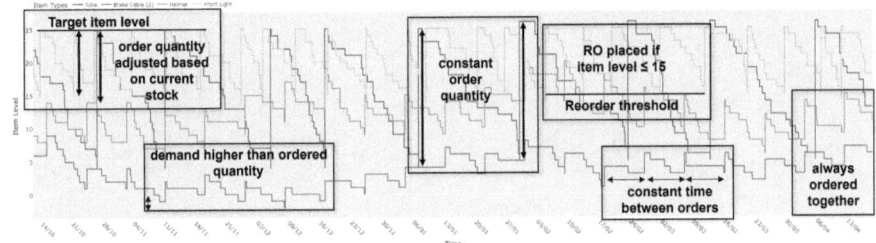

Fig. 5. Quantity State Development of QEL reveals relevant behaviour for the logistics domain.

ery, the frequency of active quantity operations between events of an activity and a cp is not considered – one occurrence in the log is enough for the arc to be added. The current framework is also incapable of detecting or displaying quantity-dependent behaviour (P2 and P3) as it does not consider connections between activities and cps beyond quantity changes, and the quantity state does not restrict the model's behaviour compared to OCPN.

Despite the limitations of the current framework, we now demonstrate the additional process intelligence that can be obtained from the QEL using QRPM and, thereby, emphasise the potential of this framework. On the one hand, including the quantity state allows insights into executed logistics practices such as replenishment policies [3]. Figure 5 shows the planning system's item levels for selected item types. Considering the quantity state, we can see that ROs for tubes and front lights are placed whenever their item level falls below 5 or 15, respectively, indicating a quantity dependency in the execution of the event (P2). We can also spot a quantity dependency in the number of ordered items (P3): While the number of ordered tubes is fixed, the front lights are ordered in varying quantities depending on the item level when the RO is placed, so a target stock level of 25 is achieved. Furthermore, Fig. 5 shows that helmets and brake cables are always ordered and delivered at the same time, independent of their item levels – in fact, the time between orders is constant. As the count of brake cables temporarily sinks below zero, we can deduce that the demand for COs exceeded both the available item level and the reordered quantity. This example shows that when using a QEL, relevant process elements in the logistics domain can now be captured and analysed.

On the other hand, the quantity state offers an additional perspective for determining patterns in the control flow. Figure 5 shows an indication of stock-based triggering of "place RO", which could not be seen without the item levels. The item levels of the vendor-managed inventory and of selected item types of the physical warehouse (Fig. 6) provide further indicators of quantity dependent behaviour. As these cps represent the stock levels of physical warehouses, none of the item levels falls below zero – however, products can be out of stock. Inspecting stock-outs reveals that whenever boxes are out of stock, the stock levels of all products in both warehouses do not decrease until boxes are available again (grey overlay in Fig. 6). Using QRPM to filter for executed events in this

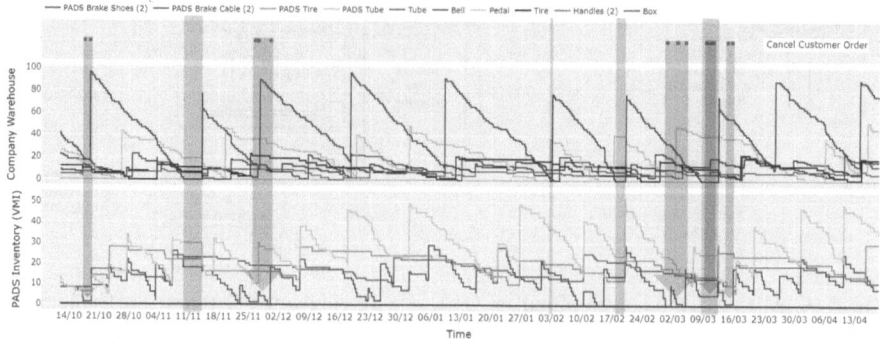

Fig. 6. Dependencies of event executions on stock levels of the physical warehouses. Grey highlighting: periods of box stock-outs, blue-green arrows: cancellations of COs. (Color figure online)

state, we can see that no event of "pick and pack" is among them – this indicates a dependency on the availability of boxes. The top chart in Fig. 6 shows the COs' cancellation, which coincides with stock-outs of the vendor's brake shoes (blue-green arrow). The only deviations occur during the stock-out of boxes, where the availability of five items remains unchanged. An incoming delivery lifts the item level to twelve, which rapidly decreases (by five) to seven. Using QRPM, we can see that the COs for these removals were registered before the cancellations. Finally, we use QRPM to consider the quantity states during the events of "pick and pack" for those COs with multiple executions of this activity (not represented in the Figure). As in the example shown in the introduction, the item level of at least one item type is zero in the company warehouse after every first iteration. In every second iteration, there are only active quantity updates for item types unavailable after the first event.

While standards such as ISA-95 and case studies using inventory data indicate the availability of relational data for creating a QEL, QRPM's practical feasibility remains an open question. Furthermore, we have shown the QEL's capability to convey different kinds of quantity dependency, yet an analyst must still support their detection. The log used in this section is noise-free and perfectly describes the intended behaviour; hence, the presented use case is purely academic and only shows the theoretical possibilities of this framework. However, this work's aim was not the analytical detection of these patterns but to introduce the necessary foundation for doing so. This we have done – by showing that the properties of quantity-related processes can be captured in the proposed QEL and providing a concept, a QEL and an implementation as a basis for further research.

5 Related Work

Several approaches discuss the problems in applying PM techniques to warehouse management processes and introduce methods to overcome this problem.

In all of the proposed methods, the addition of items to a warehouse and the removal of items from a warehouse are integrated into the event log as dedicated activities, thereby allowing for value stream mapping [8], the calculation of additional KPIs [11], or checking the conformance to First-in-First-out principles [4]. The overall state of the involved warehouses is not explicitly considered, and any analysis of the involved material movements requires domain knowledge to identify the relevant activities. The authors of [13] address the need to include additional information into an event log for PM to support the detection of material flows. They advocate the explicit inclusion of locations and introduce the combination of the control flow perspective with the location perspective in separate models. In a previous publication [6], we, rather informally, introduced the idea of including collection points and item types into an event log and suggested a different version of a q-net. In that work, no implementation nor formal definitions and requirements for the detection of the quantity state or the discovery of q-nets were provided.

Processes describing the batched execution of activities or subprocesses are another form of quantity-related process. Several works have addressed the discovery of various types of batched activities [10,12], as well as the detection and modelling of batched sub-processes using BPMN [9]. These works successfully detect this particular type of quantity-dependency without requiring the counting entity and the quantity updates to be provided explicitly. However, they require the batched objects to be uniquely identifiable without allowing for varying quantities or counting types of entities. The authors of [16] address the problem of modelling batched processes, as batched processes exceed the notion of a workflow-like process in which all executions are independent. As in [9] the batched process elements are modelled in a different style to indicate their dependency on other process executions. However, in [16] the process model depicts multiple workflows and shares the batched activities among them to indicate the number of dependent executions and includes data attributes in the semantics of the model.

6   Conclusion

In this work, we introduced a framework for the integration of a quantity state to PM by introducing quantity event logs (QEL) and process models capable of representing counts of items. We have shown the capability of QELs to include typical quantity dependencies of IMPs with a use case and an open-source implementation for a QEL's analysis. While still limited in expressiveness, the proposed extension to OCPNs allows for the representation of an activity's impact on a process' quantity state and the connection of quantity-related subprocesses. Apart from extracting the required data and evaluating the framework's robustness, the detection and modelling of quantity dependencies are areas for future work. Additionally, the consideration of implicit quantity dependencies, as opposed to counts explicitly provided in the log, also poses research questions to be pursued. Overall, this work lays a solid foundation for advancing PM techniques to better support logistics and inventory management domains by explicitly incorporating quantity-related data.

Acknowledgements. Funded by the Deutsche Forschungsgemeinschaft (DFG, German Research Foundation) under Germany's Excellence Strategy - EXC-2023 Internet of Production - 390621612. We also thank the Alexander von Humboldt (AvH) Stiftung for supporting our research.

References

1. Berti, A., et al.: OCEL (Object-Centric Event Log) 2.0 Specification (2024)
2. Berti, A., van Zelst, S., Schuster, D.: PM4Py: a process mining library for Python. Softw. Impacts **17**, 100556 (2023)
3. de Kok, T., et al.: A typology and literature review on stochastic multi-echelon inventory models. Eur. J. Oper. Res. **269**(3), 955–983 (2018)
4. Er, M., Astuti, H.M., Wardhani, I.R.K.: Material movement analysis for warehouse business process improvement with process mining. In: Asia Pacific Business Process Management, vol. 219, pp. 115–127. Springer (2015)
5. Garcia, C.D.S., et al.: Process mining techniques and applications – a systematic mapping study. Expert Syst. Appl. **133**, 260–295 (2019)
6. Graves, N., Koren, I., Rafiei, M., van der Aalst, W.M.: From identities to quantities. In: Process Mining Workshops, vol. 503, pp. 462–474. Springer (2024)
7. Jacobi, C., Meier, M., Herborn, L., Furmans, K.: Maturity model for applying process mining in supply chains. Logist. J. (12) (2020)
8. Knoll, D., Reinhart, G., Prüglmeier, M.: Enabling value stream mapping for internal logistics using multidimensional process mining. Expert Syst. Appl. **124**, 130–142 (2019)
9. Martin, N., Pufahl, L., Mannhardt, F.: Detection of batch activities from event logs. Inf. Syst. **95**, 101642 (2021)
10. Martin, N., et al.: Retrieving batch organisation of work insights from event logs. Decis. Support Syst. **100**, 119–128 (2017)
11. Paszkiewicz, Z.: Process mining techniques in conformance testing of inventory processes. In: Business Information Systems Workshops, vol. 160, pp. 302–313. Springer (2013)
12. Pika, A., Ouyang, C., Ter Hofstede, A.H.M.: Configurable Batch-Processing Discovery from Event Logs. ACM (2022)
13. van Cruchten, R.M.E.R., Weigand, H.H.: Process mining in logistics: the need for rule-based data abstraction. In: Proceedings RCIS, pp. 1–9. IEEE (2018)
14. van der Aalst, W.M., Berti, A.: Discovering object-centric petri nets. Fund. Inform. **175**(1-4), 1–40 (2020)
15. van der Aalst, W.M., Reijers, H.A., Maruster, L.: Process mining beyond workflows. Comput. Ind. **161**, 104126 (2024)
16. Wen, Y., Chen, Z., Liu, J., Chen, J.: Mining batch processing workflow models from event logs. Concurr. Comput. Pract. Exp. **25**(13), 1928–1942 (2013)

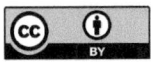

Ranking the Top-K Realizations of Stochastically Known Event Logs

Arvid Lepsien[1]([✉])[iD], Marco Pegoraro[2][iD], Frederik Fonger[1][iD],
Dominic Langhammer[3][iD], Milda Aleknonytė-Resch[1][iD],
and Agnes Koschmider[3][iD]

[1] Department of Computer Science, Kiel University, Kiel, Germany
{ale,ffo,mar}@informatik.uni-kiel.de
[2] Chair of Process and Data Science (PADS), RWTH Aachen University,
Aachen, Germany
pegoraro@pads.rwth-aachen.de
[3] Chair of Business Informatics and Process Analytics, University of Bayreuth,
Bayreuth, Germany
{dominic.langhammer,agnes.koschmider}@uni-bayreuth.de

Abstract. Various kinds of uncertainty can occur in event logs, e.g., due to flawed recording, data quality issues, or the use of probabilistic models for activity recognition. Stochastically known event logs make these uncertainties transparent by encoding multiple possible realizations for events. However, the number of realizations encoded by a stochastically known log grows exponentially with its size, making exhaustive exploration infeasible even for moderately sized event logs. Thus, considering only the top-K most probable realizations has been proposed in the literature. In this paper, we implement an efficient algorithm to calculate a top-K realization ranking of an event log under event independence within $O(Kn)$, where n is the number of uncertain events in the log. This algorithm is used to investigate the benefit of top-K rankings over top-1 interpretations of stochastically known event logs. Specifically, we analyze the usefulness of top-K rankings against different properties of the input data. We show that the benefit of a top-K ranking depends on the length of the input event log and the distribution of the event probabilities. The results highlight the potential of top-K rankings to enhance uncertainty-aware process mining techniques.

Keywords: Event Data · Uncertainty · Top-K Ranking · Algorithm

1 Introduction

Process mining is a family of techniques for analyzing event logs, providing data-driven insights and enabling objectively informed decision making [1]. However, a notable challenge arises when event logs contain events affected by uncertainty [9]. This uncertainty can emerge for various reasons, such as through

A. Delgado and T. Slaats (Eds.): ICPM 2024 Workshops, LNBIP 533, pp. 350–362, 2025.
https://doi.org/10.1007/978-3-031-82225-4_26

systems applying probabilistic models for activity recognition [3,10]. To manage this uncertainty, stochastically known event logs have been introduced [5], which encode multiple possible realizations for each of their events. Despite this, most current process mining techniques do not account for this uncertainty, and instead rely only on the most probable (top-1) interpretation of the events.

To illustrate this, let us consider an example process of patient treatment in a hospital where activities are extracted from medical note systems and handwritten notes. Techniques such as handwriting recognition and natural language processing are used to detect these activities (e.g., [8]). Table 1 shows an example of a stochastically known event log from this setting. In this example, the physician begins the treatment by establishing the medical history of the patient (activity H). The log then shows uncertainty regarding the diagnosis of either light pain (activity L) or severe pain (activity S). Similarly, there is uncertainty in the subsequent event, where either ibuprofen (activity I) or opiates (activity O) were prescribed. Table 2 lists all possible realizations of this log with their realization probabilities. While the most probable realization $\langle H, L, I \rangle$ complies with the hospital's guidelines, the second and third most probable realizations $\langle H, L, O \rangle$ and $\langle H, S, I \rangle$ – which in sum are more probable than the first realization – both hint at compliance issues. If only the most probable log realization was considered, these issues would be overlooked.

While the complete set of possible realizations can be calculated efficiently for this log with few uncertain events, the computational effort grows exponentially with the size of the event log. This raises the need for efficient techniques to prioritize the realizations of uncertain logs. One initial approach suggests considering only the top-K most probable log realizations [5]. However, neither an efficient algorithm to calculate the top-K realizations of a stochastically known log nor an evaluation demonstrating the feasibility of top-K rankings for uncertainty-aware process mining techniques have been presented yet. These issues are addressed in this paper, guided by the following research questions (RQs):

- **(RQ1)** How to efficiently calculate top-K rankings?
- **(RQ2)** What is the benefit of top-K rankings over top-1 interpretations in terms of covered probability mass?
- **(RQ3)** How well can top-K rankings represent the variability of the possible log realizations encoded by a stochastically known log?

To answer these RQs, we design a basic top-K algorithm for stochastically known logs. This algorithm is based on a generalized procedure that iteratively partitions the set of possible log realizations [7]. We then apply the algorithm to simulated stochastically known logs to evaluate the potential of top-K rankings to improve the understanding of uncertainty-aware event data.

The remainder of the paper is structured as follows. Section 2 introduces the basic notations. Section 3 discusses related literature. The algorithm to produce the top-K realizations of a stochastically known event log is presented in Sect. 4. Then, the efficiency of this algorithm and the general potential of top-K rankings to improve the understanding of stochastically known event logs are evaluated in Sect. 5. The paper concludes with a summary and an outlook in Sect. 6.

Table 1. Exemplary stochastically known event log

Event	Case	t	Activity
1	1	1	H
2	1	2	{(L, 0.7), (S, 0.3)}
3	1	3	{(I, 0.6), (O, 0.4)}

Table 2. Possible realizations of the log shown in Table 1 with their realization probabilities

L	$P(L)$
$\langle H, L, I \rangle$	0.42
$\langle H, L, O \rangle$	0.28
$\langle H, S, I \rangle$	0.18
$\langle H, S, O \rangle$	0.12

2 Preliminaries

In this section, the definitions and notations used in the paper (mostly based on [14]) are summarized. First, the universes are defined, which are then used to formally define event logs.

Definition 1 (Universes [14]). *Let $\mathcal{U}_I$ be the universe of event identifiers. Let $\mathcal{U}_C$ be the universe of case identifiers. Let $\mathcal{U}_A$ be the universe of activities and let $\mathcal{U}_T$ be the totally ordered set of timestamp identifiers.*

Definition 2 (Event, event log [14]). *We denote with $\mathcal{E}_C = \mathcal{U}_I \times \mathcal{U}_C \times \mathcal{U}_T \times \mathcal{U}_A$ the universe of deterministic events. A deterministic event log is a set of events $L_C \subseteq \mathcal{E}_C$ such that every event identifier in L_C is unique.*

Next, the notion of an event is extended to encode uncertainty by replacing the single deterministic activity with a partial function matching multiple alternative activities and their corresponding confidence.

Definition 3 (Stochastically known event, stochastically known event log [14]). *We denote with $\mathcal{E}_W = \{(e_i, c, t, f) \in \mathcal{U}_I \times \mathcal{U}_C \times \mathcal{U}_T \times (\mathcal{U}_A \nrightarrow [0,1]) \mid \sum_{a \in dom(f)} f(a) = 1\}$ the universe of stochastically known events. A stochastically known (event) log is a set of stochastically known events $\tilde{L} \subseteq \mathcal{E}_W$ such that every event identifier in $\tilde{L}$ is unique.*

An example case of a stochastically known log is shown in Table 1. We use a tilde to distinguish between stochastically known events, event logs and their deterministic counterparts (e.g., $\tilde{e}_i \in \tilde{L}$ vs. $e_i \in L$). Next, the realizations of stochastically known events and event logs are defined.

Definition 4 (Realizations). *For a stochastically known event $\tilde{e}_i = (i, c, t, f)$, the set of realizations is defined as $R(\tilde{e}_i) = \{(i, c, t, a) \mid a \in dom(f)\}$. For a stochastically known log $\tilde{L} \subseteq \mathcal{E}_W$, the set of realizations is defined as $R(\tilde{L}) = \prod_{\tilde{e}_i \in \tilde{L}} R(\tilde{e}_i)$.*

The realizations of the exemplary stochastically known event log are shown in Table 2. In the following, a tilde over a deterministic event is used to refer to the stochastically known event it stems from, e.g., $e_i \in R(\tilde{e}_i)$ with $\tilde{e}_i \in \tilde{L}$. Finally, the probability of event and log realizations is defined.

Definition 5 (Realization probability). *Let $\tilde{e}_i = (i, c, t, f)$ be a stochastically known event and $e_i \in R(\tilde{e}_i)$ be a realization of $\tilde{e}_i$. Let $\tilde{L}$ be a stochastically known log and $L \in R(\tilde{L})$ be a realization of $\tilde{L}$. Then, the probability of the event realization e_i is defined as $P_{\tilde{e}_i}(e_i) = f(e_i)$ and the probability of the log realization is defined as $P_{\tilde{L}}(L) = \prod_{e_i \in L} P_{\tilde{e}_i}(e_i)$.*

When context is clear, the subscript of the probability function may be omitted. In this paper, the realization probability is calculated under the assumption that the probability of any event realization does not depend on the realizations selected for, e.g., preceding events (*event independence* [5]). This is assumption might be required when no further information about the dependencies between events is available. In practical applications, a weaker assumption of *trace independence* – which assumes independent probabilities across cases, but allows for dependent probabilities inside cases – might be essential [5].

3   Related Work

The interest in uncertainty-aware process mining has increased in recent years. This is reflected by taxonomies classifying uncertain event data [5,14] and various approaches incorporating uncertainty into process mining [4,5,12,14]. These approaches either analyze the information of all realizations of uncertain logs, e.g., with task-specific aggregations such as lower and upper bounds for directly-follows relation frequencies [12], or they select a single representative realization and thus recover a deterministic trace [2]. Stochastically known event logs have been considered in analogy to probabilistic databases where uncertainty can be managed by considering the K most important answers or possible interpretations of the uncertain data [5,16]. For instance, Soliman et al. [16] present an efficient algorithm for top-K queries on probabilistic databases that considers *generation rules* in the form of mutually exclusive tuples. Besides, top-K rankings have also proven to be useful in additional applications, e.g., for search engine results [15], or combinatorial optimization [7,11]. While it has been proposed in the literature [5], to the best of our knowledge, no top-K algorithm specifically designed for stochastically known logs has been presented yet. The work of Pegoraro et al. [13] could be implicitly considered as a computation for the top-K realizations of a trace, but in essence it is an inefficient brute force method. Gal proposed an efficient top-K ranking algorithm for stochastically known logs relying on [7], where a generalized top-K ranking procedure for combinatorial optimization problems is presented. Bogdanov et al. [2] present SKTR, a technique that retrieves a top-1 realization of a stochastically known trace using a specially constructed graph where the paths correspond to the realizations of the stochastically known trace and the edge weights are determined based on a cost function that considers (dependent) event realization probabilities and conformance to a reference process model. The application of a K shortest paths algorithm (e.g., [6]) on the graph could result in top-K ranking on the trace level. More generally, a wide range of existing top-K algorithms for various combinatorial problems could be adapted for uncertain event data by mapping it to structure of such problems, e.g., as has been suggested for assignment ranking algorithms [5].

4   Top-K Realization Ranking

To investigate the potential of top-K rankings for uncertainty-aware process mining, we first design an algorithm to efficiently calculate the top-K realization of a stochastically known event log. An intuitive approach is to first calculate all possible realizations, and then sort the results by probability to retrieve the top-K realizations. However, since the number of possible realizations grows exponentially with the number of events in the log, this approach is affected by exponential complexity. Another approach would be adapting one of the approaches summarized in Sect. 3. These approaches impose constraints in terms of dependent probabilities, generation rules or reference process models. These constraints generally make the resulting top-K rankings more accurate because they exclude realizations that are irrelevant or meaningless in the analysis context, and thereby concentrate the probability mass among fewer realizations, which is highly beneficial for using the resulting rankings. However, in this paper, we employ a basic algorithm operating under the assumption of event independence. This is done to explore the general utility of top-K rankings for uncertain event data. Our goal is to demonstrate that even under the independence assumption, top-K rankings outperform top-1 interpretations – this would also indicate that approaches that produce more refined top-K rankings will likely offer further advantages.

In the following, we present an efficient algorithm which is based on a generalized ranking procedure from the literature [7], addressing **RQ1**. This algorithm is then used to evaluate the benefit of the produced top-K rankings to address **RQ2** and **RQ3**.

4.1   Top-K Ranking Algorithm

First, the generalized terms for top-K problems from [7] are introduced. Hamacher and Queyranne [7] define a top-K ranking as follows:

Definition 6 (Top-K ranking). *Let $\mathcal{D}$ be a set. Let $K \in \{1, \dots, |\mathcal{D}|\}$. Let $c : \mathcal{D} \to \mathbb{R}$. Then, $D_1, \dots, D_K$ is a top-K ranking iff $\forall_{D \in \mathcal{D} \setminus \{D_1, \dots, D_K\}} \, c(D_1) \leq \dots \leq c(D_K) \leq c(D)$.*

Based on this, Hamacher and Queyranne define the general structure of a top-K problem as a set of feasible solutions:

Definition 7 (Feasible solutions [7]). *Let E be a finite set and let $\mathcal{D} \subseteq 2^E$ be a set of subsets of E. We refer to the elements $e \in E$ as choices, and to the elements $D \in \mathcal{D}$ as (feasible) solutions. For any $I, O \subseteq E$ with $I \cap O = \varnothing$, $\mathcal{D}_{I,O} = \{D \in \mathcal{D} \mid I \subseteq D \wedge D \cap O = \varnothing\}$ is the set of feasible solutions restricted by I and O.*

Hamacher and Queyranne present a generalized algorithm, called the BST procedure, that iteratively partitions the set of possible log realizations [7]. This reduces the problem to a set of sub-problems, for which two auxiliary algorithms are required: (1) `ALG-1P` that yields the globally best solution and (2) `ALG-R2P` that yields the (locally) second best solution within a restricted solution set $\mathcal{D}_{I,O}$. We apply this procedure to design an algorithm for the top-K realizations problem for stochastically known logs, which is defined as follows.

Definition 8 (Realization ranking problem). *Let $\tilde{L}$ be a stochastically known log. Let $E = \bigcup_{\tilde{e}_i \in \tilde{L}} R(\tilde{e}_i)$ be the set of choices, and $\mathcal{D} = R(\tilde{L})$ be the set of feasible solutions of the top-K realizations problem. Then, $L_1, \dots, L_K$ is a top-K ranking iff $\forall_{L \in \mathcal{D} \setminus \{L_1, \dots, L_K\}} P(L_1) \geq \dots \geq P(L_K) \geq P(L)$, with L_i being the realization having rank i.*

Because the goal of our algorithm is to *maximize* the realization probability the comparison operators in the ranking are flipped with respect to Definition 6. Next, `ALG-1P` and `ALG-R2P` algorithms for the realization ranking problem are presented. Under *event independence*, the globally best log realization $L_1 \in R(\tilde{L})$ is the log realization where each stochastically known event $\tilde{e}_i \in \tilde{L}$ is realized as its most probable alternative [2], so $\text{ALG-1P}(\tilde{L}) = \bigcup_{\tilde{e}_i \in \tilde{L}} \arg\max_{e_i \in R(\tilde{e}_i)} P(e_i)$. For `ALG-R2P`, the following property of the realization ranking problem is shown:

Lemma 1. *For all $\mathcal{D}_{I,O} \subseteq \mathcal{D}$, if a second best solution $L_q^2 \in \mathcal{D}_{I,O}$ with $q \in \{1, \dots, K\}$ exists, there always exists a second best solution $L' \in \mathcal{D}_{I,O}$ that is different from the best solution $L_q \in \mathcal{D}_{I,O}$ in exactly one element, i.e., $|L' \setminus L_q| = |L_q \setminus L'| = 1$.*

Proof. Let $L_q \in \mathcal{D}_{I,O}$ be a best solution in a restricted set of feasible solutions, and $L_q^2 \in \mathcal{D}_{I,O}$ be a second best solution with $|L_q^2 \setminus L_q| = |L_q \setminus L_q^2| > 1$. Without loss of generality, selecting any $e_i' \in L_q^2 \setminus L_q$ enables constructing a new solution $L' = (L_q \setminus \{e_i\}) \cup \{e_i'\}$, where clearly $|L' \setminus L_q| = |L_q \setminus L'| = 1$. Because it is constructed only out of choices from the valid solutions

---

Algorithm 1: ALG-R2P

Data: $\tilde{L}, I, O, L_q$
Result: L_q^2

1 $\rho_{max} \leftarrow 0$
2 **for** $e_i \in L_q \setminus I$ **do**
3 $\quad$ $e_i' \leftarrow \text{next}_{\tilde{L}}(e_i, \tilde{e}_i)$
4 $\quad$ **if** $e_i' \in R(\tilde{e}_i) \setminus O$ **then**
5 $\quad\quad$ $\rho_i \leftarrow \dfrac{P(e_i')}{P(e_i)}$
6 $\quad\quad$ **if** $\rho_i > \rho_{max}$ **then**
7 $\quad\quad\quad$ $\rho_{max} \leftarrow \rho_i$
8 $\quad\quad\quad$ $e_{max} \leftarrow e_i$
9 $\quad\quad\quad$ $e_{max}' \leftarrow e_i'$
10 $\quad\quad$ **end**
11 $\quad$ **end**
12 **end**
13 $L_q^2 \leftarrow (L_q \setminus \{e_{max}\}) \cup \{e_{max}'\}$
14 **return** L_q^2

L_q and L_q^2, L' is also valid in $\mathcal{D}_{I,O}$. The constructed solution L' substitutes one element in L_q, so $P(L')$ can be rewritten as $P(L') = P(L_q) \cdot \dfrac{P(e_i')}{P(e_i)}$. As $e_i \in L_q$ is a choice within the best solution, it is the most probable event realization, i.e., $P(e_i) \geq P(e_i')$, which implies $P(L_q) \geq P(L')$. By substituting the other elements out of $L_q^2 \setminus L_q$, the solution $(L_q \setminus (L_q \setminus L_q^2)) \cup (L_q^2 \setminus L_q) = L_q^2$ can be constructed step-wise from L_q. Through transitivity this implies $P(L_q) \geq P(L') \geq P(L_q^2)$.

Using Lemma 1, the set of candidates for a restricted second best solution can be limited to the solutions in $\mathcal{D}_{I,O}$ that are different from the best solution in exactly one choice. This is used to devise an algorithm ALG-R2P (where for any $\tilde{e}_i \in \tilde{L}$, $\text{next}_{\tilde{l}}(e_i, \tilde{e}_i)$ returns the next best event realization that is allowed in the current $\mathcal{D}_{I,O}$), which is shown in Algorithm 1. ALG-R2P compares the candidate solutions by (1) selecting an event realization e_i in the best solution L_q, (2) retrieving its next best realization $e_i' \in R(\tilde{e}_i)$, and (3) calculating the substitution probability ratio $\rho_i = \frac{P(e_i')}{P(e_i)}$. Then, the second best solution L_q^2 is the candidate solution with the highest substitution probability ratio ρ_i.

These auxiliary algorithms are used with the BST procedure from [7] to calculate the top-K realizations of stochastically known logs. Note that this algorithm combining event realizations under event independence is practically identical to an algorithm combining trace-level top-K rankings into a log-level top-K ranking under trace independence. Thus, it could also be used to join the results of more refined trace-level top-K techniques.

5   Evaluation

We evaluate the efficiency of the algorithm and the benefit of the top-K rankings it produces in the following steps:

- **EVAL1** (Efficiency): Does the algorithm improve the complexity bound, and which parameters affect the execution time? (**RQ1**)
- **EVAL2** (Sensitivity Analysis): How are the results affected by different properties of the input data? (**RQ2, RQ3**)

5.1   EVAL1: Efficiency

For EVAL1, we formally prove an upper bound for the complexity of the algorithm, starting with the auxiliary algorithms.

Lemma 2. *ALG-1P is bounded by* $O(|\tilde{L}|)$

Proof. ALG-1P selects the most probable realization for each stochastically known event $\tilde{e}_i \in \tilde{L}$, so it performs $|\tilde{L}|$ selections. As the event realizations are sorted by probability, each selection is in $O(1)$, so ALG-1P is bounded by $O(|\tilde{L}|)$.

Lemma 3. *ALG-R2P is bounded by* $O(|\tilde{L}|)$.

Proof. For each stochastically known event in $\tilde{e}_i \in \tilde{L}$, so $|\tilde{L}|$ times, ALG-R2P (1) retrieves the next best event realization with $\text{next}_L(e_i, \tilde{e}_i)$, (2) calculates ρ_i ($O(1)$) and (3) compares ρ_i to ρ_{max} ($O(1)$). Consequently, the ALG-R2P is bounded by $O(|\tilde{L}| \cdot M)$ where M is the complexity of $\text{next}_L(e_i, \tilde{e}_i)$. Because the event realizations are ranked by probability, the next best event realization is simply the next element in this events' list of realizations, making $M \in O(1)$. Then, algorithm ALG-R2P is bounded by $O(|\tilde{L}|)$.

Lemma 4. *The top-K realizations algorithm is bounded by $O(K \cdot |\tilde{L}|)$.*

Proof. Hamacher and Queyranne show that the complexity of an algorithm derived from the BST procedure is in $O(C(m)+(K-1)\cdot B(m))$ where $C(m)$ is the complexity of `ALG-1P` and $B(m)$ is the complexity of `ALG-R2P` [7]. With Lemmas 2 and 3 follows that the full algorithm is in $O(|\tilde{L}| + (K-1) \cdot |\tilde{L}|) = O(K \cdot |\tilde{L}|)$.

This proof formally shows the efficiency of the algorithm compared to the exponential complexity of a brute force solution. Notably, the runtime is affected only by the number of events $|\tilde{L}|$ and the number of realizations to calculate K.

5.2   EVAL2: Sensitivity Analysis

In EVAL2, we analyze the benefit of top-K rankings over top-1 interpretations. For this, the effect of different properties of the stochastically known event logs on the distribution of probabilities in the ranking (**RQ2**) and the variability of the calculated realizations (**RQ3**) is analyzed. The implementation of the algorithm and the code to reproduce the evaluation results are available on GitHub[1].

Simulation. To examine the effect of different properties of the input data, stochastically known event logs are simulated based on a modified version of the simulation procedure from [4]. First, n_{events} events with random activity labels are generated. Then, uncertainty is introduced into $\lfloor r \cdot n_{events} \rfloor$ randomly selected events. Each uncertain event is simulated by picking n_{act} alternative activity realizations, and assigning probabilities based on the parameter β. The probability of the first activity p_1 is set to 1, and the following probabilities are generated recursively with $p_{i+1} = p_i \cdot \beta \cdot rand_i$ where each $rand_i$ is a uniformly random value in the range $[0.9, 1.1]$. Finally, the probability values are normalized to have a sum of 1 for each event.

Effect of the Simulation Parameters. This simulation procedure is used to evaluate the effect of a varying degree of uncertainty in the input data on the resulting top-K ranking. To characterize a top-K ranking, the following measures are used:

Definition 9 (Measures). *Let $L_1, \ldots, L_K$ be a top-K ranking. Then, $F_K(k) = \sum_{i=1}^{k} P(L_i)$ is the cumulative probability, and $d_{avg} = K^{-1} \cdot \sum_{L \in \{L_2,\ldots,L_K\}} |L \backslash L_1|$ is the average number of choices different to the best realization.*

Additionally, the run-time of the algorithm t is measured in seconds. In the following, the effect of the different simulation parameters (properties of the input event logs) and values of K on these measures is evaluated. This is done systematically by varying each parameter separately while keeping the other parameters fixed. All tests were executed on a computer with an Apple M2 Pro and 16 GiB memory, and the measures were averaged over 10 runs.

---

[1] https://github.com/arvidle/topK_realizations.

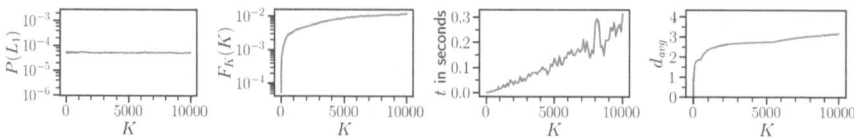

Fig. 1. Ranking measures $P(L_1)$, $F_K(K)$, t and d_{avg} for varying K. ($n_{events} = 100$, $r = 0.3$, $n_{act} = 3$ and $\beta = 0.3$; log-scaled y-axis for $P(L_1)$ and $F_K(K)$)

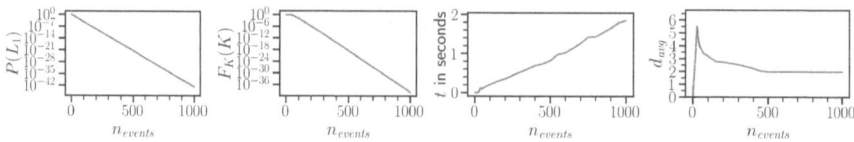

Fig. 2. Ranking measures $P(L_1)$, $F_K(K)$, t and d_{avg} for varying n_{events}. ($r = 0.3$, $n_{act} = 3$, $\beta = 0.3$ and $K = 10^4$; log-scaled y-axis for $P(L_1)$ and $F_K(K)$)

First, the effect of K is examined by fixing $n_{events} = 100$, $r = 0.3$, $n_{act} = 3$ and $\beta = 0.3$ (Fig. 1). Because K is not a simulation parameter, $P(L_1)$ is constant except for small variations due to noise occurring during simulation. The cumulative probability of the ranking $F_K(K)$ first increases sharply with K, but because the probabilities in the ranking are monotonically decreasing, the growth of $F_K(K)$ slows considerably with increasing K. The run-time of the algorithm scales linearly with K. The average difference d_{avg} also increases first, but slowly converges to a value just above 3. At certain points, almost all realizations different to the top-1 realization in 1, 2 and 3 choices are contained in the ranking. This causes sudden increases of the growth of d_{avg}.

Next, the effect of n_{events} is evaluated with $n_{act} = 3$, $r = 0.3$, $\beta = 0.3$ and $K = 10^4$ (Fig. 2). Both the top-1 probability $P(L_1)$ and cumulative probability $F_K(K)$ decrease exponentially with increasing values of n_{events}. The run-time t increases linearly with increasing n_{events}. The average difference d_{avg} spikes at $n_{events} = 31$, then decreases and plateaus around a value of 2. A low number of events forces the algorithm to choose more different realizations because the realizations which are similar to L_1 are exhausted. This effect changes if more events are affected by uncertainty since the number of highly similar realizations increases rapidly with event log length. The increase of the uncertainty threshold r results in the same effects as varying n_{events}. Thus, a separate evaluation of the effect of varying r is omitted.

Then, the number of alternatives for each stochastically known event n_{act} is evaluated for $n_{events} = 100$, $r = 0.3$, $\beta = 0.3$ and $K = 10^4$ (Fig. 3). Both $P(L_1)$ and $F_K(K)$ decrease with increasing values of n_{act}. Because the probabilities inside each event must sum up to 1, with higher number of alternatives, the probability is distributed among more alternatives (and the number of possible realizations increases significantly), making all outcomes less probable. The run-time of the algorithm is constant with respect to n_{act}. For lower values of n_{act},

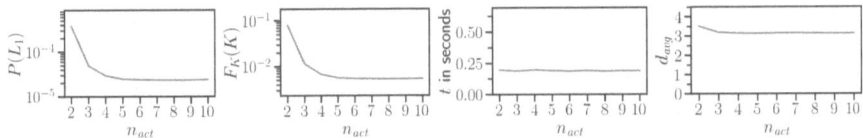

Fig. 3. Ranking measures $P(L_1)$, $F_K(K)$, t and d_{avg} for varying n_{act}. ($n_{events} = 100$, $r = 0.3$, $\beta = 0.3$ and $K = 10^4$; log-scaled y-axis for $P(L_1)$ and $F_K(K)$)

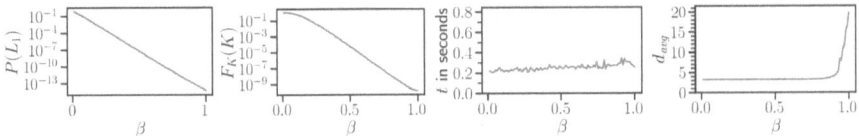

Fig. 4. Ranking measures $P(L_1)$, $F_K(K)$, t and d_{avg} for varying β. ($n_{events} = 100$, $r = 0.3$, $n_{act} = 3$ and $K = 10^4$; log-scaled y-axis for $P(L_1)$ and $F_K(K)$)

d_{avg} slightly elevates because it is more likely that the alternatives of an event have all been picked and thus another event needs to be changed to generate new candidates for the next best solution.

Finally, the effect of β is evaluated with $n_{events} = 100$, $r = 0.3$, $n_{act} = 3$ and $K = 10^4$ (Fig. 4). $P(L_1)$ and $F_K(K)$ both decrease for increasing values of β, i.e., less skewed event probability distributions. The run-time of the algorithm is largely constant with respect to β. The average difference d_{avg} is unaffected up to $\beta = 0.8$ and then increases sharply. Because the probability values of the event alternatives are very similar at this point, there are many different realizations having nearly equal probabilities.

5.3   Discussion

Overall, the sensitivity analysis confirms that the run-time of the algorithm scales linearly with both n_{events} and K. Even for larger optimization problems ($n_{events} = 1000$, $K = 10^4$), the algorithm calculates a top-K ranking in around 2 s, confirming its efficiency. To further evaluate the efficiency of the algorithm, it was applied to two uncertain event logs presented in [3]. The calculation of the top-10^4 realizations took 0.366 and 0.505 seconds respectively (33.5 and 43.16 seconds for top-10^6). For comparison, we implemented a baseline approach as described in Sect. 4. While this baseline algorithm performs reasonably well for smaller logs (e.g., $5.7s$ for $n_{events} = 40$, $n_{act} = 3$, $K = 10^4$), its run-time and memory requirements scale exponentially, making its application infeasible for larger input logs. In fact, the baseline algorithm was unable to calculate rankings for the logs from [3] because of memory limitations. Generally, additional realizations can be produced significantly faster by our algorithm than they can be processed, e.g., using process discovery algorithms. Thus, the algorithm shows how top-K rankings can be calculated efficiently, giving an answer to **RQ1**.

Regarding **RQ2**, we evaluated the top-1 probability $P(L_1)$ and the cumulative probability $F_K(K)$. Both decrease rapidly with increasing uncertainty and size of the input event log. Consequently, a direct application of the top-K algorithm to cover a representative set of the realizations by probability is only sensible for small log sizes (see Fig. 2b). For instance, a top-10^4 ranking of event logs simulated with $n_{events} = 50$, $n_{act} = 3$, $\beta = 0.3$ and $r = 0.3$ on average covers about 53% of the realizations by probability with 0.07% of the $1.43 \cdot 10^7$ possible realizations. However, even for larger and more uncertain event logs, top-K interpretations are beneficial over the most probable realization, with $F_K(K)$ being consistently larger than $P(L_1)$ by around 3 orders of magnitude for $K = 10^4$. From this, we conclude that the challenge of exponentially decreasing probabilities is not specific to top-K interpretations, but rather a general challenge when handling uncertain event data. The diminishing returns for $F_K(K)$ with increasing K constitute another challenge – an increase in uncertainty or size of the input event log cannot be compensated with a proportional increase of K.

For **RQ3**, we observe that low values result for d_{avg} (≤ 4 for sensible parameters). Because the realizations of even a small event log (e.g., 100 events) differ only slightly, the information gain of a top-K ranking in terms of the variability of the realizations appears limited for sensible values of K.

In summary, the benefit of top-K realizations is most pronounced for smaller event logs and logs with low degrees of uncertainty. However, even for larger event logs, top-K rankings consistently provide a benefit over top-1 interpretations.

6   Conclusion

In this paper, we presented an algorithm to compute the top-K most probable realizations of stochastically known event logs. We also evaluated the benefit of top-K rankings against top-1 interpretations of stochastically known event logs. We formally proved that our algorithm operates within a computational complexity of $O(K \cdot |\tilde{L}|)$ (see EVAL1), which builds a foundation for future research on uncertainty-aware process mining techniques. We also showed that top-K interpretations of stochastically known event logs provide a benefit over using the single most probable realization, especially for smaller logs or isolated cases of larger event logs with moderate incidences of uncertainty (see EVAL2).

To allow wider application of top-K rankings in process mining on uncertain event data, the incorporation of more complex event and trace dependencies into our algorithm constitutes an avenue for future research. Secondly, in order to improve the variability of the realizations, the algorithm could be extended with techniques to diversify its outputs [15].

Acknowledgments. This project has received funding from the Federal Ministry for Economic Affairs and Climate Action under the Marispace-X project grant no. 68GX21002E, the State of Schleswig-Holstein under the Datencampus project grant no. 220 21 016, and from the German Research Foundation (DFG) for the SPP 2422. The project ProcessPig is funded by the European Union within the framework of the European Innovation Partnership (EIP-AGRI) and the state program rural areas of the state Schleswig-Holstein (LPLR) (www.eip-agrar-sh.de). We thank the Alexander von Humboldt (AvH) Stiftung for supporting our research. We thank Dr. med. Volker Kattner for the inspiration of the introductory example.

References

1. van der Aalst, W., et al.: Process mining manifesto. In: BPM 2011 Workshops. LNBIP, vol. 99, pp. 169–194. Springer, Heidelberg (2012)
2. Bogdanov, E., Cohen, I., Gal, A.: SKTR: trace recovery from stochastically known logs. In: ICPM 2023, Rome, Italy, pp. 49–56. IEEE (2023)
3. Engelberg, G., et al.: An uncertainty-aware event log of network traffic. In: BPM 2023 Demos, vol. 3469. CEUR-WS.org (2023)
4. Felli, P., et al.: Multi-perspective conformance checking of uncertain process traces: an SMT-based approach. Eng. Appl. Artif. Intell. **126**, 106895 (2023)
5. Gal, A.: Everything there is to know about stochastically known logs. In: ICPM 2023, Rome, Italy, pp. xvii–xxiii. IEEE (2023)
6. Gao, J., et al.: Fast top-k simple shortest paths discovery in graphs. In: CIKM 2010, Toronto, Canada, pp. 509–518. ACM (2010)
7. Hamacher, H.W., Queyranne, M.: K best solutions to combinatorial optimization problems. Ann. Oper. Res. **4**(1), 123–143 (1985)
8. Kecht, C., et al.: Event log construction from customer service conversations using natural language inference. In: ICPM 2021, Eindhoven, Netherlands, pp. 144–151. IEEE (2021)
9. Koschmider, A., et al.: Process mining for unstructured data: challenges and research directions. In: Modellierung 2024, Bonn. LNI, vol. P348, pp. 119–136. GI (2024)
10. Lepsien, A., Koschmider, A., Kratsch, W.: Analytics pipeline for process mining on video data. In: BPM 2023 Forum. LNBIP, vol. 490, pp. 196–213. Springer, Cham (2023)
11. Pascoal, M., Captivo, M.E., Clímaco, J.: A note on a new variant of Murty's ranking assignments algorithm. Q. J. Belg. Fr. Ital. Oper. Res. Soc. **1**(3), 243–255 (2003)
12. Pegoraro, M.: Probabilistic and non-deterministic event data in process mining: embedding uncertainty in process analysis techniques. In: CAiSE 2022 Doctoral Consortium. CEUR-WS, Leuven, Belgium, vol. 3139, pp. 37–46. CEUR-WS.org (2022)
13. Pegoraro, M., Bakullari, B., Uysal, M.S., van der Aalst, W.M.P.: Probability estimation of uncertain process trace realizations. In: ICPM 2021 Workshops. LNBIP, vol. 433, pp. 21–33. Springer, Cham (2022)
14. Pegoraro, M., Uysal, M.S., van der Aalst, W.M.P.: Conformance checking over uncertain event data. Inf. Syst. **102**, 101810 (2021)
15. Qin, L., Yu, J.X., Chang, L.: Diversifying top-k results. Proc. VLDB Endow. **5**(11), 1124–1135 (2012)
16. Soliman, M.A., Ilyas, I.F., Chang, K.C.C.: Probabilistic top-k and ranking-aggregate queries. ACM Trans. Datab. Syst. **33**(3), 13:1–13:54 (2008)

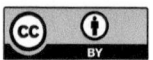

Framework for Extracting Real-World Object-Centric Event Logs from Game Data

Lukas Liss[1]([✉])(iD), Nico Elbert[2](iD), Christoph M. Flath[2](iD),
and Wil M. P. van der Aalst[1](iD)

[1] RWTH Aachen University, Aachen, Germany
{liss,wvdaalst}@pads.rwth-aachen.de
[2] Julius Maximillians Universität Würzburg, Würzburg, Germany
{nico.elbert,christoph.flath}@uni-wuerzburg.de

Abstract. In recent years, process mining has shifted towards an object-centric perspective on processes, considering interacting sub-processes that operate on objects from different types. Since businesses are hesitant to publicly share such event data that may expose business internals, there is a lack of public real-world object-centric event logs. We propose a novel approach to use publicly accessible game data as a large-scale data source for object-centric event logs. The contributions of this paper include (1) a framework to extract object-centric event logs from real-time strategy game data, (2) an application of that framework for the game Age of Empires II, (3) a published Python library to automatically transform Age of Empire gameplays into an object-centric event log, (4) a publicly accessible object-centric event log extracted from 325,398 gameplays, and (5) an evaluation of the published *aoe2pm* library. The evaluation shows that the extracted event logs can be used by state-of-the-art applications to generate relevant behavior insights that require an object-centric perspective. The size and attribute richness of the object-centric event log motivate future research questions in the field of object-centric process mining.

Keywords: Object-centric Event Data · Data Extraction · Process Mining

1 Introduction

Publicly accessible datasets are essential for process mining research [20]. Process mining analyzes event data to generate insights into processes. Typical process mining pipelines span discovery, conformance checking, and enhancement. Event data are an essential input for most process mining algorithms in each of these steps. The recent increased interest in machine learning applications in the field of process mining amplifies the need for even larger datasets further [5,11].

In recent years, a new perspective on processes gained traction in process mining research, namely object-centric process mining [22]. In object-centric

A. Delgado and T. Slaats (Eds.): ICPM 2024 Workshops, LNBIP 533, pp. 363–375, 2025.
https://doi.org/10.1007/978-3-031-82225-4_27

process mining a process can consist of interacting sub processes that operate on multiple objects of different types. In a hospital process, for example, an object-centric process can contain the behavior of the patients as well as the behavior of the doctors. Where some events like an *operation* involve both doctor and patient objects, other events like *sit in waiting room* may only involve objects of type patient. Traditional process mining assumes a single case identifier, limiting the perspective to one entity, for example, the patient or the doctor.

To support a holistic object-centric perspective on processes, new data formats like OCEL 2.0 [3] or event graphs [9] for object-centric event logs have been proposed. Because of this holistic view, companies may hesitate to publish real-world object-centric event logs possibly revealing process internals. Due to this and the novelty of object-centric event log formats, real-world object-centric event logs are very limited.

As further elaborated in Subsect. 3.2, real-time strategy (RTS) games share many characteristics that are essential for business processes like goal orientation, competitive behavior, efficient resource utilization, striving for automation, and human errors [8]. Thus, we advocate the use of RTS game data to close the gap of missing object-centric event data. This game category includes popular games such as *Starcraft 2*, AOE2, *Northgard*, or *Dune: Spice Wars*. Most games allow the export of gameplays, and there exist special community-driven websites where players publish their game data to compare themselves with other players.

Individuals are more willing to share their process data publicly than companies are, especially in the context of games, which is why multiple research domains like machine learning utilized game data as a source for large-scale datasets and scalability research [7]. To the best of our knowledge, game data has not yet been used to create object-centric event logs.

Since process mining is especially interested in the dynamic behavior between people, objects, and systems, publicly accessible object-centric event logs with real human involvement are essential for developing and evaluating process mining methods. Event logs from RTS game data can contribute to this.

This paper presents five contributions to enable the usage of game data in object-centric process mining. First, we propose a framework to extract object-centric event logs from RTS games. Second, we apply the framework to the game *Age of Empires II* (AOE2). Third, we provide a publicly accessible python library ($aoe2pm^1$) that transform exported AOE2 game data to object-centric event logs. Fourth, we published an object-centric event log[2] extracted from 325,398 AOE2 matches sourced from community websites. Fifth, we perform a quantitative and qualitative evaluation of the framework using *aoe2pm*, showing that the object-centric event logs are compatible with academic and commercial state-of-the-art object-centric algorithms, resulting in relevant process insights.

---

[1] https://github.com/nicoelbert/aoe2PM/releases/tag/v1.0.1.

[2] https://doi.org/10.5281/zenodo.11506365.

2   Related Work

Process mining analyzes event data to provide process-related insights. This spans process discovery, conformance checking, and enhancement [20]. The starting point for most process mining approaches is an event log that captures the events happening in the context of a given process. Traditional process mining assumes a single case identifier for a process, limiting the perspective to the chosen case identifier. Real-world processes tend to consist of multiple sub process that interact with each other and involve multiple object from various types. To represent these interacting multi-object processes, process mining shifted towards object-centric process mining in recent years [22]. Object-centric process mining allows events to involve multiple objects of different types. There are object-centric event formats like event graphs [9] and OCEL 2.0 [3].

Currently, there are two types of object-centric event data extractors. Some work on relational databases commonly used in ERP systems [16,23], and others take traditional event logs and transform them into object-centric event logs [18]. Both approaches do not work on game data logs. Also, both approaches are not designed to add the relevant game logic-based events, which are missing in the gameplay exports as described in Subsect. 3.2. Thus, even when transforming the input format, resulting event logs would be limited to player-based events only. To overcome this limitation, we propose a framework to extract object-centric event data from real-time strategy (RTS) games.

Another approach to creating event logs is to use process simulation [17, 19]. For traditional process mining, there exist multiple approaches that use simulation to create event logs [13,21]. Esser and Fahland [9,10] and Rebmann et al. [18] transformed traditional event logs into object-centric representations. Knopp et al. proposed an approach to create object-centric simulation models [14]. However, simulated event logs can only recreate behavior and do not contain real-world behavior directly.

To overcome the challenges posed by the limited data availability, researchers increasingly leverage competitive online games as an alternative source. Such game data offer large-scale publicly available data that captures human behavior within a naturalistic setting [6]. Driven by personal and intrinsic motivation, players exhibit highly rational decision-making and develop behavioral patterns that are adapted to changing environments. Players engage in long-term skill learning to optimize their performance [12]. Given the setting, they collaborate within intricate organizational and social structures and take on specialized roles essential for individual or collective success. Approaches to utilize this source of process data are so far missing.

3   Background

This section describes object-centric event logs and RTS games that serve as the background for the proposed framework.

3.1 Object Centric Event Data

We use the OCEL 2.0 standard for object-centric event data [3]. Once the process is stored in that format, a variety of tools using that standard can be applied for the analysis [1,4]. Events are activities that happen at a timestamp for a set of objects of different types. $\mathbb{U}_{event}$ is the universe of event identifiers. The universe $\mathbb{U}_{act}$ contains all visible activities. $\mathbb{U}_{type}$ is the universe of all object types. The universe of objects is $\mathbb{U}_{obj}$. Each object has exactly one type associated with it $\pi_{type} : \mathbb{U}_{obj} \to \mathbb{U}_{type}$. The universe of qualifiers for object-to-object relations is $\mathbb{U}_{qual}$. $\mathbb{U}_{time}$ is the universe of all timestamps. Objects have attributes that can change their values over time. Definition 1 describes the minimal set of features needed for our object-centric event logs. Note that additional OCEL 2.0 features are not considered here.

Definition 1 (Object-Centric Event Log). $L = (E, O, OT, O2O, \pi_{act}, \pi_{obj}, \pi_{time})$ *is an object-centric event log where:*

- $E \subseteq \mathbb{U}_{event}$ *is a set of events,* $O \subseteq \mathbb{U}_{obj}$ *is a set of objects,*
- $OT = \{\pi_{type}(o) | o \in O\}$ *is a set of object types,*
- $O2O \subseteq \{(o_1, o_2, q) | q \in \mathbb{U}_{qual} \land o_1, o_2 \in O \land o_1 \neq o_2\}$ *is the set of qualified object to object relations,*
- $\pi_{act} : E \to \mathbb{U}_{act}$ *maps each event to an activity,*
- $\pi_{obj} : E \to \mathcal{P}(\mathbb{U}_{obj}) \setminus \{\emptyset\}$ *maps each event to at least one object,*
- $\pi_{time} : E \to \mathbb{U}_{time}$ *maps each event to a timestamp*

3.2 Real-Time Strategy Games

In this subsection, we show why the structure of RTS games naturally facilitates in object centric processes and discuss to what extent RTS games can serve as an approximation for business processes.

In their complexity, RTS interactions are comparable to many real-world problems [2] and allow the observation of human behavior in a naturalistic environment over extended time periods [6]. Business processes are goal-orientated sequences of actions that utilize resources to reach their goal. They often strive for continuous improvement under the constraints of compliance with regulatory rules [8]. This is similar in RTS games, where players must organize and build a micro economy with the goal to outperform their opponents. They have a finite set of actions they can strategically perform and the conditions for winning are well-defined. Players are bound to the rules of the games, but driven by competitive motivation [12], they strive to optimize their performance and decision-making and thus their process. Therefore, similar KPIs are relevant for business processes and RTS games. As stated in Sect. 1, the waiting time of resources and the degree of automation are examples of that. In addition, both business processes and RTS games are based on human behavior and thus incorporate for example human errors. This makes them interesting to investigate from a behavioral point of view.

RTS games have a common structure of game objects and event types, shown in Fig. 1. Each match consists of multiple players that orchestrate working units to create structures and collect natural resources. A session is connected to all events happening on a player's computer in one match. Players create and manage their micro organization of structures and units with the goal of producing more resources than their opponents. The process of creating and managing this micro organization involves multiple objects of different types. Players strive to analyze and optimize this process to outperform their opponents. Popular games following this RTS game structure include, for example, *Starcraft 2*, AOE2, *Northgard*, or *Dune* with millions of players. Unlike turn-based games like chess, RTS games operate on a continuous time granularity [15]. There are player-based events that are triggered by the player and game logic-based events that are triggered by the game. Both types of events can contain multiple game objects of different types. For example, one player can use three units to build a structure. To represent these object interactions and avoid information loss due to convergence, divergence, or deficiency, an object-centric process notion is required [22].

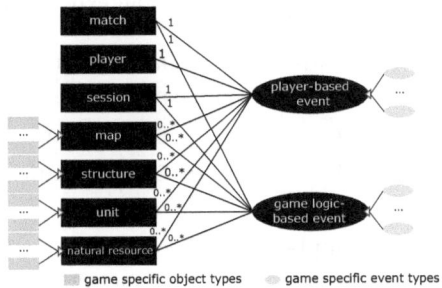

Fig. 1. Object types (boxes) and event types (ellipses) in RTS games.

3.3   Game Export Format

Each match is exported separately in a so called compressed action log file. To save memory, this file only contains player-based events since game logic-based events can be recreated by the game engine. The file contains the user inputs and relates them to involved objects. Each RTS game with an export function must export at least this information to be able to replay the game. Figure 2 shows an example exported compressed action log for AOE2 showing the user input. The event and object information from Fig. 2 are structured and summarized in Table 1.

Input(timestamp='0:0:30', type='Queue', param='Villager', payload={'building_id': 70, 'object_ids': [1001, 1002, 1003], 'amount': '3'}, player=P1, position=(x=30, y=50))

Input(timestamp='0:1:05', type='Build', param='House', payload={'object_ids': [1001, 1004], 'building': 'House'}, player=P1, position=(x=45, y=60))

Input(timestamp='0:1:20', type='Gather Point', param='Wood', payload={}, player=P1, position=(x=25, y=55))

Fig. 2. Example of an exported compressed action log from AOE2.

Table 1. Example of an exported compressed action log from AOE2.

Player ID	Timestamp	Action	Object ID	Position
1	00:00:30	Queue Villager	1001, 1002, 1003	(30, 50)
1	00:01:05	Build House	1004, 1001	(45, 60)
1	00:01:20	Set Gather Point		(25, 55)

An example of such a compressed action log for the game AOE2 can be seen in Table 1. There, player 1 first queues three villagers, who are the workforce resource in AOE2, then builds a house with one of the villagers and sets a gather point. These gather points in AOE2 are a way to automatically assign tasks to idle villagers to go and gather wood. To investigate relevant process KPIs like waiting time of resources or degree of automation, accessing only the player related events is not enough. For example, in Table 1, the waiting time of a villager before building a house seems to be 35 s. However, resources like villagers are not immediately available after being queued. Villagers are created (spawned) one by one after 30 s each by the game engine. Since that event is triggered by the game engine and not the player, it is not recorded in the compressed action log. The correct waiting time for the resource villager before building the house would be 5 s, but to be able to correctly detect that, the game logic-based events are also required. Table 2 shows the desired object-centric event log for the example in Table 1 with the game logic-based events highlighted by colors. Without the game logic-based events, many relevant business process KPIs are misleading. Another example of that is the degree of automation. Without the game logic-based events, the degree of automation would always be 0 because we only see events that involve the player. Thus, players who use automation mechanisms like gathering points cannot be distinguished from players who do not. Therefore, extending the compressed action logs and then transforming them to an object-centric event data format is necessary to enable insightful process mining on game data.

Table 2. Desired object-centric event log for the example game recording in Table 1. Game logic-based events are colored based on our framework's type of game rule used to add them (orange = construction time, blue = unit queries, green = automation).

event id	activity	timestamp	object types			...
			player	villager	house	
e1	Queue Villager	17:00:30	p01	v01, v02, v03		
e2	Spawn Villager	17:01:00		v01		
e3	Command Build House	17:01:05	p01	v01	h01	
e4	Set ·Gather Point	17:01:20	p01			
e5	Spawn Villager	17:01:30		v02		
e6	Gather Wood	17:01:31		v02		
e7	Spawn Villager	17:02:00		v03		
e8	Gather Wood	17:02:01		v03		
e9	Complete House	17:06:05		v01	h01	

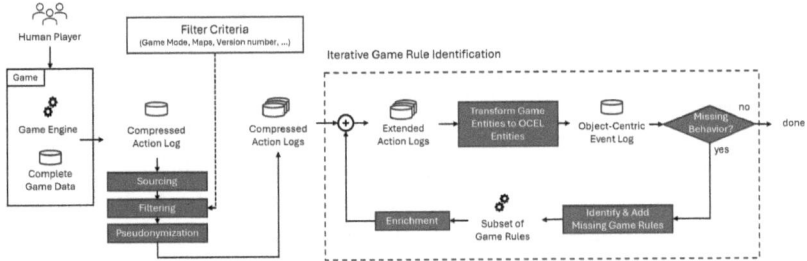

Fig. 3. Overview of the framework transforming RTS game data to object-centric logs.

4   Framework

This section outlines the framework for extracting object-centric event logs from RTS games, exporting gameplays in a compressed action log format that only contains player-based events. Figure 3 provides an overview.

Gameplay and Exporting: RTS game data originates from player interactions, resulting in compressed action logs, capturing real-world human behavior that shares key characteristics with business processes. RTS games export game interactions as compressed action logs that only contain player-based events to save memory as described in Subsect. 3.3.

Sourcing: To transform exported compressed action logs into an object-centric event log, game exports must first be collected. This sourcing step can be done through user studies, where selected participants play a controlled game setting, minimizing external influences but limiting event log size. Alternatively, pre-existing large-scale data from online communities, accessible via web scraping, can be used. There exist multiple community websites where RTS games upload game exports automatically or players upload them to compare themselves with others. Utilizing publicly available data enables the creation of large-scale event logs, capturing diverse player behaviors and strategies. The data source should be clearly indicated in the log metadata [6].

Filtering: Games vary in versions and settings, necessitating filtering of exported data to ensure consistent settings. Filter criteria should be documented.

Pseudonymization: In line with responsible data science, personal data in game replays must be pseudonymized, including clear text names and tags.

Enrichment: After filtering and pseudonymization, game data is enriched with inferred game logic-based events. This process involves iteratively adding game rules until the desired level of detail is achieved in the object-centric event log. Game rules are functions that extend action logs with game logic-based events such that the returned extended action log contains more events than before. The added game-logic based events are based on the player-based events. We identified three types of game rules: construction time rules, unit queue rules, and automation method rules. Additionally, game-specific extra rules can exist. Construction rules add events for structures that do not involve the player, for example when the construction is finished by the working units (see the orange events in Table 2). Units can be ordered in batches but are created (spawned) one after each other based on a production queue. These spawning events are added by unit queue rules that simulate the queuing (see the blue event in Table 2). RTS games offer automation methods that for example allow to assign idling units tasks automatically. For example, in AOE2, by setting gather points, which automatically sends workers to gather wood when they are free (see the green events in Table 2). The extended action logs are then transformed to an object-centric event log as described in the next step. If the resulting log contains all desired behavior, the framework ends, otherwise missing game rules are identified and added in each iteration until all desired behavior is covered.

Identify and Extract OCEL-Specific Entities and Relations: This step takes multiple action logs and returns an object-centric event log. This involves identifying events, objects, and their relationships in the game data, including event-to-object relations and object-to-object relations. The final output is an OCEL 2.0 format log, compatible with tools like pm4py [4] and ocpa [1]. The game-specific identification utilizes domain knowledge. For example, in AOE2, the activity name is split in the compressed action log. The first stored user input in Fig. 2 shows type *Queue* and param *Villager* which combined gives the activity name. Since identifiers for the events and objects are only unique within one action log, new globally unique identifiers are assigned to merge them into the object-centric event logs events E and objects O. The activity, object, and time mappings π_{act}, π_{obj}, and π_{time} for the events are adapted to the global identifiers. This mapping allows combining action logs into one cohesive OCEL 2.0 event log capturing all matches.

5   Implementation and Resulting Log for AOE2

This section describes the implementation of the framework for the game AOE2 and the resulting object-centric event log.

We applied our framework to the game AOE2, which resulted in a publicly accessible Python library *aoe2pm*. We chose AOE2 because it is one of the most established RTS games with well-organized community websites with publicly accessible compressed action logs (called .aoe2record files in AOE2). The library development followed the iterative framework presented in Fig. 4 to identify a suitable set of game rules for an authentic game state representation. For example, the initial iteration revealed missing behaviors for the working unit *villagers* as explained in the example in Subsect. 3.3. Thus, an according game rule was added to *aoe2pm* such that related game logic-based events are included in the resulting object-centric event log. The sum of all the added game rules allows *aoe2pm* to create logs that contain the desired game logic-based events that are highlighted by color in Table 2 and are required for meaningful insights.

Using a web scraper, we sourced 325,398 compressed action logs from AOE2 community websites. To keep the matches comparable, we filtered for uniform game versions and match settings, which resulted in 1,000 matches. Using our *aoe2pm* library, we processed these .aoe2record files into an object-centric event log in the OCEL 2.0 format that is publicly accessible. The event log consists of 262,994 events from 494 event types and 40,625 objects from 27 object types. Due to space limitations, we do not cover the concrete event types and their meaning in detail here. But the online description of the publicly accessible object-centric event log contains a detailed list with explanations.

6   Evaluation

First, we evaluate quantitatively the performance and correctness of the framework implementation for AOE2. Showing that *aoe2pm* is suitable for creating large scale event logs that can be used in research and industry tools. Second, we evaluate the usability of the resulting object-centric event log qualitatively. We compare the insights from the object-centric event log resulting from our framework, which contains game logic-based events, with the insights for a pure player-based event log. This shows the qualitative improvement for extracting RTS game logs with our approach over state of the art object-centric extractors that are limited to the directly logged player-based events.

Using the sourced AOE2 compressed game logs, we evaluated the runtime of *aoe2pm*. The runtime grows approximately linear with the number of compressed game log files. The average runtime was 6 s for 1 file, 74 s for 100 files, and 801 s for 1000 files on a machine with an Apple M3 processor and 16GM RAM, tacking the times five times per number of files. We imported the created event logs in pm4py [4] and ocpa [1] to validate the compatibility with state-of-the-art research libraries. As shown in Fig. 4, we uploaded the log to Celonis to validate the compatibility with industry tools using a publicly accessible upload script[3]. This shows that correctly formatted large-scale object-centric event logs can be created with *aoe2pm* on consumer hardware.

For the qualitative evaluation, we focused on two process metrics, namely the waiting time and the degree of automation. For both, we evaluate the importance of the game's logic-based events. An important object-centric process metric is the waiting time of resources before they are used. In AOE2, villagers are a good example of that because players want to utilize them as efficiently as possible to build as many structures like *Houses*, *Barracks*, or *Blacksmiths* as possible. Using discovery in Celonis, we created the object-centric directly follows graph one can see in Fig. 4. It shows the average waiting time of villagers before they start building structures. One can see that the two events before a villager starts building a structure are both game logic-based, namely *Start Queue Villager* and *Complete Queue Villager*. Thus, missing game logic-based events would lead to an overestimation of waiting time before building structures. For the given log, the waiting time of villagers would be overestimated by 4.72 min on average.

---

[3] https://github.com/Javert899/ocel20-celonis-connector.

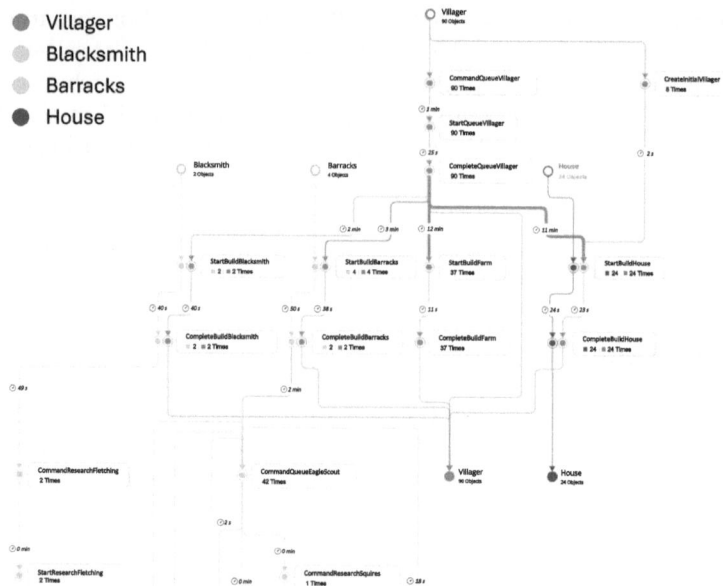

Fig. 4. Screenshot of the object-centric process explorer in Celonis loaded from an object-centric event log created from an AOE2 gameplay export with *aoe2pm*. The graph is filtered for the object types and activities visible in the screenshot. The directly following relations are annotated with the average throughput times.

The degree of automation (see Definition 2) describes how many events happen without player involvement but that belong to the same game session, so the degree of events that are part of the player's economy but do not directly involve the player. This is an important metric for players since the more automated their micro economy functions, the more time they have for advancing and extending their economy.

Definition 2 (Degree of Automation). *Given object-centric event log $L = (E, O, OT, O2O, \pi_{act}, \pi_{obj}, \pi_{time})$, player p, and session s, the degree of automation up to timestamp $t \in \mathbb{U}_{time}$ is:*

$$\frac{|\{e \in E | s \in \pi_{obj}(e) \wedge p \notin \pi_{obj}(e) \wedge \pi_{time}(e) \leq t\}|}{|\{e \in E | s \in \pi_{obj}(e) \wedge \pi_{time}(e) \leq t\}|}$$

Without the involvement of game logic-based events, which is what current state-of-the-art extractors are limited to, the degree of automation would falsely always be identified as 0%. In the published event log, we showed that the degree of automation rises over time and that players differ in how automated they play, as one can see in Fig. 5. This matches the domain knowledge of how people interact with the game. Making it an interesting metric for user behavior analysis, enabled by the added game logic-based events.

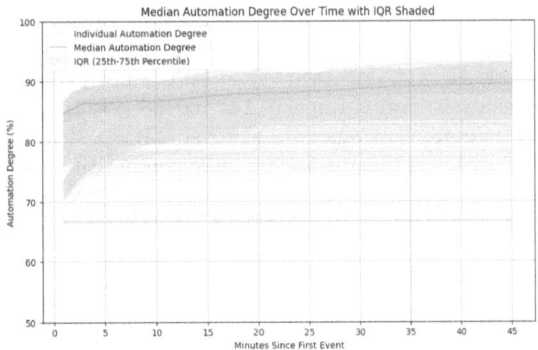

Fig. 5. Degree of automation players reach over the passed game time.

All in all, the qualitative evaluation showed that game logic-infused game logs give indeed better process mining insights than pure player-based ones. The quantitative evaluation shows that large-scale event logs can be created without intensive hardware requirements.

7   Conclusion

In this paper, we proposed a framework to extract object-centric event data from game data and applied it to AOE2, resulting in the Python library *aoe2pm*. We sourced 325,398 AOE2 matches and created a publicly accessible object-centric event log. We performed an evaluation of the framework, demonstrating its ability to create relevant object-centric event logs suitable for object-centric process mining methods like discovery and metric computation. Thus providing a new large-scale source for object-centric event data.

The framework is currently tailored for RTS games and requires adaptation for other game types as future research. Additionally, applying the framework demands domain knowledge, particularly in selecting suitable game rules. Future work includes extending the framework to other games. There is also potential to deepen the object-centric analysis. For instance, there exist community drive best practices for the games, so called build orders which can be used as normative models for object-centric conformance checking. The published event log also motivates reproducibility studies and new research into complex user behaviors.

Acknowledgments. The authors gratefully acknowledge the financial support by the Federal Ministry of Education and Research (BMBF) for the joint project Bridging AI (grant no. 16DHBKI023).

SPONSORED BY THE

Federal Ministry
of Education
and Research

References

1. Adams, J.N., Park, G., van der Aalst, W.M.P.: ocpa: a python library for object-centric process analysis. Softw. Impacts **14**, 100438 (2022)
2. Bayrak, A.E., McComb, C., Cagan, J., Kotovsky, K.: A strategic decision-making architecture toward hybrid teams for dynamic competitive problems. Decis. Support Syst. **144**, 113490 (2021)
3. Berti, A., Koren, I., Adams, J.N., et al.: OCEL (Object-Centric Event Log) 2.0 Specification (2023)
4. Berti, A., van Zelst, S.J., Schuster, D.: PM4Py: a process mining library for python. Softw. Impacts **17**, 100556 (2023)
5. Bozorgi, Z.D., Teinemaa, I., Dumas, M., La Rosa, M., Polyvyanyy, A.: Process mining meets causal machine learning: discovering causal rules from event logs. In: ICPM, pp. 129–136. IEEE (2020)
6. Chen, J., He, S., Yang, X.: Platform loophole exploitation, recovery measures, and user engagement: a quasi-natural experiment in online gaming. Inf. Syst. Res. **35**(4), 1609–1633 (2023)
7. Churchill, D., Buro, M.: Build order optimization in starcraft. In: AAAI, vol. 7, pp. 14–19 (2011)
8. Dumas, M., Rosa, L.M., Mendling, J., Reijers, A.H.: Fundamentals of Business Process Management. Springer (2013)
9. Esser, S., Fahland, D.: Multi-dimensional event data in graph databases. J. Data Semant. **10**(1–2), 109–141 (2021)
10. Fahland, D., Esser, S.: Event graph of bpi challenge 2017. tu.researchdata.dataset (2021). https://doi.org/10.4121/14169584.v1
11. Gal, A., Senderovich, A.: Process minding: closing the big data gap. In: BPM. LNCS, vol. 12168, pp. 3–16. Springer (2020)
12. Huang, Y., Jasin, S., Manchanda, P.: "level up": leveraging skill and engagement to maximize player game-play in online video games. Inf. Syst. Res. **30**(3), 927–947 (2019)
13. Khodyrev, I., Popova, S.: Discrete modeling and simulation of business processes using event logs. In: ICCS. Elsevier (2014)
14. Knopp, B., Pourbafrani, M., van der Aalst, W.M.: Discovering object-centric process simulation models. In: ICPM, pp. 81–88. IEEE (2023)
15. Lara-Cabrera, R., Cotta, C., Fernández-Leiva, A.J.: A review of computational intelligence in RTS games. In: FOCI, pp. 114–121. IEEE (2013)
16. Li, G., de Murillas, E.G.L., de Carvalho, R.M., Van Der Aalst, W.M.: Extracting object-centric event logs to support process mining on databases. In: CAiSE Forum. Springer (2018)
17. Martin, N., Depaire, B., Caris, A.: The use of process mining in a business process simulation context: overview and challenges. In: CIDM, pp. 381–388. IEEE (2014)
18. Rebmann, A., Rehse, J.R., van der Aa, H.: Uncovering object-centric data in classical event logs for the automated transformation from XES to OCEL. In: BPM. LNCS, vol. 13420, pp. 379–396. Springer (2022)
19. Tumay, K.: Business process simulation. In: WSC, pp. 93–98. IEEE Computer Society (1996)
20. van der Aalst, W.M.P.: Process mining. Commun. ACM **55**(8), 76–83 (2012)
21. van der Aalst, W.M.P.: Process mining and simulation: a match made in heaven! In: SummerSim, pp. 4:1–4:12. ACM (2018)

22. van der Aalst, W.M.P.: Object-centric process mining: dealing with divergence and convergence in event data. In: SEFM. Springer (2019)
23. Xiong, J., Xiao, G., Kalayci, T.E., Montali, M., Gu, Z., Calvanese, D.: A virtual knowledge graph based approach for object-centric event logs extraction. In: ICPM Workshops. Springer (2022)

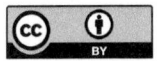

Object-Centric Local Process Models

Viki Peeva$^{(\boxtimes)}$, Marvin Porsil$^{(\boxtimes)}$, and Wil M. P. van der Aalst$^{(\boxtimes)}$

Chair of Process and Data Science, RWTH Aachen University, Aachen, Germany
{peeva,wvdaalst}@pads.rwth-aachen.de, marvin.porsil@rwth-aachen.de

Abstract. Process mining is a technology that helps understand, analyze, and improve processes. It has been present for around two decades, and although initially tailored for business processes, the spectrum of analyzed processes nowadays is evermore growing. To support more complex and diverse processes, subdisciplines such as object-centric process mining and behavioral pattern mining have emerged. Behavioral patterns allow for analyzing parts of the process in isolation, while object-centric process mining enables combining different perspectives of the process. In this work, we introduce *Object-Centric Local Process Models* (OCLPMs). OCLPMs are behavioral patterns tailored to analyzing complex processes where no single case notion exists and we leverage object-centric Petri nets to model them. Additionally, we present a discovery algorithm that starts from object-centric event logs, and implement the proposed approach in the open-source framework ProM. Finally, we demonstrate the applicability of OCLPMs in two case studies and evaluate the approach on various event logs.

Keywords: Local process models · Behavioral patterns · Pattern mining · Object-centric process mining · Object-centric event logs

1 Introduction

Process mining takes event data generated as a byproduct of organizations' operations and provides insights and improvements of the analyzed process. This is achieved by automatically discovering process models, computing conformance checking metrics, or enhancing the model with concrete KPIs. Traditional process mining considers the process from start to end and uses a single case notion. However, in reality, the process interacts with various entities, in the community known as object types or artifacts. There exist different strategies how to connect or model such entities together with the control-flow of the process. In our work, we focus on *object-centric process mining* as described in [2] and *Object-Centric Event Logs* (OCELs) [14]. Moreover, process issues like delays, high costs, etc., almost never occur on a global level but in specific subcontexts, requiring pattern mining. Pattern mining is a known discipline in data science and the concept has also been established in the area of process mining with

We thank the Alexander von Humboldt (AvH) Stiftung for supporting our research.

© The Author(s) 2025
A. Delgado and T. Slaats (Eds.): ICPM 2024 Workshops, LNBIP 533, pp. 376–388, 2025.
https://doi.org/10.1007/978-3-031-82225-4_28

works for discovering frequent subsequences [6], episodes [18], and local process models [23]. While end-to-end process models describe the entire process, process or behavioral patterns only explain (match) particular sub-behaviors of the process. In particular, the proposed approach focuses on *Local Process Models* (LPMs), which are a type of behavioral pattern, allowing for constructs such as sequence, choice, concurrency, and loop.

To combine the two areas, in this paper, we define *Object-Centric Local Process Models* (OCLPMs) as a behavioral pattern alternative for object-centric process mining. Additionally, we build a framework around an already existing LPM discovery approach to discover such OCLPMs. The discovery approach is built upon the formalisms of Petri nets, and as a result, the discovered OCLPMs are represented as object-centric Petri nets (OCPNs). Specifically, we list the following contributions:

(1) Adapting existing LPM discovery approach for OCLPM discovery.
(2) Implementing the algorithm in the publicly accessible framework ProM.
(3) Demonstrating feasibility and applicability in real-world scenarios.

The rest of the paper is structured as follows. First, we illustrate the necessity for OCLPMs in Sect. 2. Then, we present related work in Sect. 3, and give the necessary background to follow the rest of the paper in Sect. 4. In Sect. 5, we describe the proposed framework and all the surrounding details, after which, Sect. 6 covers the experiments demonstrating its applicability. In Sect. 7, we discuss the strengths and weaknesses of the proposed approach. Finally, in Sect. 8 we conclude the paper and offer an outlook on possible extensions.

2   Motivating Example

The necessity of pattern mining for processes has been demonstrated and discussed in previous works [22,23]. Challenges like spaghetti and flower process models make behavioral patterns even more attractive. However, current pattern representations lack the ability to model the process from multiple viewpoints. We use the example depicted in Fig. 1 to show the benefits of having patterns that are object-centric aware. The excerpt event log is for an order management process and includes ten events of five different activities and three object types. To discover traditional LPMs on such object-centric event logs, we would choose one object type and focus on the viewpoint of the chosen object type. From the perspective of each item, the process starts with *Place order*. However, in the process, one *Place order* is executed for more items, meaning one *Place order* event is followed by multiple *Pick item* and *Pack item* events. This can not be caught by the model because of replicating events, also called *convergence*. Moreover, for each item, first *Pick Item* and then *Pack Item* occurs. However, from the perspective of the package, it would appear there are random interleaving of the two activities. Therefore, resulting in unconnected loops in the model, see *lpm2* in Fig. 1, called *divergence*.

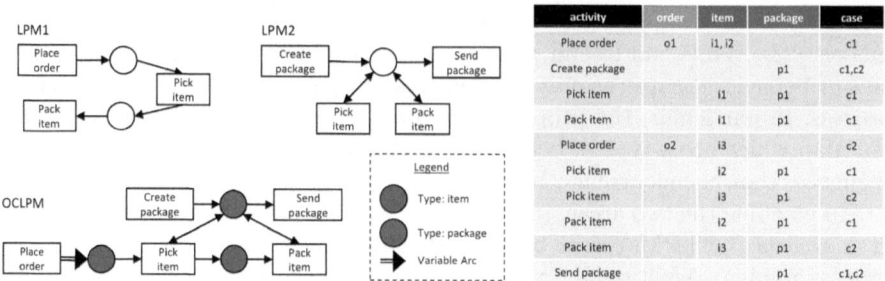

Fig. 1. Event log excerpt with example LPMs from the perspectives of the items (*lpm*1) and packages (*lpm*2) and one OCLPM depicting both perspectives.

By using OCLPMs and modeling the multiple perspectives together resolves the aforementioned problems. Consider the OCLPM in Fig. 1. The execution of *Place order* resulting in multiple items is clearly depicted with the variable arc between *Place order* and *Pick item*, solving the convergence problem. Additionally, the order of *Pick item* and *Pack item* is explicitly represented in the OCLPM, avoiding divergence. Considering this, we conclude that OCLPMs are valuable for processes with multiple object types.

3   Related Work

Object-Centric Modeling. As indicated in the introduction, there exist multiple strategies for modeling control-flow together with the associated data participators. Artifact-centric approaches [7,9,20] model the business process in terms of business artifacts. Such artifacts contain data and change states. A state change can result because of a step in the process, or it can trigger an advance in the process. Flexible case modeling [16,17] breaks the process into a domain model defining the participating entities, object lifecycles, process fragments to model the control-flow, and a goal state. Proclets [1,11] model the control flow from the perspective of the different object types and can have synchronization points between them. The synchronization points allow for one-to-one and one-to-many relationships. Although powerful, not many techniques in process mining are able to work with such models. Event-knowledge graphs and object-centric process models [2,13] are newer paradigms that put the control-flow in the main focus, but now from the perspective of multiple key entities, known as object types. For more information regarding the different modeling strategies, we refer to [2,11]. However, the more involved modeling strategies can be quite complex, and the ones focusing on control-flow can result in spaghetti models.

Behavioral Patterns. All modeling strategies above, represent the entire process in one model. However, processes can be complex, resulting in complicated over-fitting, spaghetti, models or simple, but under-fitting, flower, models. Some approaches, alleviate the complexity by introducing scenarios or fragmenting the process [12,15]. However, these still have the goal of representing the entire process. Behavioral patterns, like sequences, episodes, and local process models [4,6,8,21–23], deal with complexity by modeling subparts of the process and ignoring the rest. This makes them suitable for a spectrum of applications and not only modeling the process (see [22]). An alternative are declarative process modeling languages [3] that instead of using the activities to model control-flow, they define a set of constraints between the activities, like precedence or response. There also exist object-centric extensions for declarative constraints [19], where constraints are related to object types. However, with this work, we extend local process models as in [22] to be object-centric [2].

4 Preliminaries

We define sets $(X = \{a, b\})$, multisets $(M = [a^2, b^3])$, sequences $(\sigma = \langle a, b, c \rangle$ where $\sigma_1 = a)$, and tuples $(t = (a, b, c))$. Given a set X, $\mathcal{P}(X)$ is the power set of X, and X^* represents the set of all sequences over X. We use $f(X) = \{f(x) \mid x \in X\}$ $(f(\sigma) = \langle f(\sigma(1)), f(\sigma(2)), \ldots, f(\sigma(n)) \rangle)$ to apply the function f to every element in the set X (the sequence σ). Finally, we write $f_{\restriction X}$ $(\sigma_{\restriction X})$ to denote the projection of the domain of function f (the sequence σ) onto X.

Event Logs. Collected data used for process analysis is transformed into *event logs*. In Definition 1, we define events, and in Definition 2, we formally define *event logs* that can be used for both traditional and object-centric processes.

Definition 1 (Event). *Let* $\mathcal{U}_{ev}$ *be the universe of events,* $\mathcal{U}_{ot}$ *the universe of object types, and* $\mathcal{U}_{oi}$ *the universe of object identifiers. We define the event* $e = (ei, act, time, omap, vmap)$, *such that* $\pi_{ei}(e) = ei$ *is the event id,* $\pi_{act}(e) = act$ *is the event activity,* $\pi_{time}(e) = time$ *is the timestamp of the event,* $\pi_{omap}(e) = omap$ *(omap* $\in \mathcal{U}_{ot} \rightarrow \mathcal{P}(\mathcal{U}_{oi}))$ *is a function mapping each object type to the objects involved in the event, and* $\pi_{vmap}(e) = vmap$ *is a function assigning values to each of the event attributes.*

Definition 2 (Event Log [2]). $L = (E, \preceq_E) \in \mathcal{U}_L$ *is an event log with* $E \subseteq \mathcal{U}_{ev}$ *and* $\preceq_E \subseteq E \times E$ *such that:*

- $\preceq_E$ *defines a partial order (reflexive, antisymmetric, and transitive)*
- $\forall_{e_1, e_2 \in E} \pi_{ei}(e_1) = \pi_{ei}(e_2) \implies e_1 = e_2$, *and*
- $\forall_{e_1, e_2 \in E} e_1 \preceq_E e_2 \implies \pi_{time}(e_1) \leq \pi_{time}(e_2)$.

We use OT_L *to denote all object types in* L.

In process mining, the concept of process executions is essential for many techniques. Depending on the complexity, process executions are represented as totally or partially ordered events. For example, in traditional process mining, event logs are represented as a set of traces, where each trace is a sequence of events. Here, we call such event logs *simple event logs* and write $L_S \in \mathcal{P}(\mathcal{U}_{ev}^*)$.

To obtain a simple event log L_S from $L = (E, \preceq_E) \in \mathcal{U}_L$, we group the events on a certain object type $ot \in \mathcal{U}_{ot}$ and order them. For this, we use $flat \in \mathcal{U}_L \times \mathcal{U}_{ot} \rightarrow \mathcal{P}(\mathcal{U}_{ev}^*)$ such that $flat(L, ot) = \{\rho_{cid} \in \mathcal{U}_{ev}^* \mid cid \in \bigcup_{e \in E} \pi_{omap}(e)(ot) \wedge \forall_{e \in E}(cid \in \pi_{omap}(e)(ot) \implies e \in \rho) \wedge \forall_{1 \leq i < j \leq |\rho|}(\pi_{time}(\rho_i) \leq \pi_{time}(\rho_j))\}$. In case two events have the same timestamp, we assume some order.

Process Models. The behavior recorded in logs can be modeled using different notations, such as DFG, process trees, BPMN, Petri nets, etc. In this work, we focus on Petri nets, and more precisely on *labeled Petri nets* which we define in Definition 3 and *object-centric Petri nets* as defined in Definition 4.

Definition 3 (Labeled Petri Net). *A labeled Petri net is a tuple $N = (P, T, F, l)$ with P the set of places, T the set of transitions, such that $P \cap T = \emptyset$, $F \subseteq (P \times T) \cup (T \times P)$ the flow relation and $l \in T \rightarrow \mathcal{A} \cup \{\tau\}$ a labeling function.*

Definition 4 (Object-centric Petri nets). *An Object-centric Petri net is a tuple $ON = (N, pt, F_{var})$ where $N = (P, T, F, l)$ is a labeled Petri net, $pt \in P \rightarrow \mathcal{U}_{ot}$ maps places onto object types, and $F_{var} \subseteq N.F$ is the subset of variable arcs.*

Generally, process models define a language, commonly used in process mining to measure how well the model aligns with the collected event data. For both labeled and object-centric Petri nets, exist notions like tokens and markings, necessary to define their language. Because of space restrictions, we refer to [2] on how the language is obtained.

In this work, we consider LPMs as labeled Petri nets and OCLPMs to be OCPNs. However, LPMs and OCLPMs do not cover the entire event log, since they do not represent the entire process. Therefore, we define $E_{oclpm} \subseteq E$ to be the events in the event log $L = (E, \preceq_E)$ that are covered by the OCLPM *oclpm*. More details about how LPMs are matched to event logs, can be found in previous works [22,23].

5   OCLPM Discovery

In this section, we present a two-phase discovery approach for OCLPMs given an OCEL. In Fig. 2 we visualize the two phases of the approach: *preparation* and *discovery*, together with the input, output, and the intermediate results. In Algorithm 1.

5.1   Preparation (Phase 1)

The preparation covers the first two lines in Algorithm 1. As previously discussed, the discovered OCLPMs should describe local patterns occurring in the process but also incorporate object interactions. Therefore, with the preprocessing, we extract dominant local dependencies between activities for each object type (place net discovery) on the one hand, and identify meaningful object interactions (event log transformation), on the other.

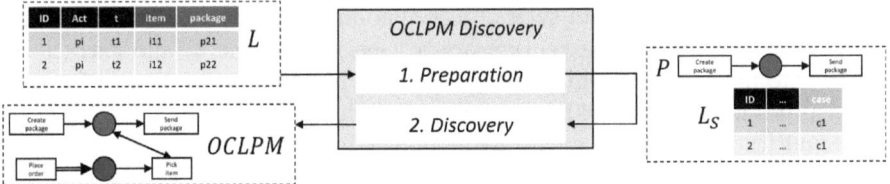

Fig. 2. Overview of the steps in the OCLPM framework, depicted with their inputs and outputs.

Algorithm 1: Discovery algorithm for OCLPMs.

---

input : $L = (E, \preceq_E)$
1 // Preparation (Phase 1)
2 $PT \leftarrow \bigcup_{ot \in OT_L} \mathtt{po}(\mathtt{flat}(L, ot)) \times \{ot\}$;
3 $L_S \leftarrow \mathtt{flat}(\mathtt{peo}(L))$;
4 // Discovery (Phase 2)
5 $P \leftarrow \{N_p \mid (N_p, ot) \in PT\}$;
6 $LPM \leftarrow \mathtt{lpmd}(L_S, P)$;
7 $OCLPM \leftarrow \emptyset$;
8 **for** $lpm \in LPM$ **do**
9 $\quad pt \leftarrow \{(p, ot) \mid p \in lpm.P \wedge (lpm_{\restriction_p}, ot) \in PT\}^1$;
10 $\quad F_{var} \leftarrow \mathtt{vararc}(lpm, pt, L_S)$;
11 $\quad OCLPM \leftarrow OCLPM \cup \{(lpm, pt, F_{var})\}$;
12 **return** $OCLPM$

Place Net Discovery. We model local dependencies between activities by using place nets, i.e., the simplest LPMs containing only one place (see output of *Preparation* in Fig. 2). To obtain local dependencies for each object type, we flatten the event log for each object type (using *flat* from Sect. 4) and execute a place net oracle *po* on the flattened event log. As a place net oracle, we can use any discovery algorithm that returns a Petri net or a set of place nets. However, algorithms unrestricted to end-to-end trace fitness, as discussed in [22], are more suitable when we are interested in local dependencies. The result is the set *PT*, a set of place nets together with the object type for which they were discovered (Line 2 in Algorithm 1).[2]

Event Log Transformation. To focus on object interactions, we enhance the event log with a new object type, used to group interacting objects, whose goal is to mimic the case notion from traditional event logs. Each object of the new object type represents a group of original objects that have met during the process. By then flattening the event log on the newly added object type, we extract process executions representing the process from the viewpoint of the interacting objects.

---

[2] $lpm_{\restriction_p} = (\{p\}, T_p, F_p, l_p)$ such that $T_p = \{t \in lpm.T \mid (t, p) \in lpm.F \vee (p, t) \in lpm.F\}$, $F_p = \{(x, y) \in lpm.F \mid x = p \vee y = p\}$, and $l_p = lpm.l_{\restriction_{T_p}}$.

In Algorithm 1, we compute such object type and enhance the event log with it, by assuming a process execution oracle (see *peo* in Line 3) and extract the process executions by flattening (see *flat* in Line 3). One way of discovering such object types and extracting process executions has been proposed in [5]. There are a multitude of ways one can define object interactions. One example is to consider sharing an event an interaction. Moreover, the new object type must not combine all interacting objects. It is up to the process execution oracle to decide what is an interaction and where to put the boundaries between the interacting objects. By abstracting from the concrete computation, we allow flexibility when it comes to which object interactions are meaningful.

5.2   Discovery (Phase 2)

In the discovery step, the event log given as input and the intermediate results from the preparation are used to build OCLPMs. First, we discover traditional LPMs (LPM discovery), and then construct the OCLPMs by enhancing the discovered LPMs with place to object type mapping (object type annotation) and variable arcs (variable arc identification). Below, we describe each in more detail and finish the algorithm by returning the set of computed OCLPMs.

LPM Discovery. We discover traditional LPMs on the simple event log we created by utilizing an existing LPM discovery technique [22]. The technique used, starts with a precomputed set of local dependencies, represented as place nets (Line 5 in Algorithm 1), and merges those into larger LPMs only when there is evidence in the provided event log that the LPM occurs in the process. Additionally, the occurrence of the LPM should be for interacting objects. Let us consider the OCLPM in Fig. 2. A claim that the OCLPM occurred in the event log means it occurred for related packages and items, and not random pairs of items and packages. The discovered set of LPMs *LPM* (Line 6 in Algorithm 1) satisfies this requirement because the simple event log focuses on interacting objects as explained above.

Object Type Annotation. An important advantage of OCLPMs is depicting object type interactions. Therefore, for each place of an LPM, we identify the object type they represent. Since we used the computed place nets for each object type P as a starting point for the LPM discovery, we use the original place net to object type mapping PT to compute the place to type mapping (Line 9 in Algorithm 1).

Variable Arc Identification. Variable arcs allow for modelling many-to-one interactions between objects of different types. Therefore, the final step is for each LPM to identify the variable arcs. In our approach, we identify variable arcs as proposed in [2]. More concretely, given an LPM (which is a labeled Petri net) $lpm = (P, T, F, l)$, we define $F_{var} = \{(p,\ \text{t}) \in F \cap (P \times T) \mid score(l(t), pt(p)) < \tau\} \cup \{(t,\ \text{p}) \in F \cap (T \times P) \mid score(l(t), pt(p)) < \tau\}$, where $score \in \mathcal{A} \times \mathcal{U}_{ot} \nrightarrow [0, 1]$ computes the fraction of events of the specified activity that contain exactly one object of the object type in question, as defined below, and τ is a user-defined threshold.

$$score(act, ot) = \frac{|\{e \in E_{oclpm} \mid \pi_{act}(e) = act \wedge |\pi_{obj}(e)(ot)| = 1\}|}{|\{e \in E_{oclpm} \mid \pi_{act}(e) = act\}|}$$

Note, for the variable arc computation, we use E_{oclpm} since OCLPMs do not cover all events in an event log. Finally, the *vararc* in Line 10 returns F_{var} computed as described before.

With this we covered all steps of the discovery algorithm.

6   Evaluation

In this section, we evaluate the proposed approach qualitatively and quantitatively. First, we demonstrate applicability on two case studies. Then, we report runtime statistics and count of discovered models for different event logs. This is the first method for discovering OCLPMs, so we are unable to compare with previous work. All experiments are performed using the open-access implementation we provide in the ProM framework[3]. As a place net oracle, we use the SPECpp plugin in ProM[4], and as an LPM discovery approach we use the approach from [22] also available in ProM[5]. For each event log, we build OCLPMs between 2 and 7 places, 3 and 10 transitions, all activities and discovered place nets, and window size 7.

6.1   Case Studies

BPI Challenge 2017. The event log is recorded from a loan application process of a Dutch financial institute [10]. It involves objects of types *application* and *offer*. The event log is available in both traditional xes and OCEL format, hence we use it to compare OCLPM discovery to LPM discovery on the same event log.

We discover LPMs using [22] on the traditional event log, and OCLPMs on the available OCEL with the proposed approach. In Fig. 3, we display two OCLPMs and two LPMs. The OCLPM at the top depicts how after an application is created and then accepted, a new offer is created and sent. The interaction between the application and offer object types is clearly shown in the discovered OCLPM. The highest-ranked LPM also shows the move from application to offer, denoted with activity names prefixed with A and O. However, this is achieved with preprocessing of the event log. Emphasizing object types visually and treating them as first-class citizens gives a much clearer picture of what the pattern is describing. Moreover, it is not just the visual appeal that is gained with OCLPMs, but also expressiveness. This is illustrated with the help of the

---

[3] https://github.com/promworkbench/ObjectCentricLPMs.
[4] https://github.com/promworkbench/SPECpp.
[5] https://github.com/promworkbench/LocalProcessModelDiscoveryByCombiningPlaces.

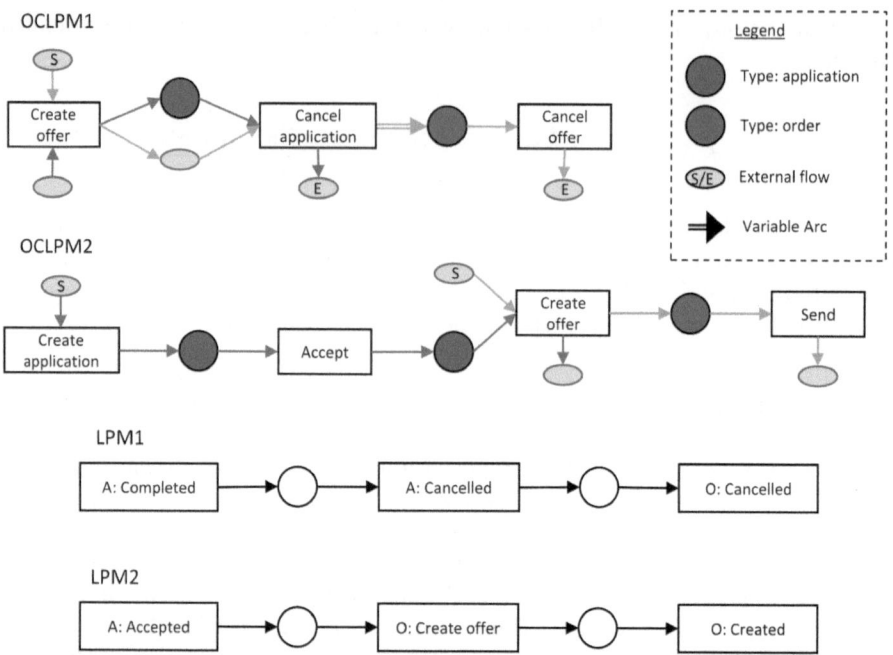

Fig. 3. Discovered OCLPMs with the proposed approach and LPMs with [22] on the BPIC2017 event log. In OCLPMs, we model external flow of the objects with elipses, where S/E denote object Start/End position.

OCLPM and LPM concerned with a cancellation of application. The shown OCLPM, with the help of variable arcs, clearly illustrates that one application might connect to multiple offers. Meaning, once the application is cancelled, all of the offers should be cancelled as well. The discovered LPM, although depicting that offer should be cancelled after an application is cancelled, does not contain information on whether one or multiple offers are cancelled.

Order Management. The event log, as its name hints, describes a process for managing orders in which objects of types *order, item, package, customer*, and *product* are involved. The main flow of the process is that a customer places an order, which is then confirmed by an employee, continuing into two disentangled subprocesses. On the one hand, we have, collecting order items, packing them, and sending the package (possibly multiple times if the deliveries have failed) until a successful delivery, and on the other hand, paying the order and possibly sending multiple reminders before the payment was completed.

The approach proposed run about 40 s and discovered in total 375 models. We show the highest ranked OCLPM in Fig. 4b. The model clearly shows the relationship between orders, customer, and items. One order is made by one

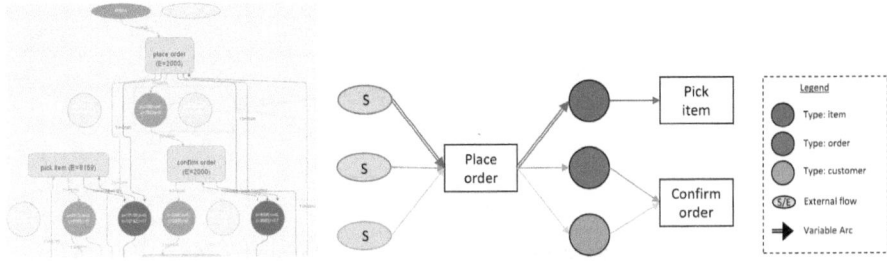

(a) Part of the full end-to-end process model describing the same behavior as the OCLPM.

(b) Discovered OCLPM showcasing the interactions between items, orders, and customers, focusing on the activities *place order*, *pick item*, and *confirm order*.

Fig. 4. Part of the end-to-end model and one OCLPM for the Order Management event log.

Table 1. Event log description with number of discovered OCLPMs and runtime (https://www.ocel-standard.org/1.0/#eventlogs).

Name	Events	Objects	Object Types	Models	Runtime(s)
Order Management	22367	11521	5	846	161
O2C	98350	107767	19	1046	258
P2P	24854	74489	8	2923	195
Transfer	10319	2500	5	8	6
Recruiting	6980	1505	6	109	43
Github	1798	532	3	2314	92
BPIC2017	31203	8416	2	918	16

customer, and one order can correspond to multiple items. Furthermore, it shows that *place order* is a starting activity for orders, customers, and items.

The end-to-end process model discovery took about 4 s to discover the original model. Although, the process itself is not too complex, the model was very cluttered and spaghetti like. In Fig. 4a, we show a part of the end-to-end process model. We had to filter on the orders, customers, and items object types, the activities, and discard most of the paths, to spot the relationships described by the OCLPM in Fig. 4b, despite it being frequent and highly-ranked. The approach returned additional 374 OCLPM, bringing valuable information that otherwise would have been lost in the complexity of the end-to-end model.

6.2 Results for Other Event Logs

In this section, we report different statistics regarding the discovery of OCLPMs on various OCEL. In Table 1 we list the event logs used in this part of the evaluation together with the number of events, objects, and object types they include. We run the *Object-Centric Local Process Model Discovery given OCEL*

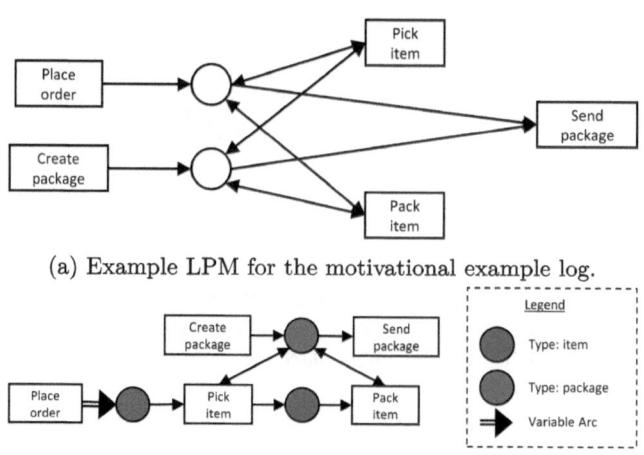

(a) Example LPM for the motivational example log.

(b) Example OCLPM for the motivational example log.

Fig. 5. Example LPM and OCLPM for the motivational example log.

plug-in in *ProM* with default parameters. In Table 1, we report the number of models discovered and the time necessary to do so for each of the event logs. The three largest event logs *Order Management, O2C,* and *P2P* have the highest running time. We can also note that usually the runtime proportionally increases with the number of models built. One exception is the *Github* event log, that has more OCLPMs discovered in less time, compared to the *O2C* and the *Order Management* event logs. However, *Github* has significantly fewer events and objects than those two event logs.

7   Discussion

In this section, we cover the strengths and weaknesses of the proposed approach. An alternative to our approach, would be to directly use traditional LPM discovery on the flattened version of the event log and skip all the other steps we presented. In Fig. 5 we show one LPM and one OCLPM discovered for the event log given in Sect. 2. The obvious arguments in favour of OCLPMs, also exhibited in the evaluation of the approach, are the explicitness of object types and the expressiveness of the variable arcs. However, examining further, we compare both models from the perspectives of convergence and divergence. First, note that the missing dependency between *Pick item* and *Pack item* in the LPM is present in the OCLPM. This is due to the *Preparation* step of our approach, in which we discover local dependencies per object type. Second, the improper dependency between *Place order* and *Send package* is avoided in the OCLPM, again as a result of the *Preparation* step. Both of these examples demonstrate *divergence* problems for traditional LPMs discovered for OCELs and the ability of our approach to avoid them. Additionally, the improper dependency also creates the untrue impression that for each *Place order* a *Send package* is executed, leading to *convergence* problems. In the OCLPM, the two activities are executed for different object types, allowing the OCLPM to be matched to one package and two orders as included in the log. In conclusion, the proposed approach resolves the convergence and divergence problems that would be introduced if a traditional LPM discovery was used.

8   Conclusion

In this work, we introduce OCLPMs as OCPNs, and present a discovery algorithm for building them from OCELs. We adapt and utilize existing work on computing local dependencies between activities and LPM discovery to support the OCLPM discovery. Moreover, we implement the proposed algorithm in the open-source process mining tool ProM and evaluate the usefulness of the proposed approach on one real-world and one artificial event log. Additionally, we report runtime statistics and discovered models on multiple event logs. Finally, we have discussed strengths and limitations of the proposed approach.

Next steps in this area would be to enhance the discovered OCLPMs with object and event attributes or allow for guided discovery similar to traditional LPMs. Furthermore, more elaborate filtering techniques for discarding or giving less weight on specific object types would allow more advanced discovery. Finally, exploring alternative methods for discovering OCLPMs would be valuable.

References

1. van der Aalst, W.M.P., Barthelmess, P., Ellis, C.A., Wainer, J.: Workflow modeling using proclets. In: CoopIS 2000, vol. 1901, pp. 198–209 (2000)
2. van der Aalst, W.M.P., Berti, A.: Discovering object-centric petri nets. Fundam. Informaticae **175**(1-4), 1–40 (2020)
3. van der Aalst, W.M.P., Pesic, M., Schonenberg, H.: Declarative workflows: balancing between flexibility and support. Comput. Sci. Res. Dev. **23**(2), 99–113 (2009)
4. Acheli, M., Grigori, D., Weidlich, M.: Efficient discovery of compact maximal behavioral patterns from event logs. In: CAiSE (2019)
5. Adams, J.N., Schuster, D., Schmitz, S., Schuh, G., van der Aalst, W.M.P.: Defining cases and variants for object-centric event data. In: ICPM 2022, pp. 128–135 (2022)
6. Agrawal, R., Srikant, R.: Mining sequential patterns. In: ICDE 1995, pp. 3–14 (1995)
7. Bhattacharya, K., Gerede, C.E., Hull, R., Liu, R., Su, J.: Towards formal analysis of artifact-centric business process models. In: BPM 2007, vol. 4714, pp. 288–304 (2007)
8. Brunings, M., Fahland, D., Verbeek, E.: Discover context-rich local process models (extended abstract). In: ICPM-D (2022)
9. Cohn, D., Hull, R.: Business artifacts: a data-centric approach to modeling business operations and processes. IEEE Data Eng. Bull. **32**(3), 3–9 (2009)
10. van Dongen, B.: BPI challenge 2017 (2017)
11. Fahland, D.: Describing behavior of processes with many-to-many interactions. In: PETRI NETS 2019, vol. 11522, pp. 3–24 (2019)

12. Fahland, D.: Oclets - scenario-based modeling with petri nets. In: PETRI NETS 2009, vol. 5606, pp. 223–242 (2009)
13. Fahland, D.: Process mining over multiple behavioral dimensions with event knowledge graphs. In: Process Mining Handbook, vol. 448, pp. 274–319 (2022)
14. Ghahfarokhi, A.F., Park, G., Berti, A., van der Aalst, W.M.P.: OCEL: a standard for object-centric event logs. In: ADBIS 2021 Short Papers, vol. 1450, pp. 169–175 (2021)
15. Haarmann, S., Lichtenstein, T., Weske, M.: Fragment-based service choreographies. In: IEEE SCC 2022, pp. 164–173 (2022)
16. Haarmann, S., Montali, M., Weske, M.: Refining case models using cardinality constraints. In: CAiSE 2021, vol. 12751, pp. 296–310 (2021)
17. Hewelt, M., Weske, M.: A hybrid approach for flexible case modeling and execution. In: BPM Forum 2016, vol. 260, pp. 38–54 (2016)
18. Leemans, M., van der Aalst, W.M.P.: Discovery of frequent episodes in event logs. In: SIMPDA 2014, Revised Selected Papers, pp. 1–31 (2014)
19. Li, G., de Carvalho, R.M., van der Aalst, W.M.P.: Automatic discovery of object-centric behavioral constraint models. In: BIS 2017, vol. 288, pp. 43–58 (2017)
20. Lu, X., Nagelkerke, M., van de Wiel, D., Fahland, D.: Discovering interacting artifacts from ERP systems. IEEE Trans. Serv. Comput. 8(6), 861–873 (2015)
21. Mannila, H., Toivonen, H., Verkamo, A.I.: Discovery of frequent episodes in event sequences. Data Min. Knowl. Discov. 1(3), 259–289 (1997)
22. Peeva, V., Mannel, L.L., van der Aalst, W.M.P.: From place nets to local process models. In: PETRI NETS (2022)
23. Tax, N., Sidorova, N., Haakma, R., van der Aalst, W.M.P.: Mining local process models. J. Innov. Digit. Ecosyst. 3(2), 183–196 (2016)

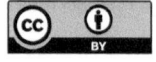

Locally Optimized Process Tree Discovery

Calvin Schröder[1(✉)], Jan Niklas van Detten[1,3], and Sander J. J. Leemans[1,2]📖

[1] RWTH Aachen University, Aachen, Germany
`calvin.schroeder@rwth-aachen.de`
[2] Fraunhofer FIT, Sankt Augustin, Germany
[3] Celonis, Munich, Germany

Abstract. Business process optimization typically involves discovering models that are fit, precise, sound and simple. Process discovery algorithms automatically obtain these models from event logs, records of past process executions, enabling insights into the underlying process. However, event logs often contain incomplete and infrequent behaviour, which presents significant challenges for these algorithms. To address these issues, we propose a new process discovery technique called OptIMIIst, which guarantees soundness while handling both infrequent and incomplete behaviour and discovering locally optimal process trees. This technique, based on the Inductive Miner framework, operates in two steps. First, it creates candidate mining decisions for each process tree operator and then decides on the optimal decision through a local fitness and precision estimation. An experimental evaluation demonstrates that OptIMIIst produces high-quality process models and offers competitive fitness, precision, and simplicity compared to state-of-the-art techniques, while maintaining soundness.

Keywords: Process Mining · Process Discovery · Process Trees

1 Introduction

In business processes activities and resources are coordinated to achieve organizational goals. Understanding and optimizing these processes is one way to enhance efficiency. Traditionally, process analysis has relied on manual construction of models in standardized formalisms, like Petri nets. However, with the advent of digital technologies, processes generate detailed automated records of their execution, called event logs. Process discovery, a central field of process mining, aims to automatically derive process models from these event logs.

For a process model to effectively aid the analysis of the underlying process, it must meet certain quality criteria, evaluated using four dimensions. Fitness measures how well the model captures the actual behaviour recorded in the event log, while precision ensures the model accurately represents only the observed behaviour, avoiding unnecessary generalisation. In addition to these quantifiable metrics, soundness ensures that the model is behaviourally correct [2,15,18], while simplicity, though not directly measurable, keeps the model straightforward and easy to understand.

A. Delgado and T. Slaats (Eds.): ICPM 2024 Workshops, LNBIP 533, pp. 389–401, 2025.
https://doi.org/10.1007/978-3-031-82225-4_29

Key challenges in process discovery include infrequent and incomplete behaviour, both of which affect the quality of models [16]. Infrequent behaviour refers to behaviour rarely observed in the log, such as noise resulting from data entry errors or rarely happening exceptions. On the one hand, process discovery techniques must avoid noisy elements to avoid overfitting and focus on capturing the "core" process. On the other hand, discovery techniques must be robust against incompleteness as we cannot assume to have recorded all behaviour that is possible in the process in the event log.

The Inductive Miner (IM) [10] is a process discovery algorithm that recursively decomposes an event log into smaller logs to construct a process tree, which can be transformed into sound workflow nets. However, balancing the remaining model qualities fitness, precision, and simplicity while handling incomplete and infrequent behaviour is particularly challenging. If no cut can be found, IM needs to resort to fallthroughs, which sacrifice precision for fitness. Existing approaches such as the Probabilistic Inductive Miner (PIM) [5] and the Approximate Inductive Miner (AIM) [7] attempt to address these issues by filtering out infrequent behaviour before applying heuristics, which deviate from formal cut definitions. While the Inductive Miner Incomplete (IMc) [12] only handles incomplete behaviour. This highlights a gap for a process discovery technique that manages both infrequent and incomplete behaviour simultaneously, while adhering closely to the formal cut definitions.

In this paper, we propose a new process discovery technique that guarantees soundness and addresses both infrequent and incomplete behaviour, by generalising the cut definitions of the IM framework. First, we choose one candidate cut for each process tree operator that is locally optimal with respect to the generalised cut definition. Second, we use an estimation of local fitness and precision to choose the best of the candidate cuts. We call our new discovery technique the Opt-IM-II-st (Optimization-InductiveMiner-Infrequent-Incomplete-eSTimation). We evaluate the model quality of OptIMIIst with respect to other state-of-the-art algorithms using real-world event logs, which shows that OptIMIIst has a competitive performance.

The paper is structured as follows: Sect. 2 introduces relevant related work, Sect. 3 introduces the basics of process trees and IM. Section 4 details OptIMIIst and its implementation. Section 5 benchmarks and evaluates OptIMIIst. Finally, Sect. 6 summarizes our findings and presents final thoughts.

2   Related Work

The Inductive Miner employs a recursive approach to process discovery, limiting itself to mining process trees. Although the IM introduces a representational bias, it offer the advantage of ensuring soundness when converted to Petri nets [10]. Several discovery algorithms implemented the IM, to address specific challenges. A common way to handle infrequent behaviour is employing filtering, for example in the Inductive Miner infrequent (IMf) [11]. Through the optimization, OptIMIIst, specifically targets and "filters" only the violating behaviour, thereby minimizing information loss in comparison to frequency-based filtering. IMc focuses on incomplete event logs, but its application can be infeasible [12]. The Evolutionary Tree Miner (ETM) [6] employs a genetic algorithm and evaluates the entire process trees based on fitness and precision, guiding the evolution of the population accordingly, but as an optimization meta-heuristics does not guarantee optimality. In contrast, OptIMIIst estimates fitness and precision at a local level, focusing on optimizing individual partitions rather than the entire tree. The Indulpet Miner [13] is a combination of four process discovery techniques including ETM and IM. The most closely related versions to the OptIMIIst are AIM [7] and PIM [5], both of which handle infrequent and incomplete behaviour through quality measures. While PIM searches all possible cuts for the best cut, AIM uses a clustering approach. For its filtering OptIMIIst implicitly filters during optimization while PIM employs a similar filtering as IMf. AIM handles filtering at the activity level through parameter optimization. Besides OptIMIIst other techniques also use optimization as a tool for process discovery but do not guarantee soundness [4,17,19].

In literature, a manifold of other techniques for process discovery have been introduced. For a review of earlier advancements in the area of process discovery and a comprehensive comparison, we refer to [3]. Newer approaches include the eST-Miner mining Petri nets by searching for fitting places [14].

3   Preliminaries

An event log L is a record of traces σ, where each trace $\sigma = \langle a_1, \ldots, a_n \rangle$ is a sequence of activities ordered by their occurrence. A trace where activity a precedes activity b is denoted by $\langle a, b \rangle$, while an empty trace is denoted by ϵ. The alphabet Σ is the set of activities in L. With $\text{START}(L)$ and $\text{END}(L)$, we denote the set of activities at the start or end of traces in the log and with $\text{start}(L, a)$ and $\text{END}(L, a)$ how often activity a is a start or end activity in L. $\mathcal{V}$ denotes the set of unique trace variants, the sequence of activities in a trace. We use the silent activity τ to denote the absence of an activity.

A follows relation exists between two activities in a log if there is a trace in which one is followed by the other. The common directly-follows relationship $a \rightarrow b$ holds if $\exists \sigma \in L | \sigma = \langle \ldots, a, b, \ldots \rangle$ and the eventually-follows relation $a \rightarrow^+$ holds if $a \rightarrow b \vee \exists \sigma \in L | \sigma = \langle \ldots, a, \ldots, b, \ldots \rangle$. From these relations, we derive the directly-follows-graph (DFG) and respectively the eventually-follows-graph (EFG). The nodes in these graphs represent the activities of a log while the edges represent the presence of follows relations. The edge weights, denoted as $|a \rightarrow b|$, indicate the number of times a relation is observed in the log.

Process Trees. Process trees are tree-structured process models where leaf nodes are labelled with elements from $\Sigma \cup \{\tau\}$, and inner nodes are labelled with an operator $\oplus$. These trees guarantee translatability into sound workflow nets when turned into Petri nets. Without loss of generality, we focus on binary process trees, where each operator node has exactly two children [9].

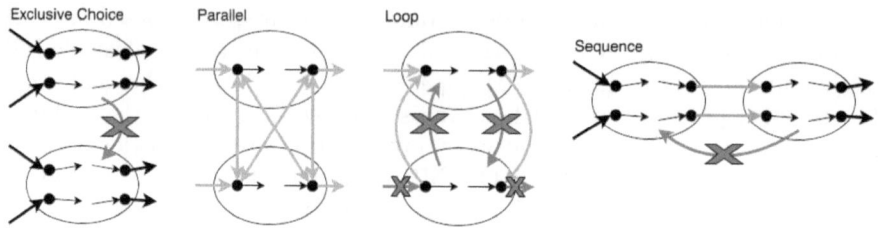

Fig. 1. Visual representations of binary IM cut profiles

The tree leaves are labeled with either an activity $a \in \Sigma$ or τ, representing the execution of an activity or the absence thereof. The operators for inner nodes consist of $\{\rightarrow, \times, ||, \circlearrowleft\}$. The sequence operator $\rightarrow$ mandates that the left child sub-tree be executed before the right. The exclusive choice operator $\times$ allows only one of the children to be executed. The parallel operator $||$ signifies the independent parallel execution of the children. Lastly, the loop operator $\circlearrowleft$ requires an initial execution of the left child, the body part, and permits its repetition after each execution of the right child, the redo part. For formal semantics of process trees, we refer to [9].

Inductive Miner. The Inductive Miner (IM) framework uses a recursive approach to construct a process tree from an event log. At each recursion IM finds a maximal non-trivial cut. This involves determining an operator and partition Σ_1 and Σ_2 of activities in the log and subsequently splitting the log into L_1 and L_2 to continue the recursion on the sublogs. This mining decision of operator and partition is called a cut. The base cases of the algorithm generate a τ or a single activity leaf if the event log contains no activities or only a single class of activities.

If no cut and no base case are found, a fall-through method is applied. These methods include structures like τ-skips, enabling optional behaviour, and τ-loops, allowing for arbitrary repetition of behaviour. A flower model is the usual last resort, which is a structure enabling the arbitrary execution of activities in the log, which often comes at the cost of precision. Each cut must adhere to its definitions as detailed in [10], with visual representations provided in Fig. 1. A *sequence cut* requires that eventually follows relations are only present from the first part to the second, not the other way around.

$$\forall_{a \in \Sigma_0, b \in \Sigma_1} a \twoheadrightarrow^+ b \land b \not\twoheadrightarrow^+ a \tag{1}$$

For an *exclusive choice* cut, activities are partitioned as such that no directly follows relations exist between the partitions:

$$\forall_{a \in \Sigma_0, b \in \Sigma_1} a \not\twoheadrightarrow b \land b \not\twoheadrightarrow a \tag{2}$$

In a *parallel cut* the partitions must be fully interconnected, and must both contain start and end activities.

$$\forall_i \Sigma_i \cap \text{START}(L) \neq \emptyset \wedge \Sigma_i \cap \text{END}(L) \neq \emptyset \tag{3}$$

$$\forall_{a \in \Sigma_0, b \in \Sigma_1} a \twoheadrightarrow b \wedge b \twoheadrightarrow a \tag{4}$$

Lastly, a *loop cut* restricts start and end activities to the body part. With directly follows relations between the partitions only being permitted from the end activities of the body to the start of the redo part, and from end activities of the redo part to the start activities of the body part.

$$\Sigma_0 \supseteq \text{START}(L) \cup \text{END}(L) \tag{5}$$

$$\forall_{a \in \Sigma_0} \exists_{b \in \Sigma_1} b \twoheadrightarrow a \Rightarrow a \in \text{START}(L) \tag{6}$$

$$\forall_{a \in \Sigma_0} \exists_{b \in \Sigma_1} a \twoheadrightarrow b \Rightarrow a \in \text{END}(L) \tag{7}$$

4 Opt-IM-II-st

OptIMIIst extends IM by applying a custom fallthrough function. The implementation of it is outlined in Algorithm 1 and visualised in Fig. 2. First, the FINDCUTS$_{\text{OPTIMIIST}}$ function finds potential cuts for each operator based on relaxations of the cut definitions, creating a set of cut candidates. In a second step, EVALUATECUT evaluates the candidates, including τ-loop and τ-skip, by estimating the local fitness and precision of the candidates selecting the best to apply. OptIMIIst as such always returns a suitable cut and maintains the same rediscoverability guarantees as IM, a fact demonstrated regardless of the fall-through methods employed [9].

4.1 FindCuts for Each Operator

The FINDCUTS$_{\text{OPTIMIIST}}$ function returns optimal partitions for each of the four operators $\{\rightarrow, \times, ||, \circlearrowright\}$. To achieve this, we formulate and solve a separate Integer Linear Programs (ILP) for each operator. Shared structures between all ILPs are the binary decision variables $x_a \forall a \in \Sigma$, each variable determining whether an

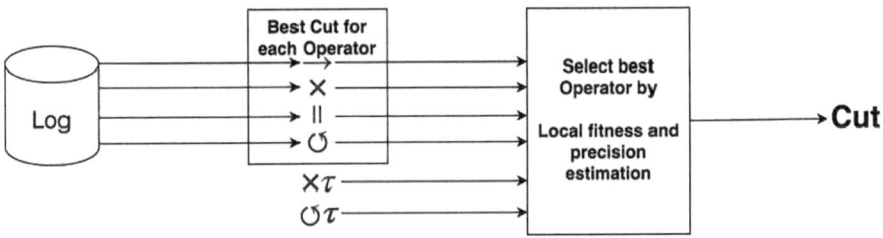

Fig. 2. Top-Level overview of OptIMIIst

Algorithm 1. Opt-IM-II-st Fallthrough

1: **function** FALLTHROUGHOPTIMIIST(L)
2:    $C \leftarrow \{\text{FINDCUTSOPTIMIIST}(L)\} \cup \{(\times, L, \emptyset), (\circlearrowleft, L, \emptyset)\}$
3:    $(\oplus_{res}, L_{res1}, L_{res2}) \leftarrow \underset{(\oplus, L_1, L_2) \in C}{\text{argmax}} \text{ EVALUATECUT}((\oplus, L_1, L_2))$
4:    **return** $\oplus_{res}(\text{IM}(L_{res1}), \text{IM}(L_{res2}))$
5: **end function**

---

activity is assigned to the left ($x_a = 1$) or right leaf of the operator node, and constraints (9) and (10), ensuring that neither partition is empty. The formal cut definitions from [10] are relaxed in the ILPs by constructing objective functions that maximize conforming behaviour while penalizing behaviour that violates the cut definitions.

Starting with the *sequence cut*, definition (1) requires that the eventually follow relations between partitions are unidirectional, from part 1 to part 2. To relax this constraint, we allow behaviour in both directions but penalise any flow from part 2 to part 1 in the objective function (8).

$$\text{maximize} \quad \sum_{a \in \Sigma} \sum_{b \in \Sigma} |a \twoheadrightarrow^+ b| \cdot (x_b - x_a) \tag{8}$$

$$\text{subject to} \quad \sum_{a \in \Sigma} x_a \geq 1 \tag{9}$$

$$\sum_{a \in \Sigma} (1 - x_a) \geq 1 \tag{10}$$

$$x_a \in \{0, 1\} \qquad\qquad \forall a \in \Sigma \tag{11}$$

Definition (2) of the *exclusive choice cut* allows for no behaviour between the partitions. In a relaxed version of the definition, we aim to minimize the total flow between the partitions in the objective function (12). We introduce a new set of binary auxiliary variables $z_{a,b}$ in (15), which through (13) and (14) function as a relaxed logical exclusive or between x_a and x_b, meaning $z_{a,b}$ is set to 1 if the activities are in different partitions.

$$\text{minimize} \quad \sum_{a \in \Sigma} \sum_{b \in \Sigma} |a \twoheadrightarrow b| \cdot z_{a,b} \tag{12}$$

$$\text{subject to} \quad (9) \wedge (10) \wedge (11)$$

$$z_{a,b} \geq x_a - x_b \qquad\qquad \forall a, b \in \Sigma \tag{13}$$

$$z_{a,b} \geq x_b - x_a \qquad\qquad \forall a, b \in \Sigma \tag{14}$$

$$z_{a,b} \in 0, 1 \qquad\qquad \forall a, b \in \Sigma \tag{15}$$

For the *parallel cut*, definition (4) requires the partitions to be interconnected, which relaxed translates into maximizing the flow between the two partitions. We use the $z_{a,b}$ variables as a xor with (13), (14), (17) and (18). According to definition (3), we also expect both partitions to contain start and end activities.

To include this in the objective function (16) we additionally aim for an even distribution of these activities between the partitions. We introduce a new variable $b \in \mathbb{N}$, calculated in (19)[1] as the difference of the number of start and end activities between the parts, subtracting it from the objective.

$$\text{maximize} \quad \sum_{a \in \Sigma} \sum_{b \in \Sigma} z_{a,b} \cdot |a \twoheadrightarrow b| - b \tag{16}$$

$$\text{subject to} \quad (9) \wedge (10) \wedge (11) \wedge (13) \wedge (14) \wedge (15)$$

$$z_{a,b} \leq x_a + x_b \quad \forall a, b \in \Sigma \tag{17}$$

$$z_{a,b} \leq 2 - x_a - x_b \quad \forall a, b \in \Sigma \tag{18}$$

$$b \geq |\Sigma_{a \in \Sigma} \text{END}(L, a) - 2 \cdot \Sigma_{a \in \Sigma} x_a \cdot \text{END}(L, a)| \tag{19}$$
$$+ |\Sigma_{a \in \Sigma} \text{START}(L, a) - 2 \cdot \Sigma_{a \in \Sigma} x_a \cdot \text{START}(L, a)|$$

$$b \in \mathbb{N} \tag{20}$$

The *loop cut* allows flow from the end activities of the body part to the start activities of the redo part and from the redo part to the start activities of the body part, as defined in (6) and (7). This flow is maximised in the objective function (21), using auxiliary variables $v_{a,b}$ and $w_{a,b} \in \{0, 1\}$ set through constraints (22)–(31), using $\mathcal{X}$ as the indicator function in some of the constraints. The auxiliary variables re_a and rs_a are used for activities which are start and end activities of the redo part. Any partition-crossing behaviour that does not originate from the end activities or does not end in the start activities is considered a violation of (6) and (7) and is represented by the auxiliary variables $f_{a,b} \in \{0, 1\}$, set in constraint (32), and are subtracted from the objective function. Additionally as defined in (5), any start or end activities of the log present in the redo part are also in violation and subtracted from the objective.

$$\text{maximize} \quad \sum_{a \in \Sigma} \sum_{b \in \Sigma} (v_{a,b} \cdot |a \twoheadrightarrow b| + w_{a,b} \cdot |a \twoheadrightarrow b|) \tag{21}$$

$$- \sum_{a \in \text{START}(L) \cup \text{END}(L)} (1 - x_a)$$

$$- \sum_{a \in \Sigma} \sum_{b \in \Sigma} f_{a,b} \cdot |a \twoheadrightarrow b|$$

$$\text{subject to} \quad 9 \wedge 10 \wedge 11$$

$$\text{rs}_a \leq (1 - x_a) \qquad\qquad \forall a \in \Sigma \tag{22}$$

$$\text{re}_a \leq (1 - x_a) \qquad\qquad \forall a \in \Sigma \tag{23}$$

$$\text{rs}_b \geq (x_a - x_b) \cdot a \twoheadrightarrow b \qquad \forall a \in \text{END}(L) \tag{24}$$

$$\text{re}_a \geq (x_b - x_a) \cdot a \twoheadrightarrow b \qquad \forall b \in \text{START}(L) \tag{25}$$

$$w_{a,b} \geq \text{rs}_b + \mathcal{X}_{\text{END}(L)}(a) - 1 \qquad \forall a, b \in \Sigma \tag{26}$$

$$w_{a,b} \leq \text{rs}_b \qquad\qquad \forall a, b \in \Sigma \tag{27}$$

---

[1] In a practical implementation the absolute value would need to be split into multiple constraints, making use of additional auxiliary variables.

$$w_{a,b} \leq \mathcal{X}_{\text{END}(L)}(a) \qquad\qquad \forall a,b \in \Sigma \quad (28)$$

$$v_{a,b} \geq \text{re}_a + \mathcal{X}_{\text{START}(L)}(b) - 1 \qquad \forall a,b \in \Sigma \quad (29)$$

$$v_{a,b} \leq \text{re}_a \qquad\qquad\qquad \forall a,b \in \Sigma \quad (30)$$

$$v_{a,b} \leq \mathcal{X}_{\text{START}(L)}(b) \qquad\qquad \forall a,b \in \Sigma \quad (31)$$

$$f_{a,b} \geq |(x_a - x_b)| \cdot a \twoheadrightarrow b - w_{a,b} - v_{a,b} \qquad \forall a,b \in \Sigma \quad (32)$$

$$f_{a,b}, v_{a,b}, w_{a,b} \in \{0,1\} \qquad\qquad \forall a,b \in \Sigma \quad (33)$$

$$\text{rs}_a, \text{re}_a \in \{0,1\} \qquad\qquad\qquad \forall a \in \Sigma \quad (34)$$

4.2   Operator Selection by Local Fitness and Precision Estimation

When approaching the task of choosing the best cut from the candidate set, the objective values produced by the ILPs are incompatible due to the different underlying measurements. Instead OptIMIIst uses local precision and fitness estimation unique for each operator. For fitness we measure the amount of behaviour in the log that is not replayable after applying the cut, while for precision, we propose frequency-based approaches. Constructing expected probability distributions of the model and comparing them with the observed behaviour using the mean absolute error (MAE), calculated as:

$$\text{MAE}(P_{\text{Observed}}, P_{\text{Expected}}) = \frac{1}{|P_{\text{Expected}}|} \sum_{i=1}^{n} |P_{\text{Observed}_i} - P_{\text{Expected}_i}|$$

For the fitness of the *sequence cut*, violating edges are those arcs in the directly follows graph that cross from part 2 to part 1. Those not being replayable after applying the cut. We define the fitness as the fraction of the frequency of those violating edges to the frequency of all crossing edges. For the precision measure, we assume that the probability of transitioning from any $a \in \text{END}(L_1)$ to any $b \in \text{START}(L_2)$ is uniform. And calculate the MAE between these probabilities with the observed transition probabilities in the log.

$$F_{seq} = 1 - \frac{\Sigma_{a \in \Sigma_2} \Sigma_{b \in \Sigma_1} |a \twoheadrightarrow b|}{\Sigma_{a \in \Sigma_2} \Sigma_{b \in \Sigma_1} |a \twoheadrightarrow b| + \Sigma_{a \in \Sigma_1} \Sigma_{b \in \Sigma_2} |a \twoheadrightarrow b|} \qquad (35)$$

$$P_{seq} = 1 - \text{MAE}(P_{Observed}, P_{Expected}) \qquad (36)$$

For the *exclusive choice cut*, fitness is calculated as the fraction of existing directly follows edges to the total possible edges between activities from different partitions. While precision is always 1, as an exclusive choice cut does not introduce any additional behaviour.

$$F_{xor} = 1 - \frac{\Sigma_{a \in \Sigma_2} \Sigma_{b \in \Sigma_1} a \twoheadrightarrow b + \Sigma_{a \in \Sigma_1} \Sigma_{b \in \Sigma_2} a \twoheadrightarrow b}{2 \cdot |\Sigma_1| \cdot |\Sigma_2|} \qquad (37)$$

The fitness of a *parallel cut* is always 1, as it guarantees that all possible interleaved combinations of traces from the sub-logs can be replayed. For precision, we estimate the expected number of variants by calculating $2^{\text{AVGLEN}(\mathcal{V}_1) + \text{AVGLEN}(\mathcal{V}_2)}$, where $\text{AVGLEN}(\mathcal{V}_1)$ and $\text{AVGLEN}(\mathcal{V}_2)$ are the average trace lengths of the sub-logs $\mathcal{V}_1$ and $\mathcal{V}_2$, respectively. This expected number of variants, V_{exp}, is then compared to the observed number of variants, $|\mathcal{V}|$, to compute the precision as:

$$P_{and} = \frac{|\mathcal{V}|}{V_{\text{exp}}} \tag{38}$$

For the *loop cut* fitness, start and end activities will not be replayable after applying the cut. As such, we calculate the fitness as the fraction of such activities in part 2. For precision we assume that both partitions are independent of each other and the transition probabilities from end activities of the body part to the start activities of the redo part as well as the transition probabilities from the end activities of the redo part to the start activities of the body part are uniform. We calculate the MAE between these probabilities and the observed transition probabilities in the log.

$$F_{loop} = 1 - \frac{|\text{START}(L_b)| + |\text{END}(L_b)|}{|\text{START}(L)| + |\text{END}(L)|} \tag{39}$$

$$P_{loop} = 1 - \frac{\text{MAE}(P_{obsA \to B}, P_{expA \to B}) + \text{MAE}(P_{obsB \to A}, P_{expB \to A})}{2} \tag{40}$$

To get a single comparison measure we calculate the F1-score, defined as $F_1 = 2 \times \frac{fitness \times precision}{fitness + precision}$, and select the candidate with the highest F1-score to apply. For the τ-skip and τ-loop, we use proxy measures from [7].

5   Evaluation

In this section, we evaluate OptIMIIst against other state-of-the-art discovery algorithms. Additionally, we discuss some limitations of OptIMIIst.

Setup. To compare OptIMIIst with other discovery algorithms, we select three existing algorithms. We use IMf as a baseline comparison, with a filter setting of 0.2, AIM, and the ILP-Miner. The latter an approach outside the IM framework. For our evaluation, we utilize public event logs from the BPI Challenges of 2012[2] 2013[3] 2017[4] and 2020[5] as well as the Sepsis log[6] We split each log into a train/test split with 80% of cases in train and 20% of cases in the test split. Models were mined on the train logs and alignment-based fitness [8] was evaluated on the test logs. Additionally, alignment-based precision [1] of the models was measured with the full logs. We also assessed the size of the resulting Petri nets (number

---

[2] BPIC$_{12}$ http://doi.org/10.4121/UUID:3926DB30-F712-4394-AEBC-75976070E91F.

[3] BPIC$_{13}$ http://doi.org/10.4121/UUID:A7CE5C55-03A7-4583-B855-98B86E1A2B07.

[4] BPIC$_{17}$ http://doi.org/10.4121/UUID:5F3067DF-F10B-45DA-B98B-86AE4C7A3 10B.

[5] BPIC$_{20}$ http://doi.org/10.4121/UUID:52FB97D4-4588-43C9-9D04-3604D4613B51.

[6] Sepsis http://doi.org/10.4121/UUID:915D2BFB-7E84-49AD-A286-DC35F063A460.

of places, transitions, and arcs), the number of activities in the models, recorded the frequency of fallthrough occurrences in the OptIMIIst and the runtime of each miner. To mitigate the effect of randomness in the splits, we repeated each experiment five times and averaged the results.

OptIMIIst was implemented in Python, using Gurobi[7] to construct and solve the ILPs. All tests were conducted on macOS 14.5 with an M3-Max processor, with RAM usage consistently remaining below 8GB.

Results. Table 1 presents the results. The fallthrough mechanism was triggered at least once for all logs, and more than five times for all logs except the BPIC 2013 and Sepsis logs. OptIMIIst generally outperforms the IMf in both terms of precision and fitness. While falling short of AIM archiving similar fitness scores, but consistently worse precision. The ILP-Miner, while achieving perfect fitness on most logs, produces models that are very large, in case of BPIC 2020_{TPD} almost nine times larger than those generated by the IM based Miner, and exhibits the worst precision across all logs. Although the precision issue could be partially addressed by manual optimisation the filter parameters, this manual step would likely also reduce fitness.

Comparing the model size of the IM based miners a similar picture as for fitness and precision can be seen. OptIMIIst produces, with one exception, smaller models than IMf but larger ones than AIM. Looking at the number of activities present in the model the reason for that is clearly visible. While OptIMIIst never excluded any activity, AIM performs excessive activity filtering on the activity level, trading information loss for increased precision and simpler models, which leads to a high loss of activities in logs. Like for the BPIC 2020 logs in which AIM filters almost 50% of activities, with in BPIC 2020_{DD} only exhibiting 7 of the original 17 activities. An issue not present in OptIMIIst, upholding similar fitness results to AIM.

Comparing runtimes, IMf is unsurprisingly the fastest miner as it only performs filtering. While OptIMIIst is generally faster than AIM, but slower than ILP-Miner. From a soundness perspective, the models of the IM framework miners are all sound while only 30% of the ILP-Miners models being sound.

Limitations. While our evaluation results show a promising performance of OptIMIIst, some limitations should be acknowledged. One key concern is the computational complexity of using ILPs for optimization. Although our evaluation showed promising runtimes, the approach may have non-polynomial complexity, and therefore, we cannot guarantee efficient computation in all cases.

The optimality of our approach is confined to the local decisions made during the mining process and the relaxation assumptions embedded in the ILPs and estimator. Since OptIMIIst does not employ backtracking, there is no guarantee that an optimal local cut will lead to the globally best mining decision.

---

[7] Gurobi Optimizer Reference Manual - https://www.gurobi.com.

Table 1. OptIMIIst, AIM, IMf, ILP-Miner Benchmarks

Event Log	Algorithm	Runtime (s)	Precision	Fitness	Size	Activities
BPIC 2012	OptIMIIst	80.20	0.902	0.649	198	24.0
	IMf	**5.60**	0.165	0.998	239	23.8
	AIM	244.65	**0.927**	0.592	162	21.0
	ILP-Miner	20.29	0.132	**1.000**	291	24.0
BPIC 2013$_{CP}$	OptIMIIst	0.86	0.927	0.958	36	4.0
	IMf	**0.01**	0.970	0.989	50	3.8
	AIM	10.92	**0.999**	0.771	16	3.0
	ILP-Miner	0.08	0.883	**1.000**	43	4.0
BPIC 2013$_I$	OptIMIIst	10.30	0.982	0.905	48	4.0
	IMf	**0.07**	0.843	0.964	49	4.0
	AIM	30.21	**0.995**	0.905	37	3.0
	ILP-Miner	0.87	0.684	**1.000**	39	4.0
BPIC 2017	OptIMIIst	769.24	**0.965**	0.742	186	26.0
	IMf	**20.92**	0.375	0.949	285	25.2
	AIM	655.36	**0.965**	0.643	116	21.2
	ILP-Miner	230.33	0.172	**1.000**	632	26.0
BPIC 2020$_{DD}$	OptIMIIst	15.55	0.600	0.942	122	16.8
	IMf	**0.03**	0.258	0.936	125	15.6
	AIM	38.96	**1.000**	0.910	36	7.0
	ILP-Miner	0.56	0.157	**1.000**	252	16.8
BPIC 2020$_{ID}$	OptIMIIst	32.41	0.378	0.878	269	33.6
	IMf	**0.09**	0.202	0.886	284	29.0
	AIM	66.22	**0.951**	0.882	89	14.2
	ILP-Miner	6.19	0.136	**1.000**	1213	33.6
BPIC 2020$_{PTC}$	OptIMIIst	6.53	0.294	0.872	236	29.0
	IMf	**0.04**	0.243	0.879	243	26.4
	AIM	23.55	**0.562**	0.889	107	13.0
	ILP-Miner	3.00	0.237	**0.999**	913	29.0
BPIC 2020$_{RFP}$	OptIMIIst	10.78	0.371	0.925	146	18.6
	IMf	**0.02**	0.272	0.913	157	16.4
	AIM	25.94	**0.851**	0.925	69	10.4
	ILP-Miner	0.57	0.194	**1.000**	324	18.6
BPIC 2020$_{TPD}$	OptIMIIst	66.22	0.271	0.800	453	50.4
	IMf	**0.45**	0.199	0.774	410	41.2
	AIM	84.36	**0.727**	0.800	137	18.0
	ILP-Miner	86.31	0.081	**1.000**	3019	50.4
Sepsis	OptIMIIst	3.53	0.727	0.846	113	16.0
	IMf	**0.05**	0.602	0.970	152	15.0
	AIM	16.39	**0.828**	0.890	105	14.0
	ILP-Miner	1.52	0.398	**1.000**	296	16.0

6   Conclusion

This paper introduced a novel twofold approach for identifying locally optimal process trees. Our method finds locally optimal activity partitions for each operator, while handling infrequent and incomplete behaviour. Utilizing a fitness and precision estimator to select the most suitable cut. We evaluated OptIMIIst by demonstrating its competitive performance in terms of precision, fitness and simplicity compared to the existing algorithms AIM, IMf and ILP-Miner. Notably it was competitive without excessive activity filtering. As future work, OptIMIIst could be extended with explicit filtering of activities in conjunction with the cut optimization routines. Furthermore, the ILPs could be used to find more complex structures like long-distance-dependencies and duplicated activities, for example by incorporating external data.

References

1. Adriansyah, A., Munoz-Gama, J., Carmona, J., van Dongen, B.F., van der Aalst, W.M.P.: Measuring precision of modeled behavior. Inf. Syst. E Bus. Manag. **13**(1) (2015)
2. Augusto, A., Conforti, R., Dumas, M., Rosa, M.L.: Split miner: discovering accurate and simple business process models from event logs. In: 2017 IEEE International Conference on Data Mining, ICDM 2017. IEEE Computer Society (2017)
3. Augusto, A., et al.: Automated discovery of process models from event logs: review and benchmark. IEEE Trans. Knowl. Data Eng. **31**(4) (2019)
4. Bergenthum, R.: Prime miner - process discovery using prime event structures. In: ICPM 2019. IEEE (2019)
5. Brons, D., Scheepens, R., Fahland, D.: Striking a new balance in accuracy and simplicity with the probabilistic inductive miner. In: ICPM (2021)
6. Buijs, J.C.A.M., van Dongen, B.F., van der Aalst, W.M.P.: Quality dimensions in process discovery: The importance of fitness, precision, generalization and simplicity. Int. J. Cooperative Inf. Syst. **23**(1) (2014)
7. van Detten, J.N., Schumacher, P., Leemans, S.J.J.: An approximate inductive miner. In: ICPM 2023 (2023)
8. van Dongen, B., Carmona, J., Chatain, T., Taymouri, F.: Aligning modeled and observed behavior: a compromise between computation complexity and quality. In: AiSE. Cham (2017)
9. Leemans, S.J.J.: Robust Process Mining with Guarantees - Process Discovery, Conformance Checking and Enhancement. LNBIP, vol. 440. Springer (2022)
10. Leemans, S.J.J., Fahland, D., van der Aalst, W.M.P.: Discovering block-structured process models from event logs - a constructive approach. In: Petri Nets. LNCS, vol. 7927 (2013)
11. Leemans, S.J.J., Fahland, D., van der Aalst, W.M.P.: Discovering block-structured process models from event logs containing infrequent behaviour. In: BPM Workshops - BPM. LNBIP, vol. 171 (2013)
12. Leemans, S.J.J., Fahland, D., van der Aalst, W.M.P.: Discovering block-structured process models from incomplete event logs. In: Petri Nets. LNCS (2014)
13. Leemans, S.J.J., Tax, N., ter Hofstede, A.H.M.: Indulpet miner: combining discovery algorithms. In: On the Move to Meaningful Internet Systems. OTM 2018 Conferences. Cham (2018)

14. Mannel, L.L., van der Aalst, W.M.P.: Finding complex process-structures by exploiting the token-game. In: Petri Nets. Lecture Notes in Computer Science, vol. 11522. Springer (2019)
15. Murata, T.: Petri nets: properties, analysis and applications. Proc. IEEE **77**(4) (1989)
16. Sani, M.F., van Zelst, S.J., van der Aalst, W.M.P.: Repairing outlier behaviour in event logs. In: Business Information Systems. Lecture Notes of Business Information Systems, vol. 320 (2018)
17. Solé, M., Carmona, J.: Encoding process discovery problems in SMT. Softw. Syst. Model. **17**(4) (2018)
18. Weijters, A.J., Van der Aalst, W.M.: Rediscovering workflow models from event-based data using little thumb. Integr. Comput.-Aided Eng. **10**(2) (2003)
19. van der Werf, J.M.E.M., van Dongen, B.F., Hurkens, C.A.J., Serebrenik, A.: Process discovery using integer linear programming. In: Petri Nets. Berlin, Heidelberg (2008)

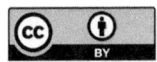

A Framework for Advanced Case Notions in Object-Centric Process Mining

Jan Niklas van Detten[1,2]([✉]), Pol Schumacher[2], and Sander J. J. Leemans[1,3]

[1] RWTH Aachen University, Aachen, Germany
n.vandetten@bpm.rwth-aachen.de
[2] Celonis Gmbh, Munchen, Germany
[3] Fraunhofer, Sankt Augustin, Germany

Abstract. Real-life processes involve interacting business objects of different types. Object-centric event logs capture the execution of activities in such processes. An important step in the analysis of such logs is the identification of sets of objects which characterize an execution of the process, called a case. Given a case notion, visualizations can be constructed to display the relations between the executed activities and the involved business objects. Depending on the utilized case notion, these visualizations can quickly become excessively complex, impeding human analysis, or may oversimplify the underlying process, inducing flawed insights. To combat these issues, new case notions are needed to reduce complexity while representing relevant structures of the underlying business process correctly. In this paper, we propose continuous measures to quantify how correctly an object-centric case notion adheres to a given log and how complex the resulting visualizations are. These measures allow us to conceptualize the search for new object-centric case notions as a joint optimization problem among the two quality dimensions of correctness and simplicity. As a result, we can provide a new case notion that significantly reduces complexity in comparison to existing techniques, while preserving relevant object interactions. To evaluate our approach, we apply it to a range of real-life logs and find that major complexity reductions can be achieved without causing excessive correctness issues.

Keywords: process mining · object-centric · case notions · visualizations

1 Introduction

The research area of process mining provides techniques to analyze business processes based on digital execution track records, called event logs. These logs contain sequences of events with the labels of executed activities. For analytical purposes, it is important to visualize the relation between these activities.

Traditionally, process mining techniques have been used to study processes in isolation. For this purpose, all events associated to one particular object, like a loan application for example, are considered an execution of the process, called a case. However, real-life business processes rarely exist in such a single-object

© The Author(s) 2025
A. Delgado and T. Slaats (Eds.): ICPM 2024 Workshops, LNBIP 533, pp. 402–414, 2025.
https://doi.org/10.1007/978-3-031-82225-4_30

vacuum. Instead, processes often involve multiple business objects that might interact in shared events. A loan application might, for example, lead to the creation of a loan contract and require multiple payments to be issued.

Object-centric process mining techniques address this reality by considering anything that participates in a process as an object. Object-centric event logs are sequences of events with activities associated to sets of objects. To study the interactions between objects, the traditional single-object case notion is not sufficient. The events associated to a payment might, for example, be influenced by the events of the preceding loan application. Therefore, it would be insufficient to exclusively focus on a single object. Instead, a set of objects with a set of associated events characterizes an execution, i.e. a case, of such processes.

The division of object-centric event logs into cases of associated objects and event sets can induce unintended side effects when done incorrectly, such as duplicated events, lost events or incorrect relationships between them [1]. Existing work to guarantee the absence of such phenomena has been proposed in [3]. However, these techniques do not take the effect of the selected case notion on the complexity of corresponding visualizations into account. As a result, practitioners are currently faced with the choice between two extreme options. That is, they either use the traditional case notion, which may induce severe correctness issues in the object-centric setting, or apply the approach from [3], which produces only few, large cases for processes with many object interactions.

In this paper, we propose an evaluation framework to conceptualize the simplicity and correctness of object-centric case notions as continuous quality measures. Additionally, we introduce a new object-centric case notion that significantly reduces the complexity of case visualizations, while preserving their ability to represent large parts of the underlying business process correctly. We apply our approach to a range of real-life logs and find that major complexity reductions can be achieved without causing excessive correctness issues.

2 Preliminaries

In this section, we summarize required background information on object-centric event logs, existing case notions and common correctness criteria for them.

2.1 Object-Centric Event Logs

An object-centric event log is an ordered sequence of events $\langle (a_1, O_1), \ldots, (a_n, O_n) \rangle$ with activities a_i and sets of objects O_i. We write Σ, Θ and Ω for all activities, objects and object types in such a log respectively. Each object is associated to its object type with the injective type function $\omega : \Theta \mapsto \Omega$. An object set O can be projected onto the subset of objects with the type $ot \in \Omega$ with $O|_{ot}$.

Table 1 shows an example log of a loan application process. It involves applications (a), loans (1) and payments (p) in addition to three employees (e) and a software system (s). Applications are submitted to be checked by an employee,

Table 1. Object-centric event log of a loan application process.

⟨SUBMIT $\{a_1, s_1\}$,	CHECK $\{a_1, e_1\}$,	SUBMIT $\{a_2, s_1\}$,	DENY $\{a_1, e_1, s_1\}$,
SUBMIT $\{a_3, s_1\}$,	CHECK $\{a_2, e_1\}$,	GRANT $\{a_2, e_1, s_1, l_1\}$,	CHECK $\{a_3, e_1\}$,
PAY $\{l_1, p_1, e_1, e_2\}$,	DENY $\{a_3, e_1, s_1, \}$,	SUBMIT $\{a_4, s_1, \}$	PAY $\{l_1, p_2, e_1, e_2\}$,
CHECK $\{a_4, e_1\}$,	GRANT $\{a_3, e_1, s_1, l_2\}$,	PAY $\{l_2, p_3, e_1, e_3\}$	PAY $\{l_2, p_4, e_1, e_3\}$⟩

which can reject it or grant a loan based upon it. Associated payments are subsequently payed, with a second employee checking the correctness of each payment. The system tracks which applications are submitted, rejected and granted.

An object-centric event log can be interpreted as an undirected bipartite graph structure. For this purpose, every object and event is conceptualized as a node. An arc between them indicates that the object is involved in the event.

We refer to such a graph as a log graph for a given object-centric event log $L = \langle (a_1, O_1), \ldots, (a_n, O_n) \rangle$. Formally, a log graph $L_G = (E, O, A)$ consists of event nodes $E = \{\bullet_i \mid 1 \leq i \leq n\}$ and object nodes $O = \{\bullet_o \mid o \in \Theta\}$, which are connected with the undirected arcs $A = \{(\bullet_i, \bullet_o) \mid o \in O_i\}$. Figure 1 shows the log graph for our example log from Table 1, with colors indicating object types.

2.2 Object-Centric Case Notions

A case notions projects object-centric event logs onto associated event and sets of objects. Each of these object-event combinations represents an independent execution of the process. In this paper, we consider this a division operation on the log graph of a given object-centric event log.

Formally, an object centric case notion is a projection of a given log graph on a set of subgraphs. For a given log L with the log graph $L_G = (E, O, A)$,

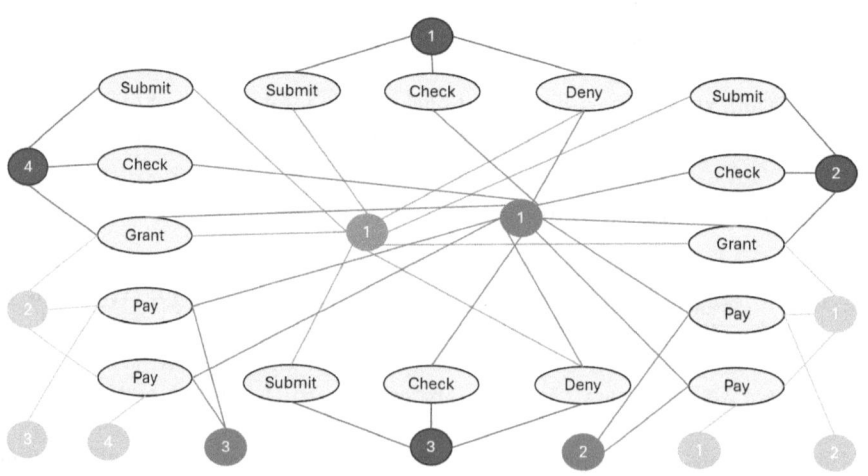

Fig. 1. Visualization of the log graph for the example log in Table 3 with applications (blue), loans (yellow), payments (violet), employees (red) and systems (green). (Color figure online)

a case notion c is any method that projects L_G on a set of subgraphs, i.e. $c : (E, O, A) \mapsto \mathbb{P}(\{E', O', A' \mid E' \subseteq E \land O' \subseteq O \land A' = A \cap (E' \times O')\})$. Note that such a case notion, without further restrictions, might duplicate or drop event or object nodes of the original graph and the edges between them.

2.3 Traditional Case Notion

The traditional case notion evolves around individual objects of the same type and their respective events. Given a log graph and an object type, each case only has a single object of this type and all the event nodes connected to it.

Formally, the results of the traditional case notion c_{ot} for an object type $ot \in \Omega$ and the log graph $L_G = (E, O, A)$ are given by the subgraphs $c_{ot} = \{(E', O', A') \mid O' = \{\bullet_o\} \land \omega(o) = ot \land E' = \{\bullet_e \mid \exists(\bullet_o, \bullet_e) \in A\} \land A' = O' \times E'\}$.

Note that the results of the traditional case notion heavily depend on the selected object type. For the example log graph in Fig. 1 and the object types of the involved employees, the resulting cases can be seen in Fig. 2

The usage of the traditional case notion can cause three correctness issues, known as divergence, convergence and deficiency [1]. Convergence and deficiency refer to events being associated to multiple cases or no case at all. Divergence describes the assignment of events to the same case without including the involved objects in which they differ. In our example we can observe convergence, since the payment events are duplicated among the two employees. Deficiency occurs, because the submission events are not related to any employee. Divergence occurs since the events of different applications involve the same employee.

For the scope of this paper, we formally consider divergence, convergence and deficiency at the level of activities and object types. That is, we speak of convergence of $ot \in \Omega$ and $a \in \Sigma$ if $\exists(a, O) \in L$ with $|O\lfloor_{ot}| > 1$. Similarly, we refer to deficiency of $ot \in \Omega$ and $a \in \Sigma$ if $\exists(a, O) \in L$ with $|O\lfloor_{ot}| < 1$. Divergence occurs for a and ot if $\exists(a, O), (a, O') \in L : O \neq O' \land (O \cap O')\lfloor_{ot} \neq \emptyset$.

2.4 Connected Component Case Notion

The correctness issues of divergence, convergence and deficiency in object-centric case notion have been addressed in literature. The approach in [3] proposes to

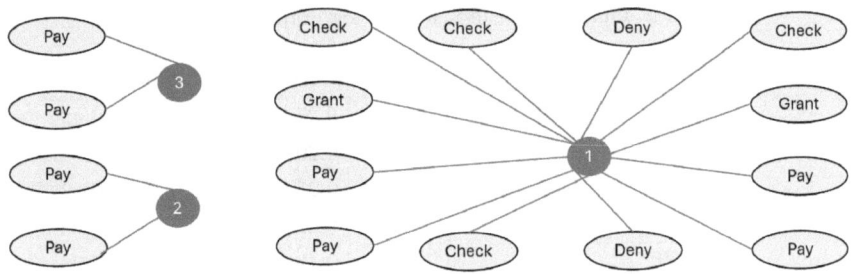

Fig. 2. Visualization of the cases resulting from the application of the traditional case notion on the log graph in Fig. 1 for the object types of employees (red). (Color figure online)

use each connected component in the log graph of an object-centric event log as a case. The approach proves that this strategy is the only one that can guarantee the absence of correctness issues due to divergence, convergence and deficiency.

For our example log graph in Fig. 1, the connected component case notion results in a single case that contains the entire log graph. The reason for this phenomenon are highly connected objects, such as the employee and the system.

3   Optimization Framework

In this section, we present our evaluation framework for object-centric case notions. First, we propose continuous measures for the correctness and simplicity of a given case notion in Sect. 3.1 and 3.2 respectively. Then, we sketch how these measures can be used to conceptualize new object-centric case notions as an optimization problem across the two quality dimensions in Sect. 3.3.

3.1   Graph-Based Correctness Measures

Our correctness criteria for object-centric case notions focus on the correct and lossless division of objects, events and the relations between them. With regards to the graph-based interpretation, these criteria correspond to the required absence of duplicated or missing nodes and edges of the log graph. Our measures are backwards compatible to existing correctness notions, i.e. a case notion with perfect scores is free of any issues due to divergence, convergence and deficiency.

Formally, for a given case notion c and log graph $L_G = (E, O, A)$, an object node $\bullet_o \in O$ adheres to the correctness criteria of the case notion, if it appears in exactly one case, i.e. $|\{(E', O', A') \in c(L_G) \mid \bullet_o \in O'\}| = 1$. We write O_c for all objects nodes that adhere to the case notion. Similarly, we define the adherence of an event node $\bullet_e \in E$ to the correctness criteria of a case notion c with $|\{(E', O', A') \in c(L_G) \mid \bullet_e \in E'\}| = 1$. We write E_c for the set of adhering event nodes. Analogously, we define the set of adhering edges of the log graph for the case notion c with $A_c = \{a \in A \mid |\{(E', O', A') \in c(L_G) \mid a \in A'\}| = 1\}$.

Based upon the notion of adhering nodes and edges, we define the correctness measures for a given log graph and case notion as the average value of $|O_c| \cdot |O|^{-1}$,

Table 2. Quality measures for the log graph from Fig. 1.

Notion	$|O_c| \cdot |O|^{-1}$	$|E_c| \cdot |E|^{-1}$	$|A_c| \cdot |A|^{-1}$	Correctness	Simplicity	Total
$c_{employee}$	0.21	0.50	0.35	0.35	0.79	0.49
$c_{payment}$	0.29	0.25	0.09	0.20	0.93	0.34
c_{system}	0.07	0.50	0.17	0.25	0.70	0.37
c_{loan}	0.14	0.38	0.13	0.22	0.87	0.35
$c_{application}$	0.29	0.75	0.26	0.43	0.87	0.58
c_{cc}	1.00	1.00	1.00	1.00	0.00	0.00

$|E_c| \cdot |E|^{-1}$ and $|A_c| \cdot |A|^{-1}$. More sophisticated aggregation methods will be investigated in future work. Table 2 shows the correctness measures for the graph in Fig. 1 and the case notions explained in Sect. 2.3 and Sect. 2.4.

3.2   Graph-Based Simplicity Measures

The complexity of case visualizations is strongly connected to the number of objects and events per case. Therefore, we use the average number of nodes in each case identified by a given case notion as a proxy measure for the complexity of the corresponding visualizations. To again have a measure on a scale from zero to one, we set that number into relation with the overall size of the log graph.

Formally, for a given log graph $L_G = (E, O, A)$ and case notion c, we first determine the average case size with $S(L_G, c) = \sum_{(E',O',A') \in c(L_G)}(|E'| + |O'|) \cdot |c(L_G)|^{-1}$. Based upon the resulting value, we subsequently define the simplicity measure for the case notion and the log graph as $1 - S(L_G, c) \cdot (|E| + |O|)^{-1}$. Table 2 shows the simplicity of existing case notions on the log graph from Fig. 2.

3.3   Graph Based Optimization

Given a set of potential case notions, we can use the measures proposed in the previous sections to select the case notion that hits the best trade off between correctness and simplicity. For this purpose, we need to combine the two quality dimensions into a single, overall score. For the scope of this paper, we utilize the harmonic mean between the correctness and simplicity for this purpose, similar to the commonly used F1-score in process mining.

For the existing case notions with the corresponding measures in Table 2, we can use this accumulation to decide which of those is best to use for the example log graph in Fig. 1. However, note that even the best case notion, which is the traditional case notion for applications, only achieves 0.58 as a total score.

4   Object-Centric Case Notions

In this section we motivate and formalize a new case notion to optimize the balance between simplicity and correctness of object-centric process visualizations

4.1   Resource-Like Business Objects

Considering the correctness and simplicity of existing case notions in Table 2, two patterns become apparent. The traditional case notions for individual object types are simple, but ignore many objects and events that refer to different object types. In contrast, the connected component case notion is correct, but excessively complex, due to some highly connected objects in the log graph. These objects are often of resource-like nature, interacting with many objects that would traditionally be considered as individual cases. Therefore, we propose a new object-centric case notion, that determines the connected components in a log graph but does not consider connections that arise from resource-like objects.

Algorithm 1. Advanced Object-Centric Case Notion

---

function $c'_{ot}((E, O, A), div)$

  $result \leftarrow \{\}$

  for $\bullet_o \in \{\bullet_o \in O \mid \omega(o) = ot\}$ **do**

    $O', O'', E', E'' \leftarrow \{\bullet_o\}, \{\bullet_o\}, \{\}, \{\}$

    while $O'' \neq \emptyset \lor E'' \neq \emptyset$ **do**

      $E'' \leftarrow \{\bullet_e \in E \setminus E' \mid \exists \bullet_o \in O'' : (\bullet_e, \bullet_o) \in A\}$

      $O'' \leftarrow \{\bullet_o \in O \setminus O' \mid \exists \bullet_e \in E'' : (\bullet_e, \bullet_o) \in A \land \omega(o) \notin div(\bullet_e) \cup \{ot\}\}$

      $O''' \leftarrow \{\bullet_o \in O \setminus O' \mid \exists \bullet_e \in E'' : (\bullet_e, \bullet_o) \in A \land \omega(o) \in div(\bullet_e) \setminus \{ot\}\}$

      $E', O' \leftarrow E' \cup E'', O' \cup O'' \cup O'''$

    $result \leftarrow result \cup \{(E', O', A')\}$

  return result

4.2 Advanced Case Notion

Similar to the traditional case notion, we use a given object type as a starting point for the construction of the cases. For each individual object of this type, we add all related events to the same case. Then we utilize the idea of the connected components and repeatedly add objects and events to the case that are transitively related to the starting object. However, if the path to an object node leads through an event node with an activity on which this object's type diverges, we stop. As a result, connections caused by resource-like business objects are not followed when constructing a case. Algorithm 1 shows the code for our advanced case notion with a given start type. The auxiliary function div maps each event node to its diverging object types. After determining the advanced case notion for each object type, we again use our framework to pick the best one. Applying this strategy to our running example, results in a case notion with 0.80 as the total score. Figure 3 shows the resulting cases for our example.

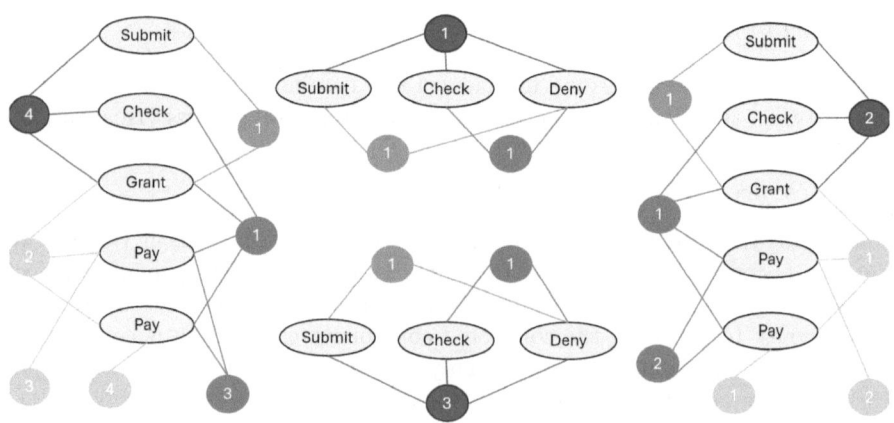

Fig. 3. Advanced case notion with applications as the starting object type.

5   Evaluation

In this section, we evaluate the technique proposed in this paper. For this purpose, we prototypically implemented our approach in Python. We utilize a large
range of synthetically generated and real-life object-centric event logs that are
publicly available and shown in Table 3. We apply our approach to these logs
and observe the runtime required to apply our framework to evaluate its computational feasibility. Additionally, we investigate how well our proposed case
notion from Sect. 3.3 performs quantitatively in comparison with the existing
notions from Sect. 2.4 and Sect. 2.3. Lastly, we perform a qualitative comparison
by manually investigating the visualizations of the different case notions.

5.1   Runtime Efficiency

To evaluate the computational feasibility of our framework, we measured the
time needed to determine and evaluate the traditional, connected component
and advanced case notion respectively. The traditional and advanced case notion
iterate over all possible start object types to determine the best one. All case
notions used the same data structure for the representation of the log graphs.
All experiments were performed on a consumer grade laptop with an Intel-Core
i5-8265U processor with exclusive access to 16GB of working memory. We set a
runtime limit of one hour per object-centric event log and case notion.

The resulting runtime measurements can be seen in Table 3, illustrating the
computational feasibility of our framework and the advanced case notion. Across

Table 3. Statistics of utilized object-centric logs and measured framework runtime for
the traditional (TD), connected component (CC) and advanced (AD) case notion.

Log	Objects	Types	Events	Activities	TD (s)	CC (s)	AD (s)
BPIC15$_1$ [8]	1269	4	52217	289	11	9	46
BPIC15$_2$ [8]	859	4	44354	304	8	6	40
BPIC15$_3$ [8]	1465	4	59681	277	12	10	53
BPIC15$_4$ [8]	1084	4	47293	272	11	8	43
BPIC15$_5$ [8]	1202	4	59083	285	13	10	55
BPIC17 [8]	106162	4	1202267	26	140	t/o	451
BPIC19 [8]	330685	4	1595923	42	336	t/o	2171
Github [10]	28317	2	27842	67	68	87	1941
O2C [4,10]	107767	19	98350	23	50	208	105
P2P [4,10]	74489	8	24854	32	11	27	44
HR [10]	1505	6	6980	16	2	1	5
Logistics [10]	11521	5	22367	11	10	18	77
Transfers [10]	2500	5	10319	3	3	2	7
MIMIC [7]	3007	3	13410	3	2	3	4

all logs and case notions, we only observed two time outs. All of them occurred during the connected component based approach. Upon closer investigation, we found this was caused by large connected components in the corresponding log graphs. While this is not a problem for the detection of connected components, it increases the runtime for the implementation of our measures drastically. The traditional and advanced case notion did not suffer from the same issue, having maximal runtime values of 6 and 37 minutes respectively. As expected, the traditional case notion outperformed the advanced case notion on all logs, since it only needs to consider object nodes of a single type, leading to smaller cases.

5.2   Case Notion Performance

Next, we investigate how well the traditional, connected component and advanced case notions perform on the logs from Table 3. For this purpose we measure simplicity, correctness and overall score as specified in Sect. 3.

The resulting scores can be seen in Table 4, confirming the pattern motivated in our running example. For most logs, the traditional case notion results in almost perfect simplicity scores, but suffers from correctness issues. Reversely, the connected component notion guarantees perfect correctness, but suffers from poor simplicity. However, the advanced notion successfully balances the two quality dimensions, resulting in the best overall score for 12 out of 14 logs.

Table 4. Measured scores for the simplicity and correctness of the traditional (TD), connected component (CC) and advanced (AD) case notion respectively.

Log	Simplicity			Correctness			Total		
	TD	CC	AD	TD	CC	AD	TD	CC	AD
BPIC15$_1$ [8]	0.99	0.00	0.95	0.73	1.00	0.98	0.84	0.00	0.97
BPIC15$_2$ [8]	0.99	0.00	0.85	0.73	1.00	0.99	0.85	0.00	0.92
BPIC15$_3$ [8]	0.99	0.00	0.99	0.73	1.00	0.99	0.84	0.00	0.99
BPIC15$_4$ [8]	0.99	0.00	0.99	0.74	1.00	0.99	0.85	0.00	0.99
BPIC15$_5$ [8]	0.99	0.00	0.99	0.73	1.00	0.98	0.84	0.00	0.99
BPIC17 [8]	0.99	0.00	0.99	0.50	1.00	0.53	0.66	0.00	0.69
BPIC19 [8]	0.99	0.00	0.99	0.67	1.00	0.99	0.80	0.00	0.99
Github [10]	0.99	0.00	0.81	0.47	1.00	0.95	0.64	0.00	0.87
O2C [4, 10]	0.99	0.99	0.99	0.26	1.00	0.39	0.41	0.99	0.56
P2P [4, 10]	0.99	0.99	0.99	0.44	1.00	0.80	0.61	0.99	0.89
HR [10]	0.99	0.00	0.99	0.61	1.00	0.71	0.76	0.00	0.83
Logistics [10]	0.99	0.00	0.98	0.53	1.00	0.99	0.69	0.00	0.99
Transfers [10]	0.99	0.8	0.99	0.58	1.00	0.94	0.74	0.88	0.96
MIMIC [7]	0.99	0.5	0.99	0.76	1.00	0.99	0.86	0.66	0.99

Two interesting outliers are the two logs describing an order-to-cash and procure-to-pay process, that were extracted from simulated SAP instances [4]. For both of these logs, the connected component approach achieves the best score, with a significant distance to our proposed case notion. Upon closer investigation of these two logs, we found that these logs contain events that only have objects of diverging object types associated to them. As a result, our case notion is not able to reach those events from, otherwise optimal, starting types.

5.3   Process Visualizations

Lastly, we manually inspect an example case visualization. Figure 4 shows a case in the human resource log, identified by our advanced case notion. We cannot visualize the corresponding case of the connected component approach, since it only identified a single case in the entire log, with more than eight thousand nodes. Using the corresponding cases of the traditional case notion for isolated object type induces several correctness issues. From the perspective of individual recruiters, it is not possible to deduct that they are assigned to applications in groups of three. For isolated applications, one can not deduct that multiple applications are submitted by the same applicant. Reversely, one cannot differentiate between events of independent applications from the applicants perspective. And by only considering a vacancy, a manager, or an offer, large parts of the process become invisible. Our advanced case notion manages to avoid these problems, without the excessive complexity of the connected components. The only correctness issue caused in exchange, is that the resource-like business objects of the managers, vacancies and recruiters are involved in multiple cases simultaneously.

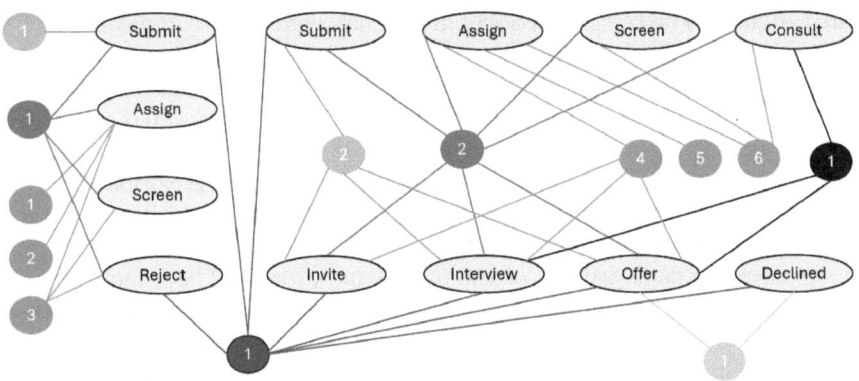

Fig. 4. Example case of the human resources log with applications (red), applicants (blue), recruiters (green), managers (black), vacancies (pink) and offers (yellow). (Color figure online)

5.4   Discussion

Our evaluation shows, that our framework for evaluating object-centric case notions is generally feasible in terms of runtime. Additionally, we found our proposed case notion to quantitatively outperform existing ones in terms of balancing simplicity and correctness. Our manual investigation example showcased that our approach offers an object-centric view on the executions of the process, without leading to excessively complex visualizations in return.

Limitations of our approach are the assumed structure of the input logs and the bias introduced by our measures. We rely on events being associated to at least one object of a non-diverging type. Approaches in literature exists to take care of situations where this is not the case, in particular by using the notion of silent objects [5] or by applying artifact-centric techniques [11]. Incorporating these approaches as a preprocessing step into our case notion might solve the issues observed on the two SAP logs, which should be subject to further research.

While our measures for correctness are well rooted in existing correctness criteria for object-centric case notions, our simplicity measure induces a selection bias. Since it measures simplicity in relation to the overall size of the log graph, large cases can still occur as long as they are small in comparison to the overall graph. Our framework could be extended with penalty measures for the absolute case size, which would however sacrifice an unknown extent of correctness.

6   Related Work

In this section, we summarize related work on object-centric case notions and their correctness. The notion of correctness criteria associated to the absence of unique case identifiers in the object-centric setting has been discussed in [1] and addressed in [2]. The key properties of divergence, convergence and deficiency are reflected in our work as well, in the sense that perfect correctness scores imply the absence of these three issues. The work in [3] proves that such guarantees can only be given if, and only if, the case notion corresponds to the connected components in the underlying log graph. Our work extents these criteria by considering them on a continuous scale to evaluate the extent to which a case notion is correct, instead of treating correctness as a binary property. Additionally, [3] explores graph isomorphism techniques to evaluate if two cases are structurally the same, i.e. represent the same variant of the underlying process. The same techniques can be applied to every case notion that follows the graph based interpretation as described in Sect. 2 and hence also to our work. The problem of excessive case complexity has so far only addressed by resorting to preprocessing steps that remove objects of highly connected object types [3]. To the best of our knowledge, our approach is the first to conceptualize object-centric case notions as a continuous optimization problem among multiple quality dimensions.

Further ideas on graph-based interpretations of object-centric event logs have been proposed in [6]. The approach has been extended with additional functionality and implementations in [9,12] and utilizes the concepts of event knowledge graphs. In contrast to our conceptualization, which only considers edges between objects and events, event knowledge graph may contain further edges of different types. These are used to represent the time-based order between events from the perspective of different objects. Additionally, relations between objects can be expressed. Our work can be applied to these graphs as well, but the quality measures should be adjusted to also account for these additional edge types.

7   Conclusion

In this paper, we introduced a novel framework to continuously evaluate object-centric case notions among the quality dimensions of correctness and simplicity. Based upon this framework, we introduced a new object-centric case notion which balances the two quality dimensions by enforcing a selection criteria on transitive relations between objects. As a result, we can construct relatively simple cases that still showcase important transitive relations between objects. We evaluated our approach threefold on a range of synthetic and real-life object-centric event logs. We found our approach to be feasible in terms of runtime, even for large input logs. Our proposed case notion quantitatively outperformed existing ones in terms of balancing simplicity and correctness. Additionally, we manually investigated some of the resulting process visualizations, exemplary confirming its qualitative advantages. Future work will be focused on providing a preprocessing pipeline to address the limitations caused by the assumptions on the input log structure, as discussed in Sect. 5.4. Additionally, further investigations should focus on the selection bias induced by our simplicity measures.

References

1. van der Aalst, W.M.P.: Object-centric process mining: dealing with divergence and convergence in event data. In: Software Engineering and Formal Methods - 17th International Conference. Lecture Notes in Computer Science, vol. 11724, pp. 3–25. Springer (2019). https://doi.org/10.1007/978-3-030-30446-1_1
2. Adams, J.N., van der Aalst, W.M.P.: Addressing convergence, divergence, and deficiency issues. In: Business Process Management Workshops - BPM 2023 International Workshops. Lecture Notes in Business Information Processing, vol. 492, pp. 496–507. Springer (2023). https://doi.org/10.1007/978-3-031-50974-2_37
3. Adams, J.N., Schuster, D., Schmitz, S., Schuh, G., van der Aalst, W.M.P.: Defining cases and variants for object-centric event data. In: 4th International Conference on Process Mining, ICPM 2022, Bolzano, Italy, 23–28 October 2022. IEEE (2022)
4. Berti, A., Park, G., Rafiei, M., van der Aalst, W.M.P.: An event data extraction approach from SAP ERP for process mining. In: Process Mining Workshops - ICPM 2021 International Workshops, Eindhoven. vol. 433. Springer (2021)
5. Jan Niklas van Detten, P.S., Leemans, S.J.: Object synchronizations and specializations with silent objects in object-centric petri nets. BPM, Proceedings (2024)
6. Fahland, D.: Multi-dimensional process analysis. In: Di Ciccio, C., Dijkman, R., del Río Ortega, A., Rinderle-Ma, S. (eds.) Business Process Management, pp. 27–33. Springer, Cham (2022)
7. Johnson, A., et al.: MIMIC-III, a freely accessible critical care database. Sci. Data 3, 160035 (2016)

8. Khayatbashi, S., Hartig, O., Jalali, A.: BPI challenge 2015-2019 (OCEL) (2023)
9. Khayatbashi, S., Hartig, O., Jalali, A.: Transforming event knowledge graph to object-centric event logs: a comparative study for multi-dimensional process analysis. In: Conceptual Modeling. Springer, Cham (2023)
10. Koren, I., Adams, N., Berti, A.: OCEL 2.0 resources - www.ocel-standard.org CoRR abs/2403.01982 (2024)
11. Popova, V., Fahland, D., Dumas, M.: Artifact lifecycle discovery. Int. J. Cooperative Inf. Syst. **24**(1), 1550001:1–1550001:44 (2015)
12. Swevels, A., Fahland, D., Montali, M.: Implementing object-centric event data models in event knowledge graphs. In: Process Mining Workshops, pp. 431–443. Springer, Cham (2024)

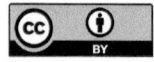

7th International Workshop on Process-Oriented Data Science for Healthcare (PODS4H 2024)

Preface

7th International Workshop on Process-Oriented Data Science for Healthcare (PODS4H 2024)

Data has become a highly valuable resource in today's world. The ultimate goal of data science techniques is not to collect more data, but to extract knowledge and valuable insights from existing data. To analyze and improve processes, event data is a key source of information. In recent years, a new discipline has emerged that combines traditional process analysis and data-centric analysis: Process-Oriented Data Science (PODS). The interdisciplinary nature of this new research area has resulted in its application to analyze processes in a wide variety of domains. This workshop had an explicit focus on healthcare.

The International Workshop on Process-Oriented Data Science for Healthcare 2024 (PODS4H 2024) provided a high-quality forum for interdisciplinary researchers and practitioners to exchange research findings and ideas on data-driven process analysis techniques and practices in healthcare. PODS4H research includes a variety of topics ranging from process mining techniques adapted for healthcare processes to practical issues related to the implementation of PODS methodologies in healthcare organizations.

The 7th edition of the workshop was organized in conjunction with the 6th International Conference on Process Mining in Copenhagen (Denmark). Similarly to last year, we allowed full papers to be either research papers or case studies. While research papers had to focus on extending the state of the art of PODS4H research, case studies had to focus on a practical application of PODS4H in a real-life context.

Each submission to our workshop was thoroughly reviewed by experts from our Program Committee such that each submission got three reviews. After the review process, 6 full papers were accepted. The distinction between research papers and case studies was also reflected in the accepted papers, which consisted of 3 research papers and 3 case studies. The research papers focused on a wide range of topics: providing interactive tools to support the structuring and semantic annotation of mined clinical workflows, establishing a multi-perspective analogy-based process instance search framework that can be used for analogy-based search in healthcare, and predicting unplanned hospital readmissions using outcome-oriented predictive process monitoring. The case studies also considered different healthcare-related problems and contexts: discovering prostate cancer treatment pathways using the Cancer Registry of Rhineland-Palatinate in Germany, using explainable predictive process monitoring methods within the context of esophagogastric cancer treatment leveraging the Netherlands Cancer Registry, and analyzing disease trajectories of multimorbidity using a dataset of patients in Scotland. Besides the presentation of the full papers included in these proceedings, the workshop program also contained an interactive poster session where 8 posters were presented.

This year's edition of the workshop featured a Best Paper Award. Based on the assessment by the reviewers, the Best Paper Award was attributed to Jana Vormann, Jonas Blatt, Flavio Horbach, Nils Herm-Stapelberg, Lukas Mittnacht, Patrick Delfmann,

Tobias Walter and Sven Pagel for their paper "Case Study: Insights on Prostate Cancer Treatment Pathways using Process Discovery".

The PODS4H workshop is an initiative of the Process-Oriented Data Science for Healthcare Alliance (PODS4H Alliance) within the IEEE Task Force on Process Mining. The goal of the PODS4H Alliance is to promote awareness, research, development and education regarding process-oriented data science in healthcare. For more information, we would like to refer the reader to our website www.pods4h.com.

The organizers would like to sincerely thank all authors for their contributions to the workshop, all Program Committee members for their valuable work in reviewing the papers, and the ICPM 2024 workshop chairs and local organizers for supporting this successful event.

November 2024

Niels Martin
Carlos Fernandez-Llatas
Owen Johnson
Marcos Sepúlveda
Jorge Munoz-Gama

Organization

Workshop Chairs

Niels Martin	Hasselt University, Belgium
Carlos Fernandez-Llatas	Universitat Politècnica de Valencia, Spain
Owen Johnson	Leeds University, UK
Marcos Sepúlveda	Pontificia Universidad Católica de Chile, Chile
Jorge Munoz-Gama	Pontificia Universidad Católica de Chile, Chile

Program Committee

Davide Aloini	University of Pisa, Italy
Robert Andrews	Queensland University of Technology, Australia
Iris Beerepoot	Utrecht University, The Netherlands
Elisabetta Benevento	University of Pisa, Italy
Daniel Capurro	University of Melbourne, Australia
Marco Comuzzi	Ulsan National Institute of Science and Technology, South Korea
Jonas Cremerius	HPI – University of Potsdam, Germany
Benjamin Dalmas	Computer Research Institute of Montreal, Canada
René de la Fuente	Pontificia Universidad Católica de Chile, Chile
Claudio Di Ciccio	Utrecht University, The Netherlands
Onur Doğan	Izmir Bakırçay University, Turkey
Carlos Fernandez-Llatas	Universitat Politècnica de València, Spain
Roberto Gatta	Università Cattolica del Sacro Cuore, Italy
Joscha Grüger	Universität Trier, Germany
Emmanuel Helm	University of Applied Sciences Upper Austria, Austria
Owen Johnson	Leeds University, UK
Felix Mannhardt	Eindhoven University of Technology, The Netherlands
Ronny Mans	Philips Research, The Netherlands
Niels Martin	Hasselt University, Belgium
Renata Medeiros de Carvalho	Eindhoven University of Technology, The Netherlands

Jorge Munoz-Gama	Pontificia Universidad Católica de Chile, Chile
Simon Poon	University of Sydney, Australia
Ricardo Quintano	Philips, The Netherlands
Hajo A. Reijers	Utrecht University, The Netherlands
Eric Rojas	Pontificia Universidad Católica de Chile, Chile
Gema Ibañez Sanchez	Universitat Politècnica de València, Spain
Fernando Seoane	Karolinska Institutet, Sweden
Marcos Sepúlveda	Pontificia Universidad Católica de Chile, Chile
Minseok Song	Pohang University of Science and Technology, South Korea
Alessandro Stefanini	University of Pisa, Italy
Emilio Sulis	University of Turin, Italy
Pieter Toussaint	Norwegian University of Science and Technology, Norway
Vicente Traver	Universitat Politècnica de València, Spain
Zoe Valero Ramón	Universitat Politècnica de Valencia, Spain
Wil van der Aalst	RWTH Aachen University, Germany
Rob Vanwersch	Maastricht University Medical Center, The Netherlands
Mathias Weske	HPI – University of Potsdam, Germany
Moe Wynn	Queensland University of Technology, Australia

Predicting Unplanned Hospital Readmissions Using Outcome-Oriented Predictive Process Mining

Abdulaziz Aljebreen[1]([⊠]) [iD], Allan Pang[1,2] [iD], Marc de Kamps[1] [iD],
and Owen Johnson[1] [iD]

[1] University of Leeds, Leeds, UK
{ml17asa,ugm5a2p,m.dekamps,o.a.johnson}@leeds.ac.uk
[2] Royal Centre for Defence Medicine, Birmingham, UK

Abstract. Many hospitals in the world are under pressure to improve their efficiency and effectiveness so that they can achieve better health outcomes with limited resources. One common measure of performance is the rate of unplanned hospital readmissions (UHRs) within 30-days. Emergency readmissions for the same disease can be assumed to indicate inappropriate discharge or poor planning, are costly, increase patients' mortality risks and put additional pressure on bed capacity. Data Mining (DM) techniques have been used to predict UHRs based on clinical and demographic features, but these ignore the process perspective. Predictive Process Monitoring (PPM) is a process mining technique using completed traces to make predictions for in progress cases with machine learning (ML) algorithms. The Outcome-Oriented PPM (OOPPM) is a sub-technique of PPM focusing on predicting categorical outcomes of process. Adaptation of OOPPM in healthcare settings has been limited to date. Here, we illustrate how to implement OOPPM in a healthcare context through an application of an OOPPM pipeline to hospital admissions using the open access MIMIC-IV dataset. Clinical, demographical and process features were used to build an extended event log, which was then employed for UHRs prediction. Results show prediction using OOPPM techniques outperformed traditional DM techniques. OOPPM tests using tree-based ML algorithms achieved better results compared to OOPPM tests using other ML algorithms. Our results suggest OOPPM can make a significant contribution to better understanding of hospital performance.

Keywords: Predictive Process Monitoring · Unplanned Hospital Readmission · 30-days Hospital Readmissions · Discharge Decisions · Process Mining · Healthcare · Electronic Health Record · EHR · MIMIC-IV

1 Introduction

Hospitals can be seen as highly complex health systems tasked with the delivery of high-quality healthcare services to their users using standardised processes, procedures, technologies, and medicines. Many hospitals in the world are under pressure to improve

© The Author(s) 2025
A. Delgado and T. Slaats (Eds.): ICPM 2024 Workshops, LNBIP 533, pp. 421–433, 2025.
https://doi.org/10.1007/978-3-031-82225-4_31

their efficiency and effectiveness so that they can achieve better health outcomes with limited resources. One common measure of the performance of hospitals is their rate of unplanned hospital readmissions (UHRs) within a defined period, with 30 days being commonly adopted [1]. UHRs happen when a patient returns to hospital through emergency services for the same medical condition causing disruption to normal operations and distress to patients. UHRs indicate inappropriate discharge or poor planning. UHRs leads to more premature discharge decisions due to pressure on hospital, creating more UHRs [2]. A vicious cycle that merits further research.

UHRs within 30 days represent 20% of total UHRs was accounting for $17.4 billion of additional hospital payments in USA in 2021 and add pressures onto hospital systems by increasing demand on hospital services with poor mortality outcomes [1, 2]. While the causes of UHRs are multifactorial, we hypothesise that decisions during the hospital admissions may contribute to UHRs. UHRs have been shown to be potentially avoidable if proper healthcare service would have been provided [1]. If such UHRs could be predicted and highlighted to the medical team, these could influence decision making to prevent future UHRs. Previous attempts to predict UHRs have included the use of statistical analysis [3], machine learning (ML) [4], deep learning (DL) [5] and Natural Language Processing (NLP) [6]. Our literature search found that none of the existing work included process data (e.g., event sequences) for the prediction.

Process Mining (PM) main techniques such process discovery and conformance checking has been adopted in healthcare domain to analyse compliance with guidelines. Healthcare process represented through a group of events, include its activities, time, and objects. Following a process view of a patient's clinical pathway through hospital we can define a typical pathway from admission to discharge as a *case*. For example, Fig. 1 below illustrates a simplified clinical pathway with possible UHR as an outcome, indicating multiple opportunities for better prediction before the discharge event.

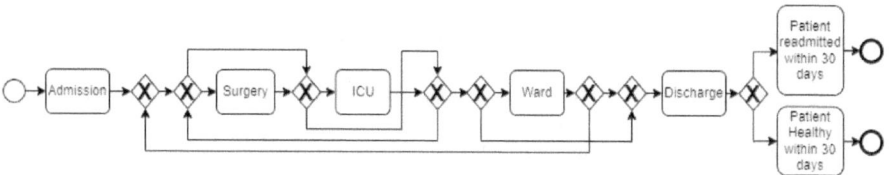

Fig. 1. Hospital admission process shows UHRs probability as an outcome.

Predictive (business) process monitoring (PPM) technique offers prediction ability to ongoing cases at different points throughout the process [7]. Predictions could be the outcome of a case; next activity/activities; execution time or expected load on a resource. Prediction in PM for healthcare (PM4H) has been considered a challenge by the PM4H community under *Challenge 2: discover beyond discovery* [8]. One PPM technique that focuses on predicting categorical case outcomes is called Outcome-Oriented PPM (OOPPM). Here, we are interested in the prediction of UHRs as an outcome but recognise that the approach should be generalisable to other outcomes and activities. OOPPM has been used in healthcare to support clinical decisions such as predicting of discharge location for patients [9]. OOPPM has also been used to predict unplanned Intensive

Care Unit (ICU) readmissions where it surpasses the baseline of Data Mining (DM) techniques [10]. From our review of the literature, we believe our work is the first work that utilises OOPPM technique to predict UHRs.

The rest of this paper is structured as follows: Sect. 2 gives background on the concepts and related work on OOPPM, Sect. 3 illustrates the OOPPM framework, Sect. 4 describes our implementation of using OOPPM for UHRs prediction and present the results, and Sect. 5 discuss and conclude our findings and future work.

2 Background

2.1 MIMIC-IV

Our data is drawn from Medical Information Mart for Intensive Care IV (MIMIC-IV), a widely used, open-access Electronic Healthcare Record (EHR) database [11]. We have selected MIMIC-IV to apply OOPPM in response to a challenge identified by PM4H community *Challenge 4: Deal with Reality* specifying the importance of using real life data [8]. MIMIC-IV includes anonymised, detailed data for patients who were admitted to an ICU or Emergency Department (ED) at Beth Israel Deaconess Medical Centre in Boston, USA. It contains information on more than 380,000 patients receiving care between 2008 to 2019. The MIMIC-IV database is rich with event data, making it an appropriate choice for process mining [8].

2.2 UHRs Prediction

UHR prediction is a complex task as it requires multiple data features to make the prediction. Prediction of UHRs can be implemented for a specific cohort (e.g., heart failure patients) or more broadly for all patients. In [3], statistical analysis using logistic regression was applied to identify variables associated with UHRs on older adult patients in Sweden. Multiple ML algorithms were used by [4] to predict UHRs in MIMIC-III (an earlier, smaller version of the MIMIC-IV dataset) using demographics, aggregated vital signs and diagnoses. DL algorithms such as Artificial Neural Networks (ANNs) and Convolutional Neural Networks (CNNs) were used to predict UHRs for pneumonia patients in Taiwan [5]. Clinical notes from MIMIC-III were able to predict UHRs successfully using NLP techniques [6]. None of the previous work considered process control-flow and the events order as a feature to be used for prediction.

2.3 Prediction in PM for Healthcare

Several methodologies are available for process mining projects. The Process Mining Project Management PM^2 [12] is a generic method contains six stages, where the use of ML is included in step 4 named Mining & Analysis. An extension of PM2 is the *ClearPath* method which was developed for clinical pathway discovery and incorporates process simulation approach [13]. The L^* life-cycle method included the prediction as part of last stage Operational Support [14]. Current PM methodologies do not provide explicit support for the detailed implementation of predictions within process mining context. However, it should be possible to incorporate PPM as a dedicated method to make predictions within these existing process mining methodologies.

2.4   Outcome-Oriented Predictive Process Monitoring

OOPPM, like other PM approaches, uses *event logs* where the *case_id*, *activity* and *timestamp* must be present. However, this information is not enough for OOPPM to make predictions and more data is needed to create *extended event logs*. We can augment event log with *event attributes* (dynamic) or *case attributes* (static). These attributes can be categorical (e.g. a patient's ethnicity), numerical (e.g. patient age) or textual (e.g., clinical note). In healthcare, data types such as age, are a case attribute since age will not vary as a result of the execution of activities during a hospital admission while data types such as Blood Pressure (BP) is a value which will change during patient hospitalisation due to multiple BP readings.

The collection of sequenced events produced by a case is called *trace*, where a trace can contain all or part of a case events. Each possibility of sequenced events represents a complete or part of a trace is called *prefix*. OOPPM uses prefixes for prediction, since the ongoing cases (e.g., incomplete traces) are employed for prediction. To make predictions, trace prefixes should be encoded into a feature vector so that it can be labelled for use in classifiers (e.g., a decision tree) [7].

The use of OOPPM in healthcare to predict process outcomes has been described in the literature. The closest to our work is the prediction of the unplanned ICU readmissions likelihood before discharging patient from ICU using control-flow with clinical metrics like laboratory tests [10]. Jonas et al. employed OOPPM using demographic, lab test values and stay information to predict where a heart failure patients should be discharged to, since the discharge location is strongly associated with UHRs [9]. OOPPM and Time-Oriented Predictive Process Monitoring (TOPPM) was used to predict next activity and its timestamp prediction for ED patients after surgery in Norway [15]. It is to be noted not all the above works followed the framework of OOPPM as described Sect. 3.

3   Methodology

In our work, we used OOPPM to predict UHRs within 30-days. We have selected the OOPPM framework suggested by [7] after they conducted a systematic literature review on OOPPM, where two phases are implemented: offline phase used for learning (see Fig. 2) and online phase for testing and application (see Fig. 3).

3.1   Extracting and Filtering Prefixes

In OOPPM, where prefix logs are extracted from event logs, classifiers use prefix logs to make predictions. This is since OOPPM when applied in the online phase, it will consume incomplete traces in order to make predictions for them as early as possible. So, the use of prefix log will provide us with training data that will match the data we want to test. However, considering all possible prefixes will raise challenges by increasing classifiers learning time and bias toward cases with longer traces as they will produce more prefixes.

There are several methods to filter prefixes, one of them is by limiting the length of the prefix to a certain number of events only [7]. Instead of fixing one prefix length, gaps can be identified to have prefixes with different lengths using a base number (e.g., 1) then add gaps accordingly (e.g., for gap = 3, we will have 1, 4, 7, 10 prefix length). Another method is to define execution time of prefix so only events in prefixes within the execution time will be considered [10].

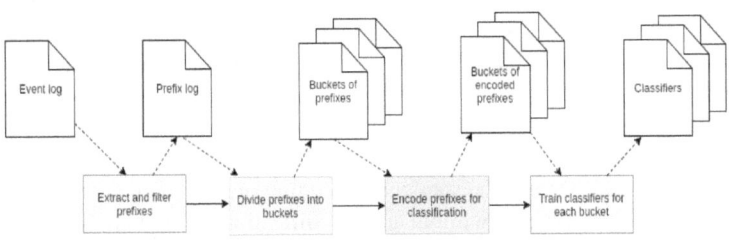

Fig. 2. OOPPM offline phase. [7]

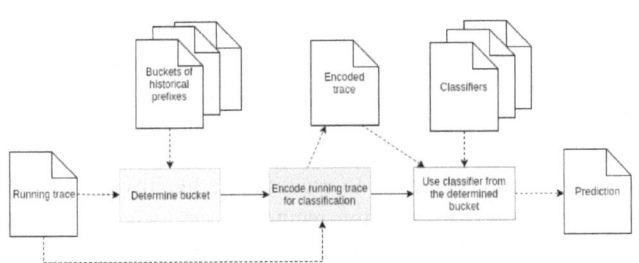

Fig. 3. OOPPM online phase. [7]

3.2 Divide Prefixes into Buckets

At this stage, the prefix log needs to be divided into *buckets*, where each bucket will have a dedicated classifier. During the online phase, cases will be assigned to a similar bucket based on its prefix to make the prediction. There are several bucketing approaches used in OOPPM. The first approach is "single bucket" or "no bucket" where all prefixes are kept in one bucket, leading to having one classifier only [10]. The second approach is to use "process states" or "decision points" available in process model based on event log and train a classifier for each state [16]. The prediction for ongoing cases will be based on the state of process they are in regardless of the followed path. The third approach is to cluster similar encoded prefixes using ML clustering algorithms (e.g., DBScan), which might ignore process structure, and then build classifier for each cluster [16]. The fourth method is to bucket the prefixes based on length, and classifiers are trained accordingly [17]. The last approach is to utilize domain knowledge by manually establishing rules for bucketing prefixes (e.g., execution stages) through consultation with domain experts [7].

3.3   Encode Prefixes for Classification

The input for classifiers should be in fixed size vectors representation, so we need to encode all bucketed prefixes' traces. This raises complications since moving forward in a case execution will add more information, but the number of features in the prefix should not increase. The solution is by applying sequence encoding which is a combination of trace abstraction and feature extraction methods [7]. At this stage, a compromise between generalisation of method (i.e., applicability for all prefixes) and information lost is to be considered. We will discuss sequence encoding methods application on numerical and categorical attributes of case and events, as unstructured textual attributes are outside the scope of our work.

For case attributes, we use the sequence encoding method named *static,* by directly adding them to feature vector without any modifications [7]. If the case attribute is categorical, then we use a baseline approach known as "one hot encoding" to convert the categorical feature into multiple binary vectors based on number of distinct categorical values. This method is to be used on conjunction with other sequence encoding methods, since these methods are concerned with event attributes.

First event attributes sequence encoding method named *Last State,* where both case and event attributes of the recent state is included in one feature vector [16]. Last event numerical attributes will be added as it is, hot encoding will be applied on this event categorial attributes and control-flow, while remining attributes for other events will be zeros. The last state method enables us to use different lengths of prefix traces buckets.

The second event sequence encoding method is *aggregation.* In this method, we aggregate all events from the start of the case in one feature vector regardless of events order, so we avoid losing of information from previous states while maintaining fixed size feature vector. Aggregation of control-flow can be achieved by counting executed activities, or to indicate whether a certain activity has been executed or not [16]. Numerical event attributes could be aggregated using statistics functions (e.g., average, or max), while categorical event attributes are hot encoded then their frequency will be accumulated. The aggregation method presents a way to preserve all the trace data but with the price of losing control-flow relationships and patterns. The aggregation method can also be applied to traces with different lengths.

Index is the third event sequence encoding method proposed by [17] to overcome the partial information loss of events order in aggregation method. This is achieved by creating a single feature in the feature vector for each event attribute executed in the trace. Encoding of control-flow and categorical event attributes is done through hot encoding and numerical event attributes will be included as it is. The issue with this method is the feature vector length depends on number of executed events, putting restriction on its use with heterogenous buckets with different traces length. With comparison to the previous two methods, the index method will create large dimensional feature vector when there are long traces leading to classifiers training complications.

3.4   Train Classifiers for Each Bucket

The problem in classification in OOPPM can be related to the problem of early sequence classification in ML literature [7]. In addition to the *accuracy, precision, recall,* and *f-1* metrics used to evaluate ML classification models, *earliness* and *computation time* are an importation evaluation metrics for OOPPM classification model, as it is designed to work in an online mode with ongoing cases. ML algorithms including logistic regression (LR), Support Vector Machines (SVM), decision tree (DT), random forest (RF), and Gradient Boosted Machines (GBM) can used in OOPPM in addition to DL algorithms like neural networks (NN) [7, 10].

4   Predicting UHRs Using OOPPM

In this section, we will discuss the implementation for our work for each stage of OOPPM. Our experiments were run on Google Colaboratory using Python 3.4.

4.1   Creating Extended Event Log

In our work, we utilised data available in MIMIC-IV dataset to create an extended event log for hospital admissions with labels. OOPPM does not consider the creating of event log as a main step. However, creating event log and extending it with useful features to be used for prediction is a crucial stage which requires more attention.

Data Filtering. We started with reading the *admissions* table since it contains basic information about hospital admissions and their unique id (*hadm_id*). We grouped admission types from nine different types into *elective* and *emergency*. There are four possible outcomes of interest – death in hospital, no further hospital admissions, emergency readmission within 30 days and subsequent readmissions that were planned or unplanned but after 30 days. For this case study we focussed on outcome concerned with readmissions. To identify patients who have been readmitted within 30-days, we sorted the table based on patient id *subject_id* and hadm_id, added a new column to record next visit admission time, subtracted next admission day from current visit discharge day, checked if the next visit was within 30 days and of emergency type, then label the patients *readmission* status accordingly. We got 350,579 admissions followed by UHR and 80,652 admissions who were not followed by UHR. We filtered out patients who had only single admission (= 101,198) and admissions were a patient died in hospital (= 8,772). This has left us with total admissions of 325,119, where 244,607 admissions (75%) were not followed by UHR and 80512 followed by UHR (25%).

Extracting Data Features. After identifying the study cohort, we started working on preparing features to be used for prediction. These features were divided into demographic, clinical and process related features. For demographic, we selected age, gender, insurance, ethnicity, and marital status. Patients age values are distributed from 18 to 91, where patients older than 91 are anonymised as 91 by MIMIC-IV [11]. To enhance the prediction results, we grouped patients into eight groups represent a ten-year age band starting from 18, 28 etc. with last group being patients who are 88 and over. MIMIC-IV has two genders available (male and female), and three types of insurance known as: Medicaid (public), Medicare (public) and Other (private, military, cash payment, ...). MIMIC-IV holds 31 different ethnicity types for patients, which we grouped into eight main groups based on ethnicity name. For marital status, there are five values: single, married, widowed, divorced and unknown.

MIMIC-IV is rich with clinical data, so the selection of clinical features was built on previous studies and clinical knowledge where such features were important for UHR prediction. The patient history was considered by calculating total number of previous UHRs and add this information for each hospital admission. Patients who were admitted through emergency department were flagged. The available patient body mass index (BMI) values were extracted and categorise into four categories: underweight, normal weight, overweight, and obese. Lab tests are important indication for patient health, so we have calculated the number of abnormal lab tests of patient per admission. It is important to identify whether a patient is having chronic diseases, so we have used chronic diseases codes developed by AHRQ to calculate how many chronic diseases the patient have. Number of Medications given to patients during their hospitalisation was included as it is an important representation of treatment provided.

Patients' diagnosis in MIMIC-IV are coded using two versions of the International Classification of Diseases (ICD) which are (ICD-9) and (ICD-10). MIMIC-IV covers patient data from 2008 to 2019 and initially used ICD-9 but switched to ICD-10 when it was implemented in the hospital systems. To overcome this challenge, we used the 18 categories of diseases defined in ICD-9 (e.g., respiratory) and for each patient calculated the number of diseases per category diagnosed within each admission. The same task was done with patients having their diagnoses registered in ICD-10, considering the changes in diagnoses codes and re-arrangement of categories. This approach allowed us to work with 18 diagnosis categories without adding the complexity of encoding the ICD codes for patient into thousands of dimensions and helped to improve the prediction accuracy and reduce the computation significantly.

Data features to be used for OOPPM should include control-flow information as this is the driving concept of OOPPM. However, other process related features can be considered as well to maximise classifiers learning and ensure better use of process-oriented data. We have looked at several process aspects of hospital admissions in terms of time, process context and number of events. For time, we calculated the length of stay (LOS) (i.e., process completion time), grouped the LOS into 4 quartiles to reduce the outliers' effect, and calculated time spent in ICUs during the admission. We also investigated process context from geographical view, where admission and discharge locations were considered. There are many events registered for patients in MIMIC-IV and we selected data on how many times a patient was admitted to ICU and number of surgeries per admission. We end up with 18 data features to be used in classifiers.

Extracting Events. Before building the extended event log to be used by OOPPM, we must also identify suitable events for our purpose. MIMIC-IV has multiple different events, making it challenging to choose appropriate events without complicating the following stages. The events selection for OOPPM should be different from other process mining tasks like process discovery, since including less-informative events will add more dimensions which will complicate the classification task. On the other hand, we should include as much information as possible about different events to ensure that processes are considered in prediction. For this case study we considered events available in the *transfers* table which shows when and where patients were admitted, transferred to within hospital and discharge. The transfer events enable us to look at the process through the eyes of a patient's experience, reflecting one of the key challenges for PM4H [8]. Other events were considered in the prediction as high-level data features (e.g., surgeries total) but not in the same detail as complete events.

The transfer events in MIMIC-IV are categorised into 77 different events (38 different events for admitted to a clinical unit, 38 different events for transferred to a clinical unit and 1 discharge event). We removed events with activities named "admitted into Unknown" or "transferred to Unknown". We grouped all admission events into one event "Admission" except for admission to ICU or surgery, all admission and transferred to ICU under one event "ICU", all admission and transferred to a surgery unit to be "Surgery", all the remaining "transferred to" became "Ward" and we renamed the discharge event. We end up with an extended event log contains 942,368 events categorised into 2423 trace variants. For result comparison purpose, we kept another copy of the event log with original events without grouping to be tested.

4.2 Implementation of OOPPM

Extracting and Filtering Prefixes. Healthcare processes are known for their heterogeneity [8], and with the high number of cases we used for training in our case study, it was essential to make the prefix logs smaller. We have considered only transfer events and aggregated them to help reduce prefix log size, removed cases with data quality issues (e.g., started with discharge event) and fixed decision point (i.e., prediction place) to be before the discharge time. However, with the 2423 trace variants we had, it was a challenge to apply any method to filter prefixes, so we chose to use all traces without filtering, taking into consideration the effect on the classifiers. Complete prefixes were used during the offline phase to train the classifiers, while in online phase we removed the discharged event from prefixes log.

Divide Prefixes into Buckets. In our work, we experimented using single cluster approach. We have also implemented clustering algorithm (K-Mean) with 3 clusters to create prefixes buckets, after testing best performing clustering algorithms and clusters number. Since our prediction place cannot be fixed in a specific state during process (e.g., patient get discharged from ICU without transfer to ward), the process state clustering method is not applicable. With the high number of heterogeneous prefixes we had, application of prefix length was excluded. Although with domain expert involvement in our work, we did not see the need to bucket prefixes based on domain knowledge in this case study.

Encode Prefixes for Classification. We used static encoding for all case attributes, while for event attributes we chose the aggregation approach (i.e., counting of grouped and ungrouped dataset of activities) as previous work suggests it can give better results when compared to other prefix encoding approaches [7].

Train Classifiers for Each Bucket. We have chosen to build a baseline classifier using LR algorithm. The tree-based classifiers are mostly used in OOPPM literature [7], so we tested DT, RF, and GBM. To complement our work and compare classifiers results, NN was included in our experiments. We have not applied hyperparameter tuning in our work as our goal is to test the usefulness of OOPPM with healthcare data. In addition to the common evaluation metrics used for classifiers, we included the area under the receiving operating characteristic curve (AUROC) as it will not be affected by our imbalanced data where 75% of the labels are 0 and 25% are 1. We did not include earliness in our evaluation since we have a fixed decision point where the prediction is required. Computing time was calculated for training and testing of the classifiers.

Execution of Offline and Online Phases. To enable us to simulate the implementation of offline and online phases, we split data into two chunks: first chunk contains 67% of data used for training classifiers (offline phase), and second chunk contains 33% of data used for testing and evaluating the classifiers (online phase). Since MIMIC-IV is anonymised on a temporal level, the splitting could not be executed on chronological order which would be ideal in this step. We have used testing data for the online phase where it was bucketed, encoded then classified.

4.3 Results

We have summarized our results in Table. 1 by mentioning the classifier name and applied approached followed: use of OOPPM, use of clustering and when the aggregated events were used. It was followed by classifiers evaluation metrics then training and predicting time in seconds. It can be noticed applying OOPPM enhanced accuracy in all cases comparing to DM approach. Clustering step did not show effect on the results, while the use of aggregated events has slightly affected results positively or negatively comparing to original events without aggregation. RF models has achieved the highest accuracy and precision, NN models scored best AUROC and F1 values, and DT gained best Recall. DT models were the fastest to learn and predict followed by GBM and RF, then NN and LR. The work done by [4] to predict 30-days UHRs using several ML models using DM approach in MIMIC-III where the RF model was the best achieving AUROC 0.66 and accuracy of 0.65 which is lower than our results in term of accuracy for all classifiers and in AUROC except for our baseline LR classifier.

5 Discussion and Conclusion

Our implementation of OOPPM was challenging due to the nature of healthcare processes and our aim to predict UHRs on hospital level for all patients instead of choosing a cohort of patients with specific disease. We had many prefixes in testing data with only one event, which has limited the learning from control-flow chances, suggesting more work on prefix filtering is needed. A limitation in our work was to ensure the patient is readmitted for the same disease, since MIMIC-IV is not providing this information clearly [11]. Even if the clinical decision was to discharge the patients with high probability of UHR instead of keeping them in hospital, predicting UHRs could help clinicians in reviewing delivered treatment, highlight potential corrections, and indicate more care is need for a patient after their discharge. It was noticed the patient history (i.e., number of previous admissions) and diseases diagnosed within the admission was the most informative features for the classifiers.

Table 1. Summary of classifiers results.

Classifier	OOPPM	Clustering	Events Aggregated	Accuracy	AUROC	Precision	Recall	F1	Learning Time	Prediction Time
Logistic Regression	No	–	–	0.76	0.55	0.69	0.54	0.53	103.68	0.13
	Yes	No	No	0.77	0.55	0.69	0.55	0.54	128.22	0.08
	Yes	Yes	No	0.77	0.55	0.69	0.55	0.54	101.24	0.05
	Yes	No	Yes	0.77	0.56	0.70	0.56	0.55	228.4	0.14
	Yes	Yes	Yes	0.77	0.56	0.70	0.56	0.55	296.02	0.08
Decision Trees	No	–	–	0.75	0.67	0.67	0.67	0.67	3.59	0.04
	Yes	No	No	0.77	0.69	0.70	0.70	0.70	5.91	0.05
	Yes	Yes	No	0.77	0.69	0.70	0.70	0.70	13.76	0.23
	Yes	No	Yes	0.77	0.68	0.68	0.68	0.68	5.5	0.04
	Yes	Yes	Yes	0.77	0.68	0.68	0.68	0.68	8.03	0.11
Random Forest	No	–	–	0.79	0.66	0.73	0.66	0.67	52.42	4.65
	Yes	No	No	0.82	0.70	0.75	0.68	0.69	55.91	5.06
	Yes	Yes	No	0.82	0.70	0.75	0.68	0.69	96.21	4.24
	Yes	No	Yes	0.80	0.68	0.74	0.65	0.67	74.88	6.2
	Yes	Yes	Yes	0.80	0.68	0.74	0.65	0.67	71.93	5.94
Gradient Boosting Machines	No	–	–	0.79	0.66	0.72	0.65	0.67	44.13	1.77
	Yes	No	No	0.80	0.67	0.72	0.66	0.68	44.35	2.55
	Yes	Yes	No	0.80	0.67	0.72	0.66	0.68	42.97	2.67
	Yes	No	Yes	0.79	0.66	0.72	0.63	0.65	41.5	3.03
	Yes	Yes	Yes	0.79	0.66	0.72	0.63	0.65	39.18	2.6
Neural Networks	No	–	–	0.79	0.87	0.72	0.70	0.71	84.07	4.26
	Yes	No	No	0.80	0.87	0.73	0.68	0.69	89.9	4.51
	Yes	Yes	No	0.80	0.87	0.73	0.68	0.69	85.53	5.39
	Yes	No	Yes	0.80	0.87	0.73	0.69	0.70	80.04	3.88
	Yes	Yes	Yes	0.80	0.87	0.73	0.67	0.69	84.48	4.58

Features engineering for prediction in PM4H settings requires more research and recommendations from PM4H community, as they are distinguished from other domains. In our work, we used intra-case attributes for prediction, but looking into inter-case attributes where shared information about concurrent ongoing cases can be useful [7]. The integration of OOPPM in healthcare information systems (HISs) satisfy a need identified by PM4H community *Challenge 9: completement HISs with the process perspective* [11]. OOPPM has performed better than traditional DM in healthcare settings, and thus its integration into PM^2 and other PM methodologies is recommended. We urge PM4H to implement OOPPM in their research work as there is large area for enhancements.

Disclosure of Interests. The authors have no competing interests to declare that are relevant to the content of this article.

References

1. Jencks, S., Williams, M., Coleman, E.: Rehospitalizations among patients in the Medicare fee-for-service program. N. Engl. J. Med. **360**(14), 1418–1428 (2009)
2. Kalra, A., Fisher, R., Axelrod, P.: Decreased length of stay and cumulative hospitalized days despite increased patient admissions and readmissions in an area of urban poverty. J. Gen. Intern. Med. **25**, 930–935 (2010)
3. Glans, M., Kragh, A., Jakobsson, U.: Risk factors for hospital readmission in older adults within 30 days of discharge–a comparative retrospective study. BMC Geriatrics **20** (2020)
4. Assaf, R., Jayousi, R.: 30-day hospital readmission prediction using MIMIC data. In: 14th International Conference on Application of Information and Communication Technologies (AICT), pp. 1–6. IEEE (2020)
5. Tey, F., Liu, C., Chien, T.: Predicting the 14-day hospital readmission of patients with pneumonia using artificial neural networks (ANN). Int. J. Environ. Res. Public Health **18**(10) (2021)
6. Thapa, N., Seifollahi, S., Taheri, S.: Hospital readmission prediction using clinical admission notes. In: 2022 Australasian Computer Science Week Proceedings, pp. 193–199 (2022)
7. Teinemaa, I., Dumas, M., Rosa, M.: Outcome-oriented predictive process monitoring: review and benchmark. ACM Trans. Knowl. Discov. Data **13**(2), 1–57 (2019)
8. Munoz-Gama, J., Martin, N., Fernandez-Llatas, C.: Process mining for healthcare: characteristics and challenges. J. Biomed. Inform. **1**(127), (2022)
9. Cremerius, J., König, M., Warmuth, C.: Patient discharge classification based on the hospital treatment process. In: International Conference on Process Mining, pp. 314–326. Springer International Publishing, Cham (2021)
10. Chen, Q., Lu, Y., Tam, C.S.: Outcome-oriented predictive process monitoring to predict unplanned ICU readmission in MIMIC-IV database. In: ECIS (2022)
11. Johnson, A., Bulgarelli, L., Shen, L.: MIMIC-IV, a freely accessible electronic health record dataset. Sci. Data **10**(1) (2023)
12. Van Eck, M., Lu, X., Leemans, S.: PM: a process mining project methodology. In: International conference on advanced information systems engineering, pp. 297–313. Springer International Publishing, Cham (2015)
13. Johnson, O., Ba Dhafari, T., Kurniati, A.: The ClearPath method for care pathway process mining and simulation. In: Business Process Management Workshops: BPM 2018 International Workshops, pp. 239–250. Springer International Publishing (2019)
14. Van Der Aalst, W.: Process mining: discovering and improving Spaghetti and Lasagna processes. In: Symposium on Computational Intelligence and Data Mining, pp. 1–7. IEEE (2011)
15. Aravazhi, A., Helgheim, B., Aadahl, P.: Decision-making based on predictive process monitoring of patient treatment processes: a case study of emergency patients. Adv. Oper. Res. (1) (2023)
16. Di Francescomarino, C., Dumas, M., Maggi, F.: Clustering-based predictive process monitoring. IEEE Trans. Serv. Comput. **12**(6), 896–909 (2016)
17. Leontjeva, A., Conforti, R., Di Francescomarino, C.: Complex symbolic sequence encodings for predictive monitoring of business processes. In: 13th International Conference on Business Process Management, pp. 297–313. Springer International Publishing. (2015)

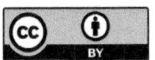

Structural and Semantic Enrichment of Models for the Interactive Discovery of Clinical Processes

Jose Luis Bayo-Montón[1] , Begoña Martínez-Salvador[1] ,
Carlos Fernández-Llatas[2(✉)] , and Mar Marcos[1(✉)]

[1] Department of Computer Engineering and Science, Universitat Jaume I,
Castelló, Spain
{jbayo,begona.martinez,mar.marcos}@uji.es
[2] SABIEN-ITACA Universitat Politècnica de València, Valencia, Spain
cfllatas@itaca.upv.es

Abstract. Process Mining (PM) is a relatively new field which provides techniques to analyze business processes in different areas. In the field of Medicine, PM seeks to infer clinical processes from the data routinely collected during healthcare activities. In most frameworks, workflows are used to represent the results obtained by PM techniques. A problem with these workflows is that their structure is complex and not always easy to understand and hence to exploit by the clinician. A different problem, related to Clinical Practice Guidelines (CPGs), is that their development is mostly manual. We posit that workflows inferred by PM techniques could be improved and enriched by providing interactive tools to support their structuring and semantic annotation by clinicians. We also postulate that these improved and enriched models can be used to facilitate the development of CPGs. In this paper we describe our approach to the interactive discovery of clinical processes as well as an implementation to support it within the PMApp PM tool.

Keywords: Interactive Process Discovery · Clinical Process Models · Model Enrichment

1 Introduction

Process Mining (PM) is a promising field with applications in numerous domains, including Medicine [9]. Healthcare institutions routinely generate large amounts of information, including data about the management and treatment of patients which are recorded in the Electronic Health Record (EHR). These data are of great value for understanding patient care processes, including the timing of interventions and their outcomes. The application of PM techniques to healthcare data can be used to infer clinical processes which can be analyzed to detect opportunities for improvement.

Workflows are the most frequent formalism used to represent the models inferred by PM techniques. The characteristics of PM techniques and the small

A. Delgado and T. Slaats (Eds.): ICPM 2024 Workshops, LNBIP 533, pp. 434–446, 2025.
https://doi.org/10.1007/978-3-031-82225-4_32

grain-size of events in the EHR often result in complex models full of states which do not always correspond with clinically significant interventions. Despite the efforts dedicated to the development of user-friendly tools, clinicians often find it difficult to understand the resulting PM models. This makes their participation in the application of PM methods difficult, and ultimately hinders the application of PM techniques and tools to the analysis and improvement of clinical (and organizational) processes. To this end, the Interactive Process Mining (IPM) paradigm [4] advocates for the participation of the clinician in the application of PM techniques. Under the umbrella of IPM, interactive process discovery techniques usually define interactive algorithms that allow clinicians to make decisions during the discovery process. As a result, two important advantages are achieved: on the one hand, the inferred model is built according to the clinician's criteria and, on the other hand, its trustworthiness increases.

In the medical domain, the standardized procedure for the diagnosis and treatment of a specific clinical condition is normally defined by Clinical Practice Guidelines (CPGs). CPGs contain recommendations elaborated by panels of experts from an analysis of the best and most up-to-date empirical evidence, or based on consensus, in case there is no evidence available. CPGs are usually text documents, often complemented with more structured information like flowcharts [8]. Developing CPGs is a difficult task, which is mostly done manually. In this context, PM techniques can be an effective tool to obtain the complementary evidence contained in EHR data [9].

The work we present in this paper is aligned with the above ideas. Like in IPM, we postulate that clinical process models resulting from the application of PM techniques can be improved by providing interactive tools to support their structuring and semantic annotation directly by clinicians. Furthermore, our goal is that Process Discovery (PD) can continue to be applied to these improved and enriched models. Ultimately, our intention is that these models could serve as a source of knowledge for the development of CPGs. This paper describes our approach to the interactive discovery of clinical processes, as well as an implementation within the PMApp IPM tool [6] to support this approach.

2   Background

2.1   Interactive Process Discovery

PM techniques use event logs and patient data associated to healthcare activities to infer the model that the patients actually follow, which can be represented graphically as a workflow [1]. During the management of patients with a particular clinical condition, the patient data and event log of the interventions and treatments carried out are recorded in the EHR. Examples are the date of the first visit to the specialist, the date and results of the diagnostic tests carried out, the date of diagnosis, and so on. PM discovery algorithms use event logs extracted from the EHR based on the registries associated with some timestamp. This timestamp allows PM algorithms to infer the sequencing of the different activities of the process along with the time in between them. In addition to sequences, PM algorithms can discover forks in the process as well as complex relationships such as loops.

The discovery of processes is a crucial stage in the implementation of a PM tool, where the understandability of the inferred model is of paramount importance for applicability. Traditional PM techniques do not always provide the best results. In this line, there are works in the literature that use interactive techniques to support the creation of more understandable models. These techniques [2,3] allow the experts to iteratively correct the structure of the workflow, with the goal of obtaining models that better fit their knowledge. For example, the interactive PD tool by Cortado [12] allows selecting the traces that infer the best workflow representing the data without noise, according to the user preferences. However, most of these techniques are based on Petri Nets, making it difficult for clinicians to directly use them. In addition, they mainly focus on clearing up the structure of the final workflow by discarding less frequent paths, in order to obtain noise-free models. This makes them not suitable for the medical domain, where it is important to gain insight into all the paths that patients follow. Finally, to our knowledge, these interactive PD techniques do not consider the integration of expert knowledge (including semantics) in the models.

2.2 The PMApp Tool

PMApp [6] is a PM tool that has been specifically designed for the clinical domain. It is a customizable tool that allows the incorporation of new modules for enabling the application of PM technologies using EHR and legacy systems in health institutions. PMApp is built according to the principles of the Process Mining for Healthcare manifesto [9], and under the umbrella of IPM for Healthcare philosophy [4]. PMApp allows the creation of specific modules for improving data preprocessing, discovery, and visualization of models. Figure 1 shows a model inferred with the I-PALIA PD algorithm [5], implemented within the PMApp tool. I-PALIA analyzes the event log extracted from the EHR and produces a model in the form of a Timed Parallel Automaton (TPA) [5]. In TPA models, actions are represented as nodes, and transitions as edges between the corresponding nodes. TPAs are a highly expressive formalism, being equivalent to safe Petri Nets but retaining the comprehensibility of automata-based formalisms. The PMApp tool and the TPA formalism constitute the framework for the implementation of our proposal.

A key component of the PMApp tool is the *Experiment Designer*, which provides a drag&drop interface to design, store and reproduce a PM experiment. It is used to create the so-called *experiment definition document* that contains detailed descriptions of all the steps involved in the discovery process, including: gathering the event logs, preprocessing them, computing the inferred models from the logs, and postprocessing them. Note that experiment definition documents contain all the elements (also the event log data) involved, such that it can be reproduced when desired. After processing the log, PMApp provides a GUI that allows the user to fine-tune the PM model to have an individualized view, for example modifying thresholds, stats and layout. It also allows visualising

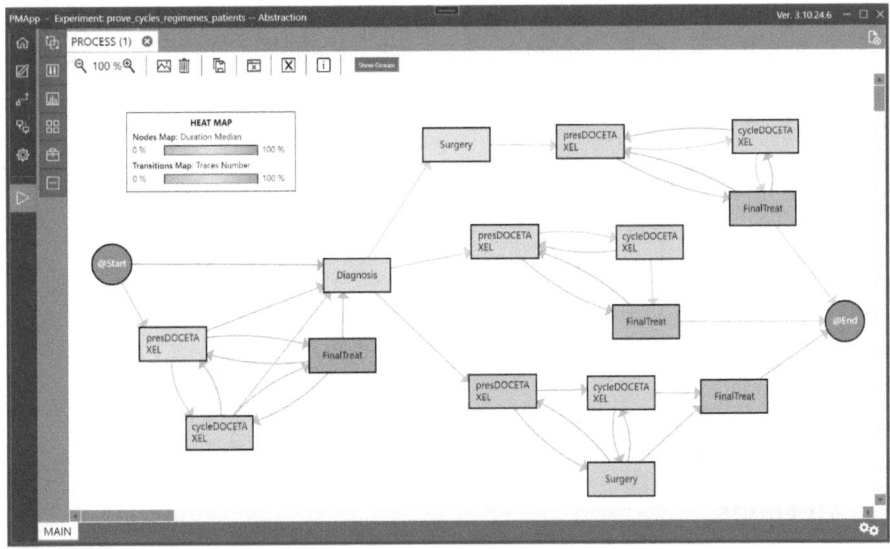

Fig. 1. Example of TPA process model: management with Docetaxel of prostate cancer patients (with three therapy paths identified using specific I-PALIA functionalities).

information of individual events related to any element of the model (nodes and edges), performing trace clustering, or creating charts, among other features.

3   Approach

Our approach consists in providing the expert with tools for the restructuring and semantic annotation of the process model obtained with the existing PMApp PD algorithms. The tools are complementary to those of PMApp, and implement operations tailored to the domain of CPGs and CPG representation languages (see Sect. 4). These operations introduce transformations in the TPA model. An example of restructuring operation is the grouping of nodes into a subprocess. In particular, the restructuring operations not only modify the model but also the data preprocessing instructions in the *experiment definition document* such that, when reproducing the experiment, the resulting model conforms to the user modifications. Moreover, the PMApp tool will be able to handle with the transformed TPA model new event logs without the need of defining additional data preprocessing instructions.

Figure 2 illustrates the proposed approach. In a first stage, an initial *experiment definition document* is created that serves to the discovery of the model from the original event log data. After this stage, the expert can improve the resulting model, according to clinical considerations, by using the restructuring and semantic tools which work on the graphical TPA model (see Sect. 5.1). Those modifications are used to automatically adapt the data preprocessing instructions that will transform the original event log data such that an improved

TPA model and associated statistics are obtained. Note that the process can be repeated until a satisfactory model is obtained, according to clinician's expectations.

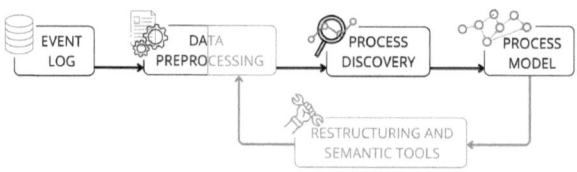

Fig. 2. Approach to the interactive process discovery of clinical processes

4   Methods

In this section we describe a set of tools to support the interactive enrichment of PM models by clinicians. The tools are inspired by the process descriptions and graphical algorithms that can be found in CPG texts [7], and are partly based on common structures found in languages for the representation of CPGs [10].

An important part of the content of CPGs are the procedures to help diagnose, treat and manage patients with a certain disease. These procedures contain knowledge that refers to the organization of the different tasks to be carried out, ranging from specific actions to more or less complex combinations of them. Kaiser and Marcos [7] analyzed the suitability of the so-called workflow control patterns, and performed a preliminary experiment confirming that real-world CPGs can be fully modeled with a small subset of these patterns, namely sequences, choices (including exclusive and multiple choices), and loops. Peleg *et al.* [11] in a use-case based analysis of CPG languages identify sequential, parallel, and iterative structures as common control structures, and add plan structures as an important instrument allowing for the nesting of elements. Decision models (choices) are also included as common structures, although with significant variation among languages. Finally, they highlight the importance of using a standardized medical concept model (terminology).

We distinguish two categories of tools for the enrichment of PM models by clinicians, according to their main purpose: 1) tools to restructure the PM model, with the aim to clarify the process flow using the above constructs; and 2) tools to support the semantic annotation of the elements of the PM model using terminologies.

4.1   Tools for the Restructuring of the PM Model

Subprocess. A subprocess is a new model element that encapsulates two or more nodes from the original model. There are several reasons why a clinician may want to encapsulate a set of interventions, such as to clarify that they are part of a more complex one, or to separate different therapeutic options. For instance, there exist different treatments for class I to class IV patients with congestive heart failure. In this case, the use of subprocesses grouping the management interventions for each class of patients may increase readability. Subprocesses are compound activities. They are depicted as a single node but contain their own process, which can be collapsed or displayed as desired.

Composition. The idea of composition is very similar to that of subprocess: several activities are collapsed in a single node representing them all. The objective is the same as in the case of subprocess, that is, to simplify the visualization of the model by hiding details. However, in the case of composition the grouped nodes are not necessary or relevant for the understanding of the model, for instance because they do not have sufficient interest or entity on their own. Therefore, composition nodes cannot be expanded again once grouped.

Decision Point. Decisions are crucial in clinical processes. The discovered PM models do not have decision nodes as such, although they are implicit every time that different paths stem from the same node. The goal of this tool is to make the decision explicit. This can be done in two ways: (1) by selecting a node and converting it to a decision (decision conversion), or (2) by introducing a new decision node in the model (decision introduction).

Cycle. Cycles (or loops) are also common in clinical processes. Consider, for example, the number of cycles of a chemotherapy treatment. A cycle is a repetition of the same action a certain number of times, or for a given period. The I-PALIA PD algorithm is able to detect this type of actions and represents them as a single node with a self-arc. Other than that, we allow the clinician to describe a cyclical action in two alternative ways: by explicitly repeating the series of nodes that make up the cyclical activity, or by encapsulating the cyclical activity in a single special node, without self-arc.

Parallelism. In this case, the clinician may want to specify that a sequence of activities in the original model is in fact a serialization of parallel activities that can be performed simultaneously. For example, administrative admission tasks could be performed in parallel with the preoperative and the anesthetist visits. Parallelism is graphically represented with two nodes, similar to BPMN parallel gateways[1], indicating the start and end of the parallel branches.

4.2 Tools for the Semantic Annotation of the PM Model

Semantic Annotation of the Elements of the PM Model. The objective is to add semantics to the PM model, preferably using a standard clinical terminology such as SNOMED CT[2]. The semantic annotation tool allows the clinician to add

---

[1] See http://www.omg.org/spec/BPMN/2.0.

[2] See https://www.snomed.org/what-is-snomed-ct.

semantics not only to the data elements on which the PM model is based, but also to all nodes in the model, including the ones that may have been introduced using the restructuring tools.

Provisions are made for two main semantic annotations, as well as for any additional annotation deemed necessary. The first annotation, *semantic tag*, serves to associate the data or node to a high level term or category, such as observable entity or procedure. The second one, *main binding*, can be used to provide a concrete terminological binding. For example, in the prostate cancer example, the age data item can be annotated as an observable entity (semantic tag) and with the SNOMED-CT term `SCTID: 424144002 | Current chronological age` (main binding). On the other hand, the node cycleDOC-ETAXEL can be annotated as a procedure (semantic tag) and with the term `SCTID: 399042005 | Chemotherapy cycle` (main binding). It is also possible to add an additional terminological binding to indicate the substance used, for example `SCTID: 386918005 | Docetaxel`.

Annotation of Transitions after a Decision Point. Normally, different paths or alternatives can be considered following a decision point. The choice of one of these paths is determined by a condition based on the result of the decision and, possibly, on some other data values. To make this explicit, the transitions after a decision can be manually annotated with the corresponding condition. A default transition can also be indicated, if necessary, which is graphically marked with (*). For example, a patient with prostate cancer may undergo a prostatectomy if his Gleason score is high and his life expectancy is good. Then, the corresponding transition can be annotated with the free-text condition *"high Gleason score==Yes and good life expectancy==Yes"*.

5   Results

5.1   Implementation

We have implemented a PMApp plugin specifically dedicated to support the restructuring of the process flow and the semantic annotation of PM models by clinical experts. This plugin, which we have named *MineGuider*, is open source and is publicly available in https://github.com/sabienitaca/MineGuider. Using *MineGuider*, the tools can be applied in a very intuitive way, by selecting the elements in the model graph. In the case of restructuring tools, right-clicking on a node displays a menu with the available options. These depend on the constraints that selected elements must meet for a proper conversion to the target element or structure.

The application of restructuring tools is subject to a number of constraints. In a *Subprocess, Composition* or *Parallelism*, the selected nodes must be a component, defined as a connected sub-graph: (1) with at least two nodes, (2) with a single (inner) entry node, and (3) with a single (inner) exit node. An exception to the latter is that there can be multiple exit nodes, as long as all of them share the same (outer) destination node. In a *Decision*, only one node must be selected and must have several output transitions. Moreover, depending on the type of decision transformation, the following restrictions apply:

- In the case of a decision conversion, the selected node cannot be itself a decision, neither can have a self-arc.
- In the case of a decision introduction, it is introduced after the selected node (preceding node). Note that output transitions must be re-distributed between the preceding node and the new decision. Then, when the preceding node has a self-arc, the number of output transitions must be at least three and the self-arc cannot be selected to be part of the decision. Otherwise, when the preceding node is a decision, the number of output transitions must be at least three and one of them must remain unchanged so that the preceeding decision still makes sense.

In a *Cycle*, the only restriction is that a single node must be selected, which must have a self-arc. Finally, in a *Parallelism*, after checking that the selected nodes are a connected component (see above), the next step is branch definition. The restrictions applied to the latter are the following: the nodes in a branch must make up a sequence, a node cannot be part of two branches, and all nodes must be in some branch.

As mentioned before, the application of restructuring tools results in modifications to the data preprocessing instructions, such that the desired effect in the model is obtained. *Composition* is translated to event merging actions that compose different events in a single one. *Subprocess* supposes tagging the events associated to the enclosed nodes, to specify that those nodes refer to the same component. *Parallelism* implies tagging the events associated to nodes of the same branch equally, and differently from those on other branches, so that subsequent PD forces the branches to be parallel. *Decision* involves tagging the concrete events associated to the node so that it is displayed with a different shape. In case a new decision node is introduced, an artificial event (with the same tag as in the previous case) is inserted after the events associated to the preceding node. Finally, *Cycles* can be collapsed or extended by merging or tagging, respectively, the associated events.

Figures 3 and 4 show the look and feel of the module. The screen is divided into two zones. On the right, the Model Visualization Area is permanently displayed. Here, the inferred model is presented, where elements can be selected to perform restructuring operations (or transformations) and the results of these operations are shown. Each time a new transformation is added, the data preprocessing instructions are modified accordingly and the transformed model is displayed. In the Model Visualization Area there is also a button to save the enriched model and to persist it as a new PMApp *experiment definition document*.

To the left of the screen there are buttons to display information about the enriched process model in the left panel. For example, it is possible to display the Transformations Tab (in Fig. 4), or the Node Annotation Tab (Fig. 3). Figure 4 shows the Transformations Tab, where the restructuring transformations are listed in order of application. They can be undone one by one in reverse order. Each time a transformation is undone, the data preprocessing instructions are

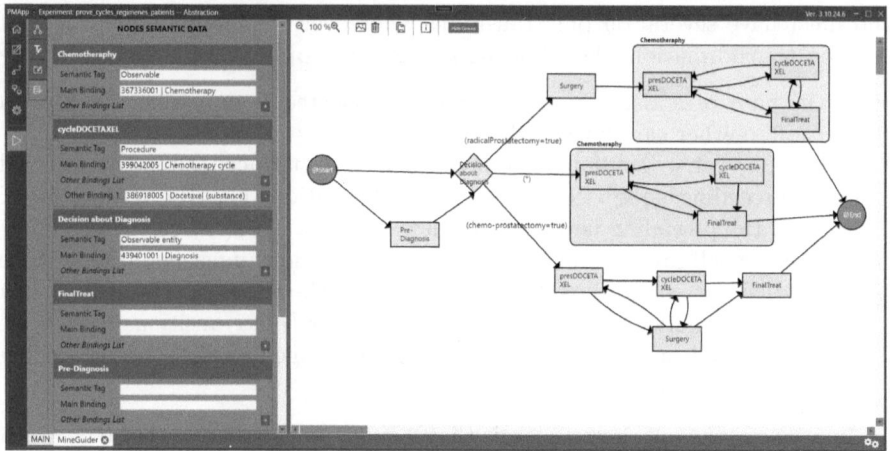

Fig. 3. *MineGuider* module: TPA model in Fig. 1 after the application of a subset of the transformations described in Sect. 5.2, with Node Annotation Tab on the left.

modified and the model is recalculated accordingly. The reason why transformations can be only undone in reverse order is that in general the data preprocessing instructions in one point depend on the preceding ones.

5.2   Use Case

As proof of concept, a subset of the proposed tools has been applied to the TPA model in Fig. 1, resulting in the model shown in Fig. 4. These models represent the treatment for patients with one single prostate cancer tumor, based on synthetic data from the Simulacrum dataset[3]. This dataset contains demographic data, information related to the tumor, the date of the diagnosis and surgery, and information about the systemic therapy prescribed. For simplicity, we have selected only patients prescribed with Docetaxel chemotherapy. The nodes in the TPA models represent the diagnosis date, the prescription of the therapy, each one of the cycles of the therapy, the end of the therapy, and the date of surgery.

As shown in Fig. 1, some patients are treated with Docetaxel therapy before the diagnosis is confirmed. After diagnosis, patients follow one of these paths: (1) surgery (prostatectomy) and then Docetaxel, (2) only Docetaxel, and (3) Docetaxel prior to or simultaneously with prostatectomy. The restructuring operations carried out are described below. Unless otherwise specified, all node references relate to Fig. 1.

First, a composition has been defined (node pre-Diagnosis in Fig. 4) grouping the nodes presDOCETAXEL, cycleDOCETAXEL and FinalTreat before the Diagnosis node. Then, a Chemotherapy subprocess has been defined grouping

---

[3] See https://simulacrum.healthdatainsight.org.uk/.

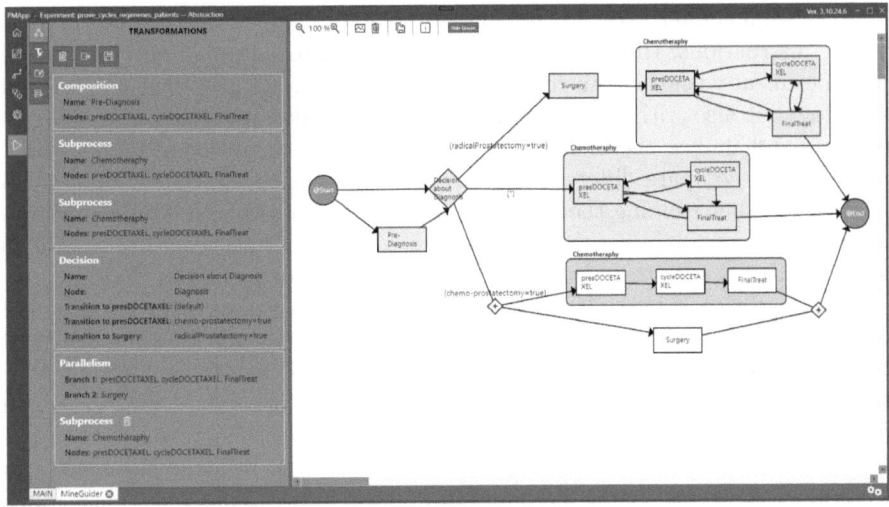

Fig. 4. *MineGuider* module: TPA model in Fig. 1 after the application of the structuring transformations described in Sect. 5.2, with a focus on Transformation Tab.

the nodes in the upper branch after Diagnosis and Surgery nodes. Similarly, the same transformation has been applied to the second branch after Diagnosis. In contrast with subprocesses (depicted as colored frames showing their content), the composition is displayed as a single node. Subsequently, the Diagnosis node has been defined as a decision node (named Decision_about_Diagnosis), and the transitions stemming from this decision have been annotated. Next, the activities in the lower branch after the previously introduced decision have been defined as parallel (see Fig. 3). Figure 4 shows the parallel branches with the appropriate delimiters. Finally, the nodes presDOCETAXEL, cycleDOCETAXEL and Final-Treat of one of the parallel branches have been grouped in a subprocess. The Transformations Tab in Fig. 4 shows the sequence of restructuring operations.

6   Discussion

In this paper we describe a novel approach to the interactive discovery of clinical processes and present the *MineGuider* module that we have implemented to support it within the PMApp IPM tool. Our approach shares the interest of previous works on interactive PD [2,3,12], but focuses on bridging the gap between the fields of PM and CPGs. We also focus on the enrichment of PM models with clinician knowledge, rather than on their simplification via abstractions used in the business process management field [13]. In the paper we also describe a use case consisting in the application of a number of restructuring and semantic annotation tools to a sample PM model related to the treatment of prostate cancer patients. Our preliminary results demonstrate the utility of our approach and developments.

Since *MineGuider* uses the model transformations to adapt the data preprocessing instructions, the PMApp tool will be able to automatically reproduce the experiment with the transformed TPA model and, not only with the original event log, but also with new event log data. This makes possible to incorporate new data and analyse them under the perspective of the transformed model, and, in general, to compare different datasets with respect to the same transformed model. Note that running the experiment with the transformed TPA model and new data can result in new model graph structures, which would be useful to identify differences with respect to the starting transformed TPA model.

One limitation is that although some of the modifications introduced by the restructuring operations, for example subprocess, are not affecting the fitness of the model, others may mean that some traces are no longer conformant with the model. For example, forcing the parallelism among several sequences can reduce the fitness of the model in situations where there exist traces that do not contain the events involved in all the parallel branches. In those cases PMApp will remove the traces in question and produce a report about rejections, which the clinician could take into consideration.

7 Conclusions

In the clinical domain, traditional PM techniques for PD are not sufficient to create models that are easy to understand and manage for clinicians, nor to incorporate their expertise. IPM techniques allow the interaction of the user with the discovered processes in order to clarify them, but in ways that are not always suitable for the clinical domain. Beyond that, we propose an approach to the interactive discovery of clinical processes that aims to improve the resulting model both structurally and semantically, by adding typical elements of CPGs and standardised term annotations. Additionally, we have implemented the *MineGuider* module to support our approach.

We have demonstrated the utility of the module by applying a number of tools to a realistic PM model related to the treatment of prostate cancer patients. The results show that the tools can be seamlessly applied to obtain a model restructured and annotated according to the knowledge of the user. An important aspect of the implementation is that, regardless of the modifications in the structure of the model, the experiment remains fully functional and thus can be reproduced without additional work. This is one of the main and distinctive features of our approach (and of the *MineGuider* tool). The other characteristic feature is that the restructuring operations have been devised with the aim of not only improving the model but also bringing it closer to the perspective of GPCs and GPC languages. Lastly, the semantic annotation is an important improvement that opens the way to new usages of the model. The possibility of making advanced queries over the data thanks to this semantic annotation might help to discover the differences among different patient cohorts in a more intuitive way.

As future work, we plan to carry out a comprehensive experiment to assess the proposed approach and tools, aimed at clinician users. Additionally, new tools can be devised to add new functionalities. For example, it could be interesting to add noise-related transformations to reduce the noise of the model by selecting or deleting actions, according to clinical criteria. In the longer term, new PM techniques and methodologies will be developed to take advantage of PM models enriched by clinicians, both to iteratively apply PM techniques and as a source of new medical evidence that can be used e.g. for the development of CPGs.

Acknowledgments. This research has been supported through project PID2020-113723RB-C21 and funded by MCIN/AEI/10.13039/501100011033.

References

1. van der Aalst, W.: Process Mining: Data Science in Action. Springer (2016)
2. Benevento, E., Dixit, P.M., Sani, M.F., et al.: Evaluating the effectiveness of interactive process discovery in healthcare: a case study. In: Business Process Management Workshops, pp. 508–519. Springer, Cham (2019)
3. Dixit, P.M., Verbeek, H.M.W., Buijs, J.C.A.M., van der Aalst, W.M.P.: Interactive data-driven process model construction. In: Trujillo, J.C., et al. (eds.) ER 2018. LNCS, vol. 11157, pp. 251–265. Springer, Cham (2018). https://doi.org/10.1007/978-3-030-00847-5_19
4. Fernández-Llatas, C. (ed.): Interactive Process Mining in Healthcare. Health Informatics, Springer, Cham (2021)
5. Fernández-Llatas, C., Burattin, A.: I-PALIA: discovering BPMN processes with duplicated activities for healthcare domains. In: International Conference on Process Mining, pp. 247–258. Springer (2023)
6. Ibañez-Sánchez, G., Fernández-Llatas, C., Valero-Ramón, Z., et al.: PMApp: an interactive process mining toolkit for building healthcare dashboards. In: International Workshop on Process Mining Applications for Healthcare 2023. Springer (2023)
7. Kaiser, K., Marcos, M.: Leveraging workflow control patterns in the domain of clinical practice guidelines. BMC Med. Inform. Decis. **16** (2016)
8. Martínez-Salvador, B., Marcos, M.: Supporting the refinement of clinical process models to computer-interpretable guideline models. Bus. Inf. Syst. Eng. **58**(5) (2016)
9. Munoz-Gama, J., Martin, N., Fernández-Llatas, C., et al.: Process mining for healthcare: characteristics and challenges. J. Biomed. Inform. **127**, 103994 (2022)
10. Peleg, M.: Computer-interpretable clinical guidelines: a methodological review. J. Biomed. Inform. **46**(4), 744–763 (2013)
11. Peleg, M., Tu, S., Bury, J., et al.: Comparing computer-interpretable guideline models: a case-study approach. J. Am. Med. Inform. Assoc. **10**, 52–68 (2003)
12. Schuster, D., van Zelst, S.J., van der Aalst, W.M.: Cortado: A dedicated process mining tool for interactive process discovery. SoftwareX **22**, 101373 (2023)
13. Smirnov, S., Reijers, H.A., Weske, M., et al.: Business process model abstraction: a definition, catalog, and survey. Distrib. Parallel Database **30**(1), 63–99 (2012)

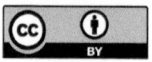

Research Paper: Enhancing Healthcare Decision-Making with Analogy-Based Reasoning

Joscha Grüger[1,2]($\boxtimes$)(ID), Martin Kuhn[1](ID), Karim Amri[1](ID),
and Ralph Bergmann[1,2](ID)

[1] German Research Center for Artificial Intelligence (DFKI), Branch Trier,
Kaiserslautern, Germany
[2] Business Information Systems II, University of Trier, Trier, Germany
grueger@uni-trier.de

Abstract. Analogy-based reasoning is often employed in the treatment
of hospitalized patients, especially when clinical guidelines or robust evidence bases are unavailable. This approach is based on the assumption
that similar patients respond similarly to comparable treatments. Traditionally, this reasoning has relied on the memory and experience of
physicians. However, the complexity of managing patient data—such
as treatment sequences and responses—presents significant challenges
without technological support. In particular, the procedural perspective
of comparing patients is especially demanding. To address these challenges, we introduce the MAPI framework, an innovative approach for
analogy-based, process-oriented search within patient data. This framework systematically manages treatment data, defines precise similarity
measures, and retrieves comparable patient cases using case-based reasoning (CBR). By integrating analogy-based reasoning, MAPI enhances
decision-making and improves the explainability of treatment choices,
offering a more reliable and transparent tool for clinical practice.

Keywords: Clinical Decision Support · Process-oriented Case-based
Reasoning · Analogy-based Reasoning · Explainable AI

1 Introduction

Clinical Decision Support Systems play a critical role in assisting healthcare
professionals with decisions related to diagnosis, treatment, and patient care
by leveraging patient data and scientific information, such as clinical guidelines. These systems are built on various technologies, focussing on different
perspectives on the patients. Addressing the procedural perspective of patient
data, often process models of clinical guidelines are used to support guideline-compliant treatments. However, the development of such process models is prone
to errors and often limited to patient cases for which guidelines exist [8, 15]. In
contrast, deep learning approaches eliminate the need for manual modeling and

© The Author(s) 2025
A. Delgado and T. Slaats (Eds.): ICPM 2024 Workshops, LNBIP 533, pp. 447–459, 2025.
https://doi.org/10.1007/978-3-031-82225-4_33

have proven highly effective in healthcare by analyzing complex and dynamic processes, allowing for the detection of intricate patterns within datasets without depending on static models [10]. Despite their high performance, these models are often criticized for their "black box" nature, which limits the explainability — a key concern in medicine, where understanding treatment rationale is essential for clinician trust and adoption [11, 16].

An alternative approach is analogy-based clinical reasoning, which offers more transparent and interpretable outcomes by drawing on similarities between cases [9]. This method is particularly used in treatment planning when clinical guidelines or evidence bases are lacking. The core idea is that patients with similar characteristics, such as diagnoses or treatment pathways, can be treated similarly. Physicians often rely on their memory to identify such similarities, a process that technology rarely supports [2]. This approach becomes especially challenging when dealing with numerous or complex characteristics, such as the procedural aspects of treatment sequences and responses. Thus, without technological assistance, quantifying these comparisons is nearly impossible for physicians

To address this problem, this paper presents the Multi-perspective analogy-based Process Instance Search (MAPI) framework. This framework is built on Case-Based Reasoning (CBR), an analogy-based artificial intelligence approach. It allows for the definition of complex and flexible similarity measures on treatment data, which can be used for analogy-based search, thereby providing decision support for patient treatment based on event logs. Thus, this framework makes physicians' analogy-based reasoning more quantifiable. The MAPI framework covers the management of procedural treatment data, defining similarity measures, and retrieving the most similar patients and their treatment processes. The framework is evaluated using a public available healthcare event log. By creating the MAPI framework, the following challenges from Munoz-Gama et al. are addressed, to advance the state-of-the-art in process mining for healthcare. First, C1 (Design Dedicated or Tailored Methodologies and Frameworks); second, C4 (Deal with Reality); and third, D8 (Consider White-box Approaches) [16]. To the best of knowledge, this is the first approach that combines CBR with process mining in the healthcare domain [7].

The remainder of the paper is organized as follows: Sect. 2 provides background information on event logs and CBR. Section 3 introduces the MAPI framework for analogy-based reasoning, while Sect. 4 presents the evaluation. In Sect. 5 the findings are discussed, and Sect. 6 concludes the paper.

2   Fundamentals

2.1   Event Logs

Event logs consist of multiple sets of cases, each case containing a sequence of events, referred to as a trace. Events represent activity executions, where a single activity can potentially refer to multiple events. Besides the control-flow, event logs can also include attributes representing various perspectives, such as the data perspective. The mathematical definitions of event logs, traces, and attributes are provided below [1].

Definition 1 (Universes). *The following universes are defined:*

- $\mathcal{C}$ *is the universe of all possible case identifiers.*
- $\mathcal{E}$ *is the universe of all possible event identifiers.*
- $\mathcal{AN}$ *is the universe of all possible attribute identifiers.*
- $\mathcal{AV}_n$ *is the universe of all possible attribute values that can be assigned to an attribute identifier* $n \in \mathcal{AN}$.
- $\mathcal{AV} := \bigcup\limits_{n \in \mathcal{AN}} \mathcal{AV}_n$ *is the universe of all possible attribute values.*

Definition 2 (Attribute). *Attributes can be used to characterize cases and events, e.g., a name can be assigned to a case or a timestamp can be assigned to an event. For any case or event identifier* $t \in \mathcal{C} \cup \mathcal{E}$ *and an attribute identifier* $a \in \mathcal{AN}$, *the value of attribute* a *for case or event* t *is denoted as* $\#_a(t) \in \mathcal{AV}$. *If the case or event* t *does not have an attribute* a, *then* $\#_a(t) = \perp$ *[1].*

Definition 3 (Trace, Case). *Each case* $c \in \mathcal{C}$ *has a mandatory attribute* $\hat{c} := \#_{trace}(c) \in \mathcal{E}^* \setminus \{<>\}$, *called trace. A trace is a finite and non-empty sequence of events where each event occurs only once, i.e.* $\forall 1 \leq i < j \leq |\hat{c}| : \hat{c}(i) \neq \hat{c}(j)$. *By* $\tau(c)$ *we denote the set* $\{(n, \#_n(c)) : n \in \mathcal{AN} \setminus \{trace\}, \#_n(c) \neq \perp\}$ *of all case attribute key-value pairs, or for short case attributes, of a case* $c \in \mathcal{C}$. *By* $\pi(e)$ *we denote the set* $\{(n, \#_n(e)) : n \in \mathcal{AN}, \#_n(e) \neq \perp\}$ *of all event attribute key-value pairs, or for short event attributes, of an event* $e \in \mathcal{E}$ *[1].*

Definition 4 (Event Log). *An event log* $\mathcal{L} \subseteq \mathcal{C}$ *is a set of cases, in the form that each event is contained at most once in the event log, i.e., in all the traces of the cases.* $\mathbb{L}$ *denotes the set of all possible event logs [1].*

2.2 Process-Oriented Case-Based Reasoning

CBR [3,13] is a problem-solving paradigm that uses the specific knowledge of previously experienced, concrete problem situations, referred to as cases. These cases are stored in a case base, which is a repository or database that stores historical cases with information about the problem solution are stored. CBR operates on the principle that problems tend to recur, and that new problems often resemble previously encountered ones. It represents a significant shift from traditional rule-based reasoning, focusing on leveraging past cases to address new problems. This approach simulates human reasoning more closely, as people often solve new problems by recalling similar experiences and adapting their solutions. CBR follows a cyclic process known as the CBR cycle. This cycle includes four main steps: *Retrieve, Reuse, Revise,* and *Retain.* First, the most relevant cases are identified and retrieved from the case base. Then, the information from these cases is applied to the new problem. The proposed solution is adapted as necessary and tested for effectiveness. Finally, the new problem and its solution are stored as a new case in the case base, ensuring continuous learning and improvement. It should be noted that in the medical domain, the focus is mostly on the retrieve step [6].

Process-oriented Case-based Reasoning (PO-CBR) [4] extends CBR methods specifically for process and workflow management. PO-CBR systems aid in the creation and adaptation of workflows or processes by leveraging experiential knowledge from past workflow modeling, execution, or monitoring activities. In these systems, a case can refer to a process schema or a particular process instance. This approach is especially beneficial in domains too complex for detailed predefined models, as it allows for flexible and adaptive workflow management. Like classical CBR, the effectiveness of PO-CBR relies on a case base, which provides the necessary data for case retrieval and reuse.

2.3   NEST Graph

In PO-CBR, workflow instances can be represented as semantically annotated graphs, called NEST graphs [5]. These graphs can be utilized to model and calculate semantic similarity measures based on graph representations. The described scheme is quite versatile, as it can represent various types of workflows. A NEST graph consists of four components: A set of nodes, a set of edges, a semantic description mapping and a type mapping.

Definition 5 (Semantic Descriptions) $\Sigma := \{(n, v) \in \mathcal{AN} \times \mathcal{AV} : v \in \mathcal{AN}_n\}$ *is the set of possible semantic descriptions, which are key-value pairs [4].*

Definition 6 (Types) *The possible types of nodes and edges are defined as* $\Omega := \{task\ node, workflow\ node, part\ of\ edge, control\ flow\ edge\}$. *In the following, the nodes and edges are explained in more detail [4].*

- *Each NEST graph consists of exactly one workflow node. The semantic description associated with a workflow node represents important general properties of the entire workflow.*
- *Each task in a workflow is represented by a task node.*
- *The workflow node is linked to each of the other nodes by a part-of edge.*
- *The control-flow among tasks is represented using control-flow edges. Such an edge connects two task nodes. An edge from node* e_1 *to* e_2 *indicates that node* e_2 *has been or must be executed after node* e_1.

Definition 7 (NEST graph) *A NEST graph* W *is a quadruple* $W = (N, E, S, T)$ *where* N *is a set of nodes and* $E \subseteq N \times N$ *is a set of edges.* $S : N \cup E \rightarrow \Sigma$ *associates to each node and each edge a semantic description from* Σ. *The function* $T : N \cup E \rightarrow \Omega$ *associates to each node and each edge a type from* Ω. $\mathbb{W}$ *denotes the set of all possible NEST graphs [4].*

3   The MAPI Framework

The MAPI Framework[1] introduces an open-source solution for conducting flexible, analogy-based searches across process instances within event logs. Specifically designed for the healthcare sector, MAPI addresses the need for effective

---

[1] https://github.com/martinkuhn94/MAPI.

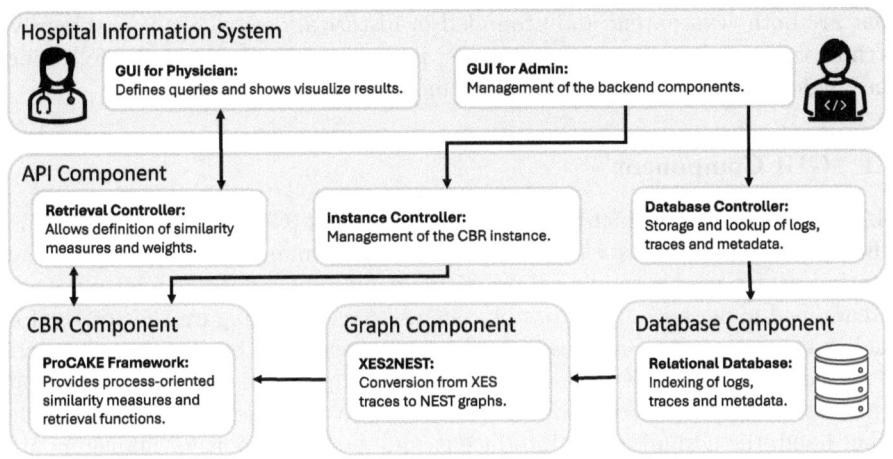

Fig. 1. Architecture of the MAPI framework, which shows the interaction of the components as well as the order in which the components are called.

and explainable treatment decisions by incorporating similarity measures tailored to specific attributes and treatment pathways. Leveraging historical patient data, the framework identifies suitable treatment strategies, thereby enhancing both decision-making and the transparency of medical choices. In this context, each case can be referred to as a trace or as a patient, where the treatment process is finished or ongoing. MAPI consists of five key components: the *GUI Component*, the *API Component*, the *Graph Converter*, the *Database Component* and the *CBR component*. The GUI Component allows physicians to visualize patient information and interact with the MAPI framework. Additionally, a dedicated GUI is provided for administrators to manage the backend functionalities. This separation ensures that each user role has a streamlined interface, displaying only the relevant information and functions needed for their specific tasks. The API Component facilitates integration with external applications, such as Hospital Information System (HIS), enabling seamless interaction with the MAPI framework within existing healthcare IT infrastructures. The Graph Converter transforms XES event logs into the NEST graph structure, enabling the integration of process mining techniques alongside CBR. The Database Component stores the case base, ensuring the persistence and accessibility of past cases. Finally, the CBR Component implements the core principles of the CBR cycle, which in the healthcare domain typically includes the retrieve and reuse steps [6]. During the retrieve step, similarity measures tailored to a process-oriented context are employed to identify the most relevant traces. In the reuse step, the retrieved similar cases are utilized to propose solutions for new cases, such as recommending new treatment strategies for patients.

By integrating these components, the MAPI framework provides a robust and adaptable approach for analogy-based reasoning in healthcare. It enables the retrieval and reuse of past cases, to assist physicians to make informed decisions, that are both transparent and grounded in historical data. This comprehensive architecture, along with its components, is depicted in Fig. 1. In the following, the single components are explained in more detail.

3.1 GUI Component

MAPI includes two distinct graphical user interfaces (GUIs) tailored to the specific needs of different user roles: physicians and administrators. The physician interface is designed with clinical practitioners in mind, offering an intuitive and streamlined experience. It allows physicians to easily configure the retrieval of similar cases from the case base, and review treatment options based on the retrieved traces. The GUI allows physicians to input patient information, configure retrieval parameters, and view results in a user-friendly format. On the other hand, the administrator interface is equipped with tools for managing and maintaining the backend functionalities of the MAPI framework. This interface enables administrators to manage essential tasks like uploading and deleting XES event logs, configuring system settings, and overseeing database operations.

3.2 API Component

The API Component, built using SpringBoot[2], serves as a RESTful service, providing multiple endpoints for interaction with the components of the MAPI framework. Through these API endpoints, users can manage backend operations, including loading new cases, deleting existing ones, administering the CBR component, and interacting with frontend features such as defining and configuring similarity measures, as well as conducting similarity-based searches. The retrieval process itself is facilitated by two primary endpoints: one for executing retrieval using a custom trace, and another for conducting retrieval with a trace from the case base as the query. The API's flexible design allows for detailed search configurations through parameters specified in the request body, including options for attribute weighting and selection of similarity measures.

3.3 Graph Converter

The Graph Converter plays a crucial role in transforming XES event logs into NEST graphs, which are essential for the ProCAKE framework's effective handling of procedural data. The converter generates individual NEST graphs for each trace within a given event log, ensuring that the procedural structure of the data are accurately represented. In this process, every trace in the event log is mapped to a corresponding NEST graph, with each event within the trace being captured as a list of attributes. These event attributes are then translated into a ProCAKE-specific format, which supports a rich, object-oriented representation. This format accommodates various attribute types, such as String,

---

[2] https://github.com/spring-projects/spring-boot.

Float, Boolean, Integer, Timestamp, and List allowing for a detailed and flexible encoding of the data. Formally, the converter is a mapping:

$$XES2NEST : \mathbb{L} \rightarrow \mathbb{W}^*.$$

Given an event log $\mathcal{L} = \{c_1, ..., c_n\}$, the converter returns a list of NEST graphs $(W_1, ..., W_n)$ where the W_i represent the i-th case and for all $1 \leq i \leq n$:

- $W_i := (N_i, E_i, S_i, T_i)$
- $N_i := \{\hat{c}_i(j) : 1 \leq j \leq |\hat{c}_i|\} \cup \{w_i\}$ is the set containing the event identifiers in $\hat{c}_i$ plus the mandatory workflow node w_i.
- $E_i := F_i \cup G_i$, where
  - $F_i := \{(\hat{c}_i(j-1), \hat{c}_i(j)) : 2 \leq j \leq |\hat{c}_i|\}$ is the set of edges between consecutive event identifiers in $\hat{c}_i$, i.e., the control flow edges.
  - $G_i := ((N_i \setminus \{w_i\}) \times \{w_i\})$ is the set of edges from all non-workflow nodes in N_i to the workflow node w_i, i.e., the part of edges.
- $S_i : N_i \cup E_i \rightarrow \Sigma, d \mapsto \begin{cases} \tau(c_i) & \text{if } d = w_i \\ \pi(d) & \text{if } d \in N_i \setminus \{w_i\} \end{cases}$ maps all case attributes of c_i to the workflow node and maps the respective event attributes to the other nodes. Note, that S_i is undefined on E_i.
- $T_i : N_i \cup E_i \rightarrow \Omega, d \mapsto \begin{cases} \text{task node} & \text{if } d \in N_i \setminus \{w_i\} \\ \text{workflow node} & \text{if } d = w_i \\ \text{part of edge} & \text{if } d \in (N_i \setminus \{w_i\}) \times \{w_i\} \\ \text{control flow edge} & \text{else} \end{cases}$

3.4 Database Component

The database component of the MAPI framework is designed to enhance efficiency by eliminating the need to re-upload logs with each engine restart. It also features a dedicated data management module. This is achieved through the integration of a MySQL database, which can be referred to as case base in this context. Logs can easily be added or deleted via API endpoints, facilitating seamless interaction and management. Upon upload, each log and trace is assigned a unique UUID, ensuring distinct identification through the API during subsequent operations. The system also automatically generates and stores metadata that describes each trace and log. This metadata not only supports current operations but also supports the development, for future enhancements, such as retrievals based on specific metadata criteria. Examples of stored metadata include the number of traces, the number of events, and the upload timestamp. Managing multiple logs is crucial in healthcare, as it enables for targeted similarity searches within specific logs. This approach improves the precision of insights and reduces computation time by focusing on relevant sub-logs.

3.5   CBR Component

For the retrieval step, the MAPI framework utilizes ProCAKE[3], a Java-based framework designed for developing structural and process-oriented CBR applications [5]. ProCAKE leverages NEST graph representations (Sect. 2.3) to incorporate a wide range of process-oriented similarity measures, making it particularly effective in comparing complex objects, including those with aggregations or lists of multiple nested attributes. This capability allows the component to handle similarity calculations during retrieval at various levels of nesting, enabling both global and local similarity measures to be applied with adjustable weights. Local similarity measures focus on evaluating individual attributes, while global similarity measures assess the overall trace, including all calculated local similarities. In this approach, local similarity measures include string similarity for comparing two strings, boolean and numeric similarity. These measures can also be combined. For example, when an event has multiple attributes—such as two string attributes and one boolean attribute—the results from the different similarity measures can be aggregated by applying weights to each attribute.

To compute global similarity, the Dynamic Time Warping (DTW) algorithm is adapted to calculate the similarity between event sequences in traces [17]. This algorithm is particularly effective in measuring the similarity between two time series by aligning them, even when they differ in length. DTW achieves this by stretching or compressing the sequences to identify the optimal alignment. The DTW algorithm computes similarity values as follows: Let $(q_1, \ldots, q_n)$ and $(c_1, \ldots, c_m)$ represent the events of traces q and c, respectively. We iteratively populate a $m \times n$ matrices, H with similarity values. For $i = 0$ or $j = 0$, the matrix value is calculated as $H_{i,j} = \text{sim}(q_j, c_i)$. For all other values of i and j, the matrix is filled as follows:

$$H_{i,j} = \max \begin{cases} H_{i-1,j-1} + 2 \cdot \text{sim}(q_j, c_i) \text{step diagonally} \\ H_{i,j-1} + \text{sim}(q_j, c_i) \text{step horizontally} \\ H_{i-1,j} + \text{sim}(q_j, c_i) \text{step vertically} \end{cases}$$

In this context, each step corresponds to a potential alignment between the events of the two sequences. The diagonal step represents aligning the current events from both sequences, which generally indicates the strongest match and is therefore weighted more heavily. The horizontal and vertical steps represent cases where an event in one sequence is aligned with a gap in the other, which might occur when one sequence has additional events that do not correspond directly to the other sequence. The value of $H_{i,j}$ is chosen as the maximum of these three options, ensuring that the algorithm always follows the path that offers the highest possible similarity score at each point in the matrix. This method allows DTW to flexibly align the sequences in a way that accounts for their differences in length and event occurrence. Once the matrices are filled, the similarity score can be computed. The similarity score is computed by dividing the value of the last element in the alignment path by the sum of the horizontal

---

[3] https://gitlab.rlp.net/procake/procake-framework.

and vertical steps and twice the number of diagonal steps, which is denoted as: $sim_{DTW} = \frac{H_{m,n}}{\sum_{(i,j)\in diag} 2*H_{i,j} + \sum_{(i,j)\in othersteps} H_{i,j}}$. Using the global similarity measure, it is possible to identify the n most similar traces according to the query trace in a case base.

4 Evaluation

Finally, we aimed to evaluate the effectiveness of the MAPI framework as a decision-making tool. We conducted a retrieval process using a partial trace from a synthetic healthcare dataset and analyzed the results. The latter events of the trace were intentionally omitted to simulate an incomplete patient case.

The dataset used as the case base is an event log comprising 25,000 synthesized cases[4], generated using the DALG tool [12] based on a process model for melanoma treatments[5] [8]. Each event in a trace represents a specific step in a patient case, which may involve a treatment, diagnostic tool usage, procedure, examination, or laboratory parameter.

For the query trace, we selected a trace from the case base and omitted the last four events (see Fig. 2). The first clinical examination (FCE) marks the beginning of the process. EXC refers to the excision of a lesion where malignant melanoma is suspected. HEX represents the histopathological examination of the excision. After melanoma is confirmed, SCE denotes the second clinical examination. DCM involves a group of diagnostic procedures to confirm metastasis. REE is a re-excision based on HEX results, while SLNB refers to a sentinel lymph node biopsy, performed to confirm or rule out the early spread of melanoma to the lymph nodes. HEXSLNB involves the examination of the biopsy, and LNS is lymph node sonography. Attributes such as float, integer, boolean, and string define these events and may change over time, as shown in Fig. 2.

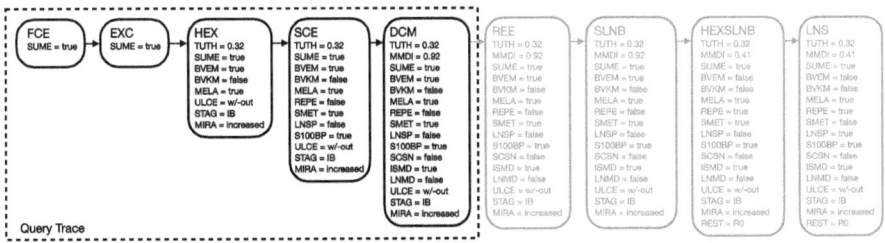

Fig. 2. Query Trace as Partial Trace from the Case Base

We aimed to utilize the MAPI framework to retrieve cases with a similar sequence of events. Specifically, the events FCE, EXC, HEX, SCE, and DCM

---

[4] https://zenodo.org/records/13828519.
[5] https://zenodo.org/records/10785431.

should not only be present but ideally appear in the same order as in the query trace. Notably, the first four events—FCE, EXC, HEX, and SCE—are consistently ordered across all traces in the case base. As a result, the fifth event, DCM, becomes critical for retrieving cases with higher similarity. To assess global similarity between traces, we employed the DTW algorithm. This algorithm aligns the query trace with the most similar subtrace of the same length from a given case. The overall similarity score is calculated as the weighted arithmetic mean of the individual similarity values for each mapped event.

To compare two events with the same "concept:name" attribute, the similarity between all their attributes is calculated and then averaged to determine an overall event similarity. For string attributes, we used a similarity measure based on the Levenshtein distance between the attribute values. For numeric attributes (either float or integer), we developed a custom similarity measure that computes the expression $\frac{b-a-|q-c|}{b-a}$, where q and c represent the query and case attribute values, and a and b define the attribute range. This range is set as a parameter before the similarity measure is applied, with 0 to 29 for integers and 0 to 8 for floats. For boolean attributes, we implemented a similarity measure that returns 1 if $(q = c)$ and 0 if $(q \neq c)$, where q and c represent the boolean input values. In cases where attributes are of different types, the similarity value defaults to 0. Additionally, we assigned a weight of 0 to the "concept:name" and "time" attributes. This is because events with different names were not compared, and the timestamp was deemed irrelevant since the sequence of events was the primary factor under consideration.

Results. The results in Table 1 show the five most similar traces and their respective similarity scores. The findings indicate that, based on the most similar traces, either a re-excision or a sentinel lymph node biopsy is suggested. Both would be guideline-compliant for the given patient, and the re-excision aligns with the original patient's treatment course. For comparison, one of the least similar traces followed the pattern FCE-EXC-HEX-SCE-LNS-REE-SLNB-HEXSLNB, with a similarity score of approximately 0.64. Not only did the fifth event not fit, but the overall event similarity was also relatively low. However, this evaluation only demonstrates usability; a separate evaluation with physicians is necessary to further assess the medical perspective.

Table 1. Most similar traces with corresponding similarity to query trace.

Trace ID	Sequence	Similarity
trace1094	FCE-EXC-HEX-SCE-DCM-SLNB-REE-HEXSLNB-REE-...	0.9908
trace18524	FCE-EXC-HEX-SCE-DCM-REE-SLNB-HEXSLNB-REE-...	0.9879
trace14454	FCE-EXC-HEX-SCE-DCM-SLNB-REE-HEXSLNB-REE-...	0.9867
trace3584	FCE-EXC-HEX-SCE-DCM-SLNB-REE-HEXSLNB-REE-...	0.9855
trace6890	FCE-EXC-HEX-SCE-DCM	0.9851

5   Discussion

The paper presents the MAPI framework, a novel approach that integrates analogy-based reasoning with process-oriented search in patient data, enhancing decision-making by offering structured methods to compare patient data. By leveraging CBR, the MAPI framework improves the reliability and explainability of decision support in healthcare settings. The framework supports event logs in XES format and allows the definition of custom similarity measures for these logs. The application supports multi-perspective, analogy-based searches of process instances within event logs, delivering results within reasonable timeframes. The framework's modular design, detailed in Sect. 3, allows for easy customization and substitution of its components as needed.

Despite its strengths, the development of the MAPI framework encountered several challenges. A key challenge was balancing the framework's simplicity with its functionality. While the framework allows for defining similarity measures at deeper levels (e.g., elements within lists), this requires creating XML configurations, which can be prone to errors, especially when performed manually. Additionally, performance issues arise as retrieval times significantly increase with larger event logs, particularly those containing a high number of traces. To address this, GPU support could be employed to accelerate the calculation of the most similar trace, as suggested by [14]. Given that real-life applications are likely to involve queries on sub-event logs, the computation times observed seem reasonable within actual treatment settings. Furthermore, the framework could be enhanced by incorporating additional similarity measures, such as those based on medical taxonomies. This would enable the semantic comparison of diseases and medical procedures based on their respective codes, further increasing its utility in healthcare contexts. This is also reflected by the evaluation.

The evaluation results should be interpreted with caution due to two main limitations: i) the case base is synthetic and may not accurately represent real-world treatment scenarios, and ii) the similarity measures and evaluations were not conducted by medical professionals. A trained clinician could apply a more nuanced weighting scheme, understanding which parameters are most critical when comparing cases. Additionally, custom similarity measures, such as those used for numerical values, can be developed to better account for the significance of these values in a clinical context.

Future work should focus on validating the approach in real-world scenarios by conducting case studies with domain experts. This would help assess and refine the framework's effectiveness. Additionally, the development of healthcare-specific similarity measures, which requires substantial domain expertise, should be prioritized to better address medical use cases.

6   Conclusion

The MAPI framework represents a significant advancement in integrating analogy-based reasoning with process-oriented patient data. By leveraging

CBR to define and apply flexible similarity measures, the framework enhances decision-making and explainability in healthcare, addressing a critical gap in medical practice where standard guidelines may be absent. Moreover, the MAPI framework effectively addresses several key challenges identified by Munoz-Gama et al. [16], pushing the boundaries of process mining for healthcare. Specifically, it addresses C1 (Design Dedicated or Tailored Methodologies and Frameworks), C4 (Deal with Reality), and the distinguishing characteristic D8 (Think about White-box Approaches). To the best of knowledge, this is the first approach that combines analogy-based reasoning methods with process mining in the healthcare domain, offering a structured and explainable method to support patient treatment decisions. Thus, the MAPI Framework holds the potential to significantly improve patient outcomes by supporting physicians with reliable, and interpretable data-driven insights.

References

1. van der Aalst, W.M.P.: Data Science in Action. Springer (2016)
2. Alsaidi, S., et al.: An analogy based framework for patient-stay identification in healthcare. In: ATA@ICCBR 2022 - Workshop Analogies: From Theory to Applications. Nancy, France (2022)
3. Bergmann, R.: Experience Management - Experience Management. Springer, Berlin, Heidelberg (January 2002)
4. Bergmann, R., Gil, Y.: Similarity assessment and efficient retrieval of semantic workflows. Inf. Syst. **40**, 115–127 (2014)
5. Bergmann, R., Grumbach, L., Malburg, L., Zeyen, C.: ProCAKE: a process-oriented case-based reasoning framework. In: 27th ICCBR Workshop Proceedings, vol. 2567, pp. 156–161. CEUR-WS.org (2019)
6. Choudhury, N., Begum, S.: A survey on case-based reasoning in medicine. Int. J. Adv. Comput. Sci. Appl. **7** (2016)
7. Grüger, J., Bergmann, R., Kazik, Y., Kuhn, M.: Process mining for case acquisition in oncology: a systematic literature review. In: Proceedings of the Conference Lernen, Wissen, Daten, Analysen. CEUR Workshop Proceedings, vol. 2738, pp. 162–173. CEUR-WS.org (2020)
8. Grüger, J., Geyer, T., Kuhn, M., Braun, S., Bergmann, R.: Verifying guideline compliance in clinical treatment using multi-perspective conformance checking: a case study. In: Process Mining Workshops, pp. 301–313. Springer International Publishing, Cham (2022)
9. Guallart, N.: Analogical Reasoning in Clinical Practice, pp. 257–273. Springer International Publishing, Cham (2014)
10. Heinrich, K., Zschech, P., Janiesch, C., Bonin, M.: Process data properties matter: introducing gated convolutional neural networks (GCNN) and key-value-predict attention networks (KVP) for next event prediction with deep learning. Decis. Support Syst. **143**, 113494 (2021)
11. Janiesch, C., Zschech, P., Heinrich, K.: Machine learning and deep learning. Electron. Mark. **31**(3), 685–695 (2021)
12. Jilg, D., Grüger, J., Geyer, T., Bergmann, R.: DALG: the data aware event log generator. In: BPM 2023 - Demos & Resources. CEUR Workshop Proceedings, vol. 3469, pp. 142–146. CEUR-WS.org (2023)

13. Kolodner, J.: Improving human decision making through case-based decision aiding. AI Mag. **12**, 52–68 (1991)
14. Malburg, L., Hoffmann, M., Trumm, S., Bergmann, R.: Improving similarity-based retrieval efficiency by using graphic processing units in case-based reasoning. In: Proceedings of the Thirty-Fourth International FLAIRS Conference (2021)
15. Mannhardt, F., Blinde, D.: Analyzing the trajectories of patients with sepsis using process mining. In: Proceedings of the 29th International Conference on Advanced Information Systems Engineering (CAiSE 2017). CEUR Workshop Proceedings, vol. 1859, pp. 72–80. CEUR-WS.org (2017)
16. Munoz-Gama, J., et al.: Process mining for healthcare: characteristics and challenges. J. Biomed. Inform. **127**, 103994 (2022)
17. Sakoe, H., Chiba, S.: Dynamic programming algorithm optimization for spoken word recognition. IEEE Trans. Acoust. Speech Signal Process. **26**(1), 43–49 (1978)

Analysing Disease Trajectories of Multimorbidity Through Process Mining Techniques: A Case Study

Daniel Petrov[1], Thu Nguyen[2], Areti Manataki[2(✉)] [iD], and Colin McCowan[2] [iD]

[1] University of Cambridge, Cambridge, UK
dp702@cam.ac.uk
[2] University of St Andrews, St Andrews, UK
{tn56,A.Manataki,cm434}@st-andrews.ac.uk

Abstract. Multimorbidity is a global public health challenge, where an individual has two or more chronic conditions, making it difficult to treat and manage illnesses. Understanding the disease trajectories of multimorbidity is crucial for providing patient-centred care. Previous research has primarily employed regression-based approaches, which don't consider the specific diseases involved and the order in which they occur. Process mining was recently proposed to address this gap, showing promising results in modelling disease trajectories across the entire spectrum of diseases. However, that study involved admissions to a single hospital, and hence the size of the dataset was much smaller than what is typically used in population-level studies on multimorbidity. In this paper, we present a case study where process mining techniques are applied to a much larger dataset of patients in Scotland. We present the disease trajectories discovered for the entire population, as well as stratified by sex. We also describe temporal patterns of disease trajectories, including trajectories with rapid progression. Finally, we discuss the experience of employing process mining within a trusted research environment, and we reflect on challenges that we faced when mining disease trajectories based on a large and complex dataset. Our main contribution involves providing additional evidence around the feasibility of disease trajectory modelling through process mining techniques, in particular when a much larger health dataset is involved.

Keywords: Multimorbidity · Disease trajectories · Process Mining

1 Introduction and Background

Multimorbidity is the co-occurrence of at least two chronic conditions in a patient and is regarded as a growing global health challenge [18]. It is associated with higher risk of mortality, poorer quality of life and increased healthcare utilisation [11,14,18,19]. Most epidemiological research on multimorbidity focuses on prevalence and disease clusters, employing a cross-sectional (i.e. 'snap-shot') rather than a longitudinal approach [3,18].

© The Author(s) 2025
A. Delgado and T. Slaats (Eds.): ICPM 2024 Workshops, LNBIP 533, pp. 460–472, 2025.
https://doi.org/10.1007/978-3-031-82225-4_34

Understanding how multimorbidity develops over time is important for developing interventions towards the prevention and management of multimorbidity, and has attracted research interest in the last few years. As revealed by a recent scoping review [3], the majority of longitudinal studies in this area employ regression-based techniques to analyse how the count of diseases or a multimorbidity index change over time for individuals. Even though this reveals certain patterns of multimorbidity, it fails to shed light on the sequence of diseases. Exploring the order in which diseases occur, in other words the disease trajectories of multimorbidity, is key to understanding multimorbidity progression and ultimately to detecting and preventing possible future diseases in individuals. Unfortunately, there is only a limited number of studies in this area [3].

Cezard et al. [4] employed sequence analysis to determine the sequencing of diabetes, cardiovascular disease and cancer in a population of 6,300 adults over a 10-year period. The main benefits of sequence analysis methods, as shown in this study, is that they can effectively capture the order of combinations of diseases, as well as timing and duration-related information. However, as soon as the number of conditions considered grows, it becomes difficult to interpret results.

Owen et al. [15] analysed a rich dataset of 1.7 million individuals in Wales to examine how psychosis, diabetes, and congestive heart failure develop over time. They employed multistate modelling to capture transitions between different combinations among these diseases, and they found that the order of disease acquisition had an important association with life expectancy. Similarly to [4], the authors recognise that increasing the number of conditions when using multistate modelling would lead to computational challenges, especially when population-level data is considered.

Xu et al. [21] analysed the progression of diabetes, heart disease, and stroke multimorbidity in middle-aged women over a 20-year period. They visualised the transitions between different combinations of the three conditions with the use of a Sankey diagram, and they also estimated the association among the three conditions using repeated measures logistic regression.

All studies discussed above focus on a small number of diseases. Jensen et al. [8], on the other hand, analysed trajectories involving the entire spectrum of diseases. This is a large-scale study on 6.2 million patients in Denmark over approximately 15 years. Their data-driven approach to identifying disease trajectories involved first identifying statistically significant, temporal correlations among pairs of diagnoses. Pairs with overlapping diagnosis were then combined to form 1,171 significant trajectories consisting of four diseases. We consider [8] to be a seminal study in this area, capturing an extremely rich set of relatively long disease trajectories. Their approach to providing an overview of this large and complex set of trajectories was through the use of clustering. Process mining is an alternative approach for mining complex trajectories.

Process mining is a set of data-driven methods for discovering, analysing and improving processes [1]. Process models are discovered based on event-based data, typically referred to as event logs. Event logs contain as a minimum a case, an activity and a timestamp for each event in the log. The discovered process models may have different forms, such as Petri Nets or Directly Follows Graphs (DFGs). These can be simulated and analysed further, for example to determine time-based performance or to detect bottlenecks. Process mining has shown promising results in several healthcare areas, including oncology, surgery and cardiology [13,16].

Process mining was recently employed to identify disease trajectories of multimorbidity for approximately 5,000 critical care patients in a hospital in the US over an 11-year period [9]. Diagnoses were considered at the level of the first 3-character ICD-9 codes. Significant trajectories were identified following the approach in [8], and then a process model was discovered with the use of the Interactive Data-aware Heuristics Miner [12]. Trajectories were analysed across different patient groups, and pairs of diseases with the quickest and slowest progression were identified. This is the first study that demonstrated the feasibility of process mining for disease trajectory modelling. One of its strengths is the fact that, similarly to [8], it covers the entire spectrum of diseases. However, the dataset upon processing was relatively small, consisting of 81 distinct trajectories for only 776 patients.

Hayward et al. [7] also employed process mining to identify trajectories of all major diseases following myocardial infarction. They considered a much larger dataset, including all NHS hospitalisations in England over a 9-year period (375,669 people with myocardial infarction). They identified 28,799 disease trajectories consisting of sequences of three-character ICD-10 codes, which were then aggregated and presented at the level of ICD-10 chapters. They also assessed the differential impact of these trajectories on long-term outcomes, including all-cause mortality. This study is effective in comprehensively describing patterns of disease accrual for myocardial infarction survivors based on large nationwide data, and it provides clear targets for public health intervention in terms of improving long-term outcomes. However, the use of process mining is rather basic, limited to the extraction of disease trajectories, without consideration of process discovery or other more advanced algorithms.

To the best of our knowledge, there is no study that employs more sophisticated process mining on a large dataset, in order to analyse trajectories across the entire spectrum of diseases. This paper aims to address precisely this research gap. Focusing on a regional Scottish population over a 21-year period, we identify the following research questions:

- RQ1: What are the most frequently followed disease trajectories of multimorbidity?
- RQ2: How do trajectories of multimorbidity differ by sex?
- RQ3: What are the temporal patterns of multimorbidity trajectories?
- RQ4: What is the value of process mining in investigating disease trajectories of multimorbidity?

2   Methodology

2.1   Data

A rich Electronic Health Record dataset was used in this study, following the entire adult population of Tayside & Fife, Scotland, from 1st January 2000 until 31 December 2021 (approx. 800,000 people). The dataset consisted of routinely collected data for general/acute and mental health hospital admissions, as well as cancer registry data, which, along with demographic information, was linked based on the Community Health Index (CHI) number, the unique patient identifier used in Scotland.

The dataset was held by the Health Informatics Centre (HIC) Trusted Research Environment at the University of Dundee. Access to data was governed by HIC Standard Operating Procedures and Polices, and ethical approval for this study was obtained by the University Teaching and Research Ethics Committee at the University of St Andrews (reference MD15619).

2.2   Method

The Process Mining Project Methodology (PM^2) [6] was followed throughout this study. Similarly to [9], the first four stages of PM^2 were deemed relevant to this project. In Stage 1 - Planning, the research questions were defined based on a literature review (as per Sect. 1 in this paper) and with input from data scientists and multimorbidity experts. In Stage 2 - Extraction, the event data was extracted (see Sect. 2.1 for scope definition).

Stage 3 - Data Processing involved generating the event log by creating the views, and then filtering and enriching them. In contrast to most related work [7–9], we decided not to aggregate diseases, as we were interested in detailed information about diseases (i.e. the entire ICD-10 codes from the International Classification of Diseases [20]) rather than disease groups. The event log was constructed by using the CHI patient identifier as the case ID, the ICD-10 diagnosis code as the activity name, and the date of admission as the timestamp. The event log was filtered to only include patients with multimorbidity, i.e. with two or more diseases from the Charlson Comorbidity Index [5] recorded as primary or secondary diagnoses. Only the first occurrence of each diagnosis for each of these patients was retained. The Charlson Comorbidity Index is a widely-used measure of multimorbidity, and diseases from this index are often the focus of longitudinal studies on trajectories of multimorbidity [3].

To create a more comprehensible process model and to account for data noise, we followed the approach by Jensen et al. [8] to retain only the most significant disease trajectories for process mining. Temporally ordered disease pairs (e.g. D1→D2) were first identified, and the relative risk (RR) for each pair was calculated by comparing the probability of disease D2 occurring with patients who did and did not have disease D1 at a previous time in the log. Similarly to [9] and unlike [8], we did not set any constraints on the time frame between D1 and D2, so as to allow for the investigation of rapidly progressing disease trajectories. Only pairs with RR > 1 were retained (i.e. where a D2 diagnosis was more present in the group with D1 diagnoses). These included cases of disease pairs, D1 and D2, in both directions (i.e. D1→D2 and D2→D1). Therefore, all pairs with RR > 1 were tested for directionality through binomial tests, so as to determine the dominant direction. The event log was filtered to retain only pairs that had dominant direction.

The event log was finally enriched with demographic information, in particular, sex, age and socioeconomic status. The latter was measured by the quintiles of the Scottish Index of Multiple Deprivation (SIMD) [17], where 1 indicates most deprived and 5 indicates least deprived.

Stage 4 - Mining and Analysis involved applying process mining techniques to answer the research questions. This included process analytics to identify the disease trajectories (equivalent to "trace variants" in process mining theory), calculate their frequency and other descriptive statistics, and produce visualisations. The Inductive Miner was used for process discovery, both for the general and the patient-stratified models, as it is guaranteed to produce sound process models with perfect replay fitness (i.e. 100% recall) [10]. Conformance checking was also carried out to calculate key evaluation metrics for the discovered models, namely replay fitness, precision, generalisation and simplicity.

Data processing and part of the analysis was carried out in Python, and the PM4Py package [2] was used for process mining.

3   Results

The research questions identified in Sect. 1 are the outcome of PM^2 Stage 1. The dataset in Stage 2 originally included data for approx. 800,000 people. This was reduced to 132,489 people with multimorbidities in Stage 3 (379,695 rows in the event log). The number of diseases in multimorbid patients is visualised in Fig. 1, and the most common diseases are presented in Table 1. The event log contained 34,592 unique disease pairs, which were tested for significance (resulting in 25,559 pairs) and directionality (yielding 642 ordered pairs out of 8,970 pairs where both directions were present). After this filtering step, the event log contained 168,448 rows for 53,230 patients, with 785 ICD-10 codes.

All disease trajectories (27,522 in total) along with their frequencies were extracted in Stage 4. Exploratory analysis revealed that 88.19% of these trajectories were only followed by one patient. This indicates a very high degree of

Table 1. Most frequently occurring diseases.

ICD-10 Code	Disease Description	Frequency
E119	Type 2 diabetes mellitus without complications	29,199
G451	Carotid artery syndrome (hemispheric)	15,724
J449	Chronic obstructive pulmonary disease	14,455
G459	Transient cerebral ischemic attack	14,344
J459	Unspecified asthma	11,842

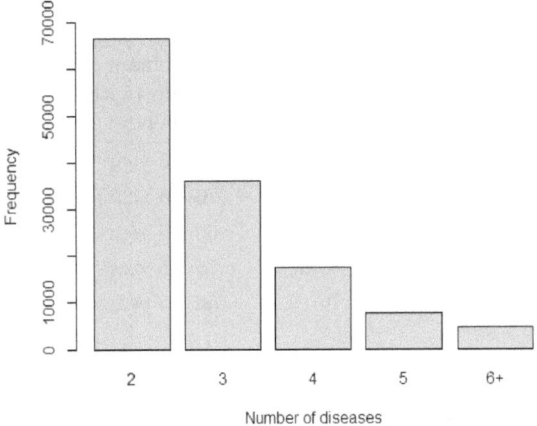

Fig. 1. Distribution of the number of diseases across the multimorbid population.

variability. We decided to exclude disease trajectories that explained a low number of patients' disease development, in order to allow for easier generalisation and computation. Setting a threshold of at least 10 patients for a disease trajectory, there were 465 such trajectories, decreasing the number of rows in the event log to 41,702, the number of patients to 20,342 and the number of ICD-10 codes to 162. Interestingly, the resulting event log only contained disease trajectories of length two or three.

3.1   Frequently Occurring Trajectories

Summary statistics were calculated for the most frequently followed disease trajectories of multimorbidity (RQ1). The most common trajectory of length two was J459→G451 (frequency 795), followed by J459→G459 (frequency 586). Table 2 shows the most common disease trajectories of length three, along with key demographic information[1]. The majority of these trajectories can be characterised as complex multimorbidity, as they contain three conditions across three body systems.

Process discovery with the use of the Inductive Miner helped generate a process model of disease trajectories in Petri Net notation. To produce visually coherent process model representations, the threshold of patients following a trajectory was increased to 20, and only patients with three or more conditions were considered. This reduced the event log to 34,823 rows, 17,317 patients, 239 trajectories, and 112 ICD-10 codes. Loosening these thresholds would produce

---

[1] ICD-10 codes not already explained: C349 (malignant neoplasm of unspecified part of bronchus or lung), C787 (secondary malignant neoplasm of liver and intrahepatic bile duct), C795 (secondary malignant neoplasm of bone and bone marrow), and N183 (chronic kidney disease, stage 3).

Table 2. Most frequently occurring disease trajectories of length three.

Disease Sequence	Frequency	Female (%)	Dominant Age Group (with frequency)	Mean SIMD (with standard deviation)
J459 → E119 → G451	35	74.29	76–85 years (11)	2.48 (1.18)
C349 → C787 → J449	28	53.57	76–85 years (10)	2.29 (1.25)
C349 → C795 → J449	23	56.52	66–75 years (12)	2.52 (1.10)
G451 → E119 → N183	21	66.67	76–85 years (12)	3.00 (1.45)
J459 → E119 → G459	21	76.19	56–65 years (6)	2.35 (1.11)

overly complex process models that are difficult to understand and would take a significant amount of time to discover.

Figure 2 presents the Directly Follows Graph (DFG) produced.[2] As seen from this graph, certain diseases (e.g. G451 and E119) were present in several trajectories. Not surprisingly, these diseases are the most frequently occurring in the multimorbid population under study. The Petri Net produced through inductive mining was similar but more complex in terms of structure, and it is therefore not included in this paper. The conformance of the discovered model demonstrated fitness = 1.00, precision = 0.60, generalisation = 0.84 and simplicity = 0.66. In the process mining community there is a recognised fitness/precision trade-off, and for the purpose of discovering disease trajectories, we prioritised fitness, to ensure that the model obtained is effective at explaining the data. The generalisation score of 0.84 indicates that the model is general enough to allow for future trajectories that are currently not observed in the data. As already mentioned, the obtained model is rather complex, hence the low simplicity score.

3.2   Trajectories Stratified by Sex

We investigated how trajectories differ between male and female patients (RQ2). The balance between the two groups (48.7% and 51.3%, respectively) is representative of the Scottish population. Many diseases may be highly dependent on the sex of the patients, leading to trajectories that are male- or female-dominated. For example, C509→ C773→G451,[3] which is the 6th most frequently occurring trajectory of length 3+, is only followed by females, which can be explained by the fact that C509 is the code for malignant neoplasm of the breast.

Setting a threshold of at least 10 male patients for a disease trajectory consisting of 3 or more diseases, we obtained 231 trajectories (7,289 patients, 105 ICD-10 codes, 15,386 rows in the event log). The most frequent trajectory was

---

[2] ICD-10 codes not already explained: C509 (malignant neoplasm of breast), I219 (acute myocardial infraction), I501 (left ventricular failure), and C779 (secondary and unspecified malignant neoplasm of axilla and upper limb lymph nodes).

[3] C773: Secondary and unspecified malignant neoplasm of axilla and upper limb lymph nodes.

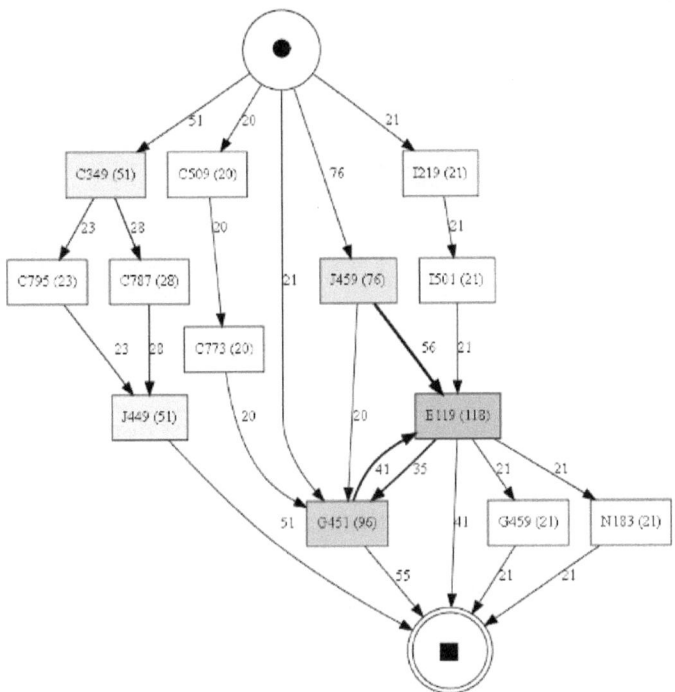

Fig. 2. Directly Follows Graph representation of disease trajectories of length three or more, with at least 20 patients following each trajectory.

I501→I252→E119, with mean duration 1,083 days (median = 112, IQR = 1534). The trajectory with the shortest duration on average was C349→C795→J449 (mean duration 38.6 days). Setting the same threshold for female patients, we obtained 278 trajectories (10,456 patients, 118 ICD-10 codes, 21,242 rows). The most frequent trajectory was J459→E119→G451, with mean duration 2,583 days (median = 2219.5, IQR = 2251.25). The trajectory with the shortest duration on average was the same as for males (mean duration 16.6 days).

We discovered the process models separately for male and female patients (containing 18 and 15 diseases, respectively), and we visualised them in DFGs and Petri Nets. Upon visual inspection, it was evident that the process model for females includes more complex relationships between diseases than the process model for males, which seems to be more structured. There were 8 diseases that were included in both models, with 10 and 7 appearing only in the male and female model, respectively. Several of the diseases that appeared in only one of the stratified models were malignant neoplasms.

3.3   Temporal Patterns of Disease Trajectories

We examined temporal aspects of all disease trajectories of length 3+ followed by at least 10 patients (RQ3), with a focus on overall duration (i.e. the time

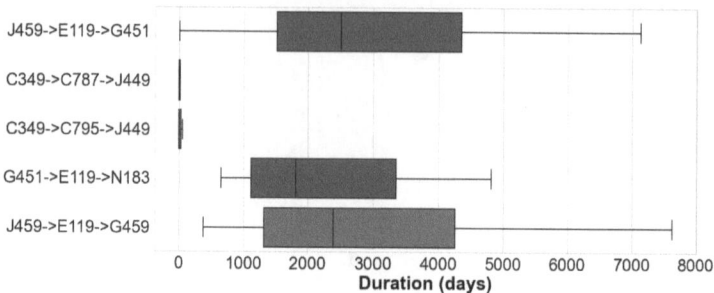

Fig. 3. Duration of 5 most frequent disease trajectories of length three or more.

difference between the diagnosis of the first and the last disease) and individual disease time distribution. There was great variability in overall duration, with some trajectories developing over the course of decades, and others consisting of diseases that were diagnosed on the same day (mean = 1,469 days; median = 782.5; IQR = 2,291.5). This variability was also evident when examining the five most frequent trajectories (Fig. 3).

We identified the trajectories with the fastest disease progression, i.e. with the lowest average duration (Table 3), many of which were cancer-related. We also examined time patterns in disease transitions (i.e. between two diseases, irrespective of overall trajectory), and we found that the fastest transitions were also cancer-related. For example, C182→C772 had mean = 0, as both diseases were diagnosed on the same day for all patients.

4   Discussion and Conclusion

In this paper, we employed process mining techniques to discover and analyse disease trajectories of multimorbidity in a Scottish population over a 21-year period based on large, routinely collected data. We identified 27,522 trajectories for 53,230 patients, but around 88% were followed by only one patient. This high degree of variability is a well-known challenge of process mining for healthcare [13] and it has been observed in other trajectory modelling studies [4,8]. Upon setting a trajectory threshold of 10 patients, we obtained 465 trajectories followed by 20,342 patients, which were analysed further. Unsurprisingly, several

Table 3. Disease trajectories with the shortest duration on average (measured in number of days).

Disease Sequence	Mean	Median (IQR)
C349 → C795 → J449	26.17	0 (25.5)
C349 → C787 → J449	34.43	0 (13.75)
G451 → C151 → C787	142.47	49 (99)

of the most frequent trajectories included diseases with high prevalence, such as diabetes and COPD. Some of the frequent trajectories identified were in line with related work (e.g. similarly to [4], we found cardiovascular disease and diabetes to frequently occur in this order), while others seemed to differ (e.g. trajectories involving COPD preceded by cancer-related diseases had a high frequency in our study, but not in [8]).

Interestingly, several of the most frequent trajectories were followed by more female than male patients, despite the sex balance in the patient cohort. This warrants further research. Sex-stratified process discovery helped reveal that trajectories for females are, overall, more complex and less structured than for males. Further research is needed to shed light on possible reasons behind this.

Temporal analysis, which is part of 'performance analysis' in process mining, revealed great variability in terms of trajectory duration, with some trajectories occurring over the course of a single day, and others taking decades for diseases to accumulate. We were also able to identify trajectories with rapid progression. To the best of our knowledge, [9] is the only other study that carried out similar analysis, but this was limited to transitions between pairs of diseases rather than longer trajectories.

In this paper, we have demonstrated how process mining can help analyse disease trajectories of multimorbidity from several perspectives, including control flow, time and patient characteristics (RQ4). This adds to the relatively small body of work that discusses the applicability of process mining for the study of disease trajectories [7,9]. Our main contribution lies in the analysis of a large and complex dataset of multimorbidity, where we go beyond basic trace extraction, to include process discovery, conformance checking and performance analysis. All this is done while considering the entire spectrum of diseases, without aggregating them in disease groups. To the best of our knowledge, this is the first study to achieve this.

Applying process mining to such a rich dataset was not without its challenges. Given the large number of diseases considered and the fact that they can be sequenced in different ways to form trajectories of variable length, the state space is huge. Following the Jensen et al. [8] approach for obtaining significant and acyclic trajectories proved invaluable for managing this complexity. To simplify further, we set a threshold of at least 10 patients for a disease trajectory, which, however, had to be increased to 20 for process discovery, which is a computationally expensive task. If we had lowered this threshold to 8, the execution time for the process discovery algorithm would have increased to approx. 5 hours, despite previous simplifications.

Analysing sensitive patient data was only possible through a Trusted Research Environment (TRE). This typically means limited computational power available, making certain kinds of analysis slow. Furthermore, TRE users may only export results of their analysis if there is no risk of revealing data of individual patients, who could potentially be identified. This makes patient-level dotted charts, which are widely used in process mining, unacceptable for export. TREs and associated data sensitivity considerations also pose constraints on the use of cloud-based process mining solutions, such as Celonis. A programmatic approach, such as PM4Py, offers a good alternative within a TRE, and we found it to work well for our analysis purposes.

Among the strengths of the paper we highlight the rich dataset that covers a large population from Scotland with comprehensive electronic health records over a long period. This is the first study to apply established process mining techniques on such a large dataset to analyse disease trajectories of multimorbidity across the entire spectrum of diseases. Nevertheless, the dataset is limited to secondary care, despite the fact that many chronic conditions are largely managed through primary care. This also means that individual diseases were allocated a diagnosis date only when recorded at hospital, while they might actually be pre-existing. This would affect the discovered trajectories, and we recognise it to be a key limitation.

Future research should investigate in more detail differences in trajectories of male and female populations, as well as the potential role of gender bias in these differences. Stratifying by age, socioeconomic status or other known risk factors, such as ethnicity, marital status and obesity, would also be advantageous. An in-depth clinical evaluation of the discovered trajectories would enhance the validity of the case study presented in this paper. The research community would also benefit from a comparative analysis of different methods (e.g. process mining, multistate modelling, Bayesian networks or even techniques from text mining) for trajectory modelling. Finally, a promising avenue for future research is the use of predictive process mining to predict disease trajectories for individual patients.

Acknowledgments. This work is independent research funded by the National Institute for Health and Care Research (NIHR, Artificial Intelligence for Multiple Long-Term Conditions (AIM), OPTIMising therapies, disease trajectories, and AI assisted clinical management for patients Living with complex multimorbidity (OPTIMAL study), NIHR202632). The views expressed in this publication are those of the authors and not necessarily those of the NHS, the National Institute for Health and Care Research or The Department of Health and Social Care. We also acknowledge the support of the Health Informatics Centre, University of Dundee for managing and supplying the anonymised data and NHS Tayside and Fife for the original data source.

References

1. van der Aalst, W.: Process mining: Overview and opportunities. ACM Trans. Manag. Inf. Syst. **3**(2) (2012)
2. Berti, A., van Zelst, S., Schuster, D.: PM4Py: a process mining library for Python. Softw. Impacts **17**, 100556 (2023)
3. Cezard, G., McHale, C.T., Sullivan, F., Bowles, J.K.F., Keenan, K.: Studying trajectories of multimorbidity: a systematic scoping review of longitudinal approaches and evidence. BMJ Open **11**(11), e048485 (2021)
4. Cezard, G., Sullivan, F., Keenan, K.: Understanding multimorbidity trajectories in Scotland using sequence analysis. Sci. Rep. **12**(1), 16485 (2022)

5. Charlson, M.E., Pompei, P., Ales, K.L., MacKenzie, C.: A new method of classifying prognostic comorbidity in longitudinal studies: development and validation. J. Chronic Dis. **40**(5), 373–383 (1987)
6. van Eck, M.L., Lu, X., Leemans, S.J.J., van der Aalst, W.M.P.: PM^2: a process mining project methodology. In: Zdravkovic, J., Kirikova, M., Johannesson, P. (eds.) Advanced Information Systems Engineering, pp. 297–313. Springer (2015)
7. Hayward, C.J., Batty, J.A., Westhead, D.R., Johnson, O., Gale, C.P., Wu, J., Hall, M.: Disease trajectories following myocardial infarction: insights from process mining of 145 million hospitalisation episodes. EBioMedicine **96**, 104792 (2023)
8. Jensen, A.B., Moseley, P.L., Oprea, T.I., Ellesøe, S.G., Eriksson, R., Schmock, H., et al.: Temporal disease trajectories condensed from population-wide registry data covering 6.2 million patients. Nat. Commun. **5**(1) (2014)
9. Kusuma, G., Kurniati, A., McInerney, C.D., Hall, M., Gale, C.P., Johnson, O.: Process mining of disease trajectories in MIMIC-III: a case study. In: Lecture Notes in Business Information Processing, pp. 305–316. Springer (2021)
10. Leemans, S.J.J., Fahland, D., van der Aalst, W.M.P.: Discovering block-structured process models from event logs containing infrequent behaviour. In: Lohmann, N., Song, M., Wohed, P. (eds.) Business Process Management Workshops, pp. 66–78. Springer International Publishing, Cham (2014)
11. Makovski, T.T., Schmitz, S., Zeegers, M.P., Stranges, S., van den Akker, M.: Multimorbidity and quality of life: systematic literature review and meta-analysis. Ageing Res. Rev. **53**, 100903 (2019)
12. Mannhardt, F., De Leoni, M., Reijers, H.A.: Heuristic mining revamped: an interactive, data-aware, and conformance-aware miner. In: 15th International Conference on Business Process Management (BPM 2017), pp. 1–5. CEUR-WS.org (2017)
13. Munoz-Gama, J., Martin, N., Fernandez-Llatas, C., Johnson, O.A., et al.: Process mining for healthcare: characteristics and challenges. J. Biomed. Inform. **127**, 103994 (2022)
14. Nunes, B.P., Flores, T.R., Mielke, G.I., Thumé, E., Facchini, L.A.: Multimorbidity and mortality in older adults: a systematic review and meta-analysis. Arch. Gerontol. Geriatr. **67**, 130–138 (2016)
15. Owen, R.K., Lyons, J., Akbari, A., Guthrie, B., Agrawal, U., Alexander, D.C., et al.: Effect on life expectancy of temporal sequence in a multimorbidity cluster of psychosis, diabetes, and congestive heart failure among 1·7 million individuals in Wales with 20-year follow-up: a retrospective cohort study using linked data. Lancet Public Health **8**(7), e535–e545 (2023)
16. Rojas, E., Munoz-Gama, J., Sepúlveda, M., Capurro, D.: Process mining in healthcare: a literature review. J. Biomed. Inform. **61**, 224–236 (2016)
17. Scottish Government: Scottish Index of Multiple Deprivation 2020. https://www.gov.scot/collections/scottish-index-of-multiple-deprivation-2020/
18. Skou, S.T., Mair, F.S., Fortin, M., Guthrie, B., Nunes, B.P., Miranda, J.J., et al.: Multimorbidity. Nat. Rev. Disease Primers **8**(1), 48 (2022)
19. Soley-Bori, M., et al.: Impact of multimorbidity on healthcare costs and utilisation: a systematic review of the UK literature. Br. J. Gen. Pract. **71**(702), e39–e46 (2021)
20. World Health Organization: International Classification of Diseases Tenth Revision (ICD-10), Sixth Edition. https://icd.who.int/browse10/2019/en
21. Xu, X., Mishra, G.D., Dobson, A.J., Jones, M.: Progression of diabetes, heart disease, and stroke multimorbidity in middle-aged women: a 20-year cohort study. PLoS Med. **15**(3), e1002516 (2018)

Predictive Insights for Personalising Esophagogastric Cancer Treatment Process - A Case Study

Mozhgan Vazifehdoostirani[1]([✉]), Andrei Buliga[2,3], Laura Genga[1], Rob Verhoeven[4,5,6], and Remco Dijkman[1]

[1] Eindhoven University of Technology, Eindhoven, The Netherlands
m.vazifehdoostirani@tue.nl
[2] Free University of Bolzano, Bolzano, Italy
[3] Fondazione Bruno Kessler, Trento, Italy
[4] Netherlands Comprehensive Cancer Organisation (IKNL),
Utrecht, The Netherlands
[5] Amsterdam UMC, location AMC, Amsterdam, The Netherlands
[6] Cancer Center Amsterdam, Cancer Treatment and Quality of Life,
Amsterdam, The Netherlands

Abstract. For metastatic esophagogastric cancer (EGC), treatments aim to extend survival time, manage symptoms, and enhance the quality of life . However, determining the best treatments for patients with EGC is challenging due to patients' variability. Personalised treatments supported by predictive models enable tailoring treatment process to individuals. Even so, traditional predictive models often neglect the interaction between treatments, limiting their utility in comprehensive planning. State-of-the-art Predictive Process Monitoring shows promising results in predicting the outcome of the treatment process but often lacks transparency. This paper investigates the potential of supporting healthcare experts in personalising the EGC treatment process, using eXplainable Predictive Process Monitoring methods. A real-world case study among 7,090 patients identifies expert needs for helpful explanations and discusses the capabilities and limitations of existing methods, suggesting future research directions. Our findings demonstrate high-quality explanations with strong *fidelity*, providing insights validated by expert knowledge. While the resulting explanations are not always actionable, experts acknowledged their value for exploratory analysis.

Keywords: Healthcare Processes · Explainable Predictive Process Monitoring · Process Pattern

1 Introduction

Stomach and esophageal cancer (combined as esophagogastric cancer, EGC) are in the top ten most common cancers worldwide [16]. The goal of palliative treatment procedures for many patients with advanced stages, including those

A. Delgado and T. Slaats (Eds.): ICPM 2024 Workshops, LNBIP 533, pp. 473–485, 2025.
https://doi.org/10.1007/978-3-031-82225-4_35

with metastatic EGC, is to extend overall survival by managing symptoms and enhancing patients' quality of life [4]. However, there is no consensus on the best treatment process. The high variability in disease aspects, patients' characteristics, desires, and dynamic conditions make it challenging for experts to determine the most effective treatments for an individual patient [15].

Predictive models can aid in personalising the treatment process and allow individualized decision-making [20]. By leveraging historical data, predictive models can identify patterns and correlations that may not be apparent to human practitioners [13]. However, traditional predictive methods often focus on the demographic and clinical characteristics of the patient and ignore the order in which the individual treatments are provided (which we refer to as the *treatment process*) [10,15,16]. As shown in [18], the impact of activities on the process outcome might vary depending on their position within the trace. Therefore, ignoring treatment orders limits the utility of previous predictive methods in comprehensive treatment planning. Additionally, considering the dynamic changes in patient conditions, practitioners require methods that enable them to monitor patient and disease progression and predict outcomes at different stages of the treatment process. Recent work in the field of Predictive Process Monitoring (PPM) provided ML-based predictive methods that consider the order in which individual treatments are provided for each patient [13]. These models have shown promise in effectively predicting the treatment process's outcome but often function as *black boxes*, offering little insight into how predictions are made or how to adjust treatment processes for a desired outcome.

This lack of transparency is a significant drawback when utilizing black box models in the healthcare domain [12]. Our healthcare partners emphasize that the prediction results must be interpretable for informed and data-driven decision-making. Furthermore, the explanations provided must be clinically sound and relevant. Recent approaches in eXplainable Predictive Process Monitoring (XPPM) aim to address these issues by promoting effective collaboration between human experts and predictive models [11].

In this paper, we aim to investigate the potential of providing practitioners with explanations of black-box predictive models to support personalising the EGC treatment process. To this end, we conducted a real-world case study to identify experts' needs for useful explanations and assess the capability of existing methods to meet these needs. Particularly, we explore the benefits and limitations of the PABLO (PAttern-based LOcal explanation) [3], a state-of-the-art XPPM technique, as the best-fitting method for this case study according to our literature review and interviews with healthcare experts.

The paper is structured as: Sect. 2 provides background, Sect. 3 outlines the methodology, Sect. 4 presents the results and discusses potentials and limitations, and Sect. 5 concludes the paper.

2   Background

Predictive Process Monitoring (PPM) aims at predicting the unfolding of ongoing process executions leveraging machine learning or deep learning models trained on event logs storing past process executions. Within PPM, there are several prediction tasks, e.g., predicting the time until the completion of an execution or the next activity to be executed. In this paper, we focus on outcome-based PPM, where we predict the outcome of ongoing trace executions. Recently, outcome-based PPM has seen growing use in healthcare, showing promising results according to various studies [1,5,13].

A pressing issue in PPM relates to the accuracy/explainability trade-off: while more complex models perform better in terms of accuracy, they often lack interpretability [11]. Therefore, prior PPM studies have utilized post-hoc eXplainable Artificial Intelligence techniques to elucidate these black-box models. Consequently, a new subfield known as eXplainable Predictive Process Monitoring (XPPM) has emerged [6]. XPPM techniques can be classified into two categories: local and global explanations. Local explainability emphasizes personalized interpretation, supporting experts in understanding *why a prediction was made for a specific trace (i.e., an "inquiry trace")*. Global explainability provides an overview of predictive models at a population level, supporting *focus on strategic decisions* [14,18]. Since this paper focuses on personalising treatment processes for individual patients, we explore local explainability methods.

Previous research has shown that process analysts frequently seek actionable insights within specific cases to achieve desired outcomes, known as counterfactual explanations [7]. This task is challenging, as the counterfactuals must conform to process constraints and closely match the inquiry trace, enabling experts to achieve desired outcomes with minimal changes. Furthermore, previous research indicates that neglecting factual explanations and concentrating on counterfactuals hinders the discovery of truly predictive process patterns [3]. To the best of our knowledge, only two methods incorporate both factual and counterfactual process-aware local explanations: the Loreley [7] and PABLO frameworks [3]. However, the Loreley method focuses exclusively on static attributes of traces and lacks control-flow-aware explanations, which are essential for practitioners when patient characteristics cannot be modified. Conversely, PABLO allows adjustments in both control flow and static attributes, offering an explanation focusing on the adjustment of treatments. Thus, in this paper, we adopt an instantiation of the PABLO framework as a best-fitting method for the goal and characteristics of the presented case study.

3 Methodology

This case study has been conducted following the PM² framework, a well-known process mining project methodology [17], outlining six steps in a process mining project: *Planning, Extraction, Data Processing, Mining and Analysis, Evaluation* and *Process Improvement and Support*. Due to space constraints, we only discuss key activities performed at each stage for the operationalisation of the PM² framework in the following sections. Note that the final step is beyond the scope of this project.

3.1   Planning

The objective of the planning step is to set up the case study and to determine the research questions. The main goal of this case study is to investigate the possibility of supporting healthcare professionals in personalising the treatment of EGC patients, leveraging predictive models and predictive insights.

Through interviews with healthcare practitioners, we identified two key limitations in deploying predictive models for treatment personalising. Since the best performing models are often black boxes, they find it essential to 1) understand the driving factors behind predictions (aka. factual explanations) and 2) learn possible factors to refine treatment plans when faced with undesirable outcomes (aka. counterfactual explanations).

Thus, we define our primary research question in this case study as: *How can we support healthcare experts with explanations of predictive models that guide them on which factors to change or retain for improved treatment outcomes?*

3.2   Data Extraction and Preprocessing

The dataset is provided by the Netherlands Cancer Registry, maintained by the Netherlands Comprehensive Cancer Organisation[1]. The dataset contains 7,090 metastatic patients between 2015–2021. We extracted data from all treatments performed on each patient after being diagnosed with EGC, including the timestamps, indicating their orders and duration. Additionally, we extracted 15 relevant patient attributes in outcome prediction reported in previous studies [16].

Data preprocessing was conducted with the guidance of healthcare professionals to ensure clinical relevance and accuracy. As part of this process, we removed 1,419 patients who had received only one treatment, focusing the analysis on those with more complex treatment histories. Additionally, we removed 553 cases where there were logging errors (e.g., patients for which the survival time was unknown) and exceptional cases, like patients who received one or multiple treatment(s) abroad. Similarly, 189 patients with too deteriorated health are removed from the dataset, as they are not fit enough to receive any treatment or to live more than 30 days. In the end, we concentrated solely on 3,217 deceased patients with observed complete survival times.

The initial log contained 161 distinct treatment codes. However, based on expert knowledge, multiple treatment codes could be grouped under common categories, reducing the complexity of the analysis. For example, 8 different types of Radiotherapy codes are relabelled to Radiotherapy. After adjusting the granularity level of the dataset, we also removed 170 patients who received a very rare treatment with lower than 0.5% frequency. The final dataset includes 3,047 patients exhibiting 807 process variants with 17 unique treatment codes.

---

[1] According to the Dutch Central Committee on Research involving Human Subjects (CCMO), this retrospective observational study does not require ethics approval from an ethics committee in the Netherlands. The scientific committee of the Dutch Upper-GI Cancer Group (DUCG) and the Privacy Review Board of the Netherlands Cancer Registry approved the use of anonymous data for this study.

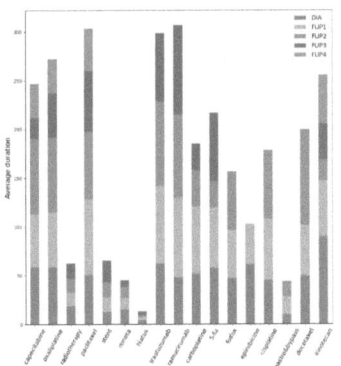
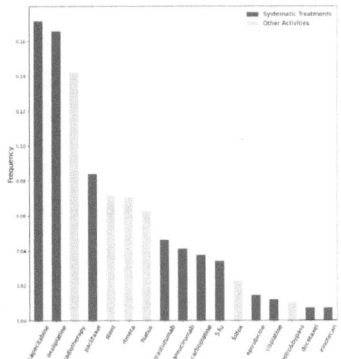

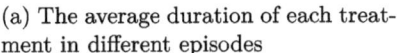

(a) The average duration of each treatment in different episodes

(b) The distribution of systematic and non-systematic treatments

Fig. 1. Frequency and duration of each treatment after preprocessing (Color figure online)

The treatment process is divided into five episodes by experts, each ending with disease progression. We imputed the missed duration of treatments for 9% of events based on their average duration in the corresponding episode. As depicted in Fig. 1a, some treatment durations vary across different episodes. We used treatment duration as a dynamic attribute for predictive models.

Eventually, we devised two scenarios based on experts' knowledge to generate life expectancy binary labels for each patient. This step is done to make the dataset compatible with existing methods, which are mainly designed for binary outcome prediction [9]. In the first scenario (L1), recorded survival times (days survived after completing the last treatment) were categorized as "Low" (162 days or fewer) or "High" (more than 162 days) based on expert knowledge, with 24% of cases labelled as "Low". In the second scenario (L2), the threshold for "Low" or "High" life expectancy varied by treatment type. Patients receiving any *systematic treatments* were classified as "Low" if their survival time was under 120 days, while those not receiving systematic treatment were classified as "Low" if their survival time was under 60 days. In this scenario, only 16% of cases were labelled as "Low". The frequency of each treatment is depicted in Fig. 1b, with systematic treatments highlighted in dark blue and other treatments shown in light blue. We will report and analyze the results of two labelling strategies in the following sections.

3.3 Mining and Analysis

Since the main research question requires a method to generate both factual and counterfactual explanations, we employ the PABLO framework (see Figure 2). In the following, we discuss the adoption of the PABLO framework for the EGC dataset according to our healthcare experts' desires and needs:

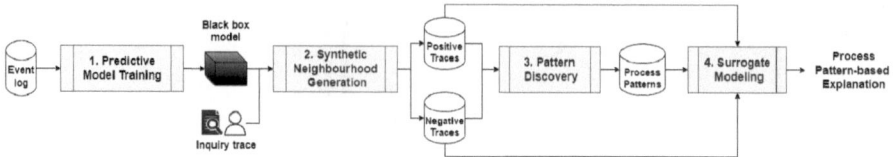

Fig. 2. The pattern-based local explanation (PABLO) framework

Predictive Model Training. We implemented the XGboost model as the black box model since it shows promising performance in previous studies [13].

To build the XGboost model, we need to encode each prefix trace in a format compatible with the model. For example, each prefix trace of length m like $\sigma =< e_1,\ldots,e_m >$ has to be represented through a feature vector F. In this case study, we used three encoding methods from PPM literature:

- In Simple-Index encoding (SI) [8], each feature corresponds to a position in the trace, with possible values being event classes, resulting in $F =< a_1,\ldots,a_m >$, where a_j is the event class a at position j.
- Simple-Trace-Index encoding (STI) [2] includes both dynamic sequence information and static trace attributes defined as $F =< s_1,\ldots,s_u,a_1,\ldots,a_m >$, where each s_u is u^{th} static feature.
- In Complex-Index encoding (CI) [8], the event classes and both static and dynamic data attributes of a trace are encoded in the vector. The resulting feature vector is $F =< s_1,\ldots,s_u,a_1,\ldots,a_m,h_1^1,\ldots,h_m^1,h_1^r,\ldots,h_m^r >$, where each h_m^r is a dynamic feature, corresponding to an event attribute.

We found the optimal XGBoost model setup for each encoding method on different prefix lengths via hyperparameter optimization using the Tree Parzen Estimator (TPE), maximizing the Area Under the Curve (AUC).

Synthetic Neighbourhood Generation. The inputs of the second component of the PABLO framework are a trained black-box predictive model and the inquiry trace as an encoded vector. The goal of this step is to generate a neighbourhood of similar cases with the same (aka, negative) and opposite (aka, positive) predicted outcomes for inquiry trace.

We used the Genetic Algorithm (GA) from [3] to generate the synthetic neighbourhood. Upon initial experiments, we found that the GA required adjustment due to the EGC dataset's unique characteristics, where longer traces often correspond to longer lifetimes (desired outcomes). As a result, the GA frequently produced impractically long counterfactual traces (in about 20% of synthetic neighbourhoods) rather than reordering treatments within shorter traces. To address this, we adjusted the GA to prioritize assigning activities to lower positions in subsequent iterations. This adjustment helps prevent the creation of lengthy traces when the inquiry trace is short. We employed two strategies to generate the synthetic neighbourhood, for different analysis purposes:

S1: In the first scenario, we synthetically generate traces with the same attributes as the inquiry case but alter the sequence of treatments to provide an actionable explanation where patient attribute changes are clinically unfeasible.

S2: In the second scenario, both treatment sequences and attributes are modified to generate the synthetic neighbourhood. Though patient attribute changes may not be clinically actionable, experts value this form of explanation for exploratory analysis.

Process Pattern Discovery. We employed IMPresseD [19] as recommended in [3] to discover outcome-oriented control-flow patterns. IMPresseD adopts a multi-objective optimization approach to discover patterns balancing between multiple interest functions [19]. We used *frequency*, *outcome*, and *likelihood* interest functions, introduced in [3]. We aim to discover patterns with high frequency and correlation with the outcome, which are obtained from traces with a high likelihood of belonging to the predicted outcome. Additionally, as experts are concerned about confounding variables, we used *case distance* interest function introduced in [19] as the fourth interest function. This metric ensures that a process pattern is genuinely discriminative by requiring a minimal distance between the initial status (attributes) of patients who received the treatment pattern and those who did not. If this distance is too large, the observed outcomes may be influenced by differences in patient characteristics rather than the pattern itself.

Surrogate Modeling. A Decision Tree (DT) is used as a surrogate model to allow us to discover a rule-based explanation using the synthetically generated neighbourhood and discovered patterns from the previous step [3]. We have also found the optimal parameter for the DT using TPE, maximizing AUC.

3.4   Evaluation

The purpose of the evaluation stage is to use the analysis results to come up with ideas that help the project's goal. To this end, we first compare the performance of the predictive models using different encoding methods w.r.t AUC. Then, to measure the quality of the generated neighbourhood, we use the following measures introduced in [2]. The distance metric (DIST) calculates the average distance between an inquiry trace and generated traces. The diversity (DIV) measures the average pairwise distance among traces in the generated neighbourhood. The implausibility metric (IMPLAUS) evaluates the distance of synthetic traces from the reference population. The sparsity (SPARS) quantifies the average number of feature changes in each synthetic trace relative to the inquiry trace. Lastly, the conformance score (CONF) indicates the ratio of synthetic traces satisfying all process DECLARE constraints, which were discovered from the traces in the training set, with a support of 50%. Due to high variability in the log, we could not discover DECLARE constraints with higher supports.

To assess the quality of the final explanation, we measure the faithfulness of the provided explanation to the original black box model using the Local

Table 1. Evaluation metrics for different labelling and encoding scenarios

labelling	Encoding	AUC	NG	LF	DIS	DIV	CONF	IMP	SPAR
L1	SI	74.12%	S1	78.12%	0.868	0.873	0.682	0.853	2.011
	STI	76.30%	S1	77.42%	0.531	0.262	0.913	1.779	2.321
			S2	87.07%	0.826	0.932	0.956	3.245	2.965
	CI	87.05%	S1	91.01%	0.911	0.104	0.875	14.04	5.584
			S2	78.40%	1.272	1.302	0.944	12.56	6.536
L2	SI	71.29%	S1	74.84%	0.852	0.858	0.844	0.600	1.714
	STI	70.43%	S1	78.08%	0.511	0.295	0.842	1.860	2.252
			S2	92.21%	0.862	0.926	0.806	1.724	3.977
	CI	85.48%	S1	82.54%	0.767	0.096	0.843	13.55	5.347
			S2	83.20%	0.917	1.021	0.919	4.795	3.690

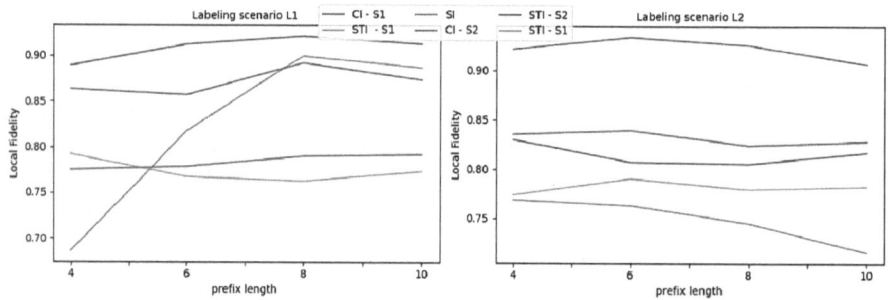

Fig. 3. Local fidelity over different prefix lengths

Fidelity (LF) measure [3]. The higher LF value indicates the higher capability of the surrogate model to mimic the behaviour of the black box model.

Additionally, we discuss the provided explanations with our healthcare partners to assess their validity and usefulness. The goal of this analysis is to determine whether the provided explanation aligns with expert knowledge. Moreover, we are interested in identifying the challenges and limitations of using the provided explanation in practice by communicating the final results to experts.

4   Evaluation Results

Table 1 shows the average values for each measurement from Sect. 3.4 across different prefix lengths, while Fig. 3 illustrates LF values by prefix length.

An initial observation from Table 1 is that CI encoding outperforms other methods in AUC due to its comprehensive attribute inclusion. The higher AUC suggests that the model is more accurate in distinguishing between patients who will benefit from certain treatments and those who will not, which is crucial for effective clinical decision-making. STI encoding's performance is close to SI encoding because STI only adds the initial state of patient attributes as static features. In contrast, CI encoding incorporates patient attributes as dynamic features and encodes all changes that occurred in the attributes through the process, leading to more precise predictions. Since the second labelling scenario (L2) depends on one group of treatments (systematic treatments) besides the remaining lifetime, the SI encoding is even slightly surpassing STI.

The first notable insight from analyzing the quality of the generated neighbourhood is a relatively high CONF measure in all scenarios (except for SI encoding in L1 labelling). Despite the 50% support for DECLARE constraints, which led to the discovery of constraints not present in all cases, GA was still able to generate highly conforming traces.

Inspecting other quality metrics for the synthetic neighbourhood, it appears that the GA method struggled to produce plausible traces using CI encoding. Despite relatively high LF values with CI encoding, the generated neighbourhood exhibited the highest IMP values, indicating a significant distance between the generated and original traces. The IMP is particularly higher for S1, where modifications are restricted to the control flow. Given that the average trace lengths are generally quite short (4 treatments), there are limited possibilities for altering the control flow, resulting in the highest IMP and lowest DIV compared to other scenarios. In contrast, in S2, where all attributes can be altered, DIV increases, but the IMP and SPAR values remain high. This indicates that the distance to the original traces is still significant (high IMP), with many changes applied to the inquiry trace to generate the neighbourhood (high SPAR).

Overall, CI encoding provides more precise predictions and high-fidelity explanations. In contrast, STI and SI encoding methods deliver more valid and less intrusive explanations, thanks to the high-quality generated neighbourhood. These findings highlight the need for further research into enhancing neighbourhood generation using dynamic attributes.

To further explore the local fidelity results, we direct your attention to Fig. 3. In L1 labelling, the combination of *CI - S1* consistently shows high fidelity, while *STI - S1* exhibits the lowest fidelity across all prefix lengths. Conversely, in L2 labelling, *STI - S2* outperforms other methods. In the L2, the rankings of the methods stay consistent across all prefix lengths. However, for L1, *SI* encoding improves significantly, going from the lowest LF at a prefix length of 4 to the second highest LF at a prefix of 10.

These contradictory behaviours between two labelling scenarios highlight the importance of defining the right outcome for a practical problem. It's worth mentioning that defining binary outcomes was challenging for experts because the final goal of the treatment process for EGC patients is to extend patients' remaining lifetime, which is, in essence, a regression problem. However, there is a lack of explanation methods designed specifically for regression problems [9], particularly when it comes to combined factual and counterfactual local explanations as needed for treatment process personalising.

4.1   Discussion

To discuss the potential and meaningfulness of the obtained explanations with healthcare practitioners, we presented explanations resulting from SI and STI

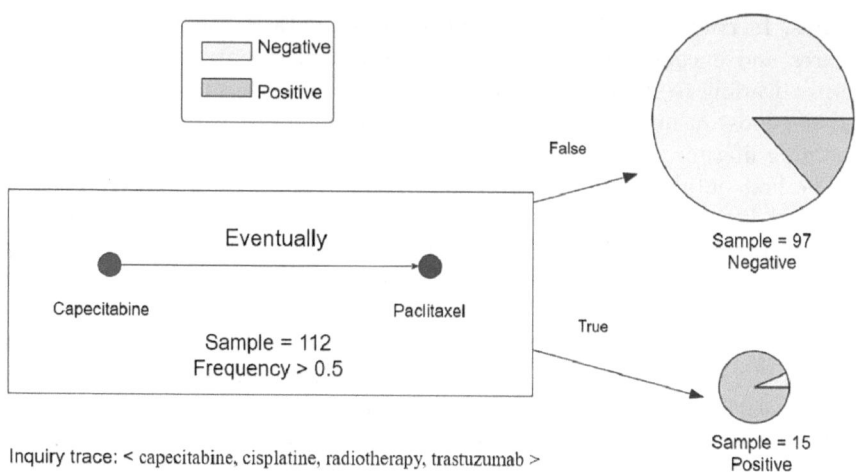

Fig. 4. Explanation example obtained from SI encoding for labelling scenario L1

encoding, which offer higher neighbourhood quality, through a workshop. In the following, we highlight two interesting examples identified in the expert review.

Figure 4 presents the explanation obtained from a patient (inquiry trace) who received four treatments shown in the figure. DT nodes represent discovered process patterns and their frequencies, edges indicate whether frequency conditions are met, and the DT leaves show the predicted outcomes for those paths. The explanation suggests that administering *paclitaxel* eventually after *capecitabine* could shift the outcome from low to high remaining life class. The expert confirmed this explanation as a clinically sound counterfactual, having observed longer survival in patients receiving these two systematic treatments. However, if the patient is not fit enough for the second treatment, this counterfactual is not actionable. Due to SI encoding limitation, which ignores case attributes, the case condition is not presented in the final explanation.

Additionally, it would be valuable to know more details about the counterfactual treatment pattern, such as the time interval between these two treatments in the process pattern, especially when we have an eventual relation. A promising direction for future work is incorporating event data, such as timestamps, to enhance the discovery of predictive process patterns.

Another explanation example is depicted in Fig. 5. With STI encoding, DT nodes may include patient attributes and their conditions or discovered patterns, similar to the previous example. The inquiry patient, in this case, received only two treatments (*hiatus* and *stent*), likely due to a bad initial health condition, as indicated by a health performance score of 3 (very poor condition). The short inquiry trace resulted in similarly short neighbourhood traces, limiting the discovery of larger process patterns. Consequently, the explanation often relies on a single treatment rather than a combination. The healthcare expert validated the relevance of the treatments provided as counterfactual for this case.

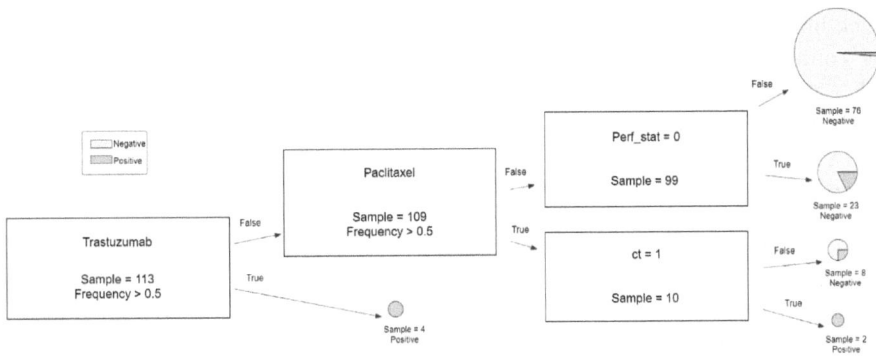

Fig. 5. Explanation example obtained from STI encoding for L2 and S2 scenarios

The counterfactual suggests that *Trastuzumab* could extend the patient's lifetime. If *Trastuzumab* is not an option, *Paclitaxel* with ct = 1 may be beneficial. If neither treatment is feasible, setting perf_stat (health performance score) to 0 (very healthy) may shift the outcome favourably. Improving health performance makes sense as the last option, however this counterfactual is not actionable for metastatic patients. This explanation is interesting and could be relevant for others where improvements in health performance through exercise and nutrition are possible. Nevertheless, such explanations can validate whether the black box model has learned from the right and meaningful features and patterns and can assist physicians in trusting the prediction made by the black box model.

While our examination of explanations with healthcare experts reveals promising insights confirmed by expert knowledge, these explanations are not always actionable in practice. For example, the discussed counterfactual scenarios highlight important considerations but also underscore the need for additional information to fully assess their applicability. Specific details, such as treatment intervals, are crucial for making these explanations more actionable.

5   Conclusion

In conclusion, our investigation into the potential of XPPM methods for supporting EGC treatment personalisation highlighted the significant promise of these methods for clinical decision-making. Our real-world case study, focusing on PABLO framework, revealed high fidelity of these explanations (nearly 90%), conforming with expert knowledge. However, further analysis showed that the provided explanations are not always actionable in real-world scenarios. This limitation underscores the need for further refinement to ensure that the explanation can be effectively translated into clinical practice. Nevertheless, our healthcare partners expressed a strong interest in exploratory explanations, which can help to discover existing relationships and support a deeper understanding of black-box models. Also, given the evolving nature of dynamic attributes, making connections between dynamic attributes and process patterns could offer richer explanations and is a promising area for future work to provide more enriched explanations.

References

1. Bekelaar, J.W., Luime, J.J., de Carvalho, R.M.: Predicting patient care acuity: an LSTM approach for days-to-day prediction. In: International Conference on Process Mining, pp. 378–390. Springer, 2022
2. Buliga, A., Di Francescomarino, C., Ghidini, C., Maggi, F.M.: Counterfactuals and ways to build them: evaluating approaches in predictive process monitoring. In: International Conference on Advanced Information Systems Engineering, pp. 558–574. Springer, 2023
3. Buliga, A., et al.: Uncovering patterns for local explanations in outcome-based predictive process monitoring. In: International Conference on Business Process Management, pp. 363–380. Springer, 2024
4. Dijksterhuis, W.P.M., et al.: Hospital volume and beyond first-line palliative systemic treatment in metastatic oesophagogastric adenocarcinoma: a population-based study. Eur. J. Cancer **139**, 107–118 (2020)
5. Dubbeldam, A.L., Ketykó, I., de Carvalho, R.M., Mannhardt, F.: Early predicting the need for aftercare based on patients events from the first hours of stay–a case study. In: International Conference on Process Mining, pp. 366–377. Springer, 2022
6. Elkhawaga, G., Abu-Elkheir, M., Reichert, M.: Explainability of predictive process monitoring results: can you see my data issues? Appl. Sci. **12**(16) (2022)
7. Huang, T.H., Metzger, A., Pohl, K.: Counterfactual explanations for predictive business process monitoring. In: EMCIS 2021, Proceedings, vol. 437, pp. 399–413, 2021
8. Leontjeva, A., Conforti, R., Di Francescomarino, C., Dumas, M., Maggi, F.M.: Complex symbolic sequence encodings for predictive monitoring of business processes. In: BPM 2015, vol. 9253, pp. 297–313, 2015
9. Letzgus, S., Wagner, P., Lederer, J., Samek, W., Müller, K.-R., Montavon, G.: Toward explainable artificial intelligence for regression models: a methodological perspective. IEEE Signal Process. Mag. **39**, 40–58 (2022)
10. Ma, X., Pierce, E., Anand, H., Aviles, N., Kunk, P., Alemazkoor, N.: Early prediction of response to palliative chemotherapy in patients with stage-iv gastric and esophageal cancer. BMC Cancer **23**(1), 910 (2023)
11. Mehdiyev, N., Fettke, P.: Explainable artificial intelligence for process mining: a general overview and application of a novel local explanation approach for predictive process monitoring. Interpret. Artif. Intell. Perspect. Granul. Comput. 1–28 (2021)
12. Munoz-Gama, J., et al.: Process mining for healthcare: characteristics and challenges. J. Biomed. Inform. **127**, 103994 (2022)
13. Pijnenborg, P., Verhoeven, R., Firat, M., van Laarhoven, H., Genga, L.: Towards evidence-based analysis of palliative treatments for stomach and esophageal cancer patients: a process mining approach. In: International Conference on Process Mining, pp. 136–143. IEEE (2021)
14. Stiglic, G., Kocbek, P., Fijacko, N., Zitnik, M., Verbert, K., Cilar, L.: Interpretability of machine learning-based prediction models in healthcare. Wiley Interdiscip. Rev. Data Min. Knowl. Discov. **10**(5), e1379 (2020)

15. van den Boorn, H.G., et al.: Source: a registry-based prediction model for overall survival in patients with metastatic oesophageal or gastric cancer. Cancers **11**(2), 187 (2019)
16. van den Boorn, H.G., et al.: Source: prediction models for overall survival in patients with metastatic and potentially curable esophageal and gastric cancer. J. Natl. Compr. Cancer Netw. **19**(4), 403–410 (2021)
17. Van Eck, M.L., Lu, X., Leemans, S.J., Van Der Aalst, W.M.: PM: a process mining project methodology. In: International Conference on Advanced Information Systems Engineering, pp. 297–313. Springer, 2015
18. Vazifehdoostirani, M., Abbaspour Onari, M., Grau, I., Genga, L., Dijkman, R.: Uncovering the hidden significance of activities location in predictive process monitoring. In: International Conference on Process Mining, pp. 191–203. Springer, 2023
19. Vazifehdoostirani, M., Genga, L., Lu, X., Verhoeven, R., van Laarhoven, H., Dijkman, R.: Interactive multi-interest process pattern discovery. In: International Conference on Business Process Management, pp. 303–319. Springer, 2023
20. Vickers, A.J.: Prediction models in cancer care. CA Cancer J. Clin. **61**(5), 315–326 (2011)

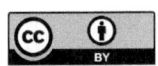

Case Study: Insights on Prostate Cancer Treatment Pathways Using Process Discovery

Jana Vormann[1]([✉]), Jonas Blatt[2], Flavio Horbach[1], Nils Herm-Stapelberg[3], Lukas Mittnacht[3], Patrick Delfmann[2], Tobias Walter[1], and Sven Pagel[1]

[1] Mainz University of Applied Sciences, Mainz, Germany
{jana.vormann,flavio.horbach,tobias.walter,sven.pagel}@hs-mainz.de
[2] University of Koblenz, Koblenz, Germany
{jonasblatt,delfmann}@uni-koblenz.de
[3] IDG Institute for Digital Health Data Rhineland-Palatinate, Mainz, Germany
{nils.herm-stapelberg,lukas.mittnacht}@idg-rlp.de

Abstract. In this *case study*, records about *prostate cancer* patients, provided by the Cancer Registry of Rhineland-Palatinate, Germany, are analyzed. The dataset is comparatively large and cases are rather complete, as they contain events gathered not only from one institution (e.g., a single hospital), but from multiple institutions along the end-to-end patient journey. The analysis, which aims at getting insights on prostate cancer treatment pathways and contributing to state-of-the-art research in the *Process Mining for Healthcare* (PM4H) field, is powered by methods and techniques from the *process mining* domain. Therefore, dealing with a process mining project, the PM^2 method was followed with the recommended phases in collaboration with the Cancer Registry of Rhineland-Palatinate, Germany. The initial analysis of $\sim$*12k cases* ($\sim$*90k events*) *recorded during 2018–2022* and considering only a small number of potential available data attributes already led to barely comprehensible spaghetti models, emphasizing the need for different views of granularity and complexity. This case study also provides results on the regular treatment pathways (such as surgery, or therapies).

Keywords: Prostate Cancer · Treatment Pathways · Process Discovery · PM4H

1 Introduction

Process mining is a continuously emerging research area that gains insights from event logs, applying "backward-looking" process discovery, conformance checking and enhancement, or "forward-looking" predictions of, for instance, possible next activities [19]. *Process Mining for Healthcare* (PM4H) is characterized by a high variability, complexity, multidisciplinarity and knowledge-intensive nature of its processes as well as a strong focus on privacy and security [5]. Though researchers are facing multiple challenges when applying process mining to healthcare processes [14], PM4H is considered a highly researched and promising domain [6].

A. Delgado and T. Slaats (Eds.): ICPM 2024 Workshops, LNBIP 533, pp. 486–499, 2025.
https://doi.org/10.1007/978-3-031-82225-4_36

With cancer being the second-leading cause of death by 9.6 million in 2020 world-wide[1] and a predicted increase of cancerous diseases to over 35 million new cases globally per year by 2050[2], oncology represents a primary research field in the PM4H domain [4]. At the same time, prostate cancer remains underrepresented in process mining research as until now it is covered only by few case studies [2,16]. Against this background, the present case study intends to contribute to the above mentioned domain while coming across several PM4H challenges outlined by Munoz-Gama et al. [14]. For this purpose, the process mining project draws on a new real-life data set of prostate cancer patients provided by the Cancer Registry of Rhineland-Palatinate (CRRLP), Germany.[3] Contrary to previous research, which considers merely single institutions and therefore does not allow to discover the end-to-end patient journey [5,13,14], this data set covers the multidisciplinary nature of cancer treatment processes by containing health records of several institutions such as the general practitioner, the pathologist, the hospital or a tumor conference. Thus, based on this data and the composed research questions (see Sect. 3.1), the resulting process models mined in this case study further aim to visualize patient's pathways and treatments.

The remainder of this paper is structured as follows. Section 2 introduces the PM^2 method applied for this process mining project. Section 3 presents the research results with a short description of each executed phase of the process mining project. Section 4 presents an overview of state-of-the-art research on PM4H and the oncology domain. Finally, Sect. 5 summarizes major contributions of this case study and relates to the aforementioned PM4H challenges.

2 Methodology

In order to conduct a process mining research project with the cancer records provided by CRRLP, we adapted the PM^2 method by van Eck et al. [21].

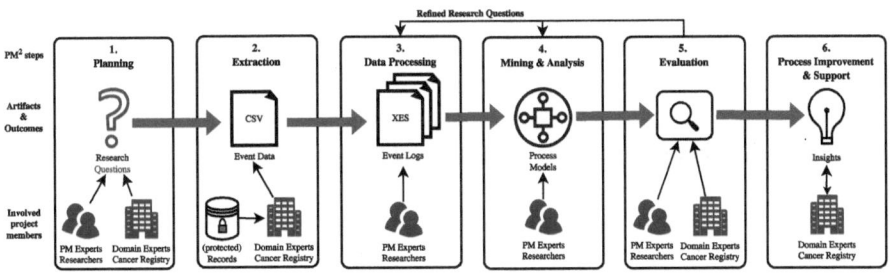

Fig. 1. Adapted PM^2 method based on van Eck et al. [21]

---

[1] https://www.who.int/health-topics/cancer (Accessed: 2024/08/13).

[2] https://www.who.int/news/item/01-02-2024-global-cancer-burden-growing--amidst-mounting-need-for-services (Accessed: 2024/08/13).

[3] https://www.krebsregister-rlp.de/ (Accessed: 2024/08/14).

Figure 1 visualizes the overview of the phases, the involved project team participants and the related artifacts. While the scientific research members contributed the methodological and technical process mining foundations, the domain experts from the CRRLP added the required oncological knowledge. In collaboration with the domain experts, multiple cycles of phases 3–5 were iteratively conducted by refining the research questions and refactoring the pre-processing and mining/analysis pipeline. Thereby, the involvement of the domain experts was strongly emphasized throughout the process mining project to prevent potential shortcomings associated with consulting domain experts at later stages [6,15]. Table 1 shortly presents inputs, outputs and activities of the PM^2 phases, which were adapted for the project. Actual outcomes are described in Sect. 3.

Table 1. Phases, Inputs, Outputs & Activities of the project, based on PM^2 [21]

#	Phase	Inputs ▷	Outputs ◁	Activities △
1	Planning	▷ Descriptions of cancer records	◁ Initial research questions	△ Set up project
				△ Determine the research question
				△ Composing project team
2	Extraction	▷ Research question	◁ Event data (multiple set of records)	△ Event data extraction
				△ Transferring process knowledge
3	Data Processing	▷ Research question ▷ Event data	◁ Event logs (sets of sequences of events)	△ Filter & repair events
				△ Creating different event logs (for different views based on the research question)
4	Mining & Analysis	▷ Research question ▷ Event logs (sets of sequences of events)	◁ Process models ◁ Statistical findings	△ Process discovery
				△ Further analysis (events per case, …)
5	Evaluation	▷ Research question ▷ Process models ▷ Statistical findings	◁ Improvement ideas ◁ Revised research question	△ Analysis of interesting & unusual results
				△ Revision of research questions
				△ Verification & Validation
				△ Map findings to project's goals, develop improvement ideas)
6	Process Improvement & Support	▷ Improvement ideas	◁ Ideas for future work	△ Elaborating future work

3   Case Study: Process Mining Project

In the years 2016–2024[4], the CRRLP collected 141,913 records (single reports submitted to the CRRLP), on a total of 22,337 distinct patients about prostate cancer cases, providing the opportunity to use this extensive data base to apply process mining techniques and to target the discovery of treatment pathways of prostate cancer patients.

---

[4] Key date: 2024/07/30.

3.1 Planning

The CRRLP in the Institute for Digital Health Data (IDG)[5] is responsible for recording every cancer case in the state of Rhineland-Palatinate in Germany. The data collection is based on the federal *Cancer Early Detection and Cancer Registries Act* (Krebsfrüherkennungs- und -registergesetz (KFRG))[6] as well as the state level *Landeskrebsregistergesetz* (LKRG)[7]. Every medical institution (e. g., hospitals, independent physicians), which is somehow related to cancer care, is obliged to send data on the diagnosis, treatment and follow-up of every cancer patient in Rhineland-Palatinate. Therefore, data is submitted via an online portal or automatically via standardized interfaces, conveying information on the patient, the attending medical institution as well as further details (e. g., the treatment or disease progression). Additionally, pathology reports, changes to personal information (name changes, relocation) as well as information on the death of a patient are available at the CRRLP. The data is sent, stored and provided in a standardized format (onkologischer Basisdatendatz[8]). Before the data is ready for scientific research analysis, it is processed and analyzed by the CRRLP. Thereby, challenges encountered during the collection and merging of cross-organizational, heterogeneous data are overcome through CRRLP's central and standardized data collection process, which is further reinforced by a binding legal foundation to be complied with by submitting institutions [8].

The initial planning phase of the project was thus driven by an intensive exchange between the researchers and domain experts to compose the joint project team, gain mutual understanding of the database, mediate required fundamental oncological knowledge and determine appropriate research questions. To ensure data minimization, relevant data items in the standardized data set were identified and denoted for extraction, while it was agreed upon omitting any personal patient data to abide by data protection laws. Though CRRLP processes data on different cancer types, prostate cancer was specifically selected for this project as no gender-specific differences apply while the high occurrence provides a large database of cancer cases [3]. Thereupon, the initial research question *"Q1: What insights can be gained from prostate cancer records using methods from the discipline of process mining?"* was formulated and iteratively refined to *"Q2: How do the typical treatment pathways look like for prostate cancer patients?"*.

3.2 Extraction

A high level of data security must be ensured when processing real patient data containing sensible personal information and health records. To achieve

---

[5] https://www.idg-rlp.de (Accessed: 2024/08/08).

[6] https://dip.bundestag.de/vorgang/gesetz-zur-weiterentwicklung-der-krebsfrüherkennung-und-zur-qualitätssicherung-durch-klinische/47081 (Accessed: 2024/08/13).

[7] https://www.landesrecht.rlp.de/bsrp/document/jlr-KrebsRegGRP2015rahmen (Accessed: 2024/08/13).

[8] https://www.basisdatensatz.de/(Accessed: 2024/08/05).

this, researchers are granted no direct access to the database storing the cancer records. Instead, the CRRLP extracts the records from the database into CSV files. Table 2 shows an overview of the CSVs with its fields and attributes, as well as the number of entries. The *event data* within these files is anonymized and contains only limited personal data (e. g., the birth month and year), which does not allow a direct link to a particular individual. Further measures to ensure anonymity include a shift of all date variables (per patient to preserve the order of events) by a random value between −183 and 183 days drawn from a uniform distribution and hashing of all identifier variables. Note, that the shifting adds limitations for the later analysis, for instance, it obstructs concept drift detection.

Table 2. Overview CSV files containing the reported data

Name	Fields & attributes	# of entries
Records (main)	patient id, tumor id, reporting date	141,913
Patient	patient id, birth & death date	22,337
Diagnosis	patient id, tumor id, icd code & diagnosis date	21,103
Histology	patient id, tumor id, histological analysis results & date	47,244
Pathology	patient id, tumor id, pathological analysis results & date	17,888
Tumor conference	patient id, tumor id, tumor conference type & date	11,687
Surgery	patient id, tumor id, surgery intention, type & date	15,702
Radiation therapy	patient id, tumor id, type, intention, end reason, start & end date	11,624
Systemic therapy	patient id, tumor id, type, intention, start & end date	9,707
Follow-up	patient id, tumor id, tumor status & date	58,840

To access and analyze the extracted data, the CRRLP provides the researchers a virtual machine, which can only be accessed in CRRLP's internal network. This encapsulated environment with no access to the internet and a restricted set of libraries and software minimizes potential data leaks, privacy breaches and ensures that no individual patient data leaves CRRLP's network. The virtual machine contains a Python environment, which is used for data processing and analysis with *PM4Py* [1] as a state-of-the-art process mining library.

3.3 Data Processing

The CRRLP provides records covering a period from 2016 to 2024, which is made available as separate CSV files, each containing information on a different type of health record (e. g., diagnostics, radiation treatments, surgeries, etc.). In order to transform the provided event data from the CSV files into event logs, we allocated (1) a *case ID* that assigns all related events to a case, (2) a *timestamp* to order events within a case and (3) an *activity* to name each event. All CSV files can be linked via the respective tumor ID, which is used as a case ID, as this attribute unites all records related to a unique cancer disease. In addition, the patient

ID for the respective patient can be used to link relevant patient data, such as the year of birth or, if applicable, the year of death. As each CSV file contains the date when a treatment or examination took place, we used this date as the event's timestamp. Some records, such as therapies, provide two timestamps, which define the start and end date of a therapy. In this case, records can be splitted into two events, for example into *Radiation Start* and *Radiation End*. Beyond that, activities can be further divided into different levels of granularity, based on additional attributes provided by the respective records. For example, the records on *systematic therapy* can be either considered as a single high-level activity or further be divided into several low-level activities (1:1 mapping) such as *hormone* or *chemo therapy, wait and see*, etc., based on an additional attribute specifying the systematic therapy type. Thus, based on the required granularity, the activity name can be defined on different levels of abstraction, challenging researchers to create a balanced ratio of increasing the log's informational value while restricting the model's complexity to a manageable level.

Various checks and evaluations are performed on the data before generating the event log. Though records are submitted in a standardized format, record completion is performed manually, leading to missing information or data inconsistencies. Since the data is filled in by doctors and administrators, implausible values sometimes occur in the data, e. g., the date of diagnosis. Traces that contain such values and do not meet the required quality are therefore removed. In doing so, we removed 2,368 traces of the initial database. The remaining 19,969 traces are further reduced to 12,210 traces as only complete traces within the years 2018 to 2022 are kept. This is due to the fact that records before 2018 are oftentimes not complete if the treatment pathway started before the recorded period. Furthermore, as cancer is considered a chronic disease, patients after 2022 are often still receiving multiple or have additional therapies planned leading to ongoing cases that cannot be taken into account for the analysis. Note, that the random shift of ±183 days is not considered.

Ultimately, we transform the event data from the CSV files into one *complete* event log that shows a high granularity for the data and is intended to provide an overall picture of the end-to-end patient pathway and a second *treatment* event log containing only treatment events such as radiation therapy, systematic therapy or surgery. The event logs are then exported as XES files that can be used for further processing in the mining and analysis phase.

3.4 Mining and Analysis

In the mining and analysis phase, process discovery was performed using the event logs processed in Sect. 3.3 and applying different process discovery algorithms in order to answer research question *Q1*. While the results of the inductive miner [11] were perceived too general, the heuristic miner [22] and directly-follows graph (DFG) [18] miner performed well when applying a limit to the number of shown variants. Unsurprisingly, considering all variants led to an indecipherable spaghetti model as depicted in Fig. 2, which does not allow useful interpretation. For further analysis, not only the *complete* event log but also the event log narrowed to *treatment* activities only was considered. Table 3 shows an overview in terms of metrics of the event logs to describe the database for the discovered process models. A limitation to top variants for #2, #3, #4 as well as additional activity filtering for #3 and #4 was chosen due to an exponentially sloping distribution of variants and to focus on main patient and treatment pathways.

Table 3. Overview of processed event logs

#	Type	Algorithm	Events	Cases	Top Variants	Cases %	Variants %	Activities
1	Complete	Heuristic	88,890	12,210	5,778	100%	100%	43
2	Complete	–	35,012	7,588	1,156	62.1%	20.0%	30
3	Treatments	DFG Frequency	18,282	9,134	50	93.79%	12.41%	5
4	Treatments	DFG Performance	18,282	9,134	50	93.79%	12.41%	5

#1: The Complete Event Log. The event log for the first analysis contains all defined activities, in total 43 distinct activities, such as the different examinations, treatments (including the start and the end of the respective activities), surgeries, or tumor conferences. Based on this event log, the first process model (Fig. 2 (#1)) was mined, considering all available events (88,890) and cases (12,210), while using the heuristic miner, to generate a heuristic map. Due to high number of variants (5,778), nearly every process instance is more or less different which, as stated above, results in a spaghetti model. This emphasizes the need to consider appropriate preprocessing to gain useful insights. It can be noted that this event log contains only a few variants with a higher frequency, however, those variants only contain a small number of events, which are usually related to diagnostic examinations.

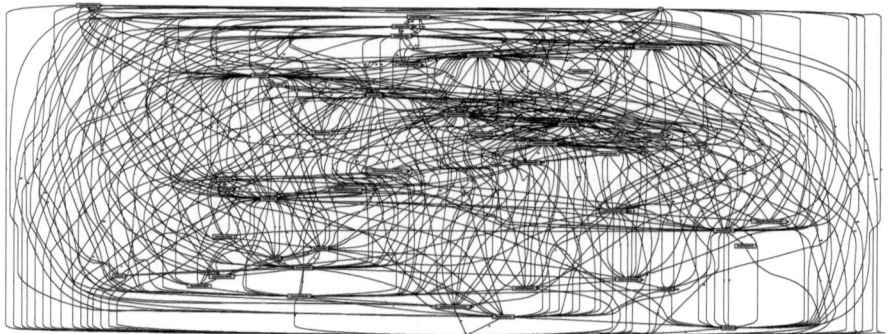

Fig. 2. Heuristic map mined from the complete event log with all variants (#1).

#2: The Main Variants. Based on these insights, this complete event log was filtered by the top 20% of the most occurring variants, retaining still 62.1% of all cases but constituting no Pareto distribution [17]. Within any arbitrary and still somewhat spaghetti-like model mined from this event log, it can be observed that the main patient pathways are related to examinations (*Diagnosis, Histological examination* and *Pathological examinations*). However, as determined in the evaluation with domain experts, many prostate cancer patients receive *Active Surveillance* as treatment, which is in reality oftentimes not reported. As a result, variants related to treatments are rather underrepresented in this process model featuring only a relatively small number of variants including radiation, chemo or hormone therapy. Moreover, further extracted from the validation with the domain experts, the activity of *Histological examination* is often part of the *Diagnosis* and the *Pathological examination*, and may not be used as a standalone activity.

Thus, based on evaluations (Sect. 3.5) of these initial results, research question *Q2* is introduced to realign the analysis towards records related to patient treatments by applying activity filtering.

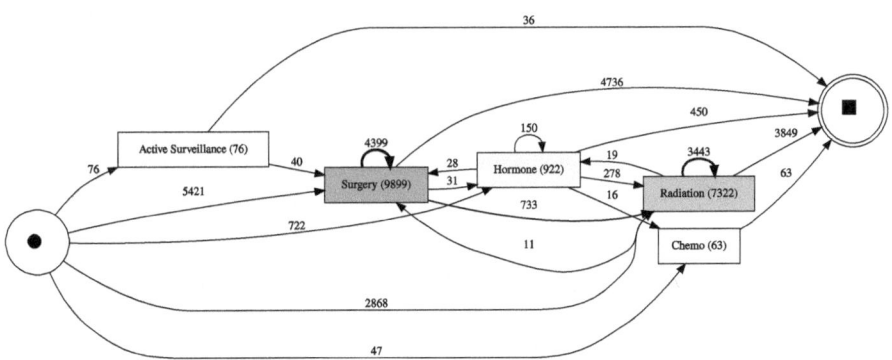

Fig. 3. Frequency DFG mined from the treatment event log filtered by the top 50 variants. (**#3**).

#3: Focus on the Frequency of Treatments. In Fig. 3 (#3), a DFG was mined based on the treatment events, namely, surgeries, radiations, and different types of systematic therapies (such as hormone, chemo or active surveillance). Thus, in a first step, we filtered for those treatment activities. Note, that in the presented model only the top 50 variants are considered to focus on the main treatment pathways. In doing so, 93.79% of the (treatment) cases are accounted for. Furthermore, only the start timestamp of the therapy records was considered, while end timestamps were discarded, being only interested in the 'directly follows'-relations of the treatments themselves. The resulting process model shows that the main treatment is surgery which may be followed by a combination with

a radiation therapy. Likewise active surveillance can be observed as a therapy, where sometimes a surgery follows if the tumor does change or progress over time. Moreover, other combinations of treatments are also possible, for instance, a treatment can start with a hormone therapy in combination with radiation. In most cases, frequent treatment pathways represent a sequential combination of different treatments rather than a single one.

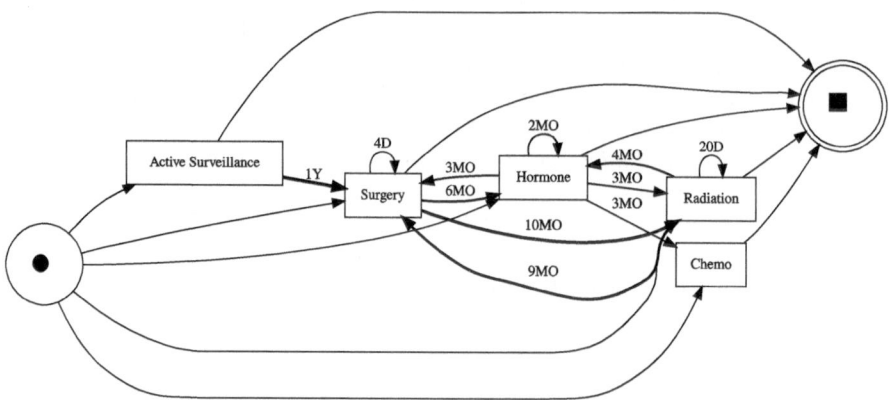

Fig. 4. Performance DFG mined from the treatment event log filtered by the top 50 variants. (**#4**).

#4: Focus on the Performance of Treatments. Lastly, Fig. 4 (#4) shows the performance DFG with the mean duration between the events. This model provides further insights on the temporal distances of prostate cancer treatments. For instance, the radiation therapy is started 10 months after the surgery on average though those average values have a high variability. Moreover, the decision, if a surgery is conducted or not, is usually taken after one year of active surveillance, e. g., if tumor progression is detected.

3.5   Evaluation

To answer research question *Q1* and further refine it to research question *Q2*, the discovered process models were evaluated in iterative cycles both from a process and oncological perspective with support of the domain experts from CRRLP. Therefore, after the first evaluation cycle, e. g., the end date of treatment activities was no longer considered as the domain experts place their emphasis rather on the fact that a patient received a treatment than on treatment duration. At the same time this leads to the limitation that insights on intervals between the end of one treatment and the start of the next treatment is lost, but might be taken up again in future research. Moreover, domain experts confirmed the observation that within the complete event log treatment activities are underrepresented in the main variants. Oftentimes, this is due to a slow progression of tumor and the advanced age of many patients and should be properly reported as treatment activities (e. g., *active surveillance*). In reality, it must be assumed that those activities are not reported in all cases thereby compromising the completeness of the data base. Lastly, the discovered models provide not only insights on treatment patterns but also on the temporal distance of treatments. Though, those temporal insights must be treated with caution as variance indicators are not considered.

3.6   Process Improvement and Support

Insights gained in Sect. 3.4 were not primarily used for process improvement and support, though researchers and domain experts should jointly seek for approaches to substitute missing data on active surveillance treatments and subsume activities that are generally performed together to increase model quality and allow mining for complete treatment patterns. Further improvement potential may be leveraged through the cross-institutional character of the database which allows for process mining from an organizational, institution-based perspective which was previously not possible when focusing on a single institution.

   Moreover, gained insights enabled researchers and domain experts to determine several future research goals. The spaghetti-model discovered in Sect. 3.4 shows the unstructured nature of the process at hand. Therefore, one major future research goal is the development of suitable *(1) preprocessing and abstraction methods* to gain insights beyond filtering on top variants (e. g., considering clustering techniques). Further analysis approaches may focus on *(2) treatment pathways in the course of time*, analyzing for example if there is a shift from surgery-oriented towards therapy-oriented treatments or vice versa. Enriching the event log by further low-level activities regarding surgery type, the *(3) role of new technologies in treatment pathways*, such as minimal invasive surgery or use of surgery robots, could be analyzed. Likewise, attributes on disease recovery, progression or death of a patient can be included and could be used combined with the identification of *(4) frequent treatment patterns* to enable feature-based *(5) treatment predictions* and *(6) recommendations* of most promising treatment pathways. As this case study solely focuses on prostate cancer, applying such treatment predictions and recommendations to other cancer types recorded by CRRLP, especially those with higher mortality rates, constitutes another future-oriented and high impact research direction. Drawing on this case study's data processing and process discovery techniques, a comparison of treatment pathways across different cancer types, e. g., through clustering, is enabled as well. Ultimately, one could consider further attributes such as the patient's PSA-value to verify the findings of Valero-Ramon et al. [16] with a new data set.

4   Related Work

Applying process mining techniques to healthcare processes is gaining not only interest but also relevance, which is evidenced by several novel literature reviews within the PM4H domain [4–6,8,13,14]. Concurrently, researchers are confronted with several challenges and characteristics of PM4H which are outlined by Munoz-Gama et al. [14] and apply to a variety of healthcare use cases such as previous research focusing on specific diseases, e. g., chronic diseases or cancer [4,7], different flow perspectives, e. g., patient, clinical or administrative pathways [2,12,23] or the integration of domain experts into the research process [15]. With regard to applied process mining techniques Dallagassa et al. [5] found that the majority of studies within PM4H focuses on process discovery, particularly on the control-flow perspective by discovering clinical pathways [4,6,8]. Furthermore, studies often consider a particular health institution, mainly single hospitals. At the same time, access to real-life data remains a major challenge within the PM4H domain, oftentimes due to the processing of sensitive personal data [14]. Distributed and privacy-preserving process mining remains rather a future research direction for the process mining domain [9]. Therefore, one of the most widely used data sets is the BPI Challenge 2011 [20] providing data from a dutch hospital on the treatment of gynaecological cancer [7]. As a result, oncology represents a primary research field in PM4H, where due to the above mentioned data set gynaecological cancer is the most studied type of cancer [4,7,10]. Although prostate cancer is the 4th most common type of cancer overall and the most common in men with more than 1.5 million new cases and nearly 400,000 deaths worldwide in 2022 [3], a very limited number of case studies deals with prostate cancer [7,10]. While Bettencourt-Silva et al. [2] and the study of Valero-Ramon et al. [16] focus on prostate cancer treatment, they only draw on data from a single hospital and lack to cover the whole patient journey.

To sum up, PM4H can be described as a highly active research field bearing not only societal value but research potential beyond process discovery [5,13].

5   Conclusion

This case study demonstrates the application of process mining to prostate cancer records provided by CRRLP. With regard to research question *Q1*, gained insights are outlined by the visualization of treatment pathways, the sequence as well as intervals between treatments in Sect. 3.4 while process improvement potentials and directions for future research are depicted in Sect. 3.6. As for research question *Q2*, typical treatment pathways for prostate cancer patients are often characterized by a sequential combination of treatments, where for example a surgery is often followed by therapy-oriented treatments. Furthermore, we outlined six future research goals in the PM4H domain.

Throughout the realization of the process mining project, several of the PM4H challenges identified by Munoz-Gama et al. [14] are addressed. The case study *deals with reality (C4)* as the data provided by CRRLP draws on a new real-life data set allowing for future research with potentially reasonable societal impact. Furthermore, though a standardized data set was used, the reporting process remains largely manual wherefore the researchers had to *pay attention to data quality (C6)* that was assessed during the data processing phase. The integration of researchers into CRRLP's organization represents a rather unique and new form of collaboration reducing the risk of data breaches while providing sufficient data access for research, thereby *taking care of privacy and security (C7)*. At last, *looking at the process through the patient's eyes (C8)* is ensured as the data is collected from multiple institutions involved in patient and treatment pathways. Dealing with the above mentioned challenges illustrates the case study's data set is highly promising to contribute to and surpass contemporary research efforts by utilizing a new real-life data set that reflects the multi-disciplinary character of cancer treatment and is ultimately able to visualize the end-to-end patient journey.

Acknowledgments. This study was funded by the Ministry of Science and Health, Rhineland-Palatinate, Germany (funding policy *Research Colleges Rhineland-Palatinate*) and supported by the Institute for Digital Health Data. The data set used in this study can be requested from IDG upon submission of a qualified research proposal.

References

1. Berti, A., Van Zelst, S., Schuster, D.: PM4Py: a process mining library for Python. Software Impacts **17**, 100556 (2023). https://doi.org/10.1016/j.simpa.2023.100556
2. Bettencourt-Silva, J.H., Clark, J., Cooper, C.S., Mills, R., Rayward-Smith, V.J., De La Iglesia, B.: Building data-driven pathways from routinely collected hospital data: a case study on prostate cancer. JMIR Med. Inform. **3**(3), e26 (2015). https://doi.org/10.2196/medinform.4221
3. Bray, F., et al.: Global cancer statistics 2022: GLOBOCAN estimates of incidence and mortality worldwide for 36 cancers in 185 countries. CA Cancer J. Clin. **74**(3), 229–263 (2024). https://doi.org/10.3322/caac.21834
4. Chen, K., Abtahi, F., Carrero, J.J., Fernandez-Llatas, C., Seoane, F.: Process mining and data mining applications in the domain of chronic diseases: a systematic review. Artif. Intell. Med. **144**, 102645 (2023). https://doi.org/10.1016/j.artmed.2023.102645
5. Dallagassa, M.R., Dos Santos Garcia, C., Scalabrin, E.E., Ioshii, S.O., Carvalho, D.R.: Opportunities and challenges for applying process mining in healthcare: a systematic mapping study. J. Ambient Intell. Humaniz. Comput. **13**(1), 165–182 (2022). https://doi.org/10.1007/s12652-021-02894-7
6. De Roock, E., Martin, N.: Process mining in healthcare - an updated perspective on the state of the art. J. Biomed. Inform. **127**, 103995 (2022). https://doi.org/10.1016/j.jbi.2022.103995
7. Grüger, J., Bergmann, R., Kazik, Y., Kuhn, M.: Process mining for case acquisition in oncology: a systematic literature review. In: Proceedings of the Conference Lernen, Wissen, Daten, Analysen, Online, 9–11 September 2020. CEUR Workshop Proceedings, vol. 2738, pp. 162–173. CEUR-WS.org (2020)
8. Guzzo, A., Rullo, A., Vocaturo, E.: Process mining applications in the healthcare domain: a comprehensive review. WIREs Data Min. Knowl. Discov. **12**(2), e1442 (2022). https://doi.org/10.1002/widm.1442
9. Khan, A., Ghose, A., Dam, H.: Cross-silo process mining with federated learning. In: International Conference on Service-Oriented Computing, pp. 612–626 (2021). https://doi.org/10.1007/978-3-030-91431-8_38

10. Kurniati, A.P., Johnson, O., Hogg, D., Hall, G.: Process mining in oncology: a literature review. In: 2016 6th International Conference on Information Communication and Management (ICICM), pp. 291–297. Hatfield, United Kingdom (2016). https://doi.org/10.1109/INFOCOMAN.2016.7784260

11. Leemans, S.J.J., Fahland, D., van der Aalst, W.M.P.: Discovering block-structured process models from event logs - a constructive approach. In: Application and Theory of Petri Nets and Concurrency, pp. 311–329 (2013). https://doi.org/10.1007/978-3-642-38697-8_17

12. Mans, R.S., Van Der Aalst, W.M.P., Vanwersch, R.J.B.: Process Mining in Healthcare: Evaluating and Exploiting Operational Healthcare Processes. SpringerBriefs in Business Process Management, Springer, Cham (2015). https://doi.org/10.1007/978-3-319-16071-9

13. Martin, N., Wittig, N., Munoz-Gama, J.: Using Process Mining in Healthcare. In: Process Mining Handbook, LNBIP, vol. 448, pp. 416–444. Springer, Cham (2022). https://doi.org/10.1007/978-3-031-08848-3_14

14. Munoz-Gama, J., et al.: Process mining for healthcare: characteristics and challenges. J. Biomed. Inform. **127**, 103994 (2022). https://doi.org/10.1016/j.jbi.2022.103994

15. Schuster, D., Benevento, E., Aloini, D., Van Der Aalst, W.M.P.: Analyzing healthcare processes with incremental process discovery: practical insights from a real-world application. J. Healthc. Inform. Res. (2024). https://doi.org/10.1007/s41666-024-00165-6

16. Valero-Ramon, Z., Fernandez-Llatas, C., Collantes, G., Valdivieso, B., Traver, V.: Understanding prostate cancer care process using process mining: a case study. In: Explainable Artificial Intelligence and Process Mining Applications for Healthcare, vol. 2020, pp. 118–130. Springer Nature Switzerland, Cham (2024). https://doi.org/10.1007/978-3-031-54303-6_12

17. van der Aalst., W.M.P.: On the pareto principle in process mining, task mining, and robotic process automation. In: Proceedings of the 9th International Conference on Data Science, Technology and Applications - DATA, pp. 5–12. INSTICC, SciTePress (2020). https://doi.org/10.5220/0009979200050012

18. van der Aalst, W.M.P.: Foundations of Process Discovery. In: Process Mining Handbook, LNBIP, vol. 448, pp. 37–75. Springer, Cham (2022). https://doi.org/10.1007/978-3-031-08848-3

19. van der Aalst, W.M.P.: Process Mining: A 360 Degree Overview. In: Process Mining Handbook, LNBIP, vol. 448, pp. 3–34. Springer, Cham (2022). https://doi.org/10.1007/978-3-031-08848-3

20. van Dongen, B.: Real-life event logs - Hospital log (2011). https://doi.org/10.4121/UUID:D9769F3D-0AB0-4FB8-803B-0D1120FFCF54

21. Van Eck, M.L., Lu, X., Leemans, S.J.J., Van Der Aalst, W.M.P.: PM^2: a process mining project methodology. In: Advanced Information Systems Engineering, pp. 297–313 (2015). https://doi.org/10.1007/978-3-319-19069-3_19

22. Weijters, A., Van Der Aalst, W., De Medeiros, A.A.: Process mining with the heuristics miner-algorithm. Technische Universiteit Eindhoven, Technical report (2006). WP **166**(July 2017), 1–34

23. Yang, W., Su, Q.: Process mining for clinical pathway: literature review and future directions. In: 11th International Conference on Service Systems and Service Management (ICSSSM), pp. 1–5. Beijing (2014). https://doi.org/10.1109/ICSSSM.2014.6943412

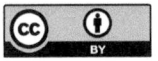

1st International Workshop on Empirical Research in Process Mining (ERPM 2024)

Preface

1st Workshop on Empirical Research in Process Mining (ERPM 2024)

Process mining, as an interdisciplinary field, has transformed various domains by enabling the comprehensive analysis and optimization of business processes. While significant advances have been made in developing algorithms for automated process discovery and quantitative process analysis, there is still a pressing need to understand the human and organizational aspects of these developments. This calls for empirical research that investigates the practical application, user interactions, and organizational impacts of process mining techniques and tools.

The *1st Workshop on Empirical Research in Process Mining* (ERPM 2024) addressed a growing demand for robust empirical studies within the field. The primary goal of ERPM was to create a high-quality forum for researchers and practitioners to share their experiences, methodologies, and findings related to empirical aspects of process mining. ERPM aimed to promote rigorous research, facilitate knowledge exchange, and encourage collaborations that advance effective and user-friendly process mining methods. The workshop was created to cover a wide range of topics, including but not limited to empirical studies on user experiences with process mining tools, case studies of the impact of process mining on organizations, human-centric methodologies for process mining, and organizational studies exploring the cultural and structural effects of process mining implementations.

The call for papers solicited two types of contributions: regular papers and "lessons learned" contributions. Regular papers were expected to make a research contribution to one of the topics listed above. They were evaluated based on their significance, originality, use of empirical methods, and potential to generate relevant discussion. "Lessons Learned" contributions were extended abstract submissions that allowed the authors to discuss ongoing work and share their experiences, challenges, and insights gained from applying empirical methods in process mining. These were not included in the proceedings.

The first edition of ERPM received 14 submissions, of which there were thirteen regular papers and one lessons-learned contribution. After thorough reviewing by the program committee members, seven regular submissions were accepted for full-paper presentation. Additionally, after careful deliberation by the workshop chairs, one additional paper was invitedfor presentation as a lessons-learned contribution alongside the formal lessons-learned submission. Below, we briefly describe the regular papers included in these proceedings.

The paper by Trottier et al. presents a case study on using process mining to enhance digital service delivery within a Canadian government department, focusing on personnel security screening. By applying process mining techniques pre- and post-intervention, the authors identified bottlenecks, such as frequent exceptional scenarios and resource allocation issues, and implemented interventions that reduced overall process time. The study emphasizes the potential of process mining as part of a digital transformation strategy to optimize service efficiency.

The paper by Shalev et al. presents a user study exploring the predictive power of facial expressions for determining process mining task performance. Using machine learning models trained on facial expression data collected via webcams, the authors demonstrated that task success can be accurately predicted early in the process. This research lays the groundwork for developing real-time support systems to assist analysts facing cognitive difficulties during process mining tasks.

The paper by Häge and Rehse proposes a taxonomy for visualizations in conformance checking, categorizing six dimensions that impact how conformance information is displayed and perceived. By systematically analyzing both academic and commercial tools, the authors aim to provide a framework that can support empirical research on visualization preferences and facilitate the improvement of process mining visual analytics.

The paper by Rothhagen et al. presents an exploratory study to assess the potential and challenges of using process mining on the manufacturing shop floor. Through interviews and a systematic literature review, the authors identify five key dimensions, including data quality and organizational factors, that influence the effectiveness of process mining in manufacturing. The study outlines future research opportunities for integrating human and technical considerations into process mining applications.

The paper by Mendling et al. integrates the Theory of Effective Use and empirical process mining research, focusing on how tool features support decision-making by process analysts. The paper addresses gaps in existing research by emphasizing the importance of theoretical cohesion and exploring how cognitive strategies of analysts can be better supported to enhance organizational performance.

The paper by Meneghello et al. applies a Hybrid Simulation Model (HSM) to a real-life purchase-to-pay process in collaboration with Ernst & Young. By combining discrete event simulation with predictive modeling, the authors demonstrate the benefits of HSM for business process analysis, identifying critical points and evaluating what-if scenarios to optimize process performance. The case study highlights HSM's potential to provide more accurate and actionable insights compared to traditional simulation methods.

Finally, the paper by Van Suetendael et al. presents an ethogram cataloging 26 distinct behaviors exhibited by analysts during exploratory process mining. Drawing from published case studies and human ethology concepts, the authors present a systematic tool to understand and record analyst behaviors. The ethogram aims to improve guidance and support for process mining analysts by providing a structured vocabulary and insights into their cognitive processes.

In addition to research contributions, the workshop featured two engaging "Lessons Learned" presentations. The first one, by Nusch et al., focused on insights from a qualitative study of process mining implementation in the German utilities sector. The presentation emphasized the importance of selecting a manageable pilot process, maintaining data quality, and addressing employee concerns transparently. The second presentation, by Kretzschmann et al., introduced an object-centric data model to optimize inventory management. Applied in a real-world case study with a pet retailer, this approach identified root causes of inefficiencies, such as overstock situations driven by supplier contract terms, and proposed adjustments to improve demand forecasting and procurement processes.

The workshop concluded with a panel discussion featuring Mieke Jans (Hasselt University), Irina Tentina (Eindhoven University of Technology), Lotte Vugs (Konekti), and Jan Mendling (Humboldt Universität zu Berlin), moderated by Kateryna Kubrak. The discussion focused on promoting empirical research within the process mining community. The panelists shared strategies to encourage more rigorous and impactful empirical studies. This was followed by an open and engaging discussion involving all workshop participants on this central theme.

We would like to thank all the members of the ERPM 2024 Program Committee for their efforts in reviewing the papers. Our sincere thanks go to all the authors and the workshop participants, who contributed with their work and the lively discussions on the workshop day. A special note of gratitude goes also to the organizing committee of ICPM 2024 for this successful edition of the conference.

November 2024

Djordje Djurica
Kateryna Kubrak
Francesca Zerbato
Amine Abbad Andaloussi

Organization

Workshop Chairs

Djordje Djurica	Vienna University of Economics and Business, Austria
Kateryna Kubrak	University of Tartu, Estonia
Francesca Zerbato	Eindhoven University of Technology, The Netherlands
Amine Abbad Andaloussi	University of St. Gallen, Switzerland

Program Committee

Han van der Aa	University of Vienna, Austria
Anti Alman	University of Tartu, Estonia
Iris Beerepoot	Utrecht University, The Netherlands
Adela Del Rio Ortega	University of Seville, Spain
Thomas Grisold	University of St. Gallen, Switzerland
Mieke Jans	University of Hasselt, Belgium
Hugo A. Lopez	Technical University of Denmark, Denmark
Jan Mendling	Humboldt Universität zu Berlin, Germany
Alexander Nolte	Eindhoven University of Technology, The Netherlands
Jana Rehse	University of Mannheim, Germany
Hajo Reijers	Utrecht University, The Netherlands
Stefanie Rinderle-Ma	Technical University of Munich, Germany
Clemens Schreiber	KIT, Germany
Pnina Soffer	University of Haifa, Israel
Bastian Wurm	University of Munich, Germany
Moe T. Wynn	Queensland University of Technology, Australia
Lisa Zimmermann	University of St. Gallen, Switzerland

A Taxonomy for Conformance Checking Visualizations

Marie-Christin Häge[✉]📵 and Jana-Rebecca Rehse📵

University of Mannheim, Mannheim, Germany
`{haege,rehse}@uni-mannheim.de`

Abstract. Conformance checking is a sub-discipline of process mining, which compares process execution data with predefined process models to identify deviations between them. Although recognized as the most important feature of process mining tools, conformance checking is currently not widely applied in practice. One reason for this lack of adoption is the absence of process-mining-specific visualizations, which can effectively communicate conformance checking results to practitioners. Although researchers have identified the need for such visualizations, they have left their development to the tool providers, such that available visualizations are highly different and difficult to compare. This inhibits the opportunities to conduct empirical research on conformance checking visualizations, which would be crucial to understanding user preferences. To address this issue and establish a foundation for future empirical research, this paper provides an overview of the existing breadth of characteristics of conformance checking visualizations in the form of a taxonomy. This taxonomy consists of six dimensions, which highlight in a structured manner what information is displayed in conformance checking visualizations and how this is visualized in different academic and commercial tools. Our research enhances the comprehension of visual analytics in process mining, particularly for conformance checking, and highlights promising avenues for future empirical research.

Keywords: Conformance Checking · Process Mining · Visual Analytics · Taxonomy

1 Introduction

Conformance checking, one of the sub-disciplines of process mining, compares process execution data with a predefined to-be process model. By analyzing intended and observed process behavior, it identifies deviations between them [1]. This can help organizations to detect violations of internal or external regulations or find process improvements [6]. These capabilities make conformance checking highly relevant in practice. This was underlined by a recent study, which found that practitioners see conformance checking as the most important feature of process mining tools and expect it to grow the fastest in the coming years [1,7].

© The Author(s) 2025
A. Delgado and T. Slaats (Eds.): ICPM 2024 Workshops, LNBIP 533, pp. 507–519, 2025.
https://doi.org/10.1007/978-3-031-82225-4_37

Despite this established relevance, conformance checking often fails to deliver the desired outcome [6] and is currently not widely applied in practice [17, p. 39]. This discrepancy in the adoption is caused by different technical and organizational aspects [5]. One of these aspects is the absence of suitable visualizations, which could help to effectively communicate conformance checking results to the user [9]. This would significantly support the analysis process by allowing users, experts and non-experts, to acquire new insights more quickly, draw conclusions more effectively, and make more knowledgeable decisions [11].

Researchers have acknowledged the need for such visualizations [9,12,16]. However, so far, their development has mostly been left to the process mining tool providers, who have developed their own visualizations, based on the context and goals of the respective tools. Consequently, the visualizations differ highly in the displayed data and their representation [16]. These differences make it difficult to compare the visualizations and generate a structured understanding. However, this is crucial to gain insights into the users, their preferences, and the effects the different visualizations have on them [8,9,16]. Such insights would enable significant improvement potential for conformance checking visualizations and, consequently, for process mining and its adoption overall.

To address these issues, this paper provides a detailed overview of the existing breadth of characteristics of conformance checking visualizations in the form of a taxonomy, i.e., a multi-dimensional classification of a set of entities that allows to better relate and structure them. We created this taxonomy through a comparative analysis of academic and commercial process mining tools that include conformance checking visualizations. It consists of six dimensions and various characteristics, which present, in a structured manner, the information that is currently depicted in conformance checking visualizations. In addition, it highlights how this information is visualized across the different tools.

In the following, the necessary background and related work are presented in Sect. 2. Section 3 outlines the method used to develop the taxonomy, which itself is introduced in Sect. 4. We discuss the results, its limitations, and future implications and conclude in Sect. 5.

2   Related Work

In this paper, we investigate visualizations in process mining and thereby connect process mining research with the field of visual analytics. In this section, we provide the relevant background information on the two research fields and elaborate on the work connecting visual analytics and process mining.

Business Process Models. Organizations typically capture business processes as business process models, which support them in communicating, analyzing, documenting, redesigning, improving, monitoring or implementing processes [4]. For this purpose, different process model notations can be used. The most common ones are DFGs (Directly-Follow-Graph), Petri Nets, and BPMNs (Business Process Model and Notation) [21]. Each notation has a different focus, leading to differences in their depiction. In Fig. 1, these process model notations are used to visualize the same process. All models show the allowed process executions for different cases. Each case is an individual occurrence of the process, which is shown in the model through a path going from start to end. Each path contains activities that can or must be completed [24]. To visualize single cases, a suitable alternative notation are chevron diagrams, which depict the sequence of executed activities [17].

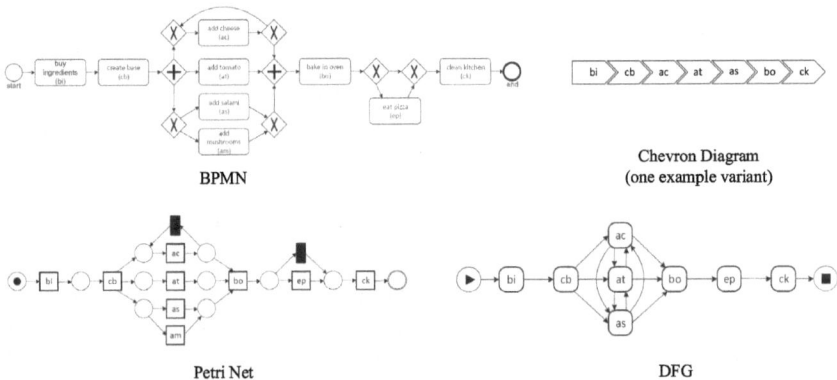

Fig. 1. Example Process depicted in All Four Process Model Notations [22, p. 10 ff.]

Although process models provide many advantages to organizations, they have certain limitations. Such challenges are the reduction of the process complexity in the models, the discrepancy between reality and the process model, the maintenance, and the restrictions of the different notations [4,21,24].

Process Mining. In order to gain data-driven insights into their processes, organizations can leverage process mining, a family of techniques aimed to analyze event data available from different information systems. The most common sub-disciplines are process discovery, conformance checking, and process enhancement [22]. They all can consider different process perspectives. The most common perspective is the control-flow, which represents the ordering of activities. Other perspectives may refer to time, data, or resources [22]. To conduct process mining, we require an event log, which is a collection of events. A single event contains at least a case identifier, an activity name, and a timestamp or another ordering mechanism. Events can also include additional attributes, such as resources or costs. A single trace is made of a sequence of events that describe a process execution. If a timestamp is available, for each trace the throughput time can be measured, which is the time from start to end. Multiple traces can follow the same activities, which can be then summarized as a variant. In the end, the results are often visualized as process models [21].

Conformance Checking. In this paper, we focus on the process mining sub-discipline of conformance checking, which considers event logs and existing process models. It aims to compare these two inputs and analyze how accurately they align. The process model usually represents the intended process, whereas the event log contains the real-world process execution. Through this comparison, deviations between them can be detected [1], which can help organizations to identify violations of internal or external regulations or find novel opportunities for process improvement [6]. There are three main conformance checking techniques: *token replay*, *rule checking*, and *alignments*. The latter two are the current state-of-the-art and can also be applied to other perspectives than the control-flow [1]. While rule checking techniques analyse if behavioural rules defined in a model are violated by certain traces in the log, alignment-based techniques differentiate between log, model, and synchronous moves. They compare a trace of an event log directly with a process execution in the model and identify possible alignments. The goal is an optimal alignment where the costs of log and model moves are kept to a minimum. To quantify the degree of conformance between a log and a model, a fitness measure is typically used, which indicates how well the model covers the recorded behavior in the event log [1].

Visual Analytics. The second relevant research area for this paper, visual analytics, can be defined as the "science of analytical reasoning facilitated by interactive visual interfaces" [20]. It aims to improve human understanding, reasoning, and decision-making with regard to provided data sets. Compared to other fields, such as information visualization, visual analytics emphasizes the importance of including the user throughout the analysis process. The goal is to achieve an intuitive and useful interpretation of the data rather than a cognitive or information overload when presenting only results [2,11]. Moreover, visual analytics always considers the task that the user wants to perform by means of the visualization, which ensures that the visualization provides the desired insights [11,13]. Through interactive capabilities, the user can see dynamics within the data, gain hidden insights, and adjust the complexity to their needs. As a consequence, they can fulfill tasks more effectively and efficiently [9,13].

To systematically evaluate visualizations, Munzner [13] defines an analysis framework with three questions: 'Why', 'What', and 'How' (Fig. 2). 'Why' analyzes the reasons for using the visualization (tool) and identifies the performed task. 'What' specifies the kind of data the users see in the visualization. 'How' describes the design of the visualization and its possible interaction options [13]. By answering these questions, a fitting visualization for a given situation can be identified.

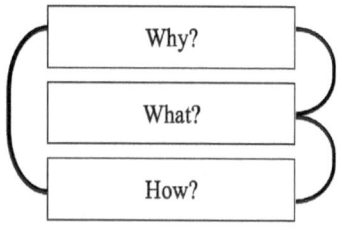

Fig. 2. Analysis Framework [13, p. 17]

Visual Analytics in Process Mining. Van der Aalst et al. [23] emphasized the relevance and opportunities of combining process mining and visual analytics already in 2011. Since then, there have been a few research initiatives in this direction. Researchers have assessed, developed, or categorized visualizations in process mining and established frameworks that consider also visual analytics [10,12,16,18]. Klinkmüller et al. [12] identified the visualizations used for different process mining domain problems, as mentioned in analysis reports. These domain problems are kept very general and represent the different process mining techniques. Rehse et al. [16] applied the three-part analysis framework by Munzner [13] to identify conformance checking tasks that are addressed by the currently available visualizations in academic and commercial tools.

Both papers find that generic visualizations are used predominantly, instead of those specific to process mining. Furthermore, the same visualizations are often used for different tasks and different information [12,16]. These findings are a starting point for improving process mining through visual analytics, but many challenges and research gaps still need to be tackled. According to Gschwandtner [9], these challenges include, among others, the visualization of time-oriented data, the question of visualization evaluation, and the issue of scalability and aggregation. On the positive side, an interplay of both research fields could provide an improved understanding of the processes and an increased support of the user's analysis process [9].

3   Method

The objective of this paper is to provide a structured overview of existing conformance checking visualizations through a taxonomy as a foundation for future research. Such a taxonomy allows the organization of knowledge and the identification of relationships among the underlying concepts. Its aim is the multi-dimensional classification of a set of entities that allows to better relate and structure them. It consists of a set of dimensions, where each dimension contains multiple characteristics. To develop such a taxonomy, we followed the iterative development method by Nickerson et al. [14], which is based on the design science paradigm in the information systems field. This structured approach suggests to develop a taxonomy over multiple iterations, following either an empirical-to-conceptual or a conceptual-to-empirical approach. An iteration with a conceptual-to-empirical approach derives the information from theory and literature, whereas an empirical-to-conceptual iteration uses empirical data. Before these iterations begin, we set the meta-characteristic that defines the goal and purpose of the taxonomy and the ending conditions that define the criteria for ending the development process. Then, in each iteration, one of the approaches is followed and the collected data will be structured, common characteristics will be identified, and lastly, grouped into dimensions for a taxonomy. This process will be repeated until the ending conditions are fulfilled [14].

Meta-characteristic and Ending Conditions. In the first step, we defined the meta-characteristic. This purpose of our taxonomy was to *identify what data and visualizations of conformance checking results are currently used in the existing process mining tools.* As ending conditions, we adopted the five objective and five subjective conditions from Nickerson et al. [14]. The objective ending conditions included that (1) no new dimensions or characteristics were added in the last iteration, (2) no new dimensions or characteristics were merged or split in the last iteration, (3) every dimension is unique and not repeated, (4) every characteristic is unique and not repeated within its dimension, and (5) each dimension consists of collectively exhaustive characteristics. Nickerson et al. [14] also suggest the ending condition that each dimension should have mutually exclusive characteristics, meaning only one characteristic per dimension is applicable when categorizing an object within the taxonomy. We excluded this condition due to the nature of visualizations and the underlying principles, e.g., visual expressiveness, which suggests the use of multiple variables. This does not completely contradict the ending condition as each combination of the characteristics and dimensions will be mutually exclusive and, therefore, unique [15,19]. The subjective ending conditions are that the taxonomy needs to be concise, robust, comprehensive, extendible, and self-explanatory [14].

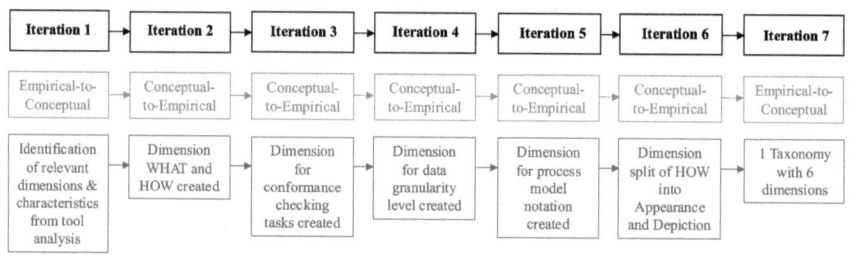

Fig. 3. Taxonomy Development Process

Iterations. We developed the taxonomy in seven iterations, outlined in Fig. 3. The identified dimensions and characteristics are described in Sect. 4. As preparation, we selected all tools supporting conformance checking from the current tool landscape [16]. In total, we were able to get access to 11 academic and commercial tools: Appian, Apromore, ARIS, Celonis, IBM, Microsoft Power Automate, mpmX analytics, ProM 'Replay a Log on Petri Net for Conformance Analysis', ProM 'Replay alignment on Performance/Conformance Checking', ProM 'Mine with Inductive Visual Miner', and SAP Signavio Process Intelligence. For mpmX analytics, we only had screenshots available. To allow a comparison between the different visualizations of these tools, we used the same data set[1]. We preprocessed it and generated a BPMN process model by applying different ProM plug-ins, allowing conformance checking in all tools.

First Iteration (Empirical-to-Conceptual). Because academic literature on conformance checking visualizations is scarce, we could not perform the more common conceptual-to-empirical first iteration. Instead, we analyzed the existing visualizations in the selected process mining tools in an empirical-to-conceptual fashion. These visualizations[2] had similar characteristics that could be clustered into groups, although each tool had a different focus when conducting conformance checking. For example, many tools used some type of process model notation, which we grouped together to process models. For each of these groups,

---

[1] Data set: Road Traffic Fine Management Process.
[2] Screenshots available upon request.

we developed fitting abstract dimensions resulting in the first version of the taxonomy that was then further specified throughout the next iterations.

Second Iteration (Conceptual-to-Empirical). Next, we applied the framework by Munzner [13], shown in Fig. 2, and added the questions 'What' and 'How' as dimensions in our taxonomy. For those dimensions, fitting characteristics were derived through the examples given by Munzner [13], which were transferred to process mining, and the characteristics that could be identified in the different tools. For the 'What', one characteristics group we identified was everything around conformity, e.g., the conformance rate. For the 'How', identified characteristics were, for example, 'Number', 'Text', or 'Table'.

Third Iteration (Conceptual-to-Empirical). Because the visualizations differed significantly, we divided them into high-level groups, according to their main purpose (the 'Why'). For the characteristics, we relied on the four conformance checking task types currently supported by process mining tools: 'Quantify Conformance', 'Break Down and Compare Conformance', 'Localize and Show Deviation', and 'Explain and Diagnose Deviation' [16].

Fourth Iteration (Conceptual-to-Empirical). In particular, the insights from literature provided by Rehse et al. [16] and others, such as De Weerdt and Wynn [3], regarding the granularity level of process mining data, were used to differentiate between the data levels used in the visualizations. This allows a better classification. In detail, process mining data can be analyzed and visualized on log, variant, deviation, deviation category, or trace level in conformance checking [16]. We conceptualized these levels as characteristics under one dimension.

Fifth Iteration (Conceptual-to-Empirical). For the task type 'Localize and Show Deviation', we recognized that the same visualization, a process model, was always used in the tools, but in different notations. Based on process modeling literature [21], we hence added this as a dimension, with DFGs, BPMNs, Petri Nets, and chevron diagrams as characteristics. While chevron diagrams only show a single trace, the others are more expressive. Nevertheless, all notations create a visualization of a process. As the other tasks do not necessarily use process models, we also added the characteristic 'No Model'.

Sixth Iteration (Conceptual-to-Empirical). Next, we went back to Munzner's framework [13], with the goal of increasing the conciseness of the taxonomy. The framework divides the 'How' into two aspects [13]: graphical elements and visual appearance. Graphical elements describe primitive objects in a visualization and are characterized through their visual appearance. Together, they define the design space of visualizations [13]. Following this, we split the 'How' dimension into two individual ones: Depiction (Marks) and Appearance (Channels). By splitting up this dimension, the taxonomy with its dimensions and characteristics increased in comprehensibility and conciseness.

Last Iteration (Empirical-to-Conceptual Approach). Finally, our goal was to verify the taxonomy with all its different dimensions and characteristics. Again, we examined the visualizations in all tools and compared them with the developed taxonomy, confirming the completeness of the different dimensions and characteristics. Throughout this process, no adaptations were made, leading to the fulfillment of the objective ending conditions. Regarding the subjective ending criteria, we did a further assessment, which showed that the taxonomy is concise and comprehensive as the dimensions and characteristics are kept to a minimum and are clearly defined. It can also be extended by adding new dimensions or characteristics with no issues. As the dimensions and characteristics are labeled precisely, as simple as possible, and on the needed differentiation level, the taxonomy appears also to be self-explanatory and robust. Hence, we concluded the development process as all subjective and objective ending conditions were fulfilled from our perspective.

4   Conformance Checking Visualization Taxonomy

The final version of our conformance checking visualization taxonomy is shown in Fig. 4. It has six dimensions, with four to 42 characteristics per dimension. In the following, we describe each dimension and its characteristics in detail.

Task Type. Any conformance checking visualization within the tools aims to achieve one of the four conformance checking tasks: *Quantify Conformance, Localize and Show Deviation, Break Down and Compare Conformance,* and *Explain and Diagnose Deviation* [16]. Even though the visualization will have one task in focus, it might also be able to support another task. Therefore, the characteristics are not necessarily mutually exclusive.

Data Granularity Level. Data is needed as input for each visualization. This data will be refined to a certain granularity level, as shown within the visualization. For conformance checking data, six granularity levels are used: *Log, Variant, Single Trace, Deviation, Deviation Category,* and *Attribute* [1,16]. Consequently, this dimension is mutually exclusive.

Process Model Notation Type. Many, but not all, conformance checking visualizations incorporate process models. Due to their dominance and importance across the different tools, this dimension includes their use and a detailed differentiation based on their notation. If a visualization does not contain a process model, it falls under the characteristic *No Model*. Otherwise, the fitting notation will be selected, which is a *DFG, BPMN, Petri Net,* or *Chevron Diagram*.

What (Data Abstraction). This dimension describes what information is shown within the visualization. As one visualization can depict multiple pieces of information, selecting multiple characteristics is possible, so they are not mutually exclusive. Due to the different information depicted across tools, this dimension includes many characteristics. To simplify this, the characteristics are clustered into several groups:

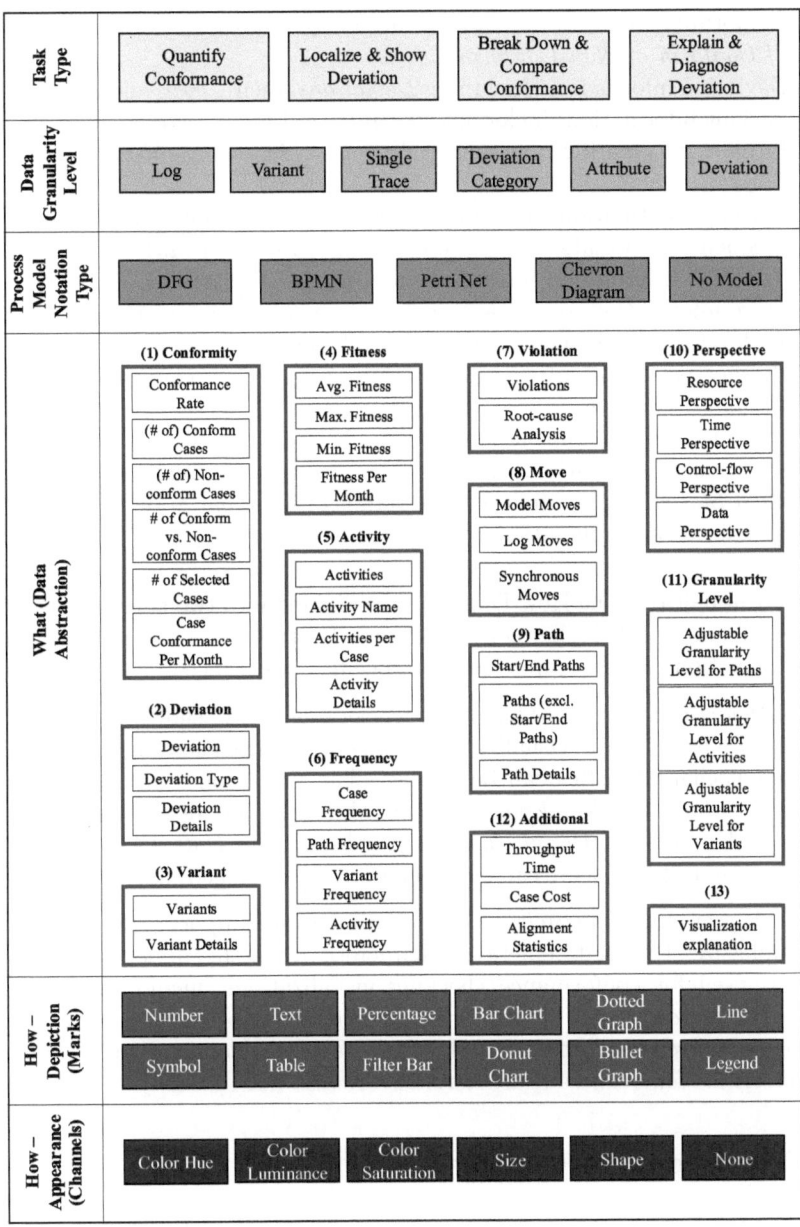

Fig. 4. Conformance Checking Visualization Taxonomy

(1) Conformity information, such as the *Conformance Rate* and the *Number of Conform or Non-Conform Cases.*
(2) Deviation information, including *Deviations*, their *Types*, and more *Details.*
(3) Variant information, including *Variants*, and more *Details.*
(4) Fitness information, including *Average, Maximum, Minimum,* or *Per Month.*
(5) Activity information, including their *Names*, and more *Details.*
(6) Frequency information, either for the *Case, Path, Variant or Activity* level.
(7) Violation information, including *Root-Cause Analysis.*
(8) Move information, if it is a *Model, Log, or Synchronous Move.*
(9) Path information, such as *Start* or *End*, and more *Details.*
(10) Perspective information, differentiating between *Control-Flow, Time, Resource*, and *Data.*
(11) Granularity level information, adjustable for *Paths, Activities*, or *Variants.*
(12) Additional information, such as *Throughput Time, Case Cost, and Alignment Statistics* providing further details on different granularity levels.
(13) Visualization Explanation.

How Dimensions. The How Dimension is divided into two sub-dimensions for a better structure and higher comprehension. However, they are interconnected, as one depiction can be supported by a specific appearance.

How – Depiction (Marks). This sub-dimension of 'How' shows what graphical elements are used for the visualization. For conformance checking visualizations, 12 different characteristics can be applied. The simple ones include a *Number, Text, Percentage, Symbol, Line,* or *Table.* More complex depictions are charts, such as a *Bar Chart* or *Donut Chart*, or graphs, such as *Dotted Graphs* or *Bullet Graphs.* As multiple of these can be selected, they are also not mutually exclusive.

How – Appearance (Channels). This sub-dimension supports the previous one and emphasizes the used depiction. Characteristics of this dimension are visual channels used for conformance checking visualizations, including *Color Hue, Color Luminance, Color Saturation, Size*, and *Shape.* However, none of these possible visual channels does not have to be used, leading to the additional characteristic *None.* These characteristics are also not mutually exclusive.

5   Discussion and Conclusion

The aim of this paper was to generate an overview of the used conformance checking visualizations, cluster the information systematically, and provide a foundation for future empirical research in order to reduce the current research gap of visual analytics in process mining. With the developed taxonomy, researchers can now categorize the visualizations they use or develop. Moreover, the taxonomy highlights how diverse and complex conformance checking visualizations are. This taxonomy is one of the first artifacts that combines the foundations of visual analytics and process mining. It provides detailed insights on the depicted conformance checking visualizations across the different tools and the visualization variables used. We hope that the developed taxonomy allows researchers to deepen their understanding of visualizations and their relevance, and helps them identify information gaps that have not been shown so far.

Our work is subject to multiple limitations. First, we focused on procedural conformance checking and excluded declarative and rule-based conformance checking visualizations, which are not used at all by industry tools. Moreover, the results are based on data acquired only during a specific time period. Therefore, all findings and information, especially from the tools, may have been subject to modifications. Furthermore, this information was gathered from a selection of tools. As we did not have access to all possible tools, important insights from these tools might be overlooked. Although the tool selection was done thoroughly, due to the fast-changing market of the tool providers, a tool might have been missed. However, with the covered tools in this paper the majority of the market for conformance checking solutions was considered. Fourth, the taxonomy only includes information on currently existing conformance checking visualizations. This means that it entails information derived from existing literature and the existing visualizations in the tools. Consequently, newly developed visualizations are not covered by this taxonomy and might include information that is not included so far. Furthermore, this also implies that it only covers what is currently available within the tools and does not cover what the user might need. In addition, the taxonomy development methodology used still leads to a certain degree of bias. Sixth, relevant literature, visualization variables, or information within the tools could have been missed and might not be included in the taxonomy, even though we conducted several iterations.

In conclusion, the taxonomy provides the foundation for future empirical research. We identified multiple potential future paths. Research should focus on developing and verifying the taxonomy further, leading to an increased objectivity and significance. It would be especially important to verify the different dimensions and characteristics through empirical data. Therefore, interviews with other experts who know either one of the research fields or both well should be conducted. Moreover, the operationalization of the taxonomy should be analyzed by applying it to further use cases. Although we tried to reduce the research gap of visual analytics in process mining, we identified further questions and problems that should be considered. First, visual analytics emphasizes focusing on the user and including them in the analysis process. However, so far, there are no user studies for visual analytics in process mining, also not for other process mining sub-disciplines. This provides an opportunity for empirical research to include the user when considering process mining visualizations and conduct research on it. Such research needs to check if the existing visualizations fulfill the users' needs for the different tasks, especially for conformance checking. Thus, future researchers could conduct experiments where users evaluate visualizations to test the user's comprehension of the process. With this knowledge, researchers could improve and standardize conformance checking visualizations.

This could also include the adaptation or new development of the underlying algorithms, precisely solving the users' needs.

Overall, this taxonomy is an important contribution, as it provides a foundation for future empirical research on conformance checking visualizations, offering an initial understanding to be elaborated on. Following this path of research would have an significant impact on the adoption of process mining and would advance the research of connecting visual analytics and process mining.

References

1. Carmona, J., van Dongen, B., Weidlich, M.: Conformance checking: foundations, milestones and challenges. In: Process Mining Handbook, pp. 155–190. Springer (2022)
2. Cui, W.: Visual analytics: a comprehensive overview. IEEE Access **7**, 81555–81573 (2019)
3. De Weerdt, J., Wynn, M.T.: Foundations of process event data. In: Process Mining Handbook, pp. 193–211. Springer (2022)
4. Dumas, M., Rosa, L.M., Mendling, J., Reijers, A.H.: Fundamentals of Business Process Management. Springer (2018)
5. Dunzer, S., Stierle, M., Matzner, M., Baier, S.: Conformance checking: a state-of-the-art literature review. In: S-BPM ONE, pp. 1–10. ACM (2019)
6. Emamjome, F., Andrews, R., ter Hofstede, A.H.: A case study lens on process mining in practice. In: OTM, pp. 127–145. Springer (2019)
7. FAU: Process mining survey (2021). https://www.processmining-software.com/wp-content/uploads/2021/FAU2021_Process_Mining_Survey.pdf
8. García-Bañuelos, L., Van Beest, N.R., Dumas, M., La Rosa, M., Mertens, W.: Complete and interpretable conformance checking of business processes. TSE **44**(3), 262–290 (2017)
9. Gschwandtner, T.: Visual analytics meets process mining: challenges and opportunities. In: SIMPDA, pp. 142–154. Springer (2017)
10. Kaouni, A., Theodoropoulou, G., Bousdekis, A., Voulodimos, A., Miaoulis, G.: Visual analytics in process mining for supporting business process improvement. In: NIDS, pp. 166–175. IOS Press (2021)
11. Keim, D., Andrienko, G., Fekete, J.D., Görg, C., Kohlhammer, J., Melançon, G.: Visual analytics: definition, process, and challenges. In: Information Visualization: Human-Centered Issues and Perspectives. Springer (2008)
12. Klinkmüller, C., Müller, R., Weber, I.: Mining process mining practices: an exploratory characterization of information needs in process analytics. In: BPM, pp. 322–337. Springer (2019)
13. Munzner, T.: Visualization Analysis and Design. CRC Press (2014)
14. Nickerson, R.C., Varshney, U., Muntermann, J.: A method for taxonomy development and its application in information systems. EJIS **22**(3), 336–359 (2013)
15. Oberländer, A.M., Lösser, B., Rau, D.: Taxonomy research in information systems: a systematic assessment. In: ECIS (2019)
16. Rehse, J.R., Pufahl, L., Grohs, M., Klein, L.M.: Process mining meets visual analytics: the case of conformance checking. In: HICSS, pp. 5452–5461. ScholarSpace (2023)
17. Reinkemeyer, L.: Process Mining in Action (2020)

18. Sirgmets, M., Milani, F., Nolte, A., Pungas, T.: Designing process diagrams–a framework for making design choices when visualizing process mining outputs. In: OTM, pp. 463–480. Springer (2018)
19. Szopinski, D., Schoormann, T., Kundisch, D.: Criteria as a prelude for guiding taxonomy evaluation. In: HICSS (2020)
20. Thomas, J., Cook, K.: Illuminating the Path IEEE. CSP (2005)
21. Van Der Aalst, W.: Foundations of process discovery. In: Process Mining Handbook, pp. 37–75. Springer (2022)
22. Van Der Aalst, W.: Process mining: a 360 degree overview. In: Process Mining Handbook, pp. 3–34. Springer (2022)
23. Van Der Aalst, W., de Leoni, M., ter Hofstede, A.: Process mining and visual analytics: breathing life into business process models. BPM **17**, 699–730 (2011)
24. Weske, M.: Business Process Management - Concepts, Languages, Architectures. Springer (2019)

Structuring Empirical Research on Process Mining at the Individual Level Using the Theory of Effective Use

Jan Mendling[1,2,3]([✉]) [ID], Mieke Jans[4,5] [ID], and Kristina Sahling[1,3] [ID]

[1] Humboldt-Universität zu Berlin, Berlin, Germany
{jan.mendling,kristina.sahling}@hu-berlin.de
[2] Wirtschaftsuniversität Wien, Vienna, Austria
[3] Weizenbaum Institute, Berlin, Germany
[4] Hasselt University, Hasselt, Belgium
mieke.jans@uhasselt.be
[5] Maastricht University, Maastricht, The Netherlands

Abstract. A growing number of empirical papers on the topic of process mining has been published in years. After a first wave of contributions on application scenarios, there has been a second wave aiming to establish theoretical insights into how process mining tools are used and how benefits unfold from this usage. Many of these papers follow an explorative, qualitative, or inductive approach. A weakness of these contributions is their theoretical cohesion and integration. This paper makes an effort to integrate them into a more holistic theory that can eventually provide a foundation for more deductive and quantitative empirical research on process mining. To this end, we build on the theory of effective use and focus on the individual effect on decision makers. We find opportunities for revision and refinement of this theory for process mining. Specifically, we discuss moving from constructs on learning to expertise, and integrating a pragmatic perspective that complements the semantic emphasis of representational fidelity.

Keywords: Process Mining · Theory of Effective Use · Empirical Research

1 Introduction

Recent years have seen process mining developing from a research domain to a category of commercial enterprise software with an increasing uptake in industry [11]. The growing usage in practice has also confronted process mining researchers with new research questions that shift from the technical level to the user level and the organizational level [7]. Many of these research questions require an empirical research agenda and a more profound treatment than many of the early empirical studies before 2018 that report which type of organization is using process mining for which application scenario [37].

A. Delgado and T. Slaats (Eds.): ICPM 2024 Workshops, LNBIP 533, pp. 520–532, 2025.
https://doi.org/10.1007/978-3-031-82225-4_38

Since 2020, a second wave of empirical works has gathered insights into how process mining contributes to organizational performance. Contributions such as [21] differ from the earlier application scenario studies in their ambition of developing a theoretical understanding of the causal chain and corresponding mechanisms from process mining adoption to usage and eventually to improved organizational performance. Much of these works use explorative, qualitative, or inductive research methods with the ambition of contributing to theory building. A diverse collection of observations and theoretical arguments on the usage and impact of process mining tools has emerged from these contributions. At the same time, this research body also exhibits weaknesses in terms of theoretical cohesion and theoretical integration of more general streams of information systems research.

This paper makes an effort to integrate into a more holistic theory that can eventually provide a foundation for more deductive and quantitative empirical research on process mining. To this end, we build on the theory of effective use and focus on the individual effect on decision makers [38]. More specifically, we use this theory to organize empirical observations on process mining. Our work contributes to the consolidation of empirical research on process mining and its integration into more general information systems theories. We also identify blind spots in the theory of effective use where empirical insights on process mining provide complementary perspectives.

The rest of the paper is structured as follows. Section 2 summarizes recent empirical work on process mining. Section 3 describes the theory of effective use and builds on it to integrate empirical process mining findings. Section 4 discusses our findings before Sect. 5 concludes with a summary and an outlook onto future work.

2   Background

This section describes the background of empirical research on process mining. Research on process mining has traditionally focused on developing new and improved algorithms for automatic process discovery, conformance checking, and process enhancement [1]. A first wave of empirical research investigates application scenarios of these algorithms and corresponding tools [37,39]. The focus of this second wave of empirical research is on the development of theoretical insights into the mechanisms of how process mining provides benefits. To this end, we discuss research that focuses on the work of the analysts and their interaction with process mining tools. Then, we describe contributions that look at the impact on organizational performance.

2.1   Analysts and Their Interaction with Process Mining Tools

Research on the impact of process mining tools on the *work of the process analyst* in various domains has been limited to exploratory studies. Early work by Ailenei et al. [2] describes 19 use cases, in essence, analysis tasks that analysts can investigate using process mining tools. They find that identifying the structure of the process, its most frequent path, the distribution of cases over paths, and the compliance with a pre-defined process models are the most relevant use cases. Interviews by Zimmermann et al. have revealed that analysts perceive challenges in conducting process mining projects [43]. From these interviews, 23 challenges of using process mining are described. What makes the analysts' work difficult appears to be essentially the access to additional information (C14), data access (C6), data extraction (C4), as much as tool knowledge (C11) and analysis focus (C17) [44]. In order to cope with these challenges, analysts apply different types of strategies to understand, plan, analyze, and evaluate their results [42]. Sorokina et al. show that effective strategies of creating process mining results lead to superior performance [35]. Much of these strategies can be related to analyst strategies described in the field of visual analytics [13] and its basic mantra of *overview first, zoom and filter, then details-on-demand* [34]. In turn, the effective use of an analytical tool then becomes an issue of how well these cognitive strategies of the analyst are readily supported by corresponding tool features.

2.2   Organisational Impact of Process Mining Adoption

Research on the impact of process mining on organizational performance has developed in recent years, mostly building on case studies and qualitative research designs. Grisold et al. conduct interviews with process managers who report difficulties in quantifying the value of process mining and issues with an increased level of transparency [21]. Eggers et al. also find a social impact of increased process transparency through process mining, but highlight its benefits for process awareness [15]. This process awareness appears to be the foundation for evidence-based decision-making and overall contributions to organizational value creation, as Badakhshan et al. emphasize [4]. However, not all process mining initiatives progress in this direction. Stein Dani et al. report issues connected with lack of expertise, lack of incentives, loss of interest, or sheer denial [36]. Mamudu et al. identify ten success factors for process mining including stakeholder support, information availability, technical expertise, team configuration, structured approach, data quality, tool capabilities, project and change management, and training [28]. Joas et al. find challenges for organizational impact of process mining with a focus on sustainability reporting in the six categories of the BPM success factors model [23]. Brock et al. develop a process mining maturity model including 23 factors grouped into the five categories organization, data foundation, people's knowledge, scope of process mining, and governance [6]. The list of these factors is extensive, yet there are no quantitative insights into the relative importance of the factors.

2.3   Theorizing the Impact of Process Mining

Some papers point to opportunities for further advancing this research area by building on theories from information systems research [7] and from cognitive research on diagrams [30]. So far, theorizing is limited to the observation that models of technology acceptance [40] and task-technology fit [19] are presumably applicable [7]. There is support from research on business intelligence systems that highlight the applicability of information systems theories including the DeLone & McLean success model, technology acceptance model, diffusion of innovation theory, and the unified theory of acceptance and use of technology [3]. Also personal factors as anxiety, absorptive capacity, self-efficacy and user involvements are discussed, as much as challenges including system acceptance, motivation, fear of losing power, or lack of knowledge [3]. The relevance of cognitive factors has been emphasized in works that build on diagram understanding [30]. In essence, this stream of research stressed the importance of understanding characteristics of analyst tasks relative to the representations that are offered to support the task at hand [27].

These theories however focus on preconditions of use, while offering little regarding how tool-supported task performance feeds back to the behaviour of the analyst. Foregrounding the dynamics of actual usage is the basis for understanding the impact that process mining tools have on the work of process analysts and their decision-making. The theory of effective use (TEU) [38] has been recently adapted for business intelligence systems, a group of systems related to process mining tools. This adaptation provides opportunities to map and integrate the different empirical studies on process mining. In the following, we will pursue this opportunity.

3 Theoretical Integration Based on Theory of Effective Use

The theory of effective use has developed from a longer debate about the relevance and characteristics of information systems use. The DeLone & McLean model of information system success had already identified the use construct as of central importance in the causal chain from information system to eventual success. However, use turned out to be difficult to specify from a theoretical angle [31]. Burton-Jones and Grange observed that use is much less of relevance than effective use. They developed their theory of effective use based on key concepts of representation theory, originally defined by Wand and Weber based on Bunge's work on ontology [33]. The original version describes effective use as a chain from transparent interaction with a system towards representational fidelity towards informed action, which all contribute to performance in terms of efficiency and effectiveness [8]. Next, we describe a recent contextualization of the theory of effective use and then use it to integrate diverse findings from qualitative studies on process mining.

3.1 Theory of Effective Use

Recently, the theory of effective use has been extended with resource-related constructs and contextualized for business intelligence (BI) systems [38]. The corresponding model describes three categories of factors with three constructs each that have a hypothetical effect on decision-making efficiency and effectiveness. We discuss these three categories in turn.

Effective Use of BI System: Constructs in this category stem from the original theory formulation of Burton-Jones and Grange, which in essence defines a causal chain from transparent interaction to representational fidelity and informed action [8]. In this context, **transparent interaction (TI)** is defined as "the extent to which a user is accessing the system's representations unimpeded by its surface and physical structures" [38]. Items of this construct relate to the system being easy to use and user-friendly, such that users do not have difficulties interacting with it. **Representational fidelity (RF)** refers to the interaction with the system and "the extent to which a user is obtaining representations that faithfully reflect the domain that the systems represent" [38]. This means in essence that the system's representations correctly represent reality. Finally, **informed decisions (IF)** as a specific type of informed action captures "the extent to which a user acts on the information/output that he or she obtains from the system to improve his or her work performance" [38].

BI Resources: The recent TEU model of Trieu et al. adds three resources to the theory at each of its three stages [38]. A hypothetical factor of transparent interaction is **BI system quality (SQ)**. This is "a measure of the performance of the BI system from a technical and design perspective" [12,18]. Representational fidelity is expected to be affected by **data integration (DI)**. "Data integration ensures that data have the same meaning and use across time and across users, making the data in different systems or databases consistent or logically compatible [20]. Finally, informed action is affected by an **evidence-based management culture (EBM)**. "An evidence-based management culture involves the use of data and analysis to support decision-making [32].

Learning Activities: The original TEU also assumes the relevance of learning activities [8]. **Learning the system (LS)** is described as a factor of transparent interaction and refers to "any action a user takes to learn the system (its representations, or its surface or physical structure)". **Learning fidelity (LF)** is described as a moderator of the effect of transparent interaction on representational fidelity. It covers "any action a user takes to learn the extent to which the output from the system faithfully represents the relevant real-world domain". The effect of representational fidelity on informed action is assumed to be moderated by **learning how to leverage output (LL)**. It refers to "any action a user takes to learn how to leverage the output obtained from the system in his/her work". Mind though that none of these learning variables were significant in the evaluation of Trieu et al. [38].

The theory of effective use and its application to business intelligence systems points to its relevance for investigating the impact of process mining systems. So far, research on process mining and on effective use have been disconnected.

3.2   Integration of Empirical Process Mining Studies

Recent empirical studies on process mining follow qualitative methods. They contribute observations on process mining use, but with little theoretical integration. The theory of effective use and its application to BI systems offers the opportunity to structure various empirical contributions on process mining. To this end, we focus on the following empirical process mining papers (*the studies* in the following):

1. Badakhshan, Wurm, Grisold, Geyer-Klingeberg, Mendling, vom Brocke: Creating business value with process mining (JSIS 2022) [4].
2. Brock, Brennig, Löhr, Bartelheimer, von Enzberg, Dumitrescu: Improving Process Mining Maturity–From Intentions to Actions (BISE 2024) [6].
3. Eggers, Hein, Böhm, Krcmar: No longer out of sight, no longer out of mind? How organizations engage with process mining-induced transparency to achieve increased process awareness (BISE 2021) [15].
4. Eggert, Dyong: Applying process mining in small and medium sized it enterprises: challenges and guidelines (BPM 2022) [16].
5. Grisold, Mendling, Otto, vom Brocke: Adoption, use and management of process mining in practice (BPMJ 2021) [21].
6. Joas, Gierlich-Joas, Bahr, Bauer: Towards Leveraging Process Mining for Sustainability – An Analysis of Challenges and Potential Solutions (BPM Forum 2024) [23].
7. Kipping, Djurica, Franzoi, Grisold, Marcus, Schmid, vom Brocke, Mendling, Röglinger: How to leverage process mining in organizations-towards process mining capabilities (BPM 2022) [25]
8. Mamudu, Bandara, Wynn, Leemans: Process Mining Success Factors and Their Interrelationships (BISE 2024) [28].
9. Sorokina, Soffer, Hadar, Leron, Zerbato, Weber: PEM4PPM: A Cognitive Perspective on the Process of Process Mining (BPM 2023) [35].
10. Stein Dani, Leopold, van der Werf, Beerepoot, Reijers: From Loss of Interest to Denial: A Study on the Terminators of Process Mining Initiatives (CAISE 2024) [36].
11. Martin, Fischer, Kerpedzhiev, Goel, Leemans, Röglinger, van der Aalst, Dumas, La Rosa, Wynn: Opportunities and challenges for process mining in organizations: results of a Delphi study (BISE 2021) [29].
12. Zimmermann, Zerbato, Weber: What makes life for process mining analysts difficult? A reflection of challenges (SoSyM 2023) [44].

We reviewed the constructs being discussed in these papers and mapped them, where possible, to constructs of the theory of effective use. We will again use the three categories of the recent version of TEU to organize this discussion.

Effective Use and Process Mining: The **transparent interaction** of a process manager with a process mining system (PMS) is mentioned as a challenge by Zimmermann et al. [44]. Kipping et al. report that a potential discrepancy between model and reality is an issue [25]. This relates to what Zimmermann et al. describe as a challenge of process mining suitability [44]. Several observations of the studies focus on the relationship between **representational fidelity** and **informed action**. First, here are observations on how this connection materializes. Both Mamudu et al. and Brock et al. emphasize the need to follow a structured approach or a systematic method [6,28]. Grisold et al. mention process selection in particular [21]. However, their arguments partially mix a) getting the PMS ready to use (planning, data extraction, project-focused) and b) actual use (analysis and evaluation). Second, Zimmermann et al. describe challenges of drawing conclusions and formulating recommendations [44]. Badakhshan et al. highlight that data-driven decision-making has to be considered separately from the actual implementation of interventions [4]. Both Mamudu et al. and Brock et al. agree that implementation requires attention to change management [6,28]. Insights do not always yield action, as Stein Dani et al. observe: stakeholders might deny the correctness of analytic insights, may have a lack of incentives to take action, or lose interest for other reasons [36]. Also Eggert and Dyong report doubts about analysis results [16]. Grisold et al. point to potential issues of coping with increased transparency along with a fear of surveillance [21]. These observations relate to what TEU describes as disturbances, i.e. external constraints affecting effective use, but without detailing them in the theory.

BI Resources and Process Mining: According to TEU, **system quality** plays an important role as a factor of transparent interaction. The studies support this view, pointing to the relevance of tool capabilities [28] such as process visualization and process analytics [4]. All studies strongly emphasize the relevance of **data integration**, not only in terms of "the same meaning and use across time and across users", but also in terms of data quality and sheer data accessibility [6,16,21,23,28,44]. Often, laborious data preparation [36] is needed to achieve data connectivity [4]. Also evidence-based management culture is mentioned. Brock et al. [6] refer to Kerpedzhiev et al. [24] who point to cultural factors including process centricity, evidence centricity, and change centricity. Martin et al. list a total of ten culture-related challenges including aversion to transparency and resistence to change [29]. Overall, the studies are consistent with TEU, partially providing a more detailed perspective on data issues and tool capabilities.

Learning Activities and Process Mining: The learning variables define the third category of factors. Though they were significant in the evaluation of Trieu et al., there was further support for their relevance in reflection interviews [38]. The studies also support their importance, a.o. by pointing to insufficient skills [23,29,44], the need to conduct training [28], and inappropriate analysis strategies [35]. **Learning the system** relates to observations about technical expertise as a prerequisite [28] and lack of expertise as a roadblock [36]. Regarding **learning fidelity**, Badakhshan et al. describe the need to perceive end-to-end process visualization and performance indicators [4]. For **learning how to leverage output**, Grisold et al. observe issues with understanding how variables inform decision-making [21]. Badakhshan et al. highlight the need to engage in sense-making of process-related information before decisions can be made [4]. Here, Zimmermann et al. identify analysis expertise as a challenges [44]. Brock et al. stress people's knowledge as a factor and point to various aspects of knowledge. They distinguish knowledge of process mining tools, technical basics, data preparation, classical data mining, process mining basics, and advanced applications [6]. Eggers et al. identify shared process awareness as a central construct [15]. In essence, they argue that process mining usage contributes to process awareness, which in turn contributes to process performance. Altogether, the studies confirm the importance of this category, but rather as a matter of skill and expertise (variables of status) instead of learning (variables of action). The study by Trieu et al. [38] partially addresses this concern by using "experience using BI" and "experience working in organization" as control variables.

Other Factors: The studies mention a number of organizational factors that are relevant for the effective use of process mining. Some of them relate to a link with **strategic objectives**. Brock et al. point to the purpose of using process mining [6] and Stein Dani et al. to incentives [36]. Potential internal resistance can be an issue [25], therefore, Mamudu et al. call for stakeholder involvement [28]. Grisold et al. and Martin et al. observe issues with justifying the business case of using process mining [21,29]. A second category relates to **governance** mentioned in [4,6,15]. Brock et al. provide the most detailed discussion. They distinguish general roles and responsibilities plus a governance of methods and tools, processes, and data [6]. Brock et al. also advocate establishing a center of excellence for process mining.

In summary, empirical studies on process mining are largely consistent with propositions of the theory of effective use. The studies provide some more detailed and nuanced perspectives on skills, culture, strategy, and governance.

4 Towards a Theory of Effective Use of Process Mining Systems

Our analysis has defined a theoretical bridge between empirical studies on process mining and the theory of effective use. While the causal path from transparent interaction to representational fidelity to informed action and eventually efficiency and effectiveness is by large consistently reflected in the studies, it is interesting to note that the studies point to those four success factors of BPM beyond the foundational method and technology category, namely strategic alignment, governance, people, and culture [14, Ch.12], also observed by Martin et al. [29]. There is potential to refine and revise the theory of effective use in each of these categories towards a theory of effective use of process mining systems. Here, we focus on relevant, but non-significant constructs of learning and the notion of process awareness.

First, a direction for further developing TEU is to move **from learning to expertise**. The non-significance together with the relevance of learning-related constructs in the study by Trieu et al. [38] points to the need for a revise the theory of effective use. We suggest refocusing on expertise instead of learning. First, the concept of learning has conceptual disadvantages. The TEU constructs refer to actions taken to acquire knowledge. This ignores the status of knowledge, and mixes in diligence and motivation. Second, information systems research has demonstrated the importance of expertise in various studies, highlighting challenges of a revision of TEU. Already in the 1980s, Vitalari identifies a catalogue of eight larger knowledge categories of a system analyst with partially up to 30 different knowledge items [41]. In relation to process mining usage, Brock et al. point to the fact that several categories of knowledge are relevant [6]. Another challenge are the dependencies between the knowledge categories. Mackay et al. find that a lack of technical usage expertise appears to be a roadblock to leveraging domain expertise [26]. Hahn and Lee discuss complications stemming from the division of labour and expertise between business and information technology units in many companies. Cross-domain knowledge turns out to be specifically important for effective collaboration.

Second, a direction for further developing TEU is to move **from semantics to pragmatics**. Zimmermann et al. mentions process domain understanding as an important factor beyond what is visible through the process mining system [44]. Trieu et al. reflect on their study and state that information provided by a system "could still be useful even when representational fidelity was low" [38]. Apparently, even when data quality is often low, managers can still draw conclusions using their business knowledge to make informed decisions. This is in line with the argument of Bera et al. that highlight the strength of pragmatics [5]. Taking pragmatics seriously requires a deeper reflection of the connection between knowledge and tasks at the individual and organizational level [27]. Indeed, Eggers et al. identify different types of use scenarios for process mining, namely explorative analysis versus monitoring, with likely implications for usage [15]. The authors also identify process awareness as a central construct on the path to organizational performance. Mind that this is not necessarily fidelity of the representations in the process mining system, but the shared understanding of the process by the process manager and involved stakeholders. Important to note is also the fact that process awareness goes beyond the ontological description of the process, but rather relates to notions of situation awareness [17] as often discussed in human factor studies. We must also acknowledge the fact that much of the work with process mining systems is rather problem solving than decision making. Both involve uncertainty, but problems are much more open. Campbell characterizes decision tasks by a number of conflicting outcomes (e.g. selecting a new employee), while problem tasks suffer from various paths to arrive at a desired outcome [9]. Chandra Kruse et al. describe various behaviours of how analysts approach such a task: understand the problem and scope, retrieve prior knowledge, look for alternatives, generate new concepts, propose solutions, and finally implement and communicate [10]. Clearly, not all of these behaviours are directly supported by systems, but much of the iterative behaviour is consistently reported in visual analytics research [13] and empirical process mining research [22,44].

In summary, the non-significance in the study of Trieu et al. [38] and the observations of empirical process mining studies highlight the potential of revising and refining the theory of effective use for process mining systems.

5   Conclusion

In this paper, we have discussed empirical research on process mining. We identified the recent contextualization of the theory of effective use for business intelligence systems as an opportunity to organize and integrate various empirical observations on process mining from twelve recent papers. Overall, we found the studies and the theory consistent in large parts, but there are also opportunities for revision and refinement. We discussed specific opportunities for moving from constructs on learning to expertise and integrating a pragmatic perspective that complements the semantic emphasis of representational fidelity. In future research, we aim to further develop our discussion into a theoretical model and make it subject to an empirical research agenda.

Acknowledgments. The research of the authors was supported by the Einstein Foundation Berlin under grant EPP-2019-524, by the German Federal Ministry of Education and Research under grant 16DII133, and by Deutsche Forschungsgemeinschaft under grants 496119880 (VisualMine) and 531115272 (ProImpact).

Disclosure of Interests. The authors have no competing interests to declare that are relevant to the content of this article.

References

1. van der Aalst, W.M.P.: Process Mining - Data Science in Action, 2nd edn. Springer (2016)
2. Ailenei, I., Rozinat, A., Eckert, A., van der Aalst, W.M.P.: Definition and validation of process mining use cases. In: Daniel, F., Barkaoui, K., Dustdar, S. (eds.) Business Process Management Workshops - BPM 2011 International Workshops, Clermont-Ferrand, France, 29 August 2011, Revised Selected Papers, Part I. Lecture Notes in Business Information Processing, vol. 99, pp. 75–86. Springer (2011)
3. Ain, N., Vaia, G., DeLone, W.H., Waheed, M.: Two decades of research on business intelligence system adoption, utilization and success-a systematic literature review. Decis. Support Syst. **125**, 113113 (2019)
4. Badakhshan, P., Wurm, B., Grisold, T., Geyer-Klingeberg, J., Mendling, J., vom Brocke, J.: Creating business value with process mining. J. Strateg. Inf. Syst. **31**(4), 101745 (2022)
5. Bera, P., Burton-Jones, A., Wand, Y.: Research note–how semantics and pragmatics interact in understanding conceptual models. Inf. Syst. Res. **25**(2), 401–419 (2014)
6. Brock, J., Brennig, K., Löhr, B., Bartelheimer, C., von Enzberg, S., Dumitrescu, R.: Improving process mining maturity–from intentions to actions. Bus. Inf. Syst. Eng. 1–21 (2024)

7. vom Brocke, J., Jans, M., Mendling, J., Reijers, H.A.: A five-level framework for research on process mining. Bus. Inf. Syst. Eng. **63**(5), 483–490 (2021)
8. Burton-Jones, A., Grange, C.: From use to effective use: a representation theory perspective. Inf. Syst. Res. **24**(3), 632–658 (2013)
9. Campbell, D.J.: Task complexity: a review and analysis. Acad. Manag. Rev. **13**(1), 40–52 (1988)
10. Chandra Kruse, L., Purao, S., Seidel, S.: How designers use design principles: design behaviors and application modes. J. Assoc. Inf. Syst. **23**(5), 1235–1270 (2022)
11. Davenport, T.H., Spanyi, A.: What process mining is, and why companies should do it. Harv. Bus. Rev. **97**(2), 2–7 (2019)
12. DeLone, W.H., McLean, E.R.: Information systems success: the quest for the dependent variable. Inf. Syst. Res. **3**(1), 60–95 (1992)
13. Du, F., Shneiderman, B., Plaisant, C., Malik, S., Perer, A.: Coping with volume and variety in temporal event sequences: strategies for sharpening analytic focus. IEEE Trans. Vis. Comput. Graph. **23**(6), 1636–1649 (2016)
14. Dumas, M., Rosa, M.L., Mendling, J., Reijers, H.A.: Fundamentals of Business Process Management, 2nd edn. Springer (2018)
15. Eggers, J., Hein, A., Böhm, M., Krcmar, H.: No longer out of sight, no longer out of mind? How organizations engage with process mining-induced transparency to achieve increased process awareness. Bus. Inf. Syst. Eng. **63**(5), 491–510 (2021)
16. Eggert, M., Dyong, J.: Applying process mining in small and medium sized it enterprises–challenges and guidelines. In: International Conference on Business Process Management, pp. 125–142. Springer (2022)
17. Endsley, M.R.: A systematic review and meta-analysis of direct objective measures of situation awareness: a comparison of SAGAT and SPAM. Hum. Factors **63**(1), 124–150 (2021)
18. Gable, G.G., Sedera, D., Chan, T.: Re-conceptualizing information system success: the is-impact measurement model. J. Assoc. Inf. Syst. **9**(7), 18 (2008)
19. Goodhue, D.L., Thompson, R.L.: Task-technology fit and individual performance. MIS Q. 213–236 (1995)
20. Goodhue, D.L., Wybo, M.D., Kirsch, L.J.: The impact of data integration on the costs and benefits of information systems. MIS Q. 293–311 (1992)
21. Grisold, T., Mendling, J., Otto, M., vom Brocke, J.: Adoption, use and management of process mining in practice. Bus. Process. Manag. J. **27**(2), 369–387 (2021)
22. Grisold, T., van der Aa, H., Franzoi, S., Hartl, S., Mendling, J., Vom Brocke, J.: A context framework for sense-making of process mining results. In: 2024 International Conference on Process Mining (ICPM) (2024)
23. Joas, A., Gierlich-Joas, M., Bahr, C., Bauer, J.: Towards leveraging process mining for sustainability - an analysis of challenges and potential solutions. In: Marrella, A., Resinas, M., Jans, M., Rosemann, M. (eds.) Business Process Management Forum, pp. 354–371. Springer, Cham (2024)
24. Kerpedzhiev, G.D., König, U.M., Röglinger, M., Rosemann, M.: An exploration into future business process management capabilities in view of digitalization: results from a Delphi study. Bus. Inf. Syst. Eng. **63**(2), 83–96 (2021)
25. Kipping, G., et al.: How to leverage process mining in organizations-towards process mining capabilities. In: International Conference on Business Process Management, pp. 40–46. Springer (2022)
26. Mackay, J.M., Elam, J.J.: A comparative study of how experts and novices use a decision aid to solve problems in complex knowledge domains. Inf. Syst. Res. **3**(2), 150–172 (1992)

27. Malinova Mandelburger, M., Mendling, J.: Cognitive diagram understanding and task performance in systems analysis and design. MIS Q. **45**(4), 2101–2157 (2021)
28. Mamudu, A., Bandara, W., Wynn, M.T., Leemans, S.J.: Process mining success factors and their interrelationships. Bus. Inf. Syst. Eng. 1–20 (2024)
29. Martin, N., et al.: Opportunities and challenges for process mining in organizations: results of a Delphi study. Bus. Inf. Syst. Eng. **63**, 511–527 (2021)
30. Mendling, J., Djurica, D., Malinova, M.: Cognitive effectiveness of representations for process mining. In: Polyvyanyy, A., Wynn, M.T., Looy, A.V., Reichert, M. (eds.) Business Process Management - 19th International Conference, BPM 2021, Rome, Italy, 06–10 September 2021, Proceedings. Lecture Notes in Computer Science, vol. 12875, pp. 17–22. Springer (2021)
31. Petter, S., DeLone, W., McLean, E.: Measuring information systems success: models, dimensions, measures, and interrelationships. Eur. J. Inf. Syst. **17**(3), 236–263 (2008)
32. Pfeffer, J., Sutton, R.I.: Evidence-based management. Harv. Bus. Rev. **84**(1), 62 (2006)
33. Recker, J., Indulska, M., Green, P., Burton-Jones, A., Weber, R.: Information systems as representations: a review of the theory and evidence. J. Assoc. Inf. Syst. **20**(6), 5 (2019)
34. Shneiderman, B.: The eyes have it: a task by data type taxonomy for information visualizations. In: The Craft of Information Visualization, pp. 364–371. Elsevier (2003)
35. Sorokina, E., Soffer, P., Hadar, I., Leron, U., Zerbato, F., Weber, B.: PEM4PPM: a cognitive perspective on the process of process mining. In: Di Francescomarino, C., Burattin, A., Janiesch, C., Sadiq, S. (eds.) Business Process Management, pp. 465–481. Springer, Cham (2023)
36. Stein Dani, V., Leopold, H., van der Werf, J.M.E., Beerepoot, I., Reijers, H.A.: From loss of interest to denial: a study on the terminators of process mining initiatives. In: International Conference on Advanced Information Systems Engineering, pp. 371–386. Springer (2024)
37. Thiede, M., Fuerstenau, D., Bezerra Barquet, A.P.: How is process mining technology used by organizations? A systematic literature review of empirical studies. Bus. Process. Manag. J. **24**(4), 900–922 (2018)
38. Trieu, V., Burton-Jones, A., Green, P.F., Cockcroft, S.: Applying and extending the theory of effective use in a business intelligence context. MIS Q. **46**(1), 645–678 (2022)
39. Van Der Aalst, W.M., et al.: Business process mining: an industrial application. Inf. Syst. **32**(5), 713–732 (2007)
40. Venkatesh, V., Thong, J.Y., Xu, X.: Unified theory of acceptance and use of technology: a synthesis and the road ahead. J. Assoc. Inf. Syst. **17**(5), 328–376 (2016)
41. Vitalari, N.P.: Knowledge as a basis for expertise in systems analysis: an empirical study. MIS Q. 221–241 (1985)
42. Zerbato, F., Soffer, P., Weber, B.: Process mining practices: evidence from interviews. In: Business Process Management: 20th International Conference, BPM 2022, Münster, Germany, 11–16 September 2022, Proceedings, pp. 268–285. Springer (2022)
43. Zimmermann, L., Zerbato, F., Weber, B.: Process mining challenges perceived by analysts: an interview study. In: Enterprise, Business-Process and Information Systems Modeling: 23rd International Conference, BPMDS 2022 and 27th International Conference, EMMSAD 2022, Held at CAiSE 2022, Leuven, Belgium, 6–7 June 2022, Proceedings, pp. 3–17. Springer (2022)

44. Zimmermann, L., Zerbato, F., Weber, B.: What makes life for process mining analysts difficult? A reflection of challenges. Softw. Syst. Model. 1–29 (2023)

Analysing and Improving Business Processes Through Hybrid Simulation Model: A Case Study

Francesca Meneghello[1,2(✉)], Massimo Coletti[3], Debora Di Marco[3],
Massimiliano Ronzani[1], Chiara Di Francescomarino[4], and Chiara Ghidini[5]

[1] Fondazione Bruno Kessler, Trento, Italy
{fmeneghello,mronzani}@fbk.eu
[2] Sapienza University of Rome, Rome, Italy
[3] Ernst & Young (EY), Rome, Italy
{Massimo.Coletti,Debora.Di.Marco}@it.ey.com
[4] University of Trento, Trento, Italy
[5] Free University of Bozen-Bolzano, Bolzano, Italy

Abstract. The increasing amount of process execution data, i.e. the event logs stored by the company, can be exploited using Business Process Simulation (BPS). BPS serves as a valuable tool for business analysts, enabling them to analyze and compare business processes and identify changes that optimize key performance measures. Especially when evaluating alternative scenarios, it is crucial to start with an accurate simulation of the current process. Recent research in the field of BPS has demonstrated that Hybrid Simulation Model (HSM) approaches reliably replicates business process behaviour, overcoming the unrealistic or over-simplified assumptions often found in traditional discrete event simulators. In this paper, we present a case study conducted in collaboration with EY, where we apply the HSM to a real-life business process log. This study demonstrates the benefits of the HSM for business process analysis and its potential to improve process performance.

Keywords: Business Process Simulation · Hybrid Simulation · Optimization

1 Introduction

Over the last few years, facilitated by the increasing amount of available data, researchers and analysts have shown interest in applying Business process simulation (BPS) techniques to real-life processes supported by ERP systems or databases. Especially in the healthcare field, numerous case studies have employed the BPS approach. For instance, it has been used to support healthcare managers in capacity management (CM) decisions [8], reduce patient waiting times through optimal physician scheduling [1], or enhance the performance of outpatient clinics by adjusting the number of receptionists, nurses, and doctors [13]. BPS [7] is a widely used and flexible technique

This work was partially supported by the Italian (MUR) under PRIN project PINPOINT Prot. 2020FNEB27, CUP H23C22000280006 and H45E21000210001 and PNRR project FAIR-Future AI Research (PE00000013), under the NRRP MUR program funded by NextGenerationEU.

A. Delgado and T. Slaats (Eds.): ICPM 2024 Workshops, LNBIP 533, pp. 533–545, 2025.
https://doi.org/10.1007/978-3-031-82225-4_39

for analyzing and enhancing business processes. It consists of simulating the behaviour of business processes by defining a simulation model, which extends a basic process model with additional probabilistic information, such as case arrival rates, activity durations, routing probabilities and resource utilisation. This enriched model enables the generation of a large number of process runs, providing valuable insights into process performance and identifying critical areas for improvement. After identifying the critical points of the process, the simulation model can be leveraged to create various what-if scenarios, allowing the assessment of the potential impact of different changes to the process.

In the current state-of-the-art research of BPS, three main approaches can be identified: DDPS (Data-Driven Process Simulation), DL (Deep Learning), and HSM (Hybrid Simulation Models). DDPS simulation models are discrete event simulation (DES) models, constructed using knowledge derived from process execution data, such as event logs [4,11,12]. While DDPS models benefit from their white-box properties and adaptability for what-if scenarios, they often involve unrealistic or oversimplified assumptions during the model-building process, due to the limited expressiveness of the DES simulator. The second group of approaches uses DL models to generate event logs trace by trace, without simulating them collectively [5]. While DL models outperform DDPS in capturing time perspectives, they are black-box models that are not suitable for analyzing simulations or creating what-if scenarios, thus limiting their usefulness for process analysts or managers. Finally, *Dsim* (DeepSimulator) [6] and RIMS (Runtime Integration Machine Learning Simulation) [9] represent hybrid simulation methods. The main idea here is to retain a white-box simulation model, as in DDPS, but enhance it with information provided by DL models. In particular, an HSM model is defined by a BPS model integrating DL models for one or more simulation parameters [9]. Finally, [6,9] demonstrate that the combinations of DDPS and DL approaches outperform the performance of each individual method.

In this paper, we present a case study conducted in collaboration with EY, where we apply the HSM approach to a real purchase-to-pay (P2P) process. Specifically, the data pertains to the *order-to-goods receipt* and *invoice-to-payment* segments of the P2P process. After extracting event logs from an ERP system based on SAP, we use them to create the HSM model. This model provides an accurate representation of the real process and enables us to analyze and evaluate potential performance improvements. The HSM model facilitates the identification of critical points in both the current process and potential overloaded scenarios, particularly in terms of waiting times. Finally, we demonstrate how the simulation model can be used to evaluate potential solutions for addressing the critical points identified in the process.

The remainder of the paper is structured as follows. First, Sect. 2 introduces the HSM approach, followed by Related Work (Sect. 3). Section 4 details the methodology applied and describes the case study. Section 5 presents the analysis and explores various what-if scenarios based on the previously defined HSM model. Finally, Sect. 6 concludes the paper.

2   Hybrid Simulation Model

A simulation model $\mathcal{M} = (\mathcal{N}, \mathcal{P})$, is composed of a business process model $\mathcal{N}$ (e.g., a BPMN), and a set of simulation parameters $\mathcal{P} = \{\mathcal{P}_R, \mathcal{P}_T, \mathcal{P}_C, \mathcal{P}_S\}$. These parameters

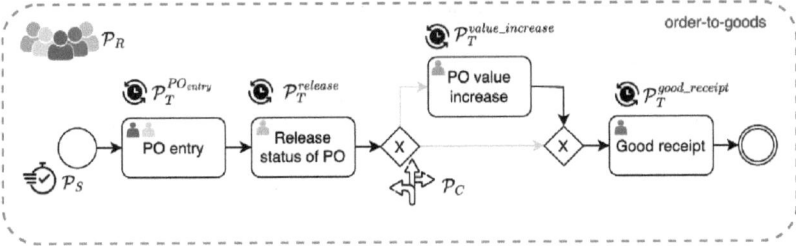

Fig. 1. Simulation model of order-to-goods process, composed of BPMN model ($\mathcal{N}$) and simulation parameters related to the resource ($\mathcal{P}_R$), time ($\mathcal{P}_T$), control flow ($\mathcal{P}_C$), and inter-arrival time ($\mathcal{P}_S$) perspectives.

address the resource, time, control flow, and inter-arrival time perspectives, respectively. Consider the simulation model in Fig. 1 of an order-to-goods process, composed of a BPMN model and the respective simulation parameters. $\mathcal{P}_R$ contains the five resources involved in the process and indicates the respective activities they can perform. For instance, the PO entry activity can be performed by gray and light green resources. The simulation time parameter, $\mathcal{P}_T$, defines the processing time needed to complete each activity in $\mathcal{N}$, such as $\mathcal{P}_T^{PO\ entry} \in \mathcal{P}_T$ which specifies the processing time for PO entry. Finally, $\mathcal{P}_S$ defines the rate at which orders arrive in the process and, $\mathcal{P}_C$ determines the path of the order, i.e., whether the PO value increase activity is executed or not.

HSM differs from DES simulation models by incorporating one or more predictive models into the simulation parameters, each addressing different aspects of the process. Predictive models are typically applied to $\mathcal{P}_T$ and $\mathcal{P}_S$ parameters [6,9], as they can capture the relationship between different trace elements and the distribution of output variables. Unlike probability distributions used in DES models, which do not consider previous activities, assigned resources or other attributes of the event, this approach aims to enhance simulation accuracy and address the often unrealistic or oversimplified assumptions of DES, which arise from the limitations of its simulation parameters.

Once $\mathcal{M}$ is defined, the traces composing a simulated log $\mathcal{L}^{sim}$ are generated by executing the model. Essentially, HSM models are discrete event simulation (DES) models that use stochastic methods to generate new traces based on inter-arrival times defined by $\mathcal{P}_S$. Each trace is simulated according to the control-flow semantics of the process model ($\mathcal{N}$) and the probabilities or predictions specified by $\mathcal{P}_C$. Events are simulated with respect to the resource allocation for all traces in execution. A task is executed only if it is enabled and a resource is available. If no resource is available, the activity waits until the required resource is released and starts immediately once it becomes available. Resource availability can also be constrained by calendars that define the resource schedules, such as Monday to Friday, 9:00–18:00. Therefore, when calendars are included in $\mathcal{P}_R$, a resource can only perform a task if it is not already busy and if it falls within the time frame designated by its calendar. Finally, $\mathcal{P}_T$ defines the processing time of each task and any potential waiting time between tasks, excluding delays caused by resource contention and the presence of resource calendars. The exe-

Table 1. Event logs.

Log	#Traces	#Events	#Activity	#Resources	#Variants	Avg. trace length	Mean case Duration	Median case Duration	Log Timeframe
$\mathcal{L}^{PO}$	425	5810	34	27	108	6.82	3.97yrs	4.4yrs	12.57yrs
$\mathcal{L}^{IN}$	2762	5470	18	18	97	1.98	2.2mths	2.25 h	12.07yrs
$\mathcal{L}^{G}$	372	3835	25	112	125	10.31	1.88yrs	6.8mths	10.92yrs

cution of each activity is recorded in $\mathcal{L}^s$ as an event that composes a trace. Finally, the cycle time of a completed trace is calculated as the difference between the timestamps of the last and first events in the trace.

3   Related Work

The BPS simulation model is a well-known method for optimizing and evaluating possible scenarios, especially in healthcare processes, where the allocation of resources during shift work plays a crucial role in minimizing waiting times for services offered. Van Hulzen et al. in [8] present a real-life case study at the radiology department of a Belgium hospital, aiming to recommend solutions to capacity management (CM) regarding the required number of radiology devices, waiting area size, and reception staffing. Similarly, [13] improves the performance of the outpatient clinic process by redesigning the resource distribution and capacity of roles. Antunes et al. [1], on the other hand, used the simulation model to evaluate the schedule derived from optimization. The approaches described in [8] and [13] are not fully automated in creating simulation models and require expert intervention during the process. However, process experts often lack complete knowledge of the process and rely on data-driven approaches to analyze and detect non-compliant behavior. In addition, the DES simulation models defined in [8,13] and [1] present several oversimplifications of the simulation parameters due to the limitations of the simulator employed. The HSM approach allows us to overcome the latter simplifications and enables the definition of the simulation model with the support of process experts or by discovering all the information directly from the data.

4   Methodology

In this section we describe the different steps of the case study as the pipeline reported in Fig. 2. The aim of the pipeline is to analyze and improve two interconnected real processes recorded from a real ERP system based on SAP. First, the pipeline starts by extracting data from the ERP system and converting it into standard event logs, as described in Sect. 4.1. Event logs are then used to create an HSM model suitable for RIMS$_{Tool}$ [10], a hybrid business process simulator. Finally, in the last step, we exploit the simulation model to analyze the process performance under heavy load and to improve it by creating various what-if scenarios (Sect. 5). While t he extraction and

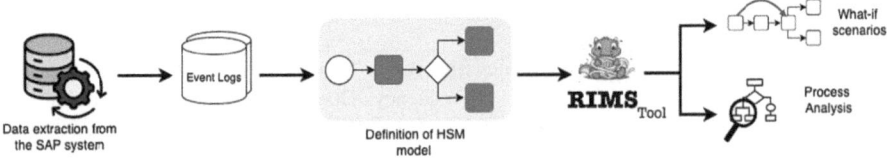

Fig. 2. Pipeline of the methodology applied to the case study

definition of the HSM with our framework can be generalized to other process models, being fully automated starting from the data, the analysis and what-if scenarios are specific of the process itself.

4.1 Data Extraction

The SAP application tracks user changes to application data, storing these records as *change documents* in the database. Each *change document* is uniquely identified and reports the changes made by a single user through a specific *transaction*, a term used in SAP to refer to an application. A *transaction* relates to a particular business object, such as vendor master data, an order, or an accounting document. Specifically, *change document* may include updates to several database tables linked to the business object, like order headers and lines. The modified field is used to assign an activity identifier to the operation. For instance, if the due date field is altered, an activity like Due date delay or Due date anticipate is assigned based on comparing the previous and new values. Finally, EY employs a non-reversible algorithm to anonymize and convert this data directly into an event log in XES format, without the need for manual processing. Anonymization is applied only to information referring to resources or companies and their descriptions. These values are replaced with random ones, maintaining a 1:1 relationship with the originals to preserve resource workloads and social networks.

The extracted event logs, denoted as $\mathcal{L}$, capture the execution of *change documents* for the business object as a series of ordered events. A trace, in turn, contains the ordered events related to the same business object, which is identified by a unique case ID. The latter may also include trace attributes, which remain constant across the events, such as the vendor code, the released value, or the order type. Events contain additional attributes that identify the timestamp and the user who performed the activities. Therefore, each event is a detailed structure that includes the activity label, its timestamp, and the resource(s) involved in the activity. In our case, the extraction process can retrieve non-instantaneous events, meaning both the start and end timestamps are recorded. This structured representation of events in the event log provides a comprehensive view of the business process execution, enabling detailed analysis and allowing us to define a hybrid simulation model.

4.2 Case Study and Data Description

The data considered in this case study pertains to the purchase-to-pay (P2P) process related to subcontracting in the construction and real estate industry. Specifically, we

Table 2. Activities descriptions

Activity	Process	Frequency	Relative Frequency	Mean Duration	Median Duration	Max Duration
PO entry	PO	425	14.63%	1.82 h	2.1 h	2.25 h
Release status of PO	PO	1507	51.87%	1.70 h	2 h	2.25 h
Good receipt	PO	828	28.5%	1.73 h	2 h	2.25 h
Invoice entry	IN	387	7.07%	2 h	2.25 h	2.25 h
Payment release	IN	1623	29.67%	1.82 h	2 h	2 h
Post clearing	IN	2779	50.8%	1.82 h	2 h	2.25 h
Due date delay	IN	138	2.52%	1.75 h	2 h	2 h

analyze three types of logs, as detailed in Table 1: one for the order-to-goods receipt part ($\mathcal{L}^{PO}$), another for the invoice-to-payment part ($\mathcal{L}^{IN}$), and a third that encompasses the entire order-to-payment process ($\mathcal{L}^{G}$). $\mathcal{L}^{G}$ is retrieved by combining the traces that are present in both $\mathcal{L}^{PO}$ and $\mathcal{L}^{IN}$, using their case IDs. Therefore, $\mathcal{L}^{G}$ in Table 1 contains only a subset of the orders, excluding the incomplete ones present in $\mathcal{L}^{PO}$ and $\mathcal{L}^{IN}$ that affect the log timeframes. Although the *PO* and *IN* processes belong to the same purchase-to-pay (P2P) process at different stages, they operate independently of each other. Therefore, we use the individual logs to discover the simulation model for each process i.e. *PO* and *IN* processes, as they contain more traces and events, as shown in Table 1. Meanwhile, we use the global log to understand how these processes interact within the overall P2P system.

Figure 3 provides a simplified representation of the main activities in the two processes, *PO* and *IN*. The *PO* process begins with the creation of a new order, represented as PO entry. The order may transit through 7 different statuses, triggered by activities such as Release status of PO changed in 0/1/2/3/4/5/6. Following this, the client or company may adjust the order's value with PO value increase. Finally, when the goods are delivered, the Goods Receipt activity is recorded. The delivery may occur in multiple instalments over time, resulting in several records of the same activity. The *IN* process starts on average one month after the order has been created and approved. In particular, different activities can be performed to finalize the order, such as Invoice entry and Payment release, to proceed with the payment, which may include deferrals or payment in instalments.

From Table 1 and Table 2, we can observe that the average case duration is on the order of years for the *PO* process and months for the *IN* process, even though the main activities last at most two hours. This suggests that the waiting times between activities significantly impact the overall cycle times. Waiting times between activities may occur for various reasons. The main causes are typically resource contention when a resource is occupied by other activities, and the work schedules of the resources themselves, as explained in Sect. 2. However, in an *PO* process like our case study, waiting times are closely tied to the size and value of the order, as well as the requests, especially when the orders concern urbanisation contracts, which may require years to complete.

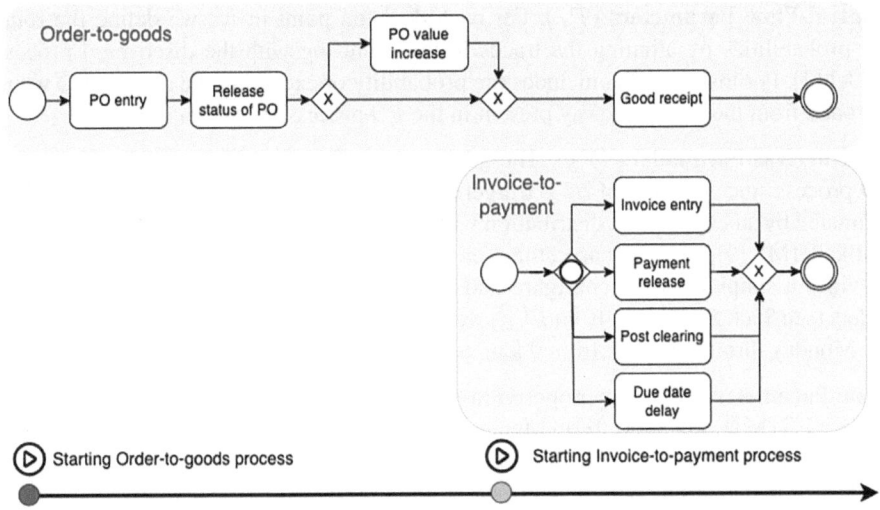

Fig. 3. Interaction between the *Order-to-goods* (PO) and *Invoice-to-payment* (IN) processes.

In the *IN* process, delays can be influenced by payment extensions, delays, or potential changes to the final invoice but also by the nature of the process itself. In fact, in the construction and real estate industry, invoices are typically closed by the customer only after verifying the proper fulfillment of various guarantees by the supplier, which generally takes a long time. Indeed, $\mathcal{L}^{PO}$ log includes only traces that began within 6 months (from February 2010 to August 2010), but 36% of these traces continue for over 5 years.

4.3 Definition of Hybrid Business Process Simulation

In this section, we describe how we define the HSM model using the extracted event logs, as detailed in Sect. 4.1. In particular, we outline the methods for discovering all elements of $\mathcal{M}$, including the process model $\mathcal{N}$ and the set of simulation parameters $\mathcal{P}$. To define the HSM model, we follow the approach proposed by RIMS [9], which is compatible with RIMS$_{Tool}$ [10] and allows us to customize the simulation parameters to properly represent our case study. Specifically, RIMS$_{Tool}$ requires as input a Petri net process model and the corresponding simulation parameters, which can be specified either through the tool's configuration or by defining specific ones.

Process Model ($\mathcal{N}$). To define $\mathcal{N}$, we first derive $\mathcal{N}^{PO}$ from $\mathcal{L}^{PO}$ and $\mathcal{N}^{IN}$ from $\mathcal{L}^{IN}$, as BPMN models, using the SplitMiner algorithm [2]. Then from $\mathcal{L}^{G}$, we identify the interactions between the two processes by the definition of the final $\mathcal{N}$. Specifically, we define when the *IN* process begins to handle the order that was processed by the first one, as shown in Fig. 3. Subsequently, the two processes continue their execution in parallel. This approach allows us to create a unified process model while maintaining the independence of each process. Finally, $\mathcal{N}$ is transformed into a Petri net model as required by RIMS$_{Tool}$.

Control-Flow Parameters ($\mathcal{P}_C$). For each decision point in $\mathcal{N}$, we define the routing probabilities by aligning the traces in the event log with the discovered process model [4]. For instance, $\mathcal{P}_C$ includes the probability of executing the activity PO value increase from the XOR gateway present in the *PO* process, as shown in Fig. 3.

Inter-arrival Parameters ($\mathcal{P}_S$). The arrival time of a new trace is defined only for *PO* process since the start of *IN* is triggered by the first. The creation of a new order is estimated by an exponential distribution with a mean of 10 hours as we observe in $\mathcal{L}^{PO}$. Unlike RIMS [9], we do not use a time series to estimate $\mathcal{P}_S$, as the distribution function provides a simpler way to configure and evaluate the process with a high volume of orders (see Sect. 5). Finally, from $\mathcal{L}^{PO}$, we also identify a calendar that restricts arrivals i.e. Monday through Friday, from 9 a.m. to 6 p.m.

Time Parameters ($\mathcal{P}_T$). As proposed in [6,9], the $\mathcal{P}_T$ parameter is defined using two distinct LSTM (Long Short-Term Memory) models: one for predicting activity processing times and another for predicting waiting times between activities. These predictions are based on the current activity (for processing times) or the next activity (for waiting times), along with additional attributes such as the timestamp of the current activity, the day of the week, and inter-case features like work-in-progress and resource occupancy.

Resource Parameters ($\mathcal{P}_R$). The resources involved in the simulation model are defined in $\mathcal{P}_R$. From $\mathcal{L}^G$, we observe that the resources involved are not shared among the two processes. Therefore, even though we define a unified simulation model, we keep the resources distinct from each other. In particular, resources are grouped into roles based on the activities they are allowed to perform by applying the method proposed in [3] to event logs. From $\mathcal{L}^{PO}$, six different roles are identified, while $\mathcal{L}^{IN}$ reveals five roles.

Finally, we set the number of traces generated in the initial HSM to 2000,[1] and the start timestamp of the simulation is aligned with that of $\mathcal{L}^{PO}$

5   Analysis and Improving

In this section, using the HSM model defined in Sect. 2, we first analyze the performance of the current process and its response to an increased order load, focusing on the waiting times, which significantly impact the cycle times in our case study. Based on the results of this analysis, we evaluate two what-if scenarios ($w1$ and $w2$) to determine whether they can reduce the process waiting times. Finally, $w1$ and $w2$ are validated by process experts as achievable what-if scenarios. For each scenario we performed 10 simulations and the reported results are the mean values from all simulations.

5.1   Analysis of Waiting Times

As mentioned in Sect. 4.2, both processes exhibit significant waiting times, as evidenced by the large final cycle times of the traces compared to the processing times of the main

---

[1] As reported in Table 1, each log contains a different number of traces. Therefore, we assume 2000 as a plausible number of traces. For the same reason, a direct comparison between $\mathcal{L}^{sim}$ and the original logs $\mathcal{L}^{PO}$, $\mathcal{L}^{IN}$, and $\mathcal{L}^G$ is not feasible.

Table 3. Analysis of the results of the increased order load.

Log	#Traces	Median Cycle Times	Mean Waiting Times	Median Waiting Times	Mean Queue	Median Queue
$\mathcal{L}^{sim}$	2000	8.10mnths	41d	0.07d	0.009	0
$\mathcal{L}^{+25\%}$	2500	8.87mnths	42d	0.065d	0.014	0
$\mathcal{L}^{+50\%}$	3000	8.41mnths	40d	0.067d	0.013	0
$\mathcal{L}^{+75\%}$	3500	8.17mnths	39d	0.071d	0.013	0

activities (Table 1 and Table 2). Before attempting to optimize process performance in terms of waiting times, we need to identify which aspects of the process can be modified to create plausible what-if scenarios. For example, waiting times caused by external factors or the processing time of activities dictated by procedures to be followed cannot be changed. In our case study, potential optimizations to reduce waiting times may involve reallocating resources to better manage congestion within the process or making minor adjustments to the control flow.

To verify that the waiting times are not due to resource contention but are inherent to the process itself, we increase the number of traces simulated in the HSM model by 25%, 50%, and 75% compared to the initial setting, by defining three what-if scenarios $\mathcal{M}^{25\%}$, $\mathcal{M}^{50\%}$ and $\mathcal{M}^{75\%}$. Table 3 compares the queue, cycle and waiting times of the resulting simulated logs. Despite the substantial increase in the number of traces handled by the process, performance remains largely unchanged (Table 3).

Therefore, to minimize the waiting times in the process, we should focus on the control-flow perspective rather than rethinking the allocation of resources within roles. To pinpoint where waiting times are most prevalent related to the control-flow, we generated the heatmap plots displayed in Fig. 4(a) and 5(a) to represent their distribution in $\mathcal{L}^{sim}$. Figure 4(a) illustrates the median waiting times, in days, between one activity and those directly following it in the *PO* process, while Fig. 5(a) does the same for the *IN* process. For instance, when Goods Receipt activity is directly followed by Change Requestor in $\mathcal{L}^{sim}$ the median for the waiting times is 156 days (Fig. 5(a)). Regarding the *PO* process we can observe that we have a strong presence of waiting times between the activity ⟨Good Receipt, Change PO requestor⟩, ⟨Good Receipt, Good Receipt⟩ and, finally, ⟨Release status of PO changed in 0, Release status of PO changed in 6⟩. For the first two pairs of activities, the waiting times are closely associated with the type of order and the specific goods requested. In contrast, the waiting times for the last pair of activities are related to the various stages the order may pass through before the goods are dispatched. On the other hand, for the *IN* process, the waiting times are more prevalent between the ⟨Payment Release, Reset Invoice Clearing⟩ and ⟨Payment Release, Post Clearing⟩ activities. Therefore, the activities that generate the most waiting times are those related to authorizing and executing payments.

5.2 Definition of What-If Scenarios

Starting from the analysis presented in Sect. 5.1, we define two what-if scenarios—one for each process—with the goal of minimizing waiting times and, consequently,

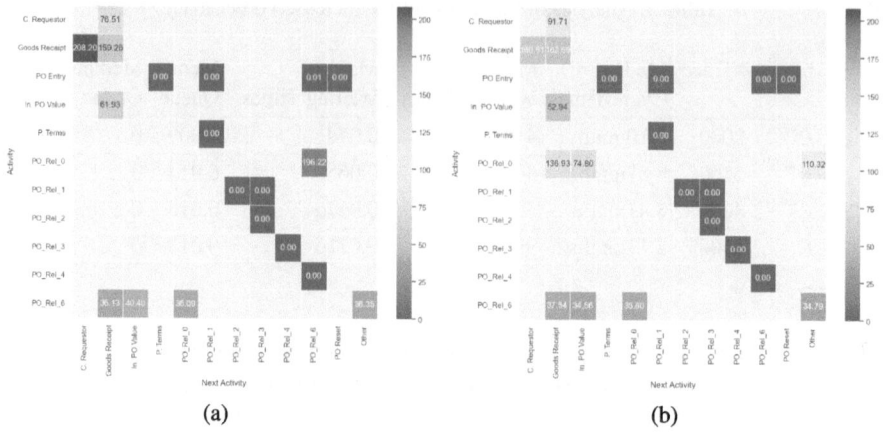

Fig. 4. Heatmap representing the median waiting times, in days, between *PO* activities performed in $\mathcal{L}^{sim}$ and $\mathcal{L}^{sim}_{w1}$.

reducing the overall cycle times of the traces. For the *PO* process, we aim to minimise the waiting time between ⟨Release status of PO changed in 0, Release status of PO changed in 6⟩, as Fig. 4(a) shows that the waiting times between ⟨Release status of PO changed in 6,Release status of PO changed in 0⟩, by contrast, are lower. Therefore, as our first what-if scenario $\mathcal{M}^{w1}$, we modified the initial simulation model to ensure that the activity Release status of PO changed in 0 is executed before the activity Release status of PO changed in 6. The simulated log $\mathcal{L}^{sim}_{w1}$ is obtained from the simulation of $\mathcal{M}^{w1}$, and the resulting waiting times are shown in Fig. 4(b).

Since the position of Release status of PO changed in 0 is modified in $\mathcal{M}^{w1}$, this activity is now followed by different ones compared to the initial simulation model $\mathcal{M}$. Indeed, Fig. 4(b) shows new directly follow relations between activities in the *PO* process, such as ⟨Release status of PO changed in 0, Goods receipt⟩, ⟨Release status of PO changed in 0, Invoice PO value⟩, and ⟨Release status of PO changed in 0, Other⟩. Specifically, for these new relations, we observe moderate waiting times, indicating that the high waiting times originally associated with ⟨Release status of PO changed in 0, Release status of PO changed in 6⟩ are redistributed. As a result, the median cycle times of traces in $\mathcal{L}^{sim}_{w1}$ remain similar to those in $\mathcal{L}^{sim}$ without any statistically significant difference, at 7.92 months and 8.10 months, respectively (see Table 3). Therefore, the application of the $w1$ what-if scenario in the real process should be evaluated by the process owner based on their preferences regarding the distribution of waiting times, taking into account factors such as client satisfaction and costs.

The second what-if scenario ($w2$) defined for the *IN* concerns the activities ⟨Payment Release, Reset Invoice Clearing⟩. In the process model $\mathcal{N}$ contained in $\mathcal{M}$, the execution of the activity Reset Invoice Clearing in $\mathcal{L}^{PO}$ is always followed by the activity Post Clearing. Thus, we hypothesise to postpone the execution of Reset Invoice Clearing with the Post Clearing activity. Specifically, whenever Reset Invoice Clearing occurs in the process, it is combined with Post Clearing and performed as a single activity, with the processing time being the sum of the individual processing times.

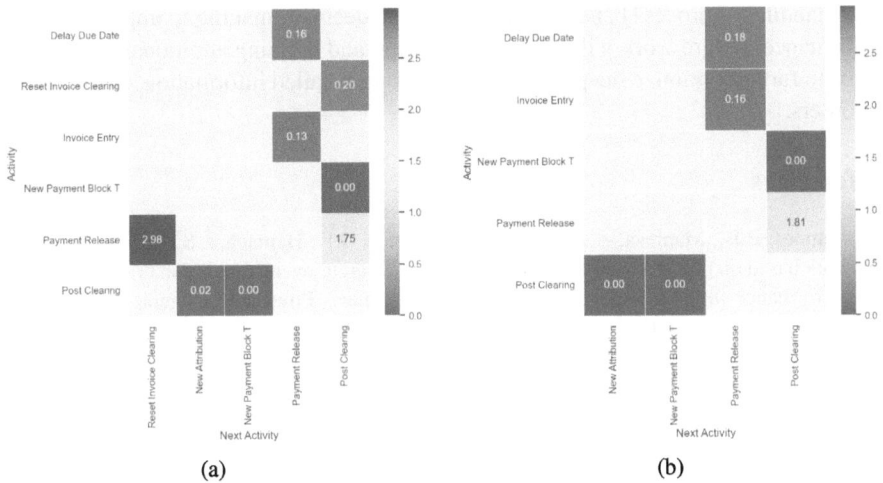

Fig. 5. Heatmap representing the median waiting times, in days, between *IN* activities performed in $\mathcal{L}^{sim}$ and $\mathcal{L}^{sim}_{w2}$.

Figure 5(b) shows the resulting waiting times in $\mathcal{L}^{sim}_{w2}$, which is generated by running $\mathcal{M}^{w2}$. With the what-if scenario $w2$ we are able to eliminate the waiting times between Payment Release and Reset Invoice Clearing without a relevant increase of the waiting times on ⟨Payment Release, Post Clearing⟩. In this case, we do not observe a reduction in the median cycle times in $\mathcal{L}^{sim}_{w2}$ because Reset Invoice Clearing is not a frequent activity and therefore does not impact most traces. However, Fig. 5(b) shows that scenario $w2$ effectively reduces waiting times, which, in turn, lowers costs and resource utilization, as the two activities are performed together.

6   Conclusion

In this paper, we present the results of a case study conducted in collaboration with EY, focusing on the application of Hybrid Simulation Model (HSM) approach to enhance the analysis and improvement of business processes within a real purchase-to-pay (P2P) process. Leveraging event logs extracted from an ERP system, we developed an HSM model that accurately reflects the actual process, without the need for prior domain knowledge. The HSM model enabled us to analyze the process and identify critical points, particularly concerning waiting times. Building on the identified weaknesses, we demonstrated how to define and evaluate two what-if scenarios to reduce these waiting times. Moreover, we demonstrated the ability and flexibility of the HSM approach to generate various what-if scenarios. This capability proved invaluable for assessing the potential impact of different changes and proposing targeted solutions to optimize performance. The limitation of our approach lies in its inability to represent external factors, as well as information absent from the event log, that influence process performance. These factors cannot be simulated and are therefore not addressable in a what-if scenario for potential optimization. Nevertheless, we show that the HSM approach offers a powerful tool for process managers and analysts, facilitating a detailed understanding of process behavior and supporting decision-making to improve process performance. Future work will focus on exploring and defining additional what-if scenarios to further optimize the process, incorporating detailed information about individual orders.

References

1. Antunes, B.B., Manresa, A., Bastos, L.S., Marchesi, J.F., Hamacher, S.: A solution framework based on process mining, optimization, and discrete-event simulation to improve queue performance in an emergency department. In: Business Process Management Workshops: BPM 2019 International Workshops, Vienna, Austria, 1–6 September 2019, Revised Selected Papers 17, pp. 583–594. Springer (2019)
2. Augusto, A., Conforti, R., Dumas, M., La Rosa, M., Polyvyanyy, A.: Split miner: automated discovery of accurate and simple business process models from event logs. Knowl. Inf. Syst. **59**, 251–284 (2019)
3. Burattin, A., Sperduti, A., Veluscek, M.: Business models enhancement through discovery of roles. In: 2013 IEEE Symposium on Computational Intelligence and Data Mining (CIDM), pp. 103–110. IEEE (2013)
4. Camargo, M., Dumas, M., González-Rojas, O.: Automated discovery of business process simulation models from event logs. Decis. Support Syst. **134**, 113284 (2020)
5. Camargo, M., Dumas, M., Rojas, O.G.: Learning accurate LSTM models of business processes. In: Business Process Management - 17th International Conference, BPM, Proceedings. LNCS, vol. 11675, pp. 286–302. Springer (2019)
6. Camargo, M., Dumas, M., Rojas, O.G.: Learning accurate business process simulation models from event logs via automated process discovery and deep learning. In: Advanced Information Systems Engineering - 34th International Conference, CAiSE 2022, Proceedings. LNCS, vol. 13295, pp. 55–71. Springer (2022)
7. Dumas, M., La Rosa, M., Mendling, J., Reijers, A.H.: Fundamentals of Business Process Management. Springer (2018)
8. van Hulzen, G., Martin, N., Depaire, B., Souverijns, G.: Supporting capacity management decisions in healthcare using data-driven process simulation. J. Biomed. Inform. **129**, 104060 (2022)
9. Meneghello, F., Di Francescomarino, C., Ghidini, C.: Runtime integration of machine learning and simulation for business processes. In: 5th International Conference on Process Mining, ICPM 2023, pp. 9–16. IEEE (2023)
10. Meneghello, F., Francescomarino, C.D., Ghidini, C.: Rims_tool: a hybrid simulator for business processes. In: van der Werf, J.M.E.M., Cabanillas, C., Leotta, F., Genga, L. (eds.) Doctoral Consortium and Demo Track 2023 at the International Conference on Process Mining 2023 co-located with the 5th International Conference on Process Mining (ICPM 2023), Rome, Italy, 27 October 2023. CEUR Workshop Proceedings, vol. 3648. CEUR-WS.org (2023)
11. Pourbafrani, M., van Zelst, S.J., van der Aalst, W.M.P.: Supporting automatic system dynamics model generation for simulation in the context of process mining. In: Business Information Systems - BIS 2020. LNBIP, vol. 389, pp. 249–263. Springer (2020)
12. Rozinat, A., Mans, R.S., Song, M., van der Aalst, W.M.P.: Discovering simulation models. Inf. Syst. **34**, 305–327 (2009)
13. Zhou, Z., Wang, Y., Li, L.: Process mining based modeling and analysis of workflows in clinical care-a case study in a Chicago outpatient clinic. In: Proceedings of the 11th IEEE International Conference on Networking, Sensing and Control, pp. 590–595. IEEE (2014)

Leveraging Process Mining on the Shop Floor: An Exploratory Study

Felix Rothhagen[1]([✉])(iD), Felix Kerst[1](iD), Eduard Kant Mandal[1](iD),
Candan Çetin[1,2](iD), and Carolin Ullrich[2](iD)

[1] Technical University of Munich, Arcisstraße 21, 80333 Munich, Germany
{felix.rothhagen,ga94tix,kant.mandal,candan.cetin}@tum.de
[2] Celonis SE, Theresienstraße 6, 80333 Munich, Germany
c.ullrich@celonis.com

Abstract. This paper explores the potential and limitations of process mining on the shop floor in the manufacturing industry. Despite its increasing popularity, the application of process mining in manufacturing remains under-explored. Through a combination of systematic literature review and interviews with 22 industry experts, academicians, shop floor workers, and production managers, we identify key areas where process mining can be leveraged on the shop floor. Our findings can be grouped into five dimensions: organizational management & human factors, data management & quality, digitalization & technology advancements, process efficiency & optimization, and production & supply chain complexity. The findings offer a comprehensive understanding of how process mining can be leveraged to improve manufacturing processes while also addressing the organizational and technical hurdles that may impede its adoption. This study contributes to the emerging field of process science by combining findings from the literature and collecting voices on and around the shop floor. The paper closes by proposing future research and practice by incorporating organizational and human insights from the shop floor.

Keywords: Process Mining · Shop Floor · Manufacturing · Interview Study

1 Introduction

Process mining lies at the intersection of process management and data science [1] and was able to demonstrate positive effects on the increase of automation and digitalization, reduction in manual rework rate and throughput times, identification of improvement opportunities, bringing transparency and other areas in organizations of various industries including manufacturing [18]. Due to rapid

---

F. Rothhagen, F. Kerst, and E. K. Mandal—These authors contributed equally to this work.

© The Author(s) 2025
A. Delgado and T. Slaats (Eds.): ICPM 2024 Workshops, LNBIP 533, pp. 546–558, 2025.
https://doi.org/10.1007/978-3-031-82225-4_40

technological advancements and globalization, the competition in the manufacturing sector is high [3]. This requires manufacturing companies to achieve optimal production efficiency and streamline processes to maintain their competitive edge [3].

To do so, manufacturing companies can use process mining to improve the organization of processes efficiently and support production planning. Specifically, an interesting area of application is on the shop floor, where the primary operational activity takes place. While some manufacturing companies have already adopted and benefited from process mining [3,7,20,21], a systematic review of its application is missing [4,6]. Still, in the last decade, the number of academic publications on the use of process mining on the shop floor has increased considerably. An examination of databases such as Scopus, EBSCO, and Web of Science reveals a marked increase in publications on this topic, with 44 new publications appearing after 2014, compared to only 4 before that year. However, compared to other industries, we see less research output for the manufacturing industry. The number of publications in the same databases for another field, like process mining in healthcare, has been over 780 in the last decade.

To better understand the current use of process mining in the manufacturing sector, this paper aims to answer the following research question: *"What opportunities does process mining bring to the operational settings on the shop floor?"*. To address the research question, we first conducted a systematic literature review, followed by qualitative research. The qualitative research was carried out through semi-structured interviews with 22 participants, who were categorized into the following personas: academicians, industry experts, shop floor workers, and production managers. The rationale for this sequence and the reasons behind our methodological choices are detailed in the methodology section. As an outcome, this paper identifies seven aggregated dimensions of process mining on the shop floor, five of which are discussed in this paper, including insights on the technologies' possibilities and limitations when applied in the industry.

The rest of the paper is structured as follows. Section 2 presents the related work. Section 3 describes and illustrates the research methodology. Section 4 presents the findings of the paper. Followed by Sect. 5, where we discuss the findings and the limitations of our work. Finally, Sect. 6 concludes the paper.

2   Related Work

Our research focuses on the application areas and challenges of process mining in manufacturing, particularly on the shop floor. We define the shop floor as the physical space where production activities occur, including assembly, machining, and material handling [9]. Despite the growing interest in process mining and interview studies [24], the literature specifically addressing its application on the shop floor remains notably limited. As the shop floor is part of an organization's production and supply chain, use cases and challenges have already been reported selectively in other papers.

One of the first publications looking into challenges in the production context is from Natschläger et al. [11]. The authors develop an innovative algorithm to address the complex data structures inherent in production lines, overcoming the limitations of existing algorithms. Subsequent research has explored diverse applications of process mining in manufacturing, with Netto et al. [12], Santos et al. [20], and Pourbafrani et al. [14] addressing maintenance prediction, failure diagnosis, and production performance respectively. These studies highlight process mining's potential to improve operations despite challenges like data complexity and real-time monitoring needs.

Stertz et al. [21] explore the implementation of process mining in small and medium-sized manufacturing companies. The paper emphasizes the need to address infrastructure and data collection challenges early in the implementation process. While Stertz et al. [21] touch upon the potential perception of process mining as a threat by shop floor workers, the literature examining the specific perspectives of these workers about process mining remains notably scarce.

Examining individual case studies reveals indications of challenges when implementing process mining in manufacturing, which are inherent in the characteristics of the shop floor environment, being fast-paced with a complex process structure and work steps executed by humans [9]. Concurrently, there is a notable accumulation of successful case studies that indicate a significant potential for process mining on the shop floor.

3   Research Method

Our methodology comprises a systematic literature review (see Fig. 1) and semi-structured interviews. The literature review synthesized existing research with a sole focus on shop floor-related operations, as highlighted in previous studies such as Natschläger et al. [11] and Stertz et al. [21]. To fill the gap in understanding the human and operational challenges faced by workers on the shop floor, we complemented this with semi-structured interviews, capturing real-world perspectives directly from industry practitioners. Each phase is conducted with an evaluation based on predefined inclusion and exclusion criteria. Additional information on the data collection and analysis can be found in the supplementary material available on Zenodo [19].

3.1   Literature

The initial step of the literature review involved forward and backward research based on Dreher et al. [6], which conducted a systematic literature review on process mining within the full supply chain. This paper was considered a key article because it includes a broad scope that allows us to identify and focus on the specific aspects of process mining relevant to the shop floor. In the backward research step, we specifically reviewed the references cited in this article that pertained to the shop floor. This step aimed to trace the foundational studies that have significantly contributed to the understanding and application of process

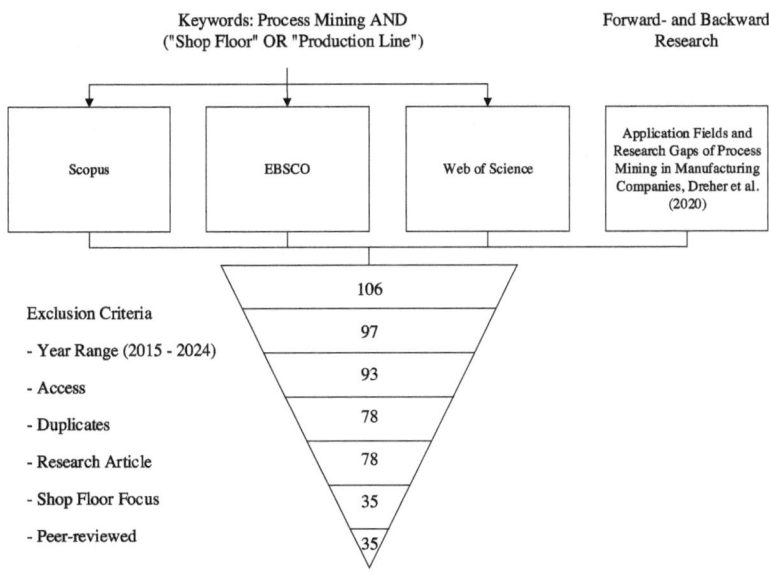

Fig. 1. Methodology for Literature Research and Interview-Based Insights

mining in the context of the shop floor. By examining these references, we identified 40 relevant articles. In the forward research step, we identified subsequent studies that have cited this key article via Google Scholar. This step focused on capturing recent developments and ongoing research trends that build upon the foundational study, resulting in an additional 21 articles. Together, this culminated in a total of 61 articles identified as relevant.

We conducted a systematic keyword-based literature review by following a scoping review. Following Paré et al. [13], we developed a review plan and research question, established a search strategy, and documented our search terms and methods. We selected the search term "process mining" AND ("shop floor" OR "production line") to reflect the most commonly used phrases for process mining in operational settings. Avoiding broader search terms such as "manufacturing" ensured that the findings remained highly relevant and specific to the shop floor activities. We excluded purchasing activities, which are part of the production process but do not directly involve shop floor operations and thus were outside this research's scope.

We searched three academic databases: EBSCO Business Source Complete, Scopus, and Web of Science. This resulted in 45 articles, increasing the total number of articles identified to 106. We filtered these articles based on exclusion and inclusion criteria. Articles published between 2015 and 2024 were included to ensure the research reflected the latest advancements in the field. Only articles accessible through institutional databases were considered, ensuring that the full text could be reviewed. Duplicate articles across different databases were identified and removed, resulting in a unique set of studies. Only peer-reviewed research articles were included to ensure the credibility of the findings. Articles specifically focusing on the shop floor within manufacturing settings were selected to maintain the research scope's relevance to the operational aspects of manufacturing. After applying these criteria, the number of articles was systematically reduced as follows: from an initial set of 106 articles, 97 articles remained after applying the year range, 93 articles after access checks, 78 articles after removing duplicates, 78 articles confirmed as research articles, and finally, 35 articles focused on the shop floor and peer-reviewed.

3.2   Interviews

We adopted a grounded theory approach to examine process mining challenges on the shop floor, using Gioia's methodology to inductively generate new insights [8]. The perception of the shop floor area was examined from multiple viewpoints during operations. These perspectives included those of academicians, industry experts, shop floor workers, and production managers, representing the four key personas in this study. We aimed to gather insights that could potentially be addressed by applying process mining techniques. For the interviews, we followed a semi-structured approach [8]. In this paper, we utilized the interviewee's work practice as a reference point to prompt participants to discuss their challenges and experiences. The semi-structured questions were divided into four sections: (i) processes and activities, (ii) challenges, (iii) strategy and communication, and (iv) goals aimed at capturing the full context of the shop floor, encompassing all its potentials and challenges.

A sampling approach was followed, with participants recruited through professional networks and via judgmental sampling [22]. We gathered data in the spring of 2024 via in-person and virtual participant interviews. Our study included interviews with two academicians, eleven industry experts, five shop floor workers, and four production managers. The interviews were transcribed using OpenAI's Whisper model [16] and manually verified against audio recordings for accuracy. On average, each interview lasted for 34 min.

The data analysis of the interview data consisted of two phases. First is discovery and narrowing, which includes reading the transcripts and defining a code book for tagging [15]. To facilitate the process of tagging, the tool Taguette was employed. Each interview was tagged by at least two authors, one present at the interview and one not, and all authors collectively participated in revising and refining the codes. The second phase is about enriching and validating the insights from the interviews. The applied Gioia method involves organizing qualitative data into a structured framework that begins with first-order concepts directly reflecting the interviewee's narrative [8]. Concepts are synthesized into theoretically focused second-order themes, which are then consolidated into broader, overarching aggregate dimensions. This hierarchical data structure supports theory development and captures core research findings, progressing from specific insights to more generalized theoretical constructs [8]. As a result, we obtained seven aggregated dimensions supported by 995 statements from the participants.

Table 1. Data Structure Excerpt: Concepts, Themes, and Aggregated Dimensions

1st order concepts	2nd order themes	Aggregated dimensions
Problem solving in cooperation with the team	Optimizations dependent on people	
Different personas think about different optimizations		Organizational management and human factors
New challenges require achieving goals without prior experience	Experimentation and risk-taking	
Shift to agile methods and fail-fast mindset		
Digitalization of end-to-end processes	Need for digitalization in production	
Important to identify gaps in terms of digitalization of processes		Digitalization & technological advancements
In the end only AI will help us to manage the amount of data	Future of AI	
Generative AI can simplify navigation of complex regulations		

4 Findings

The data analysis progressed from first-order concepts to second-order themes, yielding seven aggregate dimensions. Table 1 illustrates this progression for two dimensions. Although all aggregated dimensions provide valuable insights, this findings section concentrates on five aggregate dimensions, each accounting for 15 to 21% of the total mentions. These key aggregated dimensions will be examined in greater detail in the following subsections, presented in order of declining mention percentage. Each aggregated dimension includes representative participant quotes. Participants are identified by persona (A = Academician, I = Industry expert, S = Shop Floor Worker, P = Production manager) followed by a unique number.

4.1 Organizational Management & Human Factors

The main themes included in this aggregate dimension 'organizational management & human factors' are the importance of inter-departmental and inter-company communication, employee enablement for process mining, addressing fears of redundancy, and fostering user engagement.

One reoccurring 2nd order theme was 'Importance of Communication between departments', highlighting the need for precise, timely, and relevant information exchange, including the right information for the current situation. Starting with inter-company communication, this also extends to relationships between companies (e.g., supplier relationships) to better navigate discrepancies within the processes. Participants in our study emphasized that *"cross-functional communication is key between different departments"* (I1) and *"the supply chain needs to communicate any problems to the production so it can be adjusted in time"* (P1).

A further area of 2nd order themes within the 'organizational management & human factors' dimension reveals challenges in employee enablement for process mining, addressing redundancy fears, and fostering user engagement. The study highlights the challenge of developing effective training programs that empower employees while mitigating job security concerns. Balancing formal education with ongoing learning presents another challenge in keeping pace with industry advancements. As one interviewee noted, *"the first solution that gets implemented to the shop floor is a supporting solution"* (I2), suggesting a challenge in introducing gradual improvements. Another challenge lies in clearly communicating the benefits of human-machine interaction, as emphasized by a participant: *"the benefit of human-machine interaction needs to be clear towards the user"* (S1) to ensure engagement.

4.2   Data Management & Quality

The aggregate dimension 'data management & quality' incorporates insights regarding the topic of data quality within the shop floor area. It also stresses the need for data enrichment and interpretation, adding context to raw data to generate actionable insights for industrial business problems.

The study identifies challenges within the 2nd order themes 'data centralization across systems' and 'quality data in one place'. A key challenge lies in centralizing data from diverse systems, including both sensor-generated shop floor data and derived insights, into a single location for broader utilization. The study highlights the need to ensure data specificity, reliability, and relevance to enable accurate conclusions, which may require data-cleaning processes before centralization. Participants emphasized these challenges, with one interviewee noting that *"different data sources need to be unified"* (I3), while another stressed that *"data sets with high quality are important for process mining"* (I4). These findings underscore the complexities in achieving effective data centralization and maintaining data quality in process mining implementations.

The study identifies critical issues within the 2nd order themes 'contextualizing data information' and 'real-time data processing & insights'. A key challenge lies in integrating diverse data sources into existing streams, particularly in connecting business context and manufacturing process information for effective root cause determination. This is especially crucial for operating sequences involving human operations. Another significant hurdle emerges in real-time data processing for process mining, questioning its ability to keep pace with production processes. These challenges are highlighted by interviewees, with one emphasizing that *"contextual information is key as not everything is captured in current production spaces"* (A1), and another noting that *"real-time process mining is desirable, but real-time data processing remains challenging"* (P2).

4.3 Digitalization & Technology Advancements

The aggregate dimension of 'digitalization & technology advancements' emerged as a central theme. This dimension covers future developments in process mining and shop floor applications, emphasizing the importance of digitalization across industries. These aspects, crucial for process mining, are relevant to many digital solutions but are especially vital for advancing process mining in manufacturing.

The 2nd order theme, 'need for digitalization in production,' highlights that process mining can only be effective with digitized processes. Our research findings emphasize the importance of end-to-end digitization, which presents a significant challenge in manufacturing environments. Achieving this comprehensive digital transformation requires substantial investments in technology, training, and infrastructure. As one interviewee noted, illustrating the extent of digitization needed, *"every little parameter change is important to know"* (P3). At the same time, another stressed the prerequisite nature of digitization, stating *"manufacturing must be more digitized before using process mining"* (I5).

The study identifies opportunities and challenges within the 2nd order theme 'Future of AI' for process mining. A key area of focus is the potential role of AI in enabling non-experts to analyze data more effectively, presenting challenges in democratizing data analysis. The study highlights the potential of machine learning in identifying clusters within large data sets. Participants expressed optimism about AI's potential, with one interviewee stating that *"AI will help to improve the workplace"* (I6) and another noting that *"the potential for large language models is considerable"* (P2).

4.4 Process Efficiency & Optimization

A further aggregate dimension that emerged from the data analysis was 'process efficiency & optimization'. This dimension encapsulates the value proposition of process mining as a means of streamlining and enhancing the performance of business processes, providing insights into how organizations can identify inefficiencies, bottlenecks, and potential areas for improvement within their processes.

The 2nd order theme, 'Efficiency & Optimization Challenges in Process Mining', captures productivity problems worked on with process mining. Participants stated that increasing efficiency is a critical goal in producing industries, which can be achieved due to process mining. An interviewee highlighted that with process mining *"increased profits due to better management and planning"* (I4) are possible.

The study identifies challenges within the 2nd order themes 'Process Mining for Enhancing Visibility & Transparency'. A key hurdle lies in leveraging process mining to uncover previously hidden insights into company processes through process discovery and relationship mapping between objects and process steps. The study highlights the complexity of using process mining to *"link different processes and showing problems occurring from them"* (I5) while also *"knowing where everything is"* (I6). Another significant challenge emerges in the 2nd order theme 'Identifying & Improving Bottlenecks', which captures how to effectively identify root causes and facilitate early detection of shop floor problems.

4.5   Production & Supply Chain Complexity

The aggregate dimension 'production & supply chain complexity' encompasses themes related to maintaining a resilient, well-functioning, and uninterrupted supply chain. Additionally, it highlights how the diversity and uniqueness of production processes complicate the ease of use for process mining applications.

Despite the shop floor focus, the study identifies challenges within second-order themes related to supply chain management, including 'complexity of tracking supply chain', 'uninterrupted supply chain', and 'unflexible supply chains'. A key challenge lies in ensuring the timely availability of correct components for production, while end-to-end supply chain tracking remains difficult due to disconnected data systems. Participants emphasized these challenges, with one noting that the *"supply chain environment is complex with many people involved"* (P1) and another observing that *"problems usually come from the supply chain and not the production"* (A2).

The study identifies challenges within the 2nd order themes 'variance of production processes' and 'complexity of production & planning'. A key challenge lies in developing individual approaches for manufacturing lines while maintaining interconnected shop floor processes. Participants emphasized these challenges, with one noting that the *"shop floor is highly complex for process mining"* (I4) and another observing that *"production data variability is inherent even within the same factory for different production lines"* (I7).

In conclusion, based on 22 interviews, our study revealed different challenges, such as the need for inter-organizational and inter-departmental communication and the importance of end-to-end data capturing and centralization while highlighting the complexities of production and supply chain management, each of which must be addressed to effectively implement process mining on the shop floor.

5   Discussion

This section examines the recognized challenges, connects them with existing research, and explores potential solutions that could make the implementation of process mining on the shop floor easier.

Among our findings, a significant cluster of mentions concerns data, primarily falling into the aggregate dimension 'data management & quality', with some data gathering points in the 'digitalization & technology advancements' dimension. Building upon Netto et al.'s [12] findings, IT infrastructure limitations were not prominently mentioned in our study. Our research instead highlights the frequent mention of real-time data streaming as an enabler for expanding process mining into new use cases requiring prompt reactions, aligning with Reinkemeyer's [17] observations on dynamic process mining applications. The findings reveal challenges in implementing process mining within organizations, echoing Martin et al.'s [10] findings on the importance of team composition and requisite skills. Our study aligns with Zimmermann et al.'s findings, emphasizing that training and ongoing education within organizations and educational institutions are crucial for successfully implementing new technologies [25].

Implementing process mining on the shop floor necessitates a comprehensive change management strategy to effectively engage all stakeholders, particularly those directly impacted by the technology. This approach addresses workers' fears of job loss due to technology, promoting user engagement. This finding aligns with Bala et al.'s emphasis on involving users early in the process when introducing process mining and communicating the benefits of the technology [2]. Our findings reinforce Reinkemeyer's [17] assertion that centralizing both structured and unstructured data in one place is pivotal for successful implementation. Furthermore, we underscore the importance of reliable data input for process mining, echoing the sentiments of Hofstede et al. [23], to ensure the accuracy and reliability of analytical outcomes. This imperative extends beyond implementing organizations to encompass software and cloud providers, who are crucial in lowering the entry barriers for process mining on the shop floor.

To summarize, we discovered that various areas are essential to successfully implement process mining on the shop floor. This exploratory study has identified initial patterns, suggesting the need for broader research across diverse industries, personas, and company sizes to validate and extend these findings. We encourage future research to broaden its focus beyond technological solutions, considering the organizational and human implications, and to explore the emerging field of "Process Science" [5].

Our study has limitations typical of interview-based research. Participants might have been influenced by recency biases when reporting on the benefits and challenges of process mining. In addition, desirability bias can potentially emerge in interview studies. Researcher bias may have influenced data collection and analysis, potentially affecting the study's outcomes. Our findings from interviews with recommended participants, primarily from the German market, offer valuable insights but may not be exhaustive due to sampling biases. To enhance validity, future research should consider methodological triangulation to corroborate findings and mitigate potential biases inherent in single-method approaches.

6   Conclusion

Based on 22 interviews with representatives from academia, manufacturing and process mining experts, shop floor workers, and production managers, we identified five core aggregated dimensions around process mining on the shop floor. Our research highlights the importance of organizational and human factors as well as data management and quality for a successful process mining implementation on the shop floor. Successful implementations yield process efficiency and optimization and go hand-in-hand with digitalization and technological advancements in manufacturing companies. Meanwhile, the complex and varied nature of production and supply chain is a challenge for successfully applying process mining at scale.

Acknowledgments. We appreciate the participants' time and shared experiences in this study. We sincerely thank Celonis for their support in making this research possible and Dr. Mario Keiling from the Technical University of Munich for his valuable contributions and guidance throughout the project.

References

1. van der Aalst, W.: Process mining: overview and opportunities. ACM Trans. Manag. Inf. Syst. **3**(2), 17 (2012). https://doi.org/10.1145/2229156.2229157
2. Bala, H., Venkatesh, V.: Adaptation to information technology: a holistic nomological network from implementation to job outcomes. Manag. Sci. **62**(1), 156–179 (2016). https://doi.org/10.1287/mnsc.2014.2111
3. Bettacchi, A., Polzonetti, A., Re, B.: Understanding production chain business process using process mining: a case study in the manufacturing scenario. In: Krogstie, J., Mouratidis, H., Su, J. (eds.) CAiSE 2016. LNBIP, vol. 249, pp. 193–203. Springer, Cham (2016). https://doi.org/10.1007/978-3-319-39564-7_19
4. Birk, A., Wilhelm, Y., Dreher, S., Flack, C., Reimann, P., Gröger, C.: A real-world application of process mining for data-driven analysis of multi-level interlinked manufacturing processes. Procedia CIRP **104**, 417–422 (2021). https://doi.org/10.1016/j.procir.2021.11.070
5. Brocke, J.V., et al.: Process science: the interdisciplinary study of socio-technical change. Process Sci. **2**(1) (2024). https://doi.org/10.1007/s44311-024-00001-5
6. Dreher, S., Reimann, P., Gröger, C.: Application fields and research gaps of process mining in manufacturing companies (2021). https://doi.org/10.18420/INF2020_55
7. Duong, L.T., Travè-Massuyès, L., Subias, A., Roa, N.B.: Assessing product quality from the production process logs. Int. J. Adv. Manuf. Technol. **117**(5–6), 1615–1631 (2021). https://doi.org/10.1007/s00170-021-07764-2
8. Gioia, D.A., Corley, K.G., Hamilton, A.L.: Seeking qualitative rigor in inductive research: notes on the Gioia methodology. Organ. Res. Methods **16**(1), 15–31 (2013). https://doi.org/10.1177/1094428112452151
9. Groover, M.P.: Automation, Production Systems, and Computer-Integrated Manufacturing, 5th edn. Pearson Education (2019)
10. Martin, N., et al.: Opportunities and challenges for process mining in organizations: results of a Delphi study. Bus. Inf. Syst. Eng. **63**(5), 511–527 (2021). https://doi.org/10.1007/s12599-021-00720-0
11. Natschläger, C., Kossak, F., Lettner, C., Geist, V., Denkmayr, A., Käferböck, B.: A practical approach for process mining in production processes. In: Piazolo, F., Geist, V., Brehm, L., Schmidt, R. (eds.) ERP Future 2016. LNBIP, vol. 285, pp. 87–95. Springer, Cham (2017). https://doi.org/10.1007/978-3-319-58801-8_8
12. Kurscheidt Netto, R.J., de F. R. Loures, E., dos Santos, E.A.P.: Enabling the use of shop floor information for multi-criteria decision making in maintenance prediction. In: Tavares Thomé, A.M., Barbastefano, R.G., Scavarda, L.F., Gonçalves dos Reis, J.C., Amorim, M.P.C. (eds.) IJCIEOM 2021. SPMS, vol. 367, pp. 435–447. Springer, Cham (2021). https://doi.org/10.1007/978-3-030-78570-3_33
13. Paré, G., Trudel, M.C., Jaana, M., Kitsiou, S.: Synthesizing information systems knowledge: a typology of literature reviews. Inf. Manag. **52**(2), 183–199 (2015). https://doi.org/10.1016/j.im.2014.08.008

14. Pourbafrani, M., van Zelst, S.J., van der Aalst, W.M.P.: Supporting decisions in production line processes by combining process mining and system dynamics. In: Ahram, T., Karwowski, W., Vergnano, A., Leali, F., Taiar, R. (eds.) IHSI 2020. AISC, vol. 1131, pp. 461–467. Springer, Cham (2020). https://doi.org/10.1007/978-3-030-39512-4_72
15. Pratt, M.G., Rosa, J.A.: Transforming work-family conflict into commitment in network marketing organizations. Acad. Manag. J. **46**(4), 395–418 (2003). https://doi.org/10.2307/30040635
16. Radford, A., Kim, J.W., Xu, T., Brockman, G., McLeavey, C., Sutskever, I.: Robust speech recognition via large-scale weak supervision. arXiv abs/2212.04356 (2022). https://doi.org/10.48550/arXiv.2212.04356
17. Reinkemeyer, L.: Business view: towards a digital enabled organization. In: Reinkemeyer, L. (ed.) Process Mining in Action, pp. 197–206. Springer, Cham (2020). https://doi.org/10.1007/978-3-030-40172-6_22
18. Reinkemeyer, L.: Purpose: identifying the right use cases. In: Reinkemeyer, L. (ed.) Process Mining in Action, pp. 15–25. Springer, Cham (2020). https://doi.org/10.1007/978-3-030-40172-6_3
19. Rothhagen, F., Kerst, F., Kant Mandal, E., Çetin, C., Ullrich, C.: Leveraging Process Mining on the Shop Floor: An Exploratory Study - Supplementary Material (2024). https://doi.org/10.5281/ZENODO.13854557
20. Santos, C., Fialho, J., Silva, J., Neto, T.: Process mining in a line production. In: Arai, K. (ed.) FICC 2024. LNNS, vol. 921, pp. 241–257. Springer, Cham (2024). https://doi.org/10.1007/978-3-031-54053-0_18
21. Stertz, F., Mangler, J., Scheibel, B., Rinderle-Ma, S.: Expectations vs. experiences – process mining in small and medium sized manufacturing companies. In: Polyvyanyy, A., Wynn, M.T., Van Looy, A., Reichert, M. (eds.) BPM 2021. LNBIP, vol. 427, pp. 195–211. Springer, Cham (2021). https://doi.org/10.1007/978-3-030-85440-9_12
22. Taherdoost, H.: Sampling methods in research methodology; how to choose a sampling technique for research. SSRN Electron. J. (2016). https://doi.org/10.2139/ssrn.3205035
23. Ter Hofstede, A.H.M., et al.: Process-data quality: the true frontier of process mining. J. Data Inf. Qual. **15**(3), 1–21 (2023). https://doi.org/10.1145/3613247
24. Zerbato, F., Soffer, P., Weber, B.: Process mining practices: evidence from interviews. In: Di Ciccio, C., Dijkman, R., Del Río Ortega, A., Rinderle-Ma, S. (eds.) BPM 2022. LNCS, vol. 13420, pp. 268–285. Springer, Cham (2022). https://doi.org/10.1007/978-3-031-16103-2_19
25. Zimmermann, L., Zerbato, F., Weber, B.: Process mining challenges perceived by analysts: an interview study. In: Augusto, A., Gill, A., Bork, D., Nurcan, S., Reinhartz-Berger, I., Schmidt, R. (eds.) BPMDS EMMSAD 2022. LNBIP, vol. 450, pp. 3–17. Springer, Cham (2022). https://doi.org/10.1007/978-3-031-07475-2_1

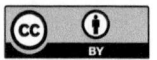

Using Facial Expressions to Predict Process Mining Task Performance

Lital Shalev[1], Irit Hadar[1](✉) ⓘ, Rotem Dror[1] ⓘ, Adir Solomon[1] ⓘ,
Elizaveta Sorokina[1], Michal Weisman Raymond[2], and Pnina Soffer[1] ⓘ

[1] University of Haifa, Haifa, Israel
hadari@is.haifa.ac.il
[2] Ben Gurion University of the Negev Beer Sheva, Beersheba, Israel

Abstract. Process mining analysis is a complex task that presents significant challenges to human analysts. To aid along this process, it is essential to identify difficulties as they occur. This study takes an initial step in this direction, by predicting the quality of task performance based on analysts' facial expressions while they are engaged in a process mining task. Data were collected using participants' webcams and the iMotions™ cloud application while they performed a process mining task. The data were then utilized to train and evaluate several machine learning classifiers, which classified participants based on the grade given to their task outcome. Our results show the high performance of these classifiers in predicting participants' success based on facial expressions. We further showed that the chosen outcome classifier could accurately classify additional participants, demonstrating its generalizability. Notably, the classifier was able to predict participants' success within a very short time frame. These findings could pave the way for developing a near-real-time support system to detect when analysts engaged in process mining may benefit from assistance.

Keywords: Process of Process Mining · Machine Learning · Facial Expressions

1 Introduction

It is commonly recognized that process mining (PM) analysts face significant challenges during their work. For example, handling different types of process variations [1] handling multiple perspectives of the same process [2] and coping with missing information in the event logs [3], to name a few. Zimmermann et al. identified as many as 23 such challenges [2].

Even though process mining analysts face these complex difficulties, research efforts in the area of process mining have so far focused primarily on the development of algorithms and approaches for specific process mining tasks, addressing each one separately from a technical perspective [4, 5]. Less attention has been given to supporting PM practitioners along the entire process of process mining (PPM). Wongsuphasawat et al. further indicate a need for analysis guidance, e.g., by augmenting tools with ready-to-use recommendations and templates [6]. To improve the understandability and usability

© The Author(s) 2025
A. Delgado and T. Slaats (Eds.): ICPM 2024 Workshops, LNBIP 533, pp. 559–571, 2025.
https://doi.org/10.1007/978-3-031-82225-4_41

of PM tools for providing better support for process miners, we first need to gain an in-depth understanding of the cognitive processes underlying the PPM. Several recent works have taken steps in this direction, showing that when analysts explore event logs, they follow different behavioral patterns and strategies to gain insights from the data, and that these may help predicting their chances of succeeding in the PM task [7, 8].

In this study we are setting a first steppingstone towards specialized online support for process mining analysts. To assist analysts, a first step is to detect when they are facing obstacles and could benefit from support. In other words, we need to predict when they are on a path that might set them up to failure. Therefore, our research question for this study was: **How can multimodal data be used for predicting process mining task success?** While attempting to make this prediction as early in the PPM as possible.

By using facial expressions data, collected from process analysts in a simple remote setting, using only the participant's webcam, we envision that a similar near-real-time analysis could be integrated into a supporting system to detect when the process miner could benefit from receiving assistance that would lead them to a more promising path.

We report on the outcomes of this study as well as share our unique dataset of mean facial expressions intensity values, collected as part of this research, with the research community to encourage other research groups in the field of process mining to use multimodal data, such as facial expressions, in their studies.

The rest of the paper is organized as follows. Section 2 presents a summary of related work. Section 3 details the research method and Sect. 4 its findings. We discuss the findings in Sect. 5 and conclude in Sect. 6.

2 Related Work

2.1 The Process of Process Mining (PPM)

Studies into the individual process of process mining (PPM) have just recently started to emerge [7, 8]. To the best of our knowledge, this research is a first attempt of applying machine learning (ML) for predicting the outcome of this process. The most closely related work we found is in the field of process modeling, where a classifier was trained to predict whether the modeler is a novice or an expert process modeler based on layout features of the model under development [9].

A different relevant line of work, related to the analysis and prediction of participants' engagement and emotions based on facial expressions, was conducted in classroom [10] and in online settings with 10 s clips [11]. Similarly, research focusing on different ML approaches aimed to predict participants' performance based on static predictive variables [12–15]. Research focusing on learning and emotions [16–18] may also inform our work, since we hypothesize that the PPM entails learning activities, i.e., learning about the process. Positive emotions affect learning by increasing students' attention and motivation [17]. Surprise, in particular, has been explored as a phenomenon that affects learning in both child development and education settings [19, 20]. Surprise has an effect on learning by requiring the individual to explain unexpected outcomes; the more unexpected the outcome is and requires more explanation, the more memorable the learning will be [16].

As PM is characterized as a knowledge-intensive and unstructured process that often yields unpredictable outcomes, it may entail varying levels of cognitive load. Cognitive load has been vastly investigated in relation to biometric sensors and multimodal data which are similar to some extent to the tools used in this study. Two ML predictive models have been trained to detect cognitive load during driving assignment based on eye measurements only [21]. In an e-learning setup, a cognitive load predictive models were developed based on eye-movements, heart rate and skin-based measures [22]. The combination of blink rate and galvanic skin response (GSR) measures were also shown to be highly distinctive features in different ML classifiers [23].

2.2 Prediction Error Minimization for the Process of Process Mining (PEM4PPM)

Results analysis in this paper will be considered in light of the PEM4PPM model, since it provides conceptualization of the cognitive process that process miners might follow. The PEM4PPM model is an adaptation of Prediction Error Minimization (PEM) to the PPM [7]. PEM is a principal within the cognitive theory of Predictive Processing (PP), viewing the brain as a sophisticated machine that attempts to predict what it will sense and to create a model of what might be causing the sensory inputs it receives. According to the PEM principal, the brain then aims to minimize the difference between its predictions and the real input as much as possible. If its predictions are already quite accurate, it might not need to change its models; if they are not, it will continue adjusting the prediction models until they are accurate enough [24].

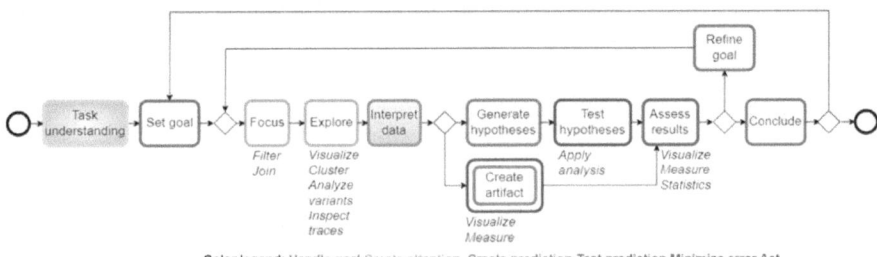

Fig. 1. The PEM4PPM model.

Figure 1 illustrates the PEM4PPM model, highlighting the sequence of steps and their corresponding cognitive operations. The PPM begins with high-level business goals, which serve as the starting point for any process mining endeavor. These goals can be decomposed or refined into more specific objectives as needed. The refinement process continues until the goals are concrete enough to be achieved through available mining operations. For example, a high-level goal can be to find how cycle times can be reduced. This goal can be refined to detection of bottlenecks in the process. To focus attention on relevant aspects of the input data, a relevant subset of the data is filtered and organized. This step enables subsequent exploration of the data to identify behavioral patterns that are of interest considering the identified goals. Based on the exploration results, concrete hypotheses are formed as predictions to be tested. For example, hypotheses can be formed about specific activities which may act as a bottleneck in the process. Predictions are tested through the creation of specific artifacts, such as discovered process models. Available PM techniques are applied to validate the hypotheses or create artifacts that support the predictions. The obtained results are assessed against the original goal or hypothesis to evaluate prediction errors and take actions for their minimization. This assessment serves as a basis for determining whether the goal has been achieved or if further refinement is needed [7]. This process is iterative in nature, and may involve additional filtering, focusing, and exploration to form new hypotheses and to test them.

Four process mining cognitive strategies have been identified and validated based on the PEM4PPM model, and their effect on the PM task performance was analyzed. The strategies are: (1) NNN - No data interpretation - No indicated hypothesis - No testing, where the conclusions of the participants were based on the data exploration stage only; (2) WNN - With data interpretation - No indicated hypothesis - No testing, where participants based their conclusions mostly on data exploration and interpretation; (3) WWN - With data interpretation - With hypothesis - No testing, where participants formulated hypotheses but did not follow a trial-and-error approach; (4) WWW - With data interpretation - With hypothesis - With testing, where participants performed all the activities of the PEM4PPM model. Analysts who followed this full WWW strategy demonstrated significantly better performance than analysts who applied other strategies [7].

In relation to learning, we posit that the PEM4PPM steps of Task Understanding, Explore, Interpret Data and Assess Results, require some extent of learning the mined process. We further speculate that the phases of Task Understanding, Focus, Generate Hypothesis, Set Goal and Refine Goal would require high cognitive load. We will analyze our findings in light of these assumptions.

3   Methods

3.1   Study Settings

The data for this research were collected from 16 B.Sc. and M.Sc. students in the Department of Information Systems at the University of Haifa, taking an advanced course in Process Mining. As facial expression recognition may involve bias in terms of gender and ethnicity [25] we note that all participants were Caucasian/Middle eastern, 13 females and 3 males. For the participation in the study, students received bonus points to their final course grade. Students who chose not to participate in the study were offered an alternative non-experimental assignemnt with the same bonus points. This study setup was approved by the IRB.

The students who chose to participate in the study were presented with the following question about the Road Traffic Fine Management (RTFM) event log, "Based on the data in the log, if the offender wants to pay as little as possible, how should they act? Suggest at least two alternative actions, show why they are fulfilling the requirement of paying as little as possible, and compare between them." Students were asked to use the Disco (Fluxicon Disco™) application and think-aloud, namely, verbally describe their thinking process when performing the task.

3.2 Data Collection

The data were collected with both iMotions™ cloud platform and Zoom application. The iMotions™ cloud platform was used to collect eye tracking data, screen recordings, and participants' face recordings. The Zoom application was used to record the think-aloud data. The data collection was done remotely, with the participants using their own computers and sharing their screens and web camera through the iMotions™ cloud platform. Figure 2 shows an example of a processed video exported from iMotions™. The video includes voice recording, participant's face recording (anonymized in the figure), screen recording with gaze path, and two graphs of selected facial expressions (further explained below).

Facial Expressions. The participants' face recordings were analyzed using AFFDEX 3.0 SDK [26, 27], a toolkit for analyzing facial expressions in real life setups. AFFDEX was used through its integration in iMotions.[1] Every 30 ms the state of the participant was recorded by iMotions and analyzed by AFFDEX, which provides detections of the following emotional expressions: Anger, Contempt, Disgust, Fear, Joy, Sadness, Surprise, Engagement, Valence, Sentimentality, and Confusion. The detection of facial Action Units is translated to facial expressions such as Chick Raise, Blink Rate, Smile, and Smirk. For each facial expression, an intensity score is provided, between 0 and 100. The higher the score, the higher the likelihood the participant is presenting that emotional expression. From iMotions™ it is possible to export all the facial expression data into a CSV file for further analysis. Figure 2 shows a screenshot taken from iMotions™, where the main part of the screen shows the participant's screen recording while using Disco. The orange circle on the Disco screen recording represents the location the participant's eyes were fixated on. The bottom part of the figures shows a graph of the AFFDEX facial expressions analyzes for Confusion and Contempt.

Think Aloud. The Zoom voice recordings of the participants describing their thought process were combined with the screen recordings from iMotions™ to generate a single video and audio recording for each participant. This combined video was then used to determine the grade for the task performance. Grades were on the scale of 0–100, considering both the provided answer, and the evidence that supported the answer. E.g. a student who provided the expected answer (the offender should wait for 90 days or pay the fine immediately), but did not analyze the data in Disco to support this answer, received a grade of 50. The recordings were viewed carefully as part of the participants' task performance evaluation in order to decide on the appropriate grade.

3.3 Data Preprocessing

We preprocessed the collected data in the following manner. First, the facial expressions data were exported from iMotions™ for each participant. Second, we set two grade groups, High Performers, participants whose grades are above 55, and Low Performers, participants whose grades are below 55. This threshold was set since grades below 55 indicate poor performance in the provided task, and since it marked a clear break between two balanced groups of 8 participants (see grades distribution in Fig. 3).

---

[1] https://imotions.com/.

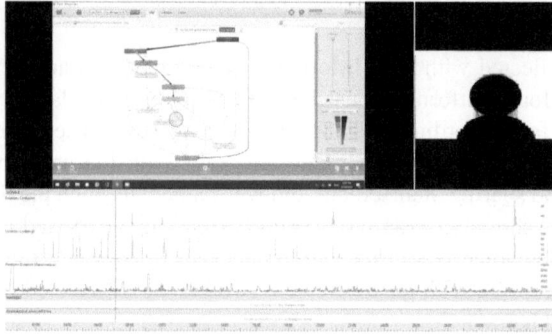

Fig. 2. Snapshot from a processed video exported from iMotions™.

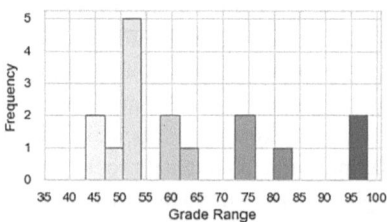

Fig. 3. Grades Distribution.

We then used a Wilcoxon statistical test for the hypothesis that there is a significant difference between the High Performers and Low Performers groups in average facial expression values. The data we used for the test were the first 10,000 samples from each participant's data, representing the first 5 min of the session. To prepare the data for the ML classifiers training, the mean value of each facial expression intensity was calculated for each participant for all the valid data points in the session.

3.4   ML Model Training

Multiple ML classifiers, including Decision Tree Classifier, Random Forest Classifier, and Naïve Bayes Classifier, were trained to predict if the participant belonged to the High or to the Low Performer groups. We chose to train a Naïve Bayes Classifier due to its ability to handle small data sets. Further, the Decision Tree Classifier was selected for its proficiency in handling non-linear relationships effectively, and its inherent ability to accommodate correlations among features, making it particularly suited for complex but small datasets. Lastly, the Random Forest Classifier was chosen due to its ensemble approach, which integrates multiple decision trees, and mitigates overfitting associated with single decision models to provide a reliable assessment of feature relevance. We used Python Sklearn package implementations of these models. Since our dataset was relatively small, with mean values for 16 participants for each facial expression, we chose to use Leave One Out Cross Validation (LOOCV) approach for the evaluation of the classifiers' performance. We then calculated the mean accuracy of each iteration, where in each, 1 participant was used as a test set and the rest of the 15 served as a train set. This approach guarantees that each participant will be in the test set only once. This approach is appropriate for small datasets such as the one we had.

3.5 Independent Temporal Data Evaluation Setting

For the temporal evaluation of the trained Random Forest classifier, we used additional data collected from 4 participants, as part of a previous data collection study, which used the same event log and asked the participants similar questions [7]. The independent data used for the evaluation were collected with Zoom application only. The Zoom video recordings were concatenated into a new video file which included only the participants' face recording. The new video file was then imported into iMotions™ and post-processed using the AFFDEX 3.0 toolkit to provide the same facial expressions data format used to train the ML classifiers. The data were then aggregated in the same way as the training data; the mean value was calculated for each relevant facial expression throughout the whole session. The trained classifier was then used to predict the grade group of the participant in different time points during the process mining task.

4 Findings

Three ML classifiers for predicting participants' task performance were trained during this study. Their accuracy was evaluated by both using the LOOCV method and additional real-world evaluation data. Figure 4 presents the mean accuracy results for the three ML classifiers with the LOOCV evaluation method. Figure 5 presents the F1-score for each classifier. The classifier that had the best performance in both the mean accuracy and F1-score metrics was the Random Forest Classifier with mean accuracy of 87.5% and F1-score micro of 88% for both classes. The Decision Tree classifier and the Naïve Bayes classifier had the same mean accuracy results of 62.5%.

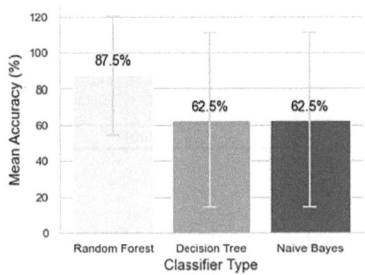

Fig. 4. Classifiers Comparison Mean Accuracy.

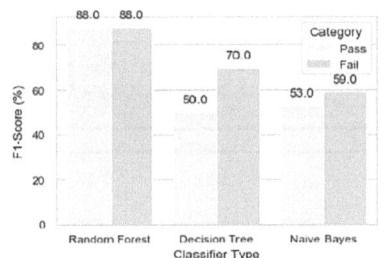

Fig. 5. Classifiers Comparison F1-score micro. Legend: Pass = High Performers group, Fail = Low performers group

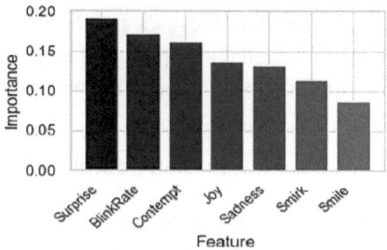

Fig. 6. Feature Importance of the Random Forest Classifier.

Figure 6 presents the features used for the Random Forest classifier and their importance. The highest importance ranks were for Surprise, Blink Rate, and Contempt, and then Joy, Sadness, Smirk, and Smile. The parameters used for the Random Forest were minimal samples split: 5, number of estimators: 200, and balanced class weight.

To explore the generalization capabilities and temporal responsiveness of the Random Forest classifier, independent data evaluation was performed for different time points during the process. Data of 4 participants from a previous study were used [7]. The focus of the previous study was not the analysis of facial expressions, hence video had to be processed for facial expressions. As a result, most of the data were partial, since the participants' faces were not clearly visible part of the time. Results are presented in Table 1. For 3 out of 4 of the participants, the classifier was able to detect correctly the class of the participant (High Performers/Low Performers) after the first minute. After 7.5 min, the classifier had accuracy of 100% for the 4 participants. For the participant with ID 2, the classification was correct for all time points except for the 5 min window. We assume that is due to the low visibility of the participant's face which resulted in lower quality of the facial expressions analysis.

Table 1. Temporal Independent Data Evaluation

ID	1 Min.	2.5 Min.	5 Min.	7.5 Min.	10 Min.	15 Min.	Full Session
1							
2							
3							
4							
Accur.	75%	75%	75%	100%	100%	100%	100%

Figure 7 shows the significant differences (p-value < 0.001 in a Wilcoxon statistical test) in the facial expression mean values between the High Performers and Low Performers groups during the first 5 min of the process mining task. Positive values in Fig. 7 show that the High Performers group had a higher mean value, and negative values indicate that the Low Performers group had higher values. It is evident that Blink Rate, Smile, and Joy had higher mean values for the High Performers group, where Contempt, Smirk and Surprise had higher mean values for the Low Performers group.

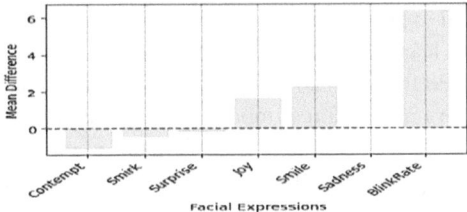

Fig. 7. Significant Differences Between the High Performers and Low Performers Groups.

5 Discussion

The presented findings show that it is possible to predict if a participant will be successful in a process mining task, solely based on facial expressions. We show that this ability remains also when the dataset is partial and generated from a regular Zoom recording with no special setup. Furthermore, the classification had 75% accuracy after only 1 min of partial data, and 100% accuracy after 7.5 min of partial data.

We hypothesize that it is possible to predict the success in a process mining task early in the process, due to the cognitive strategies the High Performers and Low Performers follow. Participants whose strategy included generating and testing hypotheses had higher rates of success [7]. We believe there are facial cues presented during the Generate Hypothesis step of the PEM4PPM model, and that they occur at an early stage of the session for most of the participants. For other participants it might take a few minutes longer to generate a hypothesis, but if it takes longer than that, they might not generate hypotheses at any time during the analysis. If this is indeed the case, it might be an explanation for the finding that after 7.5 min, the classifier was able to predict the outcome correctly for the 4 independent participants. Future research combining the settings of the two studies will enable us to test our hypothesis.

Another possible explanation could be that other PEM4PPM steps could also be reliable predictors of the process mining task outcome. These steps might be Task Understanding, Focus, Set Goal and Refine Goal which we anticipate will require higher cognitive load. Blink Rate has been indicated as a measure of cognitive load [28, 29], and, as shown in Fig. 7, it has the highest difference in the mean values between the two grade groups. The High Performers group had significantly higher mean values than the Lower performers group, which might indicate a higher cognitive load for the High Performers. Further investigation is required to validate this explanation.

The feature importance of the trained classifier resonates well with the conceptual arguments we presented, as Surprise was the feature of the highest importance. Surprise has previously been reported as being related to learning processes [16]. Since we view the PPM as partially a learning process, we expected Surprise to be one of the high importance features for a trained outcome classifier.

The additional selected features are Contempt, Joy, Sadness, Smirk and Smile. We note that the differences in the mean values showed that the Low Performers had higher negative facial expressions (Contempt and Smirk), and High Performers had higher values of positive facial expressions (Joy and Smile). It has been established that positive emotions improve learning, while negative emotions reduce it [17]. We therefore speculate that the Low Performers had less phases of learning than the High Performers.

We suggest that the random forest model outperformed other classification algorithms in predicting the success or failure of participants completing the task, because it leverages various combinations and interactions among features—in our case, the different facial expressions displayed by the participants—resulting in a more comprehensive and accurate model. As the random forest constructs an ensemble of decision trees, capturing the complex patterns and nuances in facial expressions that a single decision tree might miss. Based on these results, we recommend that researchers intending to explore the use of facial expressions in PM tasks use ensemble classifiers, as we believe that the relationships between different expressions can explain various phenomena in unique ways, making ensembles more adequate for this kind of task in this domain. We are publicly sharing the dataset and implementation of the classifiers presented in this paper, to facilitate the use of multimodal data and ML models in the research community of process mining.[2]

Threats to Validity. Several threats to the validity of the study need to be considered. First, to date, there is no agreement in the literature whether facial expressions are indications of emotions or not. This could be relevant to the conclusions we draw from the results, however, it does not present a threat to the validity of our classifier, since we record facial expressions and predict based directly on them. Our interpretations of the meaning of the facial expressions are what could be compromised. Second, the datasets we used in this study are relatively small. As this is a clear limitation of our study, it is also one of its strengths, since we were able to show that it is possible to gain reliable results and train an accurate ML classifier also with small datasets. In future research, a larger dataset would also enable to refine the binary classification of high and low performers into finer-grained performance groups. Third, the data collected in this study relate to a single PM tool and a single PM task. While this adequately addresses our research questions regarding the prediction of a PM task outcome, further studies are necessary to establish broader conclusions. In particular, different tasks (e.g., process discovery, conformance checking) should be investigated.

6 Conclusion

This research has several novel methods and findings. Firstly, we show that collecting facial expressions data in a simple remote setup, using only a webcam, can provide valuable insights for better understanding the PPM, and potentially other related tasks, e.g. process modeling and data mining. Our findings show that the intensity scores of Surprise and Blink Rate are associated with PM task performance, and that based on this association, task performance can be predicted early in the process. We hypothesize this is due to differences in cognitive load and learning-related phases during the PPM. We intend to further investigate this relationship in future research.

---

[2] https://github.com/litalshl/Facial-Expressions-Classifiers.

Secondly, we present that it is possible to train ML classifiers for process mining task performance based on a small dataset, containing data of only 16 participants. In addition, we present that it is possible to make relatively accurate predictions (75%) of students' task performance by using only 1 min of partial facial expressions data gathered from a simple Zoom recording that was post-processed by using iMotions™. After 7.5 min of data, our classifiers accuracy increased to 100%. We plan to increase our dataset to further validate these results as well as to generalize our chosen classifier for similar tasks, such as business process modeling.

Lastly, our current classifier uses only facial expressions intensity data. We view this as an advantage for remote setups and the usage of it in a future online support system for process miners. However, we believe it would be interesting and possibly beneficial to enhance this classifier with additionally collected data, such as eye tracking measurements, therefore our future research plans include that as well. We believe that once the presented classifier is appropriately generalized, it would be possible to use it for near-real-time predictions as part of a specialized support system, thereby identifying when an analyst requires support to avoid their predicted failure.

Acknowledgement. The research was funded by the Israel Science Foundation, grant no. 2005/21.

References

1. van der Aalst, W.M.P., Weijters, A.J.M.M.: Process mining: a research agenda. Comput. Ind. **53**(3), 231–244 (2004)
2. Zimmermann, L., Zerbato, F., Weber, B.: Process mining challenges perceived by analysts: an interview study. In: Enterprise, Business-Process and Information Systems Modeling, pp. 3–17 (2022)
3. Bose, R.P.J.C., Mans, R.S., van der Aalst, W.M.P.: Wanna improve process mining results? In: 2013 IEEE Symposium on Computational Intelligence and Data Mining (CIDM), pp. 127–134 (2013)
4. Augusto, A., et al.: Automated discovery of process models from event logs: review and benchmark. IEEE Trans. Knowl. Data Eng. **31**(4), 686–705 (2019)
5. Pasquadibisceglie, V., Appice, A., Castellano, G., van der Aalst, W.: PROMISE: coupling predictive process mining to process discovery. Inf. Sci. **606**, 250–271 (2022)
6. Wongsuphasawat, K., Liu, Y., Heer, J.: Goals, process, and challenges of exploratory data analysis: an interview study. arXiv [cs.HC] (2019)
7. Sorokina, E., Soffer, P., Hadar, I., Leron, U., Zerbato, F., Weber, B.: PEM4PPM: a cognitive perspective on the process of process mining. In: Business Process Management, pp. 465–481 (2023)
8. Zerbato, F., Soffer, P., Weber, B.: Process mining practices: evidence from interviews. In: Business Process Management, pp. 268–285 (2022)
9. Burattin, A., et al.: Who is behind the model? Classifying modelers based on pragmatic model features. In: Business Process Management, pp. 322–338 (2018)
10. Tonguç, G., Ozkara, B.O.: Automatic recognition of student emotions from facial expressions during a lecture. Comput. Educ. **148**, 103797 (2020)
11. Thomas, C., Jayagopi, D.B.: Predicting student engagement in classrooms using facial behavioral cues. In: Proceedings of the 1st ACM SIGCHI International Workshop on Multimodal Interaction for Education, Glasgow, UK, pp. 33–40 (2017)

12. Nespereira, C.G., Elhariri, E., El-Bendary, N., Vilas, A.F., Redondo, R.P.D.: Machine learning based classification approach for predicting students performance in blended learning. In: The 1st International Conference on Advanced Intelligent System and Informatics (AISI2015), Beni Suef, Egypt, 28–30 November 2015, pp. 47–56 (2016)

13. Joshi, A., Saggar, P., Jain, R., Sharma, M., Gupta, D., Khanna, A.: CatBoost—an ensemble machine learning model for prediction and classification of student academic performance. Adv. Data Sci. Adapt. Anal. **13**(03n04) (2021)

14. Rastrollo-Guerrero, J.L., Gómez-Pulido, J.A., Durán-Domínguez, A.: Analyzing and predicting students' performance by means of machine learning: a review. Appl. Sci. (2020)

15. Albreiki, B., Zaki, N., Alashwal, H.: A systematic literature review of student' performance prediction using machine learning techniques. Neveléstudomány (2021)

16. Foster, M.I., Keane, M.T.: The role of surprise in learning: different surprising outcomes affect memorability differentially. Top. Cogn. Sci. **11**(1), 75–87 (2019)

17. Pekrun, R.: Emotions and Learning. Educational Practices Series, vol. 24, no. 1, pp. 1–31 (2014)

18. Hökkä, P., Vähäsantanen, K., Paloniemi, S.: Emotions in learning at work: a literature review. Vocat. Learn. **13**(1), 1–25 (2020)

19. Tsang, N.M.: Surprise in social work education. Soc. Work. Educ. **32**(1), 55–67 (2013)

20. Ramscar, M., Dye, M., Gustafson, J.W., Klein, J.: Dual routes to cognitive flexibility: learning and response-conflict resolution in the dimensional change card sort task. Child Dev. **84**(4), 1308–1323 (2013)

21. Fridman, L., Reimer, B., Mehler, B., Freeman, W.T.: Cognitive load estimation in the wild. In: Proceedings of the 2018 CHI Conference on Human Factors in Computing Systems, Montreal, QC, Canada, pp. 1–9 (2018)

22. Herbig, N., et al.: Investigating multi-modal measures for cognitive load detection in e-learning. In: Proceedings of the 28th ACM Conference on User Modeling, Adaptation and Personalization, Genoa, Italy, pp. 88–97 (2020)

23. Chen, F., et al.: Robust Multimodal Cognitive Load Measurement. Springer, Cham (2016)

24. Williams, D.: Predictive processing and the representation wars. Minds Mach. **28**(1), 141–172 (2018)

25. Singh, R., Majumdar, P., Mittal, S., Vatsa, M.: Anatomizing bias in facial analysis. In: Proceedings of the AAAI Conference on Artificial Intelligence, vol. 36, no. 11, pp. 12351–12358 (2022)

26. McDuff, D., Mahmoud, A., Mavadati, M., Amr, M., Turcot, J., Kaliouby, R.E.: AFFDEX SDK: a cross-platform real-time multi-face expression recognition toolkit. In: Proceedings of the 2016 CHI Conference Extended Abstracts on Human Factors in Computing Systems, San Jose, California, USA, pp. 3723–3726 (2016)

27. Jmour, N., Masmoudi, S., Abdelkrim, A.: A new video based emotions analysis system (VEMOS): an efficient solution compared to iMotions Affectiva analysis software. Adv. Sci. Technol. Eng. Syst. (2021)

28. Magliacano, A., Fiorenza, S., Estraneo, A., Trojano, L.: Eye blink rate increases as a function of cognitive load during an auditory oddball paradigm. Neurosci. Lett. **736**, 135293 (2020)

29. Chen, S., Epps, J.: Using task-induced pupil diameter and blink rate to infer cognitive load. Hum.-Comput. Interact. **29**(4), 390–413 (2014)

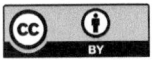

Using Process Mining with Pre- and Post-intervention Analysis to Improve Digital Service Delivery: A Governmental Case Study

Jacques Trottier[1]([✉]), William Van Woensel[2], Xiaoyang Wang[3], Kavya Mallur[1], Najah El-Gharib[3], and Daniel Amyot[3]

[1] Government of Canada, Ottawa, Canada
jacques@trottier.us
[2] Telfer School of Management, University of Ottawa, Ottawa, Canada
wvanwoen@uottawa.ca
[3] School of EECS, University of Ottawa, Ottawa, Canada
{xwang233,nelgh031,damyot}@uottawa.ca

Abstract. We present a case study of Process Mining (PM) for personnel security screening in the Canadian government. We consider customer (process time) and organizational (cost) perspectives. Furthermore, in contrast to most published case studies, we assess the full process improvement lifecycle: pre-intervention analyses pointed out initial bottlenecks, and post-intervention analyses identified the intervention impact and remaining areas for improvement. Using PM techniques, we identified frequent exceptional scenarios (e.g., applications requiring amendment), time-intensive loops (e.g., employees forgetting tasks), and resource allocation issues (e.g., involvement of non-security personnel). Subsequent process improvement interventions, implemented using a flexible low-code digital platform, reduced security briefing times from around 7 days to 46 h, and overall process time from around 31 days to 26 days, on average. From a cost perspective, the involvement of hiring managers and security screening officers was significantly reduced. These results demonstrate how PM can become part of a broader digital transformation framework to improve public service delivery.

Keywords: Process mining · government services · social network mining · process enhancement · case study

1 Introduction

Recent issues with passport processing [9] and immigration [6] highlight challenges that the Government of Canada (GC) is facing in implementing efficient business processes for delivering services to Canadians. The increasing need for digital service delivery has required governments worldwide to redesign processes that were originally geared towards pre-digital paper-based services. To support such a process redesign, Process Mining (PM) offers evidence-based and

A. Delgado and T. Slaats (Eds.): ICPM 2024 Workshops, LNBIP 533, pp. 572–585, 2025.
https://doi.org/10.1007/978-3-031-82225-4_42

data-driven technology to map current business processes, study their performance, diagnose their potential issues, and derive potential improvements.

In this paper, we demonstrate the utility of PM to improve government hiring by mining the Personnel Security Screening (PSS) process [10,12] of a particular GC department. This process is a mandatory part in the hiring and vetting of all prospective employees, and the GC processes tens of thousands of PSS transactions per year. Hence, while individual departments can choose how to implement the process, an optimized process implementation may provide insights for improving cost and hiring time efficiency across the GC.

The objectives of this case study are to (a) discover and evaluate process and handover-of-work models for PSS, analyzing process performance and bottlenecks; (b) present subsequent opportunities for process improvement; and (c) assess the results from PSS process improvements that followed from opportunities identified in (b). By using PM techniques, we were able to gain insights into the frequency of problematic scenarios (e.g., applications requiring amendment), time-intensive loops (e.g., employees forgetting tasks), and resource allocation issues (e.g., involvement of non-security personnel). Leveraging a flexible low-code digital platform, we were able to quickly guide multiple interventions to resolve these issues. We found that these interventions improved service delivery from customer (process time) and organizational (cost) standpoints: the part targeted by the interventions, namely security briefings, had its average process times reduced from about 7 days to 46 h; overall average process time was thus reduced from about 31 days to 26 days. Moreover, involvement of the hiring manager and security screening officer were significantly reduced.

Contributions of this paper include: (1) the mining of a security clearance process in the GC, with a discussion of lessons learned (during this and other case studies) on conducting PM in a government context; (2) an empirical analysis of the full process improvement lifecycle, i.e., covering both pre- and post-intervention; and (3) re-usable code for event log cleaning and transformations used in the project, which illustrates the Python library for *Process Mining – Log Filtering & Preprocessing* (logprep4pm) developed by the authors [3,14].

In this paper, Sect. 2 covers related work. Section 3 elaborates on our methodology, whose results are presented in Sect. 4 and further discussed in Sect. 5. Section 6 highlights limitations, and Sect. 7 provides conclusions.

2   Related Work

The importance of process mining in government services and digital transformation was acknowledged in a recent literature review from Rawiro et al. [8], which covered 25 papers between 2009 and 2022 that spanned 18 different countries. The papers reported case studies ranging from car registration to civil status management, procurement, and fine management, typically covering process discovery (n = 14). Most usages focused on process discovery, with a few addressing process conformance (n = 6) and enhancement (n = 5). Note that no services from Canada were discussed, and the processes covered did not include security screening. In that review [8], the paper closest to ours was the assessment of a passport application process in Uruguay by Delgado et al. [1,2], who introduced a framework for selecting and analyzing target processes, with a focus on process discovery and improvement opportunities. The framework also includes a metamodel for data integration. The authors reported the access to data, quality of event logs, and inter-organizational processes as major challenges. We also note that recent work started integrating AI into government process mining projects. For example, Nai et al. [5] recently used natural language processing for the generation and enrichment of event logs in support of the discovery and analysis of procurement processes from France, Spain, and Italy.

To our knowledge, outside of healthcare, there is a lack of case studies that cover the full process improvement lifecycle—i.e., before and after specific interventions. Zuidema-Tempel et al. [15] compare PM methodologies with PM practitioner experiences; they report that while post-analysis and monitoring in industry do happen in practice, PM methodologies lack focus on quantifying, selecting and *monitoring* improvement actions. Leemans et al. [4] focus on process compliance and performance at a Queensland Government department, but do not address actual process improvements. Park et al. [7] compare process mining vs. traditional process re-engineering in government; they shortly discuss process changes before and after interventions, but mainly focus on differences in processing times between municipalities.

3   Methodology

During the COVID-19 pandemic, a GC department[1] implemented a new PSS system, which includes an web-based portal for new/prospective employees to complete their PSS application. Its goal was to facilitate a more contactless experience while improving processing times. The PSS system was built on a low-code Business Process Management (BPM) platform, which records events throughout a case's lifecycle. As the GC processes tens of thousands of PSS applications per year, an optimized process could pave the way for large gains in hiring efficiency. These factors made it a highly suitable candidate for PM.

Our goal was to improve the *security briefing* part of PSS. Our initial research question thus revolved around finding bottlenecks from two perspectives:

- *Process time*: time for an applicant to complete the security briefing.
- *Cost*: salary implications of the GC employees involved in the briefing sessions.

Using PM, we were able to answer this question, which informed improvement interventions that were then implemented. Subsequently, our research question was refined to measure the interventions' impact on process time and cost.

The project included 3 distinct phases described in Table 1. For each phase, we applied the methodology from Table 2. Below, we discuss general aspects that apply to all phases. For the *extraction of raw event logs* step, the logs were

---

[1] Due to issues of confidentiality, we cannot identify the actual department.

Table 1. Project phases, date ranges of analyzed event data, and activities

Phase	Event Date Range	Activities
I	Jan 6–Oct 26, 2022	Initial Analysis (Process Discovery & Social Mining)
II	Jan 5–May 15, 2023	Intervention I (Group Briefing) & Subsequent Analysis
III	Jun 15–Oct 23, 2023	Intervention II (Video Briefing) & Subsequent Analysis

Table 2. Steps for the 3 phases. Steps with (*) were only conducted in Phase I.

Activity	Chosen Tools	Result/Output	Reason
Extraction of raw event logs	MS SQL Server Management Studio 18	Raw Event Log (CSV)	Compatibility with backend DB (MS SQL)
Pre-processing of the event log	`logprep4pm` [14] library Pandas library JupyterLab	Preprocessed Event Log (CSV) .ipynb notebook	`logprep4pm` and Pandas to clean and filter event logs with re-usable code JupyterLab for documenting steps
Process model discovery	Disco	Directly Follows Graph	Discover a process model from the event log data
Exporting XES event log (*)	Disco	XES file	ProM requires XES file
Social Network Model Discovery (*)	ProM	Handover-of-work model	Disco does not support social network mining

extracted from the SQL database of the PSS system. For pre-processing and event log generation, we used JupyterLab with data analysis libraries, including a Python port (`logprep4pm`) [14] of the *Cloud Pattern API for Process Mining* [3].

The `logprep4pm` library overlays filtering and pre-processing functionalities for PM on top of the popular Pandas library. An important benefit of using a code library for this purpose is code reuse: code written for complex (yet common) exploratory data analysis, filtering, and pre-processing, can be re-used across phases, and shared within the organization (e.g., GC), regardless of PM tools used. We provide abstracted and anonymized notebooks that document these exploratory data analysis, filtering, and event log pre-processing steps using the `logprep4pm` library, among other libraries, in our online appendix [12].

During the *pre-processing of event logs*, we observed 8 event classes (i.e., types of events) for which there were less than 10 occurrences; these were deleted to prevent them from cluttering the process. Also, we observed duplicate events in short succession; we attributed this to users accidentally double clicking a button. `logprep4pm` provides a function to delete duplicate events within a time threshold; we selected a time threshold of 3 min (i.e., events separated by 3 min or more were assumed to be separate actions). This seemed appropriate based on the event data and nature of the tasks, and removed most of the duplicate events (10 in total). Using `logprep4pm`, case ID numbers were also anonymized to protect privacy, and event names were renamed to user-friendly descriptions. Employee emails were replaced with the corresponding role.

For each phase, in line with the PM^2 methodology [13], we applied several iterations of *pre-processing, mining & analysis,* and *evaluation* to refine the event data and eliminate data quality issues. Throughout these cycles, our event log was exported multiple times as a CSV file from `logprep4pm` (Jupyter Notebook) and imported into the Disco PM tool. Iterations continued until we were satisfied that the discovered model accurately represented the business process with minimal noise, in collaboration with the process owner (i.e., GC department).

3.1 Phase I - Initial Process Discovery & Social Network Mining

The event logs generated shortly after the PSS launch in April of 2021 were noisy. Given the sensitive nature of PSS for higher-level clearances, this case study's scope was also limited to exploring security briefings for "reliability status", the lowest security clearance level. After filtering, this resulted in an initial case count of 273. We used the methodology from Table 2 to answer our initial research question on process time and cost for the PSS process, i.e., by discovering and studying the associated process and social network models. Whereas the process model allowed us to map the current business process, the social network helped us to understand the interplay and participation levels of stakeholders.

3.2 Phases II and III - Interventions

Two interventions were applied to the PSS process to improve processing times. We note that the original process included a one-on-one security briefing between the new employee and hiring manager (see appendix [12]). The **first intervention** replaced these one-on-one briefings with a group briefing session with the security screening officer. These group sessions were scheduled 4 times per week. This intervention took place at the end of October 2022, and the resulting process lasted until June 2023 (when the second intervention took place). We extracted all 191 cases from January 5 to May 15, 2023; as before, we chose these times to cope with bug fixes and process drift right after and before interventions.

The **second intervention** subsequently replaced these group briefings with a non-proctored video that applicants would watch by logging into the PSS web portal. Applicants would digitally attest to having watched the video and accept the conditions of their clearance. This is the solution that is still in place at the time of writing (August 2024). The intervention took place in June 2023. We extracted all 182 cases during this time period, from June 15 (considering a buffer after implementation) until October 23, 2023 (time of analysis). Log inspections confirmed that there was no overlap from different phases.

We discuss how these interventions were motivated by PM result analyses in Sect. 4. After each intervention, we refined our research question to measure the resulting process time and cost, which involved re-applying our methodology.

4   Results

4.1 Phase I - Initial Process Discovery & Social Network Mining

The initial process model is illustrated in Fig. 1. Mean and median case durations were 30.9 days and 19.9 days, respectively (this included weekends, vacations, and public holidays). We found that this process model generally complies with the standard for security screening [10]. We summarize here 3 major findings.

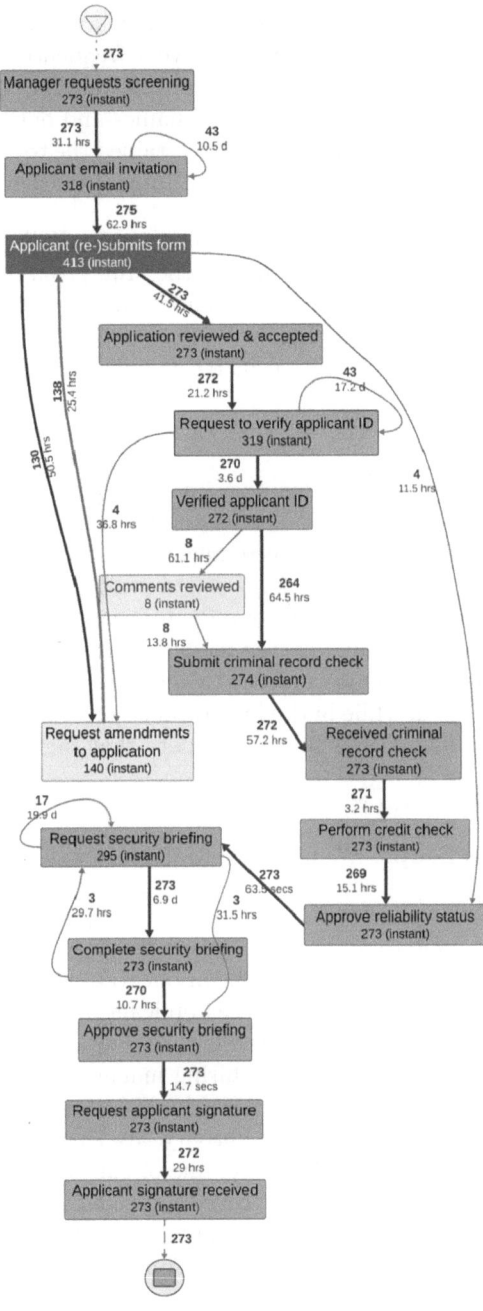

Fig. 1. Process model discovered using Disco and reformatted (Phase I). Links with two or fewer cases were left out for clarity. Exceptional activity flows mostly cover cases where other steps (e.g., "Applicant (re-)submits form" to "Approve reliability status") had already been performed. Numbers in bold indicate frequencies; numbers below them indicate durations.

Finding 1 – Data Validation. We found that scenarios involving security screening applications required amendments very frequently. In particular, 48% (130/273; Fig. 1) of security screening applications were refused after initial submission, mainly because of missing/inverted names and outdated ID issues.

Referring to the system's database, we ascertained the top five reasons why an application required amendments (in order of frequency from highest to lowest):

1. The applicant omitted their middle name from the "full given names" field.
2. The applicant included their surname in the "full given names" field.
3. The applicant had an overlap in residences and resided at more than one address during the same timeframe.
4. The applicant uploaded a scan of an ID document that was expired at the time of application.
5. The applicant did not specify information about their parents.

Other reasons for refusal included poor image quality, the applicant's mailing address not matching their driver's license, and the applicant not including their birth name. Several solutions were recommended to mitigate this issue. In the short term, the online application form was extended with tooltips (or hints) in the "full given names" field to encourage applicants to include their middle name and exclude their surname. In the medium term, name, address, and date extraction from uploaded ID documents (using optical character recognition – OCR) was recommended, while in the long term a better integration with federal and provincial systems would help pre-populate that information from reliable sources.

Finding 2 – Event Loops. We found multiple time-wasting loops in the initial process model (Fig. 1):

1. *Applicant Email Invitation:* An email is sent to the applicant requesting they register to the portal and complete the application form. In 43 instances, an email invitation had to be re-sent as the applicant had not registered yet (e.g., missed the email, went to junk folder, lack of digital competency).
2. *Request to Verify Applicant ID:* The hiring manager must verify the ID documents from the application submission. In 43 instances, the hiring manager had to be reminded to conduct this activity. We suspect this was due to the managers' busy workload and large volume of emails.
3. *Requested Security Briefing:* An approved applicant must be briefed on their security responsibilities by the hiring manager. In 17 instances, this briefing activity had to be re-requested (likely for similar reasons as above).

To partially address these issues, it was suggested that the system could automatically send daily reminders to the applicant and hiring managers to complete outstanding tasks. Some reminders were implemented after our study.

Finding 3 – Social Mining. A handover-of-work (HoW) model, as an output of social network mining, captures a relation between stakeholders X and Y when, for two sequential activities $A1$ and $A2$, X does $A1$ and Y does $A2$. This model also captures the size and influence that each stakeholder plays in a given process. Figure 2 shows the HoW model as generated by ProM and Table 3 details the stakeholders' coverage in the process.

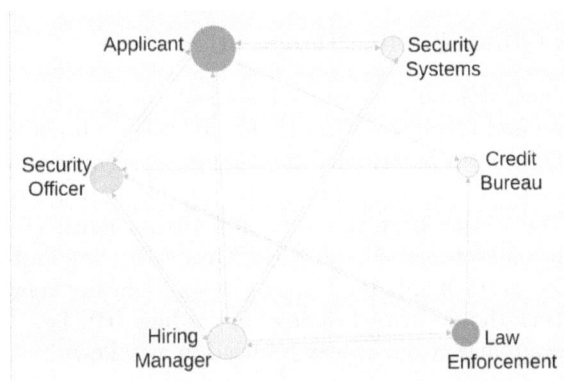

Fig. 2. Handover-of-work model for the PSS process (generated with ProM).

Table 3. Stakeholder involvement in the PSS process.

Stakeholder	Frequency	Coverage
Applicant	1277	28%
Hiring Manager	1159	26%
Security Officer	942	21%
Law Enforcement	547	12%
Security Systems	298	6.6%
Credit Bureau	273	6.1%

We found that the *Applicant* had the largest participation in the process, and the *Credit Bureau* had the least. Rather surprisingly, however, security screening resources—including *Security Officers* and *Security Systems*, which should be pivotal in the process—were only involved in 28% of the process lifecycle, while the *Hiring Manager* was involved to a similar degree (26%), although security is not their primary role. We further observe that *Security Officers* acted mainly as facilitators as all other stakeholders but one (*Security Systems*) involved handover work to the security officer. Once all necessary information had been gathered, they rendered a decision of whether to grant reliability status. This process put a large strain on *Hiring Managers*; we found that the security briefings (which last 10–15 minutes) were a major contributor to their involvement. A separate briefing had to be scheduled per *Applicant*, which delayed the process by 7 days on average (Fig. 1). We had suspected (see prior section) that their busy workload had led to process delays and time-wasting loops.

In line with this observation, two interventions were proposed by the process owner to re-organize these security briefings. Our research question was thus refined to measure process time and cost of post-intervention security briefings.

4.2   Phase II: Group Briefing Intervention

The Group Briefing intervention involved 4 weekly briefing sessions (applicants would attend one) and transferred the *Hiring Manager's* briefing-related duties to the *Security Officer* (in particular, the Security Screening Officer, SSO).

Figure 3 zooms in on part of the process model that pertains to security briefings: (A) shows the section from the original model, whereas (B) and (C) show the post-intervention sections, i.e., after the Group Briefing and Video Briefing interventions. The parts highlighted in red are specifically related to requesting and completing the security briefing. Regarding (B), i.e., Group Briefing intervention, we can answer our research question as follows:

– *Process time*: the process enters the relevant stage in (A) when the hiring manager is supposed to schedule a briefing session with the applicant; in (B), when the applicant receives an automated request to register for a group briefing. We point out that this time includes service time as well as waiting for the applicant. The mean process time was reduced from 7 to 4.6 days; the median process time however stayed more or less the same.

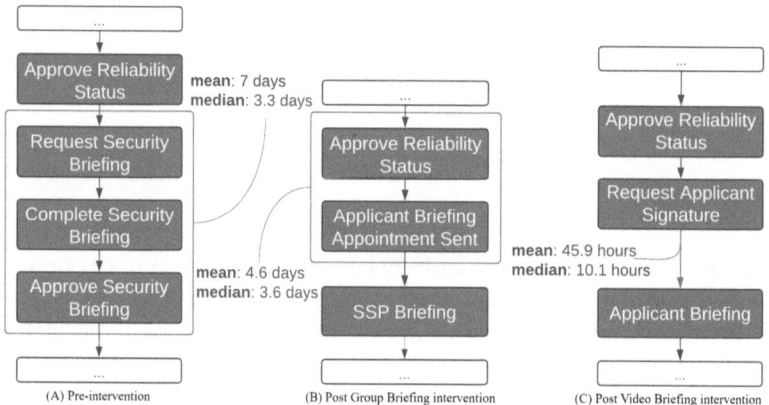

Fig. 3. Process models pertaining to security briefings.

- *Cost*: moving to group-based briefings meant a reduction from 191 sessions (1 per case) to 76 sessions (4 per week) over the time period, leading to a 60% reduction in number of sessions. Conservatively, assuming 10 min per briefing, this saves about 18 h of organizational time and associated salary over the time period. The government department performs around 3000 clearances per year (including secret and top-secret instances, not discussed in this case study); avoiding one-on-one briefings thus saves around 500 h of hiring manager time annually.

4.3   Phase III: Video Briefing Intervention

The Video Briefing Intervention, which was developed concurrently with the first intervention, replaced the Group Briefing with a non-proctored online briefing video. Hence, the intervention removed employee involvement altogether, and allowed applicants to perform the security briefing at their convenience. Figure 3 (C) shows the result of this new intervention. Regarding our research question on process times and cost:

- *Process time*: the process enters this stage when the applicant receives an automated request for watching and digitally attesting to the online video. As before, this time includes both service time and waiting for the applicant. The mean process time was reduced from 4.6 days to 45.9 h; the median process time was reduced from 3.6 days to 10.1 h. Comparing Phases I and III yields an overall time savings of around 5 days on average.
- *Cost*: as there is no more involvement required from GC employees during briefings, this removed any employee time involvement and associated salary implications. Avoiding group briefings thus saved around 35 h of SSO time annually (4 briefings for 52 weeks). The initial cost of recording the video, and updating the process on the BPM platform, was quickly amortized over time. Cumulatively, the impact of these two interventions led to approximately 535 h of departmental time savings annually.

5   Discussion and Lessons Learned

We make the following observations:

Process mining was instrumental in the problem identification. We found frequent erroneous sequences, time-wasting loops, long delays, and unexpected degrees of participation, in the PM models. While we focused on relatively basic PM techniques, they were nevertheless effective at identifying these problems. A bonus here is that the algorithms and their output are easy to understand, seeing how it was the first time that PM was applied in this government department.

PM showed a clear potential for a Return On Investment (ROI). The interventions could be seen as obvious improvements that did not necessarily require insights from PM results. In an organizational setting, however, even straight-forward improvements will involve resources for their implementation, and we found that they require a clear indication of their ROI (we revisit this issue in our conclusion). To that end, our pre-intervention analysis pointed out that process time (mean 7 days for a 10–15 minute briefing) and cost (Hiring Managers were overly involved) were problematic; and, post-intervention analysis for the Group Briefing confirmed the need for the Video Briefing intervention, as process times (similar median, 4.6 days mean) were still high.

Process time and cost were significantly reduced after the final intervention. The Group Briefing reduced the mean process times by around 2.5 days (no impact on median); the Video Briefing intervention, compared to the initial process, reduced mean process times by about 5 days (median savings of about 3 days). Regarding cost, the Group Briefing reduced the number of briefing sessions by around 60%, saving around 500 h of hiring manager time annually; the Video Briefing intervention removed employee involvement altogether.

Qualitative review of interventions applied. In terms of reducing cost and processing times, the video briefing intervention provided the most effective out-come. In turn, however, this may also mean that the briefing materials are not as fine-tuned to the applicant's needs as compared to the one-on-one briefing. Also, the applicant may not pay as close attention to the briefing materials when delivered in group format or by video. A possibility for future work is to per-form a qualitative analysis of applicant feedback on different types of security briefings to enable a cost-benefit analysis of personalized vs. standardized, and in-person vs. remote, security briefings.

Lessons learned from PM in a governmental context. We performed this case study as a centralized team of technology experts, called a "Centre of Excellence" (CoE), to collaborate with the government department. This setup is common in large organizations for a relatively novel and challenging technology. How-ever, this context gave rise to, or at least aggrevated, a number of issues. These issues were not technical, but involved the need for (a) *process selection*, i.e., prioritizing candidate processes and readiness from departments for managing risk and maximizing value; (b) *establishing value (pre- and post)*, i.e., engaging process owners a priori by presenting an ROI for resource allocation, and then measuring concrete impacts after interventions; and (c) *domain understanding*, i.e., continuous communication with process owners to understand the process and interpret analysis findings. We revisit this in the future work.

Findings from the study can be applied to other GC departments. The results applied to a single department. The GC employs over 300,000 individuals and has over 100 departments, agencies and crown corporations that implement their own version of the PSS process; applying the findings from this case study across the GC could thus yield substantial cost and time benefits. Depending on the similarities of their PSS process, findings could be directly used to improve their own process; otherwise, a methodology similar to the one presented in Sect. 3 could be used to guide potential and customized interventions.

6   Limitations

Limitations of our study include the following four items.

- *Restricted number of cases used in the study.* The sample cases (around 190 for each intervention) is only a portion of the total number of security clearance cases (3000) in the department, which is itself a fraction of the cases in the GC. The process model and performance metrics may not fully capture process variations in the entire GC, as each GC department can implement its own bespoke version of the Treasury Board of Canada's standard for security screening.
- *Potential seasonal process variations.* Different time periods may have associated differences in workload that could impact durations (e.g., process times) of security screenings. Due to time constraints, we were unable to select cases from the same annual period for the group briefings (Jan 5, 2023, to May 15, 2023) and video briefings (June 15, 2023, to Oct 23, 2023, our study endpoint).
- *Lack of event durations.* Only the start time of each event is recorded; the event duration (service time) is thus calculated as the difference between the current and next event's start times. Hence, we are unable to distinguish between the service time of an activity and the wait time to reach the next activity.
- *Limited to reliability status screening.* These findings apply to reliability status only; outcomes might differ for higher level clearances, such as secret level.

7   Conclusions and Future Work

We presented a case study of PM in government, which focused on optimizing personnel security screening from customer (process time) and organizational (cost) perspectives. We used PM to assess the full process improvement lifecycle: pre-intervention analyses pointed out initial process and performance issues; post-intervention identified the impact of interventions and further areas for improvement. Due to the use of a low-code, process-aware BPM platform, the turnaround time for interventions was relatively low. The applied interventions successfully reduced the process time from about 30.9 days down to 25.8 days on average, and removed employee involvement and associated salary implications.

The lessons learned from this case study (Sect. 5), and subsequent studies we have conducted in the meantime, will be used as a basis for a PM methodology for use in large governmental contexts. Compared to our lessons learned (Sect. 5), PM^2 [13] similarly considers PM projects from a CoE viewpoint, and discusses process selection (a) and domain understanding (c). We further found establishing value (b) to be essential.

From the GC perspective, its Policy on Service and Digital [11] emphasizes that digital transformation is ultimately focused on enhancing the customer experience. We argue that PM will play an important role in supporting this policy, by ensuring that public services are delivered in a timely and cost-effective manner, in compliance with service-level agreements. Finally, by illuminating often opaque government processes in an evidence-based way, PM has the potential to support the Open Government goals of greater openness and accountability.

Acknowledgements. This work was partially supported by GC's Innovation Funding and by the NSERC Discovery grants of W. Van Woensel and D. Amyot. We thank the process owners and department managers for their collaboration.

References

1. Delgado, A., Calegari, D.: Discovery and analysis of e-government business processes with process mining: a case study. In: 55th Hawaii International Conference on System Sciences (HICSS) (2024). http://hdl.handle.net/10125/79629
2. Delgado, A., Marotta, A., González, L., Tansini, L., Calegari, D.: Towards a data science framework integrating process and data mining for organizational improvement. In: Proceedings of the 15th ICSOFT, pp. 492–500. SciTePress (2020). https://doi.org/10.5220/0009875004920500
3. El-Gharib, N.M., Amyot, D.: Data preprocessing method and API for mining processes from cloud-based application event logs. Algorithms **15**(6) (2022). https://doi.org/10.3390/a15060180
4. Leemans, S.J., Poppe, E., Wynn, M.T.: Directly follows-based process mining: exploration & a case study. In: 2019 International Conference on Process Mining (ICPM), pp. 25–32. IEEE CS (2019). https://doi.org/10.1109/ICPM.2019.00015
5. Nai, R., Sulis, E., Genga, L.: Automated analysis with event log enrichment of the European public procurement processes. In: Sales, T.P., Araújo, J., Borbinha, J., Guizzardi, G. (eds.) CAiSE 2023. LNCS, vol. 14319, pp. 178–188. Springer, Cham (2023). https://doi.org/10.1007/978-3-031-47112-4_17
6. Osman, L.: Canada's auditor general calls on feds to create online portal for refugees amid backlogs. Global News (2023). https://globalnews.ca/news/10035790/canada-refugees-online-application-portal/
7. Park, S., Kang, Y.S.: A study of process mining-based business process innovation. Procedia Comput. Sci. **91**, 734–743 (2016). https://doi.org/10.1016/j.procs.2016.07.066
8. Rawiro, D., Gaol, F.L., Supangkat, S., Ranti, B.: Process mining applications in government sector: a systematic literature review. In: 5th European International Conference on Industrial Engineering and Operations Management, pp. 3110–3118. IEOM Society International (2022). https://doi.org/10.46254/EU05.20220617
9. Tasker, J.P.: Federal government scrambles to address hordes of passport applicants at overwhelmed offices. CBC News (2024). https://www.cbc.ca/news/politics/federal-government-passport-chaos-1.6499458
10. Treasury Board of Canada Secretariat: Standard on security screening (2014). https://www.tbs-sct.canada.ca/pol/doc-eng.aspx?id=28115
11. Treasury Board of Canada Secretariat: Policy on service and digital (2020). https://www.tbs-sct.canada.ca/pol/doc-eng.aspx?id=32603

12. Trottier, J., Woensel, W.V., Wang, X., Mallur, K., El-Gharib, N., Amyot, D.: Supplementary material (2024). https://doi.org/10.5281/zenodo.14034642
13. van Eck, M.L., Lu, X., Leemans, S.J.J., van der Aalst, W.M.P.: PM^2: a process mining project methodology. In: Zdravkovic, J., Kirikova, M., Johannesson, P. (eds.) CAiSE 2015. LNCS, vol. 9097, pp. 297–313. Springer, Cham (2015). https://doi.org/10.1007/978-3-319-19069-3_19
14. Yu, D., Trottier, J.: logprep4pm: Python library for log filtering & preprocessing of event logs (2024). https://github.com/ProcessMining-uOttawa/logprep4pm/
15. Zuidema-Tempel, E., Effing, R., van Hillegersberg, J.: Bridging the gap between process mining methodologies and process mining practices: comparing existing process mining methodologies with process mining practices at local governments and consultancy firms in The Netherlands. In: Di Ciccio, C., Dijkman, R., del Río Ortega, A., Rinderle-Ma, S. (eds.) BPM 2022. LNBIP, vol. 458, pp. 70–86. Springer, Cham (2022). https://doi.org/10.1007/978-3-031-16171-1_5

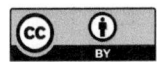

Towards an Ethogram of Exploratory Process Mining Behavior

Jessica Van Suetendael[1]([✉])[iD], Benoît Depaire[1][iD], Mieke Jans[1,2][iD], and Niels Martin[1][iD]

[1] UHasselt, Digital Future Lab, Agoralaan, 3590 Diepenbeek, Belgium
{jessica.vansuetendael,benoit.depaire,
mieke.jans,niels.martin}@uhasselt.be
[2] Maastricht University, Minderbroedersberg 4-6,
6211 LK Maastricht, The Netherlands

Abstract. Exploratory process mining aims to better understand event logs. However, this is not a clear-cut procedure and relies heavily on the analyst's cognitive skills. Research has been conducted to better understand the analyst's behavior, yet an overview of exhibited behaviors during exploratory process mining is lacking. Such an overview would not only facilitate the direct comparison of empirical findings but would also serve as a recording tool for such process mining behavior. Drawing inspiration from the field of (human) ethology, which studies behavior, this paper presents an ethogram of exploratory process mining behavior, i.e., a catalog of behaviors. Via a systematic analysis of published process mining case studies, we developed an ethogram, consisting of 26 distinct behaviors such as "Discover process model", "Define questions", and "Explore data". This ethogram provides insights into analysts' actions, contributing to a more comprehensive understanding of their role.

Keywords: Process of Process Mining · Ethogram · Exploratory Process Mining · Human Behavior

1 Introduction

Process mining (PM) aims to extract valuable insights from event logs originating from business information systems. Most endeavors of PM start with an exploratory analysis [9]. Exploratory PM is defined according to Tukey's [13] five characteristics of exploratory data analysis. These five characteristics entail a focus on understanding the data, as well as model and hypothesis building through the use of robust measures. Furthermore, graphical representations and flexibility regarding the methods used are important.

Performing exploratory PM requires a certain set of skills and knowledge, and the quality of the work depends heavily on the analyst [16]; therefore, it is vital that PM analysts receive the proper guidance and support. A better understanding of PM analysts' behavior is vital to aid them in their endeavors.

© The Author(s) 2025
A. Delgado and T. Slaats (Eds.): ICPM 2024 Workshops, LNBIP 533, pp. 586–598, 2025.
https://doi.org/10.1007/978-3-031-82225-4_43

This can be achieved by developing an ethogram, a catalog of behaviors exhibited by PM analysts [4]. Furthermore, the ethogram can also be used as a data collection and analysis tool by recording behavioral observations in a quantitative manner [6].

In this paper, an exploratory PM ethogram will be developed by systematically analyzing published PM case studies. The ethogram consists of 26 behaviors, including, "Discover process model", "Explore data", and "Define questions". This overview provides researchers with a common vocabulary of exploratory PM behavior and will aid in better understanding the task of exploratory PM. Furthermore, the ethogram can be used to analyze fine-grained behavioral data capturing exploratory PM.

The remainder of this paper is structured as follows. Section 2 discusses related work on the Process of Process Mining and human ethology. Section 3 details the methodology followed to construct the ethogram. Section 4 presents the developed ethogram of exploratory PM behavior. Section 5 discusses the ethogram, and the paper ends with a conclusion in Sect. 6.

2   Related Work

2.1   Process of Process Mining

Process of Process Mining focuses on the human aspect of PM and studies the behavior of PM analysts [16,17]. By better understanding PM behavior, improvements can be developed to better support PM analysts [9]. Areas that have already been researched include exploratory analysis [16], question development [18], and challenges that PM analysts face [19]. This research discipline employs a variety of qualitative and quantitative data-gathering techniques, such as interviews [17,18], think-aloud [16] and digital trace data [9]. Within this field, a cognitive process model (PEM4PPM) has been developed to describe how PM behavior can be analyzed in a theory-guided manner. This model can be related to our ethogram is the sense that both describe a kind of behavior. However, unlike our ethogram, the activities from this model were identified in a deductive way, which restricts unique discoveries of behaviors. Furthermore, the focus on both models is different since our ethogram is focused on exploratory PM.

While the work of Sorokina et al. [9] leans into the concept of an ethogram, the work of Capitan et al. [1] and Klinkmüller et al. [5] use a similar methodology as ours to investigate the cognitive aspect of PM. Both papers code PM case studies to find either PM operations [1] or information needs [5]. Furthermore, the work of Capitan et al. [1] identified 55 PM operations to answer performance-related questions. These operations are defined at a different granularity level than our ethogram and are focused on performance-related analysis instead of exploratory PM. In sum, no catalog of behaviors (an ethogram) exists that could support understanding exploratory PM behavior.

2.2 Human Ethology and Ethograms

Process of Process Mining can be related to human ethology, a field focused on human behavior. Like ethology, human ethology studies behavior by document-ing and analyzing it to discover patterns [4]. A commonly used method is the ethological approach developed by Lehner [6], which provides a way to gain a holistic understanding of behavior by integrating observations with experimental and theoretical perspectives.

A part of Lehner's [6] ethological approach is the development of an ethogram, a catalog of behaviors, intending to develop a better understanding of behavior displayed by a certain species. In the later stages of the approach, the ethogram is used to record qualitative data in a quantitative manner [6]. Traditionally, ethograms are developed through an observational study where all the actions of the behavior of the species in question are recorded table-wise [4]. The table consists of the name of the behavior, a description of the behavior, and, optionally, a drawing of the behavior [6]. However, ethogram development has taken a new direction, where ethograms are developed using texts describing behavior. For instance, Stanton et al. [10] used literature describing behaviors to make a standardized ethogram for the Felidae. The methodology used in this paper is based on this new direction of ethogram building.

3 Methodology[1]

Based on the coding process of Thomas [12], a six-step procedure, visualized in Fig. 1, is followed to develop our ethogram. First, relevant papers are selected and coded to find behaviors; whereafter, an ethogram is constructed. The remainder of this section describes the procedure in more detail. Further details about the methodology can be consulted in [15].

3.1 Step 1: Construct a Set of Case Studies

In the first step of the procedure, a set of published PM case studies is com-posed to extract behavior from. The following four different literature sources are identified to extract case studies from:

- 45 publicly available case studies on the IEEE Task Force of PM website.
- 36 BPI Challenge reports by professionals and academics. The reports made by students are excluded as their quality cannot be assured.
- 3 of the most recent systematic literature reviews about PM case studies [2, 3,11], containing 18, 36 and 38 case studies, respectively.
- 12 case studies discussed in the book "Process mining in Action" [7].

To qualify whether the papers from the sources are relevant, the following exclusion and inclusion criteria are established:

---

[1] Given the limited space, a separate document is provided with more detailed information [15].

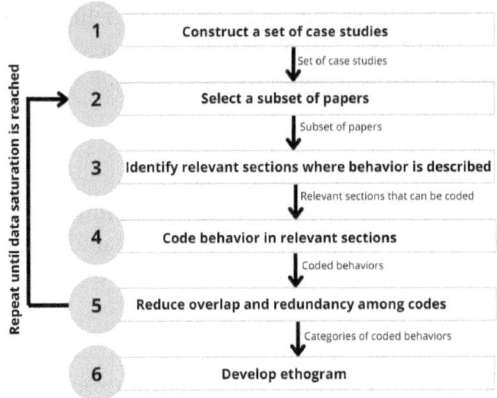

Fig. 1. Procedure that is followed in this study to construct an ethogram

- INCLUSION: A paper containing a PM case study.
- EXCLUSION: A paper not written in English.
- EXCLUSION: A paper with no online record.
- EXCLUSION: A paper that does not describe exploratory PM behavior.

The inclusion criterion requires the papers to include a PM case study. The focus on papers containing case studies is deliberate, as our study requires a description of actual PM analysts' behavior. The exclusion criteria are self-explanatory.

Exploratory analysis is iterative, starting with initial questions and evolving them as new insights emerge. Exploratory PM behavior follows this idea and is defined according to the characteristics of exploratory data analysis defined by Tukey [13], which are the following:

- a focus on understanding the data, and discovering what is going on
- graphical representations are important
- emphasis on model building and generating hypotheses
- use of robust measures, subset analysis, and reexpression
- flexibility regarding which methods are applied

Process mining practices are categorized as exploratory PM whenever the practices correspond with one of the characteristics of Tukey [13] and do not contradict any of the five characteristics. For example, process discovery is classified as exploratory because it emphasizes data understanding, uses graphical models, and applies robust measures like fitness and precision. In contrast, conformance checking is not considered exploratory, as it primarily compares logs with models rather than building new models or hypotheses.

Behavior is defined as high-level actions with specific intent. Similar behaviors are not merged if their intents differ. For instance, "Consult with experts/stakeholders" aims to extract hidden information, while "Discuss with experts/stakeholders" seeks to validate conclusions through discussion.

Applying these definitions to our inclusion and exclusion criteria, we identify 103 of 185 papers as relevant. Most papers are excluded based on a lack of describing exploratory PM behavior.

3.2   Step 2-5: Open Coding

The following steps (step 2 to 5) are performed in multiple iterations. The coding procedure is repeated until no new codes are found and data saturation is reached. Steps 3 to 5 (and 6) align closely with the steps of open coding described in [12].

Step 2: Select a Subset of Papers. For each iteration, a subset of 16 papers is selected, where four papers are selected randomly from each of the four sources. Once one of the sources is depleted, more papers are chosen from the other sources to keep the total of 16 papers per iteration constant.

Step 3: Identify Relevant Sections Where Behavior is Described. After selecting the papers for the coding iteration, relevant sections are identified within each paper. A section is deemed relevant when it describes exploratory PM behavior. These sections are used in the following steps for coding behavior.

Step 4: Code Behavior in Relevant Sections. In open coding, behaviors are labeled by examining the text line by line and marking segments where the behaviors are described. Coding involves using words or brief phrases that encapsulate the essence of each concept [8]. One person codes all the papers in Atlas.ti. Each behavior is coded independently, without the need to fit it into predefined categories. An example of this coding process applied to a segment of [14] can be found in Fig. 2. In this paragraph, six different codes are identified. Each code is assigned to a sentence or a part of a sentence. For example, the sentence "We assumed that it took place not longer than 6 months ago" is coded as an assumption due to the fact that they state "we assume".

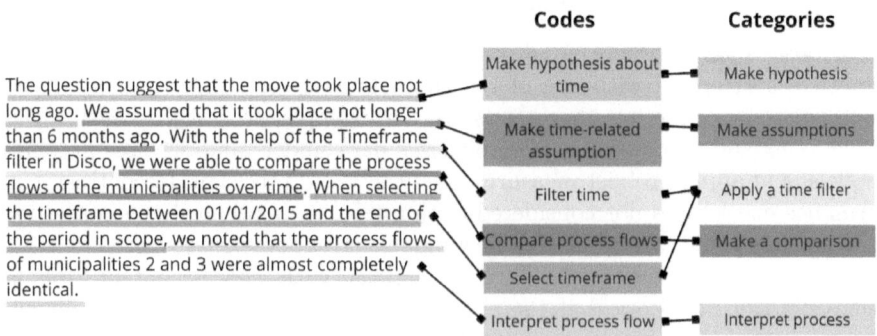

Fig. 2. Example of coding

Step 5: Reduce Overlap and Redundancy Among Codes. After all the papers are coded, the found codes are revised and combined into categories. In Fig. 2, the codes "Filter time" and "Select timeframe" are combined into one category named "Apply a time filter". The code "Compare process flows" is put into the category "Make a comparison" to make the code more general.

After step 5, a check is performed to assess whether data saturation is reached. Steps 2 to 5 are repeated until no new categories are identified.

3.3 Step 6: Develop Ethogram

To construct the ethogram, the coded categories are transformed into behaviors by grouping similar categories together, ensuring the ethogram's structure and comprehensibility. Each behavior included in the ethogram is accompanied by a clear and concise definition [6].

4 Results

This section describes the ethogram, which can be found in Table 1, which was constructed after a total of 3 iterations. After 3 iterations, data saturation was reached, and 79 coding categories were identified (75, 5, and 0 in three consecutive iterations). The 79 coding categories were grouped into 26 behaviors. The behaviors are divided into five phases: Preparation, Pre-processing, Analysis, Interpretation, and Conclusion. Note that these phases are merely introduced as a structuring element to present the ethogram in a more comprehensible way. The behaviors per phase are listed alphabetically; their order does not portray the order in which they are executed. In turn, the phases are in order of execution, although it is possible to return to a particular phase when necessary.

4.1 Phase 0: Preparation

In this phase, preparatory actions are taken for exploratory PM analysis to gain a better understanding of the context of the analysis.

Consult with Experts/Stakeholders: Consult experts/stakeholders to retrieve information that is not (easily) deductible from the data in combination with more context about the data. Furthermore, learn the expectations of the experts/stakeholders.

Define Problem Statement: Define the problem to be scrutinized with the intent of guiding what has to be analyzed and aiding the questions, scope, and strategy development. The problem statement describes the problem and the related challenges. The problem statement is often already defined.

Define Questions: Define the leading questions of the analysis to stimulate creative thinking about the application of the scope and solving the problem statement. Predefined questions are always present in exploratory process mining, even as simple as "What is going on in the data?".

Define Scope: Define the analysis scope, to set boundaries and align the analysis with its objectives. The scope determines what will be investigated and what will not. The scope should align with the problem statement and questions.

Define Strategy: Define the analysis strategy, which includes the used metrics and tools. The strategy heavily depends on the problem statement, scope, and questions. This behavior aims to provide a guide for conducting the analysis. It differs from "Define problem statement" since the focus is not on what has to be analyzed but on how to analyze it.

Examine Context: Gain a better understanding of the context of the data, which includes information about the goal of the process, the organization linked to the process, etc.

Extract Raw Data: Select and collect raw data for the analysis to create a first collection of data. This data should describe a process utilizing events. Transforming this raw data into an event log is done is the next phase (Phase 1: Pre-processing).

4.2   Phase 1: Pre-processing

The first phase entails pre-processing the data and preparing it for analysis.

Profile Data: Profile the raw data to get familiar with its content and structure. This could include calculating summary statistics or identifying data quality issues.

Remove Data: Remove data points, instances, or variables from the raw data to improve its quality. Reasons to remove data include incorrect or irrelevant data.

Transform Data: Transform the data to make it more approachable for analysis. This involves splitting, renaming, and restructuring the data. At the end, an event log should be constructed.

4.3   Phase 2: Analysis

In the second phase, the data is analyzed to discover patterns and insights.

Analyze Perspectives: Analyze the data from a specific process to gain a comprehensive understanding. Commonly used perspectives are control-flow, organizational, or time perspectives.

Apply a Filter: Focus on specific information by excluding parts of the data. A commonly applied filter is a path filter, which filters out infrequent paths. A filter will not erase data; it only temporarily excludes data.

Calculate a Metric: Calculate a previously defined metric based on the data to quantify a certain aspect of the data.

Categorize the Data: Organize the data into categories to find patterns within or across categories. These categories can be predefined or self-made by the analyst. For example, categories can be based on who executes the activity.

Create a Figure/Table: Create a figure or table to visualize patterns in the data. Examples include dotted charts and frequency tables. Process discovery is not included in this behavior since it has a different intent, namely discovering/visualizing the process instead of visualizing patterns.

Define a Metric: Define a metric to measure or describe phenomena quantitatively. This can be a more known metric or a newly defined one.

Discover a Process Model: Discover the process with a process discovery technique. The process model can represent the control flow, social network, etc. The goal of this behavior is to visualize the dynamic between activities or entities of the process.

Generate a Hypothesis: Create a testable statement or prediction that guides further analysis.

Identify an Element of Interest: Make a first observation based on the generated figure, process, table, or metric with the intent to further analyze and interpret it. This observation is a high-level observation, something that catches your eye.

Make a Comparison: Compare two or more metrics, figures, tables, or process models with one another. The goal of this behavior is to find similarities and differences.

4.4 Phase 3: Interpretation

During the third phase, the results from the analysis phase are interpreted.

Interpret Found Results: Make interpretations about the analysis results (metrics, figures, process models, etc.) to better understand them. It involves recognizing patterns, relationships, and interesting data points.

Make Assumptions: An assumption is a belief or statement accepted as true without direct evidence. An assumption is made to reduce uncertainty and ease the process of analyzing data. There is a distinction between an assumption and a hypothesis. An assumption is a belief that someone has, while a hypothesis is a prediction you make.

4.5 Phase 4: Conclusion

The last phase involves combining the interpretations that were made and drawing conclusions from them.

Answer Questions: Formulate an answer to the predefined questions using the interpretations made in the previous phase. The goal of this behavior is to provide clarity and advance the understanding of the data.

Table 1. Ethogram describing Exploratory PM behavior

Behavior	Description	Intent
Phase 0: Preparation		
Consult with experts/stakeholders	Consult experts/stakeholders to retrieve information	Retrieve information that is not (easily) deductible from the data
Define problem statement	Define the problem that will be scrutinized	Guide the analysis and aid the scope, question, and strategy development
Define questions	Define questions that need to be answered after the analysis	Stimulate creative thinking about solving the problem statement
Define scope	Define the scope of the analysis	Set boundaries and align the analysis with its objectives
Define strategy	Define the analysis strategy, such as used metrics and tools	Guide how to solve the defined questions of the analysis
Examine context	Gain a better understanding of the context of the data	Learn about the context of the data
Extract raw data	Select and collect raw data for the analysis	Create a first collection of data which will be analyzed in the later phases
Phase 1: Pre-processing		
Profile data	Profile the raw data to get familiar with it	Get familiar with the content and structure of the data
Remove data	Remove variables, instances, or data points from the raw data	Improve the quality of the data
Transform data	Apply transformations such as splitting, and restructuring	Make the data more approachable for exploratory analysis
Phase 2: Analysis		
Analyze perspectives	Analyze the process, a metric, ... from a specific perspective	Get the full picture of the process
Apply a filter	Exclude part of the data/process	Focus on specific information
Calculate a metric	Calculate a previously defined metric based on the data	Quantify a certain aspect of the process or data
Categorize the data	Organize the data/process into categories	Organize and structure the data to find patterns
Create a figure/table	Based on the data, create a figure or table	Visualize patterns in the data
Define a metric	Define a metric to measure phenomena quantitatively	Define a measure to describe a phenomena quantitatively
Discover a process model	Discover the process flow by building a process model	Visualize the sequence of a process
Generate a hypothesis	Make a hypothesis about expected outcomes	Serve as a guiding point to further analyze a certain aspect of the data
Identify an element of interest	Make an observation based on a figure, process, table, ...	Identify an interesting element which will be further analyzed
Make a comparison	Compare two or more metrics, figures, ... with one another	Find similarities and differences
Phase 3: Interpretation		
Interpret found results	Make interpretations about the results	Gain a better understanding of what is discovered during the analysis
Make assumptions	Make an assumption about the data/process	Simplify the analysis process by accepting certain conditions
Phase 4: Conclusion		
Answer questions	Formulate an answer for the questions	Provide clarity and advance the understanding of the data
Discuss with experts/stakeholders	Validate previously made assumptions	Validate assumptions through discussion
Make recommendations	Make recommendations based on the results	Provide guidance for further actions or further analysis
Revise hypothesis	Revise a previously made hypothesis	Ensure the relevance and accuracy of the created hypothesis

Discuss with Experts/Stakeholders: Validate previously made assumptions and discuss found results by consulting with experts/stakeholders.

Make Recommendations: Make recommendations based on the interpretations made in the previous phase. It gives guidance for the next steps to improve or better understand the process under analysis.

Revise Hypothesis: Revise a previously made hypothesis to ensure the relevance and accuracy of the created hypothesis. The hypothesis is not tested, since this is not a part of exploratory PM.

5   Discussion

5.1   Implications

Fine-grained activity data, such as digital trace data, has its challenges when searching for meaningful patterns and insights about the behavior described in the data. An ethogram can be used to transform such fine-grained activity data into more comprehensible behavioral data by aggregating detailed actions into broader behaviors based on their shared intent. For instance, actions like 'filter', 'select', and 'remove' related to a variable can be combined into the behavior "Remove data." This shift in granularity allows for a more meaningful analysis of PM. However, digital trace data only reveals actions, not the intent behind them. Qualitative methods such as interviews or think-aloud practices are necessary to uncover intent. These methods help clarify why certain actions were taken, providing a fuller understanding of observed behaviors. Combining quantitative data with qualitative insights is crucial for accurately interpreting behaviors.

5.2   Comparison with PEM4PPM Model

Sorokina et al. [9] developed the PEM4PPM model to describe PM behavior, similar to our ethogram but with key differences. The ethogram defines more specific behaviors, while PEM4PPM remains at a higher level. Furthermore, PEM4PPM is process-structured, whereas the ethogram categorizes behaviors into five phases. Additionally, the ethogram focuses on exploratory PM, while PEM4PPM describes theory-guided PM. Despite their differences, the PEM4PPM model and our ethogram share similarities. Nine out of ten PEM4PPM activities align with behaviors in the ethogram based on matching actions and intents. Figure 3 illustrates these connections.

The activity "Task understanding" links to Phase 0 (Preparation) and Phase 1 (Pre-processing) behaviors. It involves understanding the problem, data, and consulting experts, corresponding to the behaviors "Examine context", "Define questions", "Explore data", and "Consult with experts/stakeholders." The "Set/Refine goal" activity links to "Define strategy", focusing on deciding how to analyze data to answer predefined questions. The "Focus" activity corresponds with "Apply a filter" since both aim to focus at a specific part of the process.

The "Explore" activity aligns with Phase 2 (Analysis) behaviors, excluding "Generate a hypothesis" and "Apply a filter", illustrating PEM4PPM's higher-level definition compared to the ethogram. "Interpret results" can be linked to both "Interpret data" and "Assess results", which aim to explain insights from the analysis phase. The difference is that checking hypothesis is included in "Assess results", which is not part of exploratory PM. "Generate hypotheses" is similarly defined in PEM4PPPM and the ethogram, focusing on generating hypotheses from data insights. The "Create artifact" activity involves goal-driven object creation, aligning with "Explore" if focused on exploratory analysis but not matching any ethogram behaviors if outside this scope. Finally, the "Conclude" activity corresponds to "Answer question", focusing on addressing predefined questions.

The activity "Test hypotheses" could not be linked to the ethogram as it does not align with exploratory PM. Additionally, PEM4PMM lacks coverage of dataset preparation and omits behaviors such as "Define problem statement", "Extract raw data", "Remove data", and "Transform data". Futhermore, the behaviors "Revise hypothesis", "Discuss with stakeholders", and "Make recommendations" also have no counterparts.

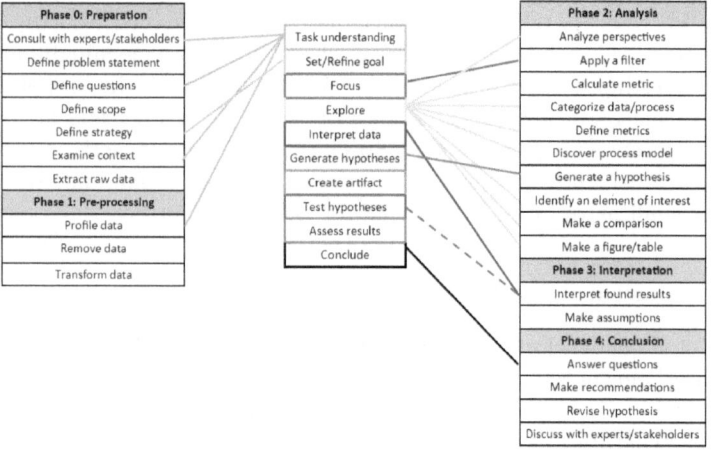

Fig. 3. Comparison between Ethogram and PEM4PPM

6   Conclusion

Analyzing exploratory PM behavior can be challenging. To aid in this endeavor, this paper developed an ethogram of 26 behaviors observed during exploratory PM, categorized into 5 phases: Preparation, Pre-processing, Analysis, Interpretation, and Conclusions. This ethogram provides a clear overview of the different behaviors and a vocabulary that can be used to analyze exploratory PM behavior. The ethogram is based purely on the behavior described in the literature; 48 case studies were investigated and coded to this end. Despite the meticulously designed research method, we acknowledge three key limitations to this research. Firstly, only selected sources of case studies have been considered. Therefore, there is a risk that not all behaviors have been identified. Secondly, as the ethogram is based on published case studies, some performed behaviors might not be explicitly or implicitly reported since some behaviors might be omitted by the authors of the case studies. Those behaviors could not be integrated as part of the ethogram. Thirdly, since coding was only performed by one person, some subjectivity is introduced into the results. Future research directions include the application of the ethogram to make fine-grained digital trace data more comprehensible for analysis purposes by linking the behaviors of the ethogram to the fine-grained actions. Another area for future research is to refine the ethogram based on interviews with PM analysts. Through interviews, the intent of the different behaviors can be further investigated. Lastly, our ethogram was tailored to exploratory PM. Ethograms describing other PM behaviors, such as predictive PM, can be developed in future research.

Acknowledgment. This study was supported by the Special Research Fund (BOF) of Hasselt University under Grant No. BOF23OWB03.

References

1. Capitán-Agudo, C., Salas-Urbano, M., Cabanillas, C., Resinas, M.: Analyzing how process mining reports answer time performance questions. In: International Conference on Business Process Management, pp. 234–250 (2022)
2. Corallo, A., Lazoi, M., Striani, F.: Process mining and industrial applications: a systematic literature review. Knowl. Process. Manag. **27**(3), 225–233 (2020)
3. Dakic, D., Stefanovic, D., Cosic, I., Lolic, T., Medojevic, M.: Business process mining application: a literature review. In: Annals of DAAAM & Proceedings, vol. 29 (2018)
4. Immelmann, K., Beer, C.: A dictionary of ethology (1989)
5. Klinkmüller, C., Müller, R., Weber, I.: Mining process mining practices: an exploratory characterization of information needs in process analytics. In: Business Process Management: 17th International Conference, BPM 2019, Vienna, Austria, 1–6 September 2019, Proceedings 17, pp. 322–337 (2019)
6. Lehner, P.N.: Handbook of ethological methods (1998)
7. Reinkemeyer, L.: Process mining in action. In: Process Mining in Action Principles, Use Cases and Outlook (2020)
8. Saldaña, J.: The coding manual for qualitative researchers (2021)
9. Sorokina, E., Soffer, P., Hadar, I., Leron, U., Zerbato, F., Weber, B.: PEM4PPM: A cognitive perspective on the process of process mining. In: International Conference on Business Process Management, pp. 465–481 (2023)
10. Stanton, L.A., Sullivan, M.S., Fazio, J.M.: A standardized ethogram for the felidae: a tool for behavioral researchers. Appl. Anim. Behav. Sci. **173**, 3–16 (2015)
11. Thiede, M., Fuerstenau, D., Bezerra Barquet, A.P.: How is process mining technology used by organizations? A systematic literature review of empirical studies. Bus. Process. Manag. J. **24**(4), 900–922 (2018)

12. Thomas, D.R.: A general inductive approach for analyzing qualitative evaluation data. Am. J. Eval. **27**(2), 237–246 (2006)
13. Tukey, J.: Exploratory data analysis (1977)
14. Van den Spiegel, P., Blevi, L.: Discovery and analysis of the Dutch permitting process (2015)
15. Van Suetendael, J., Depaire, B., Jans, M., Martin, N.: Methodology details of towards an ethogram of exploratory process mining behavior. Zenodo (2024). https://doi.org/10.5281/zenodo.13253995
16. Zerbato, F., Soffer, P., Weber, B.: Initial insights into exploratory process mining practices. In: Business Process Management Forum: BPM Forum 2021, Rome, Italy, 06–10 September 2021, Proceedings 19, pp. 145–161 (2021)
17. Zerbato, F., Soffer, P., Weber, B.: Process mining practices: Evidence from interviews. In: International Conference on Business Process Management, pp. 268–285. Springer, Cham (2022)
18. Zerbato, F., Koorn, J.J., Beerepoot, I., Weber, B., Reijers, H.A.: On the origin of questions in process mining projects. In: International Conference on Enterprise Design, Operations, and Computing, pp. 165–181 (2022)
19. Zimmermann, L., Zerbato, F., Weber, B.: Process mining challenges perceived by analysts: an interview study. In: International Conference on Business Process Modeling, Development and Support, pp. 3–17 (2022)

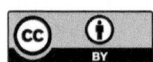

1st International Workshop on Generative Artificial Intelligence for Process Mining (GenAI4PM 2024)

Preface

1st International Workshop on Generative AI for Process Mining (GenAI4PM 2024)

The First International Workshop on Generative AI for Process Mining (GenAI4PM 2024) came at a pivotal moment, marking the convergence of two transformative fields: generative AI and process mining. While early explorations have demonstrated the potential of GenAI in process analysis, this workshop aimed to delve deeper into the methodologies, practical implementations, and long-term implications of this powerful synergy. We sought to foster a dynamic exchange between researchers developing cutting-edge techniques and organizations eager to leverage GenAI for process improvement and innovation. A key objective was to explore the integration of GenAI with other advanced technologies, paving the way for a future where processes are not just mined, but intelligently shaped and automated.

This volume presents six accepted papers that offer a diverse and insightful glimpse into the landscape of GenAI for process mining. These contributions span a range of crucial topics, from benchmarking the capabilities of LLMs in process mining tasks to developing novel frameworks for process optimization and automated process model generation.

The paper by Alessandro Berti et al. introduces PM-LLM-Benchmark, a comprehensive benchmark designed to evaluate the performance of open-source LLMs on a variety of process mining tasks. This benchmark considers both domain-specific and process-specific knowledge and explores different implementation strategies, providing valuable insights into the current capabilities and limitations of LLMs in the process mining domain.

Max W. Vogt et al. present a proof-of-concept framework that integrates LLM-based agents into process mining. This agentic approach aims to democratize access to process optimization by enabling users with limited expertise to leverage the power of process mining for process discovery, problem identification, and improvement suggestion.

Kaan Apaydin et al. explore the use of locally fine-tuned LLMs for automated business process modeling. Their proposed pipeline takes textual process descriptions as input and generates process tree representations, addressing privacy concerns associated with third-party LLMs while maintaining promising process model quality.

The paper by Nataliia Klievtsova et al. investigates the qualitative aspects of LLM-generated process models through a user survey. Their findings reveal a surprising preference for LLM-generated models over human-created models, suggesting that LLMs have the potential to meet and even exceed expert expectations in process model generation.

Andrea Cosmin Redis et al. introduce a novel approach to skill learning in LLMs by integrating process mining techniques. This integration enables flexible skill discovery, parallel execution of tasks, and improved interpretability of generated plans, addressing key limitations of current LLM-based plan generation methods.

Finally, Wesley da Silva Santos et al. address the scarcity of publicly available multi-perspective declarative process models. Their work introduces a tool for generating synthetic MP-Declare models using LLMs, providing a valuable resource for the BPM community and facilitating research on declarative process mining.

These six papers represent a significant step forward in our understanding of the potential of GenAI for process mining, laying the foundation for future research and innovation in this novel field.

October 2024

Maxim Vigdof
Alessandro Berti
Mohammadreza Fani Sani

Organization

Program Committee

Adela del Río Ortega	Universidad de Sevilla, Spain
Agnes Koschmider	University of Bayreuth, Germany
Amin Beheshti	Macquarie University, Australia
Amin Jalali	Stockholm University, Sweden
Andrea Burattin	Technical University of Denmark, Denmark
Andreas Oberweis	KIT, Germany
Arthur ter Hofstede	QUT, Australia
Arik Senderovich	University of Toronto, Canada
Boualem Benatallah	Dublin City University, Ireland
Chiara Di Francescomarino	University of Trento, Italy
Chiara Ghidini	FBK, Italy
David Chapela	University of Tartu, Estonia
Fabrizio Maria Maggi	Free University of Bozen-Bolzano, Italy
Fareed Zandkarimi	University of Mannheim, Germany
Felix Mannhardt	Eindhoven University of Technology, The Netherlands
Gabriel Marques Tavares	LMU München, Germany
Gyunam Park	RWTH Aachen University, Germany
Istvan Koren	RWTH Aachen University, Germany
Jan Mendling	Humboldt University of Berlin, Germany
Luciana Barbieri	University of Campinas, Brazil
Manuel Resinas	Universidad de Sevilla, Spain
Marlon Dumas	University of Tartu, Estonia
Majid Rafiei	SAP, Germany
Michal Sroka	Microsoft, Denmark
Kamil Żbikowski	Processifier, Poland
Karolin Winter	Eindhoven University of Technology, The Netherlands
Kleber Stroeh	Pegasystems, Brazil
Yago Fontenla-Seco	Universidad Intercontinental de la Empresa, Spain
Stefanie Rinderle-Ma	Technical University of Munich, Germany

Sven Weinzierl   Friedrich-Alexander-Universität
                              Erlangen-Nürnberg, Germany
Thomas Grisold   University of St. Gallen
Urszula Jessen   ECE, Germany

Local Large Language Models for Business Process Modeling

Kaan Apaydin[1(✉)] and Yorck Zisgen[2]

[1] Department of Computer Science, Kiel University, Kiel, Germany
kap@informatik.uni-kiel.de
[2] University of Bayreuth, Bayreuth, Germany
yorck.zisgen@uni-bayreuth.de

Abstract. Large language models (LLMs) are capable of efficiently understanding natural language by processing large volumes of text data. Natural language is also used in process descriptions, thus LLMs appear to be a suitable candidate to significantly improve business process modeling. Although plenty of third-party LLMs exist, they raise the risk of privacy disclosure, untrustworthiness, and generalizability of the results. This paper proposes a pipeline to use a local and fine-tuned LLM that expects a textual process description as input and finally generates a visual process tree representation. We instantiate our pipeline with Llama3 8B and fine-tune the LLM with a training set of 120 self-generated examples. Initial evaluation results of our LLM-based approach for automated business process modeling promise usefulness of the approach in terms of process model quality while preserving data privacy.

Keywords: Generative AI · Large Language Models · Process Modeling · Fine-Tuning · Pipeline · Process Descriptions · Dataset

1 Introduction

Large Language Models (LLMs) have gained significant attention for their ability to process text data, making them a suitable candidate for business process management tasks, particularly for business process modeling [4]. Existing LLM-based approaches for business process modeling rely on cloud-based services to generate process models from textual descriptions [1,3,7]. However, sharing sensitive data with third parties hampers data privacy and security.

This paper proposes an LLM-based processing pipeline for automatic business process modeling. Compared to existing works, the pipeline relies on fine-tuning and local deployment of LLMs. By fine-tuning an LLM, it can demonstrate competitive performance against commercial vendors like ChatGPT with GPT-4 on specific tasks [2,9], while offering an improved control over data security when employed locally.

We use prompt engineering techniques and input from process experts to generate a representative data set consisting of process trees [8] and textual process descriptions. The data set is then used to fine-tune a local LLM.

© The Author(s) 2025
A. Delgado and T. Slaats (Eds.): ICPM 2024 Workshops, LNBIP 533, pp. 605–609, 2025.
https://doi.org/10.1007/978-3-031-82225-4_44

We demonstrate the feasibility of the pipeline by implementing a tool for generating training data with scripts for fine-tuning LLMs[1] relying on our dataset[2], and providing the first fine-tuned LLM for modeling process trees when prompted with process descriptions[3].

The remainder of the paper is structured as follows. Section 2 presents a comparative analysis of related works. The LLM-based pipeline is presented in Sect. 3. The paper concludes with Sect. 4.

2   Related Work

Existing LLM-based approaches primarily use the latest versions of ChatGPT [1,3,4] and, to a lesser extent, Gemini for modeling processes based on textual descriptions [7]. Common across the approaches is the integration of definitions for process modeling languages, ensuring that the LLM response uses the expected process model notation. Additionally, few-shot learning techniques have been found to be advantageous in improving process model quality. Kourani et al. [7] further report improved results through role injection and negative prompting. However, to the best of our knowledge, there remains a gap in the literature regarding techniques that utilize locally executed LLMs and fine-tuning. Even though other authors considered fine-tuning, it is often reported as unfeasible due to the extensive datasets that are required but not available.

3   Pipeline for Process Modeling Using Local LLMs

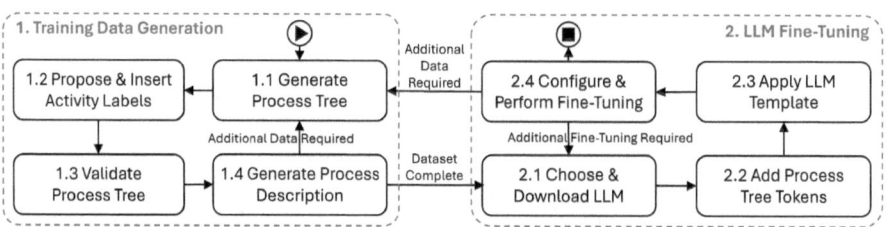

Fig. 1. Pipeline for generating training data and fine-tuning an LLM.

Figure 1 shows our pipeline, which consists of two phases: *(1) Training Data Generation* and *(2) LLM Fine-Tuning*. In the first phase, labeled process trees and their corresponding textual descriptions are generated to serve as a training data set for fine-tuning in phase 2. The first phase consists of four steps and is performed iteratively while additional data is required.

---

[1] https://github.com/ApaydinK/local-LLMs-for-process-modelling.
[2] https://huggingface.co/datasets/ApaydinK/process_trees_w_descriptions.
[3] https://huggingface.co/ApaydinK/lora_model_process_tree_generator.

1.1. Generate Process Tree: In this step the user generates a random process tree using e.g. the implementation of the framework described by [6] in PM4PY. We generated random process trees in increasing complexity. Starting with three activities and going up to nine activities while iteratively restarting the first phase. The weights for choosing operators randomly was set to sequence 0.5, choice 0.2, parallel 0.2, and loop 0.1. In this step, the activities have dummy labels. **1.2 Propose & Insert Activity Labels**: In this step, the LLM proposes concrete process activity labels to replace the dummy labels based on the process tree's control flow. Subsequently, in step **1.3 Validate Process Tree** the user validates and revises the meaningfulness of the process tree and thus can shift or rename activities and operators. Next, in step **1.4 Generate Process Description** the user manually generates a textual process description corresponding to the process tree of step 1.3. In our case, three process experts leveraged our tool (see footnote 1) to view the process tree while generating a corresponding process description.

In the second phase, the process trees and corresponding process descriptions are used to fine-tune a local LLM in four steps. **2.1 Choose & Download LLM:** First, a publicly available LLM is chosen and downloaded. We chose Llama 3 8B Instruct[4] and downloaded the LLM without quantization as it has high rankings across benchmarks on the HuggingFace LLM Leaderboard[5]. **2.2 Add Process Tree Tokens:** The string representation of the process tree's operators are then added to the tokenizer of the LLM. **2.3 Apply LLM Template:** Then, the LLM-specific template for prompts and responses is applied. This is done to ensure that the training data will be delivered to the LLM in the format that it requires, e.g. providing a system message labeling the textual description as input and defining the process tree as the desired output. **2.4 Configure & Perform Fine-Tuning:** Finally, the LLM is fine-tuned. This step can involve testing different parameter configurations. We used LoRA [5] with rank 16 for efficient fine-tuning and bfloat 16 to improve accuracy over 10 epochs.

The performance of the fine-tuned LLM was evaluated iteratively after performing both phases of the pipeline three times. For evaluation, we used one process description from the PET Dataset[6] and modeled a ground truth process tree for comparison with sequence, choice, parallel, and loop operators. We observed that after fine-tuning with 40 examples, the LLM modeled sound process trees in 11 of 15 cases. After fine-tuning with 80 examples, all modeled process trees were sound. After fine-tuning with 120 examples, the proposal of process activity labels improved further - on average, 6,66 out of the 8 expected activities were modeled successfully. However, despite these advances, challenges remained in finding the correct process model. Especially the identification of parallel activities was difficult. The average F1 score of discovered process models increased from 0.36 after the first to 0.53 after the third iteration.

---

[4] https://llama.meta.com/.

[5] https://huggingface.co/spaces/open-llm-leaderboard/open_llm_leaderboard.

[6] https://pdi.fbk.eu/pet-dataset/.

4 Conclusion

In this paper, we proposed a pipeline for fine-tuning locally deployed LLMs for modeling process trees based on textual descriptions. We demonstrated the feasibility of the pipeline by generating training data and fine-tuning a local LLM. After fine-tuning with 120 examples, the local LLM exhibited adequate performance in proposing activity labels. It consistently generated sound process trees, while the identification of parallel activities still has potential for improvement.

Future research should focus on expanding the size and diversity of the training dataset. Incorporating a wider array of process trees and using different linguistic styles for process descriptions could enhance the LLM's ability to generalize. Additionally, decomposing the modeling task into smaller steps could lead to more robust results. For instance, initially extracting activity labels followed by determining the control flow for each activity might yield improved outcomes. Finally, exploring various LLMs and fine-tuning configurations could provide further insights into optimizing performance.

Acknowledgments. This project has received funding from the State of Schleswig-Holstein under the Datencampus project grant no. 220 21 016, the Federal Ministry for Digital and Transport under the CAPTN-Förde 5G project grant no. 45FGU139 H and the German Federal Ministry of Education and Research (BMBF) for the ABBA project grant no. 16DHBKI002, 16DHBKI003, 16DHBKI004, 16DHBKI005.

References

1. Bellan, P., Dragoni, M., Ghidini, C.: Extracting business process entities and relations from text using pre-trained language models and in-context learning. In: Enterprise Design, Operations, and Computing. Lecture Notes in Computer Science, vol. 13585, pp. 182–199. Springer, Cham (2022)
2. Bucher, M.J.J., Martini, M.: Fine-tuned 'small' LLMs (still) significantly outperform zero-shot generative AI models in text classification (2024)
3. Fill, H.G., Fettke, P., Köpke, J.: Conceptual modeling and large language models: impressions from first experiments With ChatGPT. Enterp. Modell. Inf. Syst. Archit. (EMISAJ) **18**(3), 1–15 (2023)
4. Grohs, M., Abb, L., Elsayed, N., Rehse, J.R.: Large language models can accomplish business process management tasks. In: International Conference on Business Process Management, pp. 453–465. Springer (2023)
5. Hu, E.J., et al.: LoRA: low-rank adaptation of large language models (2021)
6. Jouck, T., Depaire, B.: PTandLogGenerator: a generator for artificial event data (2016)
7. Kourani, H., Berti, A., Schuster, D., van der Aalst, W.M.P.: Process Modeling with large language models. In: International Conference on Business Process Modeling, Development and Support, pp. 229–244. Springer (2024)
8. van Zelst, S.J., Leemans, S.J.J.: Translating workflow nets to process trees: an algorithmic approach. Algorithms **13**(11), 279 (2020)
9. Zhao, J., et al.: LoRA land: 310 fine-tuned LLMs that rival GPT-4, a technical report (2024)

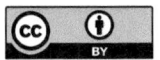

PM-LLM-Benchmark: Evaluating Large Language Models on Process Mining Tasks

Alessandro Berti[1,2](✉)(iD), Humam Kourani[1,2](iD),
and Wil M. P. van der Aalst[1,2](iD)

[1] Process and Data Science Chair, RWTH Aachen University, Aachen, Germany
{a.berti,wvdaalst}@pads.rwth-aachen.de
[2] Fraunhofer FIT, Sankt Augustin, Germany
humam.kourani@fit.fraunhofer.de

Abstract. Large Language Models (LLMs) have the potential to semi-automate some process mining (PM) analyses. While commercial models are already adequate for many analytics tasks, the competitive level of open-source LLMs in PM tasks is unknown. In this paper, we propose *PM-LLM-Benchmark*, the first comprehensive benchmark for PM focusing on domain knowledge (process-mining-specific and process-specific) and on different implementation strategies. We focus also on the challenges in creating such a benchmark, related to the public availability of the data and on evaluation biases by the LLMs. Overall, we observe that most of the considered LLMs can perform some process mining tasks at a satisfactory level, but tiny models that would run on edge devices are still inadequate. We also conclude that while the proposed benchmark is useful for identifying LLMs that are adequate for process mining tasks, further research is needed to overcome the evaluation biases and perform a more thorough ranking of the "competitive" LLMs.

Keywords: Process Mining · Large Language Models · Evaluation Strategies · LLM Benchmarking

1   Introduction

Process mining (PM) is a branch of data science aiming to derive process-related insights from the event data recorded during the execution of a process. A wide set of automated PM techniques exist for process discovery (the automated discovery of process models starting from the event data), conformance checking (comparing event data and process models), and model enhancement (annotating a process model with metrics derived from the event data). PM could benefit significantly from the provision of domain knowledge [7]. Modern Large Language Models (LLMs) have the capability to follow the instructions contained in a given prompt and are trained on large sets of generic knowledge, including process-related knowledge. The release of OpenAI's GPT-4 has been a milestone,

A. Delgado and T. Slaats (Eds.): ICPM 2024 Workshops, LNBIP 533, pp. 610–623, 2025.
https://doi.org/10.1007/978-3-031-82225-4_45

as such LLM proved capable in different PM tasks [4] including semantic anomaly detection and root cause analysis. However, GPT-4 is a commercial LLM, and open-source LLMs were significantly behind the quality of GPT-4. Recently, many companies released good-performing open-source LLMs, which in general-purpose benchmarks approach GPT-4-level quality[1]. For example, *Llama 3*[2] by Meta, *Mixtral 8x7B* and *Mixtral 8x22B*[3] by Mistral, and *WizardLM2*[4] by Microsoft are all-rounder LLMs. Also alternative commercial models have been proposed from Antrophic (*Claude AI*[5]) and Google (*Gemini*[6]), which also approach GPT-4 levels of quality.

Given the large number of commercial and open-source LLMs, benchmarks are essential to distinguish between good and bad-for-the-purpose LLMs. While many general-purpose benchmarks exist for LLMs, there is a lack of comprehensive benchmarks in process mining (PM). Several factors contribute to the difficulty of proposing such a benchmark: multiple PM artifacts exist (e.g., traditional/object-centric event logs, procedural/declarative process models, situation tables); multiple PM types exist (e.g., process discovery, conformance checking, applications of machine learning such as anomaly detection and root cause analysis, predictive analytics); multiple PM practices exist, with different pathways followed during a process mining analysis [27]; multiple PM code libraries and query languages exist, including Python (e.g., pm4py), SQL, and non-relational languages; and the ability to propose valuable answers depends on the ability of the analyst to propose valuable inquiries/hypotheses [2].

In this paper, we propose three main contributions: i) a first *comprehensive benchmark for process mining tasks executable by LLMs*, focusing on two implementation paradigms (direct provision of insights and code generation), and including several categories of "static" prompts (stored in TXT files) requiring process-mining-specific and process-specific domain knowledge; ii) a *scalable evaluation strategy* to assess the quality of the textual/coding answers provided by LLMs; iii) the *results of the application of the benchmark* on several state-of-the-art LLMs. While the benchmark provides a score useful to rank LLMs, some caveats discussed in Sect. 3 suggest avoiding comparing the scores for highly-performing LLMs. In particular, the role and limitations of LLMs as judges for PM tasks' outputs need to be discussed along with the need for ground truth in scoring the answers. Moreover, advanced implementation paradigms (RAG, agents crew, multi-stage hypothesis generation), discussed in Sect. 5, are not assessed by the benchmark.

The rest of the paper is organized as follows. Section 2 describes the related work connecting process mining and LLMs, and the evaluation of LLMs outputs. Section 3 introduces the categories of prompts included in the benchmark and the

---

[1] https://chat.lmsys.org/.
[2] https://llama.meta.com/llama3/.
[3] https://mistral.ai/news/mixtral-of-experts/.
[4] https://huggingface.co/WizardLM.
[5] https://claude.ai/.
[6] https://gemini.google.com/.

proposed evaluation strategy. Section 4 discusses the results of the benchmark on state-of-the-art LLMs. Section 5 proposes some novel scenarios requiring novel benchmarks. Finally, Sect. 6 concludes the paper.

2   Related Work

Connecting LLMs to PM: Several Business Process Management tasks have been linked with LLMs [24]. For instance, process modeling exploits LLMs to create process models starting from textual descriptions [11,15,16]. Process mining tasks have been implemented on LLMs thanks to textual description of the mainstream artifacts (event logs, process models) [4]. Three implementation paradigms are identified [3]: i) *direct provision of insights*, ii) *generation of database queries* (SQL), and iii) *autonomous hypotheses generation*. The direct provision of insights requires the provision of the necessary information to the LLM. Generating database queries [13] uses LLMs to create (SQL) statements to be executed against the data source, mitigating privacy risks but not exploiting the domain knowledge of LLMs. The autonomous formulation of hypotheses combines the two methodologies allowing the LLM to create database queries and interpret their output. In [2], the capabilities required for process mining on LLMs are described: *acceptance of long prompts*, allowing for the provision of a significant amount of information to the LLM; *acceptance of visual prompts*, as visualizations allow us to easily identify process-related patterns; *coding capabilities*, including the generation of scripts and SQL statements; and *factuality*, being able to cross-check the outputs against knowledge bases or search engines. Given the absence of process-mining-specific benchmarks, [2] suggests using general-purpose benchmarks (using traditional, domain-knowledge, visual, coding, fairness, and hypotheses generation benchmarks).

Other Benchmarks of PM on LLMs: In [13], the authors assess the LLM-based translation of process mining questions proposed in [1] to SQL statements. They found that even advanced LLMs require the provision of database-specific and process-mining-specific domain knowledge, that requires prompt injection. Moreover, the questions that could be translated to SQL statements are quantitative and do not assess the process-specific knowledge of the LLMs. In [3], an initial comparison of two LLMs (GPT-4 and Google Bard) on different process mining tasks and implementation paradigms is performed. The results lay the foundations for this paper, which proposes a much more comprehensive benchmark. In [9,10], some benchmarks covering causal reasoning and explaining decision points in business processes are proposed. In [21], benchmarks for some semantics-aware process mining tasks, i.e. semantic anomaly detection and the prediction of the next activity, are provided along with strategies to fine-tune the LLMs to improve their ability to execute the tasks. Moreover, [26] proposes a benchmark at the intersection between Robotic Process Automation and Business Process Management, evaluating the ability to exploit workflows recorded in user screenshots for Business Process Management tasks.

LLMs-as-Judges: As the outputs of LLMs are mainly textual, evaluating them in an automatic way is challenging. Some metrics have been proposed to evaluate how well an answer matches a "ground truth" provided by an human analyst[7]. However, their evaluation schema cannot be adapted to open-ended answers. Another option is to let an LLM evaluate the answer (LLM-as-a-Judge) [28]. Using LLMs as judges, the evaluation can be tailored to the desired criteria and consider open-ended answers. Some studies compared the scores given by humans and LLMs to a given set of questions/answers, finding a good alignment between humans and LLMs [23,28]. However, some studies highlighted potential weaknesses due to bias [20] and difficulty in following arbitrary evaluation directives [8]. In [22], it is shown that LLMs (as also humans) suffer from the Dunning-Kruger effect, underestimating/overestimating scores. LLMs-as-Judges can be implemented with or without the provision of a ground truth [6]. If no ground truth is provided, it is necessary that the judge LLM would be able to i) respond correctly to the given inquiry; ii) identify errors and opportunities for improvement in the provided answer. In ranking different LLMs without ground truth, there are other potential biases to consider. In [25], it is highlighted how LLMs tend to prefer answers of similar LLMs. The "egocentric bias" (LLMs preferring their own answers) is highlighted in [14].

3   Benchmark

In this section, we describe *PM-LLM-Benchmark*, which is available at the address https://github.com/fit-alessandro-berti/pm-llm-benchmark. First, in Sect. 3.1, we describe the categories of prompts included in the benchmarks. Then, in Sect. 3.2, we describe the evaluation strategy (LLM-as-a-Judge).

3.1   Categories of Tasks

Our benchmark measures how much an LLM is *knowledgeable* and *capable* in process mining. The capability is measured in the correct interpretation and production of different process mining artifacts (traditional and object-centric event logs; procedural and declarative process models). We also evaluate the ability of the LLM to autonomously formulate hypotheses over the event data or the process model. Moreover, as the goal of process mining is to assist data-driven decision-making, we aim to assess how much the LLM is able to identify biases starting from the event data. We also want to assess the ability of Large Vision Language Models (LVLMs; so LLMs supporting visual prompts) to interpret popular visualizations and process mining diagrams.

The benchmark focuses on two implementation paradigms, i.e., the *direct provision of insights* and *code generation*. Moreover, specific focus is given on process-mining-specific and process-specific *domain knowledge*, which is required for the considered prompts. Other available lists of process mining inquiries, such

---

[7] https://mlflow.org/docs/latest/llms/llm-evaluate/index.html.

Table 1. Prompts included in the benchmark.

	Prompt	Open	Requires DK	Task	Input Abstraction	Input Dataset
C1	cat01_01_variants_bpic2020_rca	X	X	RCA	Variants	BPI2020 Domestic
C1	cat01_02_variants_roadtraffic_anomalies	X	X	Semantic AD	Variants	Road Traffic
C1	cat01_03_bpic2020_var_descr	X	X	Description	Variants	BPI2020 Domestic
C1	cat01_04_roadtraffic_var_descr	X	X	Description	Variants	Road Traffic
C1	cat01_05_bpic2020_dfg_descr	X	X	Description	DFG	BPI2020 Domestic
C1	cat01_06_roadtraffic_dfg_descr	X	X	Description	DFG	Road Traffic
C1	cat01_07_ocel_container_description	X	X	Description	OC-DFG	Logistics
C1	cat01_08_ocel_order_description	X	X	Description	OC-DFG	Order Management
C1	cat01_09_ocel_container_rca	X	X	RCA	OC-DFG	Logistics
C1	cat01_10_ocel_order_rca	X	X	RCA	OC-DFG	Order Management
C2	cat02_01_open_event_abstraction	X	X	Domain Knowledge		
C2	cat02_02_open_process_cubes	X	X	Domain Knowledge		
C2	cat02_03_open_decomposition_strategies	X	X	Domain Knowledge		
C2	cat02_04_open_trace_clustering	X	X	Domain Knowledge		
C2	cat02_05_open_rpa	X	X	Domain Knowledge		
C2	cat02_06_open_anomaly_detection	X	X	Domain Knowledge		
C2	cat02_07_open_process_enhancement	X	X	Domain Knowledge		
C2	cat02_08_closed_process_mining		X	Domain Knowledge		
C2	cat02_09_closed_petri_nets		X	Domain Knowledge		
C3	cat03_01_temp_profile_generation	X	X	Process Modeling		
C3	cat03_02_declare_generation	X	X	Process Modeling		
C3	cat03_03_log_skeleton_generation	X	X	Process Modeling		
C3	cat03_04_process_tree_generation	X	X	Process Modeling		
C3	cat03_05_powl_generation	X	X	Process Modeling		
C3	cat03_06_temp_profile_discovery	X	X	Process Discovery	Variants	Road Traffic
C3	cat03_07_declare_discovery	X	X	Process Discovery	Variants	Road Traffic
C3	cat03_08_log_skeleton_discovery	X	X	Process Discovery	Variants	Road Traffic
C4	cat04_01_bpmn_xml_tasks	X	X	Task List	BPMN XML	Running Example
C4	cat04_02_bpmn_json_description	X	X	Description	BPMN JSON	CCC19
C4	cat04_03_bpmn_simp_xml_description	X	X	Description	BPMN XML (simple)	CCC19
C4	cat04_04_declare_description	X	X	Description	DECLARE	BPI2020 Domestic
C4	cat04_05_declare_anomalies	X	X	Semantic AD	DECLARE	BPI2020 Domestic
C4	cat04_06_log_skeleton_description	X	X	Description	Log Skeleton	BPI2020 Domestic
C4	cat04_07_log_skeleton_anomalies	X	X	Semantic AD	Log Skeleton	BPI2020 Domestic
C5	cat05_01_hypothesis_bpic2020	X	X	Hypothesis Generation	Variants	BPI2020 Domestic
C5	cat05_02_hypothesis_roadtraffic	X	X	Hypothesis Generation	Variants	Road Traffic
C5	cat05_03_hypothesis_bpmn_json	X	X	Hypothesis Generation	BPMN JSON	CCC19
C5	cat05_04_hypothesis_bpmn_simpl_xml	X	X	Hypothesis Generation	BPMN XML (simple)	CCC19
C6	cat06_01_renting_attributes		X	Discrimination Factors	Situation table	Renting (Fairness)
C6	cat06_02_hiring_attributes		X	Discrimination Factors	Situation table	Hiring (Fairness)
C6	cat06_03_lending_attributes		X	Discrimination Factors	Situation table	Lending (Fairness)
C6	cat06_04_hospital_attributes		X	Discrimination Factors	Situation table	Hospital (Fairness)
C6	cat06_05_renting_prot_comp	X	X	Comparison	Variants	Renting (Fairness)
C6	cat06_06_hiring_prot_comp	X	X	Comparison	Variants	Hiring (Fairness)
C6	cat06_07_lending_prot_comp	X	X	Comparison	Variants	Lending (Fairness)
C6	cat06_08_hospital_prot_comp	X	X	Comparison	Variants	Hospital (Fairness)
C7	cat07_01_dotted_chart	X	X	Description	Visual	Road Traffic
C7	cat07_02_perf_spectrum	X	X	Description	Visual	Road Traffic
C7	cat07_03_running-example	X	X	Description	Visual	Running Example
C7	cat07_04_credit-score	X	X	Description	Visual	Credit Score
C7	cat07_05_dfg_ru	X	X	Description	Visual	Running Example
C7	cat07_06_process_tree_ru	X	X	Description	Visual	Running Example

as the ones proposed in [1], are based on the generation of SQL statements but do not require process-specific domain knowledge.

Different categories of prompts (Table 1) are contained in the benchmark:

C1 General-purpose qualitative tasks: The first category assesses the ability to describe processes, detect anomalies, and analyze root causes using DFG/variants abstractions of event logs. It also includes object-centric process mining artifacts for testing object-centric comprehension.

C2 Open/closed process mining domain knowledge questions: The second category evaluates the process mining domain knowledge of the LLM, with open and closed questions about process mining and Petri nets.

C3 Process model generation: The third category tests the ability to generate procedural (process trees, POWLs [17]) and declarative process models (control-flow and temporal) for mainstream processes, and the ability to propose constraints given some process data.

C4 Process model understanding: The fourth category assesses the understanding of proposed procedural (BPMN) and declarative (Log Skeleton and DECLARE [18]) process models.

C5 Hypotheses generation: The fifth category evaluates the ability to generate hypotheses over the proposed data and process models.

C6 Fairness assessment: The sixth category tests the ability to identify event log attributes sensitive for fairness and compare protected and non-protected groups [19].

C7 Visual prompts: The seventh category assesses the visual capabilities (if supported) of the LLM/LVLM.

We tailored the benchmark to the level of comprehension and reasoning of currently available state-of-the-art LLMs (in particular, *gpt-4o-20240513* and *claude-3.5-sonnet*), which can perform the tasks satisfactorily. Some mainstream tasks (for instance, applying the Alpha Miner algorithm, or checking the soundness of a Petri nets) are still not supported effectively by state-of-the-art LLMs. Therefore, they have not been included in the current version of the benchmark, which is comprehensive but not complete. The prompts of the benchmark are "static" (i.e., stored in TXT files). The benchmark could be easily adapted in the future to contain more prompts and/or different categories of tasks.

The size of the prompt does not exceed $8K$ characters, ensuring their executability on any of the considered LLMs. Among the considered LLMs, *Llama3 70B Instruct* has the most restrictive context window (i.e., the number of tokens that can be provided). Some state-of-the-art LLMs, such as *Nemotron 340B* or *Phi-3*, only support a baseline context window of $4K$, but we choose not to support that as it is too restrictive for process mining tasks. For more difficult event logs or process models, a bigger context window ($32K$, $64K$, or $128K$) is preferable as it allows to encode more information in the prompt.

3.2 Evaluation Strategy

The challenge of evaluating textual outputs from LLMs in an objective manner is significant. Traditional metrics that compare answers to a human-provided

Table 2. Scores between 1.0 and 10.0 (*mean±stddev*) of various LLMs in the proposed benchmark (using *gpt-4o-20240513* as a judge).

Commercial LLMs	Big Open-Source LLMs	Small LLMs (≤ 8 GB)	Tiny LLMs (≤ 4 GB)
claude-3.5-sonnet 8.4 ± 0.7	Qwen v2.0 72B (instruct, fp16) 7.6 ± 1.4	Qwen v2.0 7B (instruct, Q6K) 6.5 ± 2.2	Mistral 7B v0.3 (instruct, Q3KS) 4.6 ± 2.2
gpt-4o-20240513 (self) 8.3 ± 1.0	WizardLM v2 8x22b (16b) 7.5 ± 1.7	Mistral 7B v0.3 (instruct, Q6K) 5.9 ± 2.5	Qwen v2.0 7B (instruct, Q2K) 4.6 ± 2.1
gpt-4-turbo-20240409 8.1 ± 1.0	Mixtral v0.1 8x22b (instruct, 16b) 7.5 ± 1.6	Llama 3 8B (instruct, Q6K) 5.9 ± 2.5	Gemma v1.0 2B (instruct, Q6K) 4.0 ± 2.6
claude-3-sonnet 7.8 ± 1.4	Llama 3 70B (instruct, 16b) 7.4 ± 1.5	WizardLM v2 7b (Q6K) 5.9 ± 2.3	Qwen v2.0 1.5B (instruct, Q6K) 3.8 ± 2.2
Google Gemini (20240528) 7.5 ± 1.7	Mixtral v0.1 8x7b (instruct, 16b) 6.9 ± 1.7	Gemma v2.0 9B (instruct, Q6K) 5.7 ± 2.9	Qwen v2.0 0.5B (instruct, Q6K) 3.1 ± 1.7
gpt-3.5-turbo-0125 7.1 ± 1.8	Llama 3 70B (instruct, Q4_0) 6.7 ± 2.4	CodeGemma v1.5 7B (instruct, Q6K) 4.9 ± 2.6	Qwen 4B v1.5 (text, Q6K) 2.5 ± 2.2
	Codestral 22B (Q6K) 6.7 ± 2.1	Gemma v1.0 7B (instruct, Q6K) 4.5 ± 2.6	
	Llama 3 8B (instruct, 16b) 6.6 ± 2.0		
	OpenChat 3.6 8B (16b) 6.5 ± 1.7		

ground truth are limited by their inability to be customized to specific evaluation criteria and to consider open-ended answers. This leads to the exploration of using LLMs as judges (LLMs-as-Judges), a method that offers the potential for more comprehensive evaluations.

As the output of LLMs for the proposed prompts is textual, we propose to use an advanced LLM (for instance, *gpt-4o-20240513*) as judge [28], assigning a score from 1.0 (minimum) to 10.0 (maximum) to each answer.

In this benchmark, LLMs-as-Judges are utilized without ground truth for two primary reasons:

- The open-ended nature of many inquiries, in particular *process modeling* (C3) and *automated hypotheses generation* (C5), which lack definitive answers.
- The possibility that future LLM training sets could include the benchmark inquiries and their ground truths, potentially compromising the integrity of the benchmark by allowing "cheating" during the training phase of the LLM.

Potential limitations have been summarized in Sect. 2. In particular, LLMs-as-Judges are more reliable when there is a significant performance gap in favor of the judge LLM compared to the answering LLM. Also, scoring similar-performing LLMs without ground truth is challenging and requires accounting for potential "egocentric" bias. Moreover, high-performing LLMs tend to produce verbose and detailed outputs, which can result in a bias against more concise responses from lower-performing LLMs and vice-versa.

For the evaluation, the following procedure is followed for every prompt:

1. The prompt is provided to the LLM:
   - Reported as-is for all the textual prompts.
   - For visual prompts (if supported by the given model), upload the image accompanied by the following textual prompt: *Can you describe the provided visualization?*

Table 3. Scores between 1.0 and 10.0 (*mean ± stddev*) for different model categories and question categories (using *gpt-4o-20240513* as a judge).

	Commercial LLMs	Big Open-Source LLMs	Small LLMs ($\leq$ 8 GB)	Tiny LLMs ($\leq$ 4 GB)
C1	7.6 ± 1.1	7.0 ± 1.5	5.5 ± 2.3	3.2 ± 1.6
C2	8.7 ± 0.6	8.4 ± 0.9	8.5 ± 0.9	6.5 ± 2.2
C3	7.1 ± 1.7	5.7 ± 2.0	4.7 ± 2.5	2.4 ± 1.5
C4	7.7 ± 1.5	6.7 ± 1.9	3.7 ± 2.0	2.9 ± 1.5
C5	7.8 ± 1.8	7.3 ± 1.6	6.0 ± 2.5	4.6 ± 2.2
C6	8.1 ± 1.2	7.2 ± 2.0	5.0 ± 2.2	3.1 ± 1.6
C7	8.2 ± 1.3	no supp.	no supp.	no supp.

2. The LLM's answer is persisted.
3. An expert LLM (LLM-as-a-Judge) is used to evaluate the output. Template:
   - For textual prompts, *Given the following question: . . . How would you grade the following answer from 1.0 (minimum) to 10.0 (maximum)?*.
   - For visual prompts, upload the image to the LVLM and ask *Given the attached image, how would you grade the following answer from 1.0 (minimum) to 10.0 (maximum)?*.

3.3 Benchmarking Scripts

The provided benchmark can be executed manually (first, an LLM is used to answer the questions, and its answers are evaluated by another LLM). We also provide some scripts to automate the execution of the benchmark. In particular, the Python script **answer.py** can be used to execute the prompts against any LLM supporting the OpenAI APIs, while **evaluation.py** can be used to evaluate the answers using an LLM as the judge. The configuration parameters could be set up inside the two scripts.

4 Benchmark Results

We executed the proposed benchmark against current state-of-the-art LLMs. The results are collected at the address https://zenodo.org/records/13164994.

Table 4. Scores between 1.0 and 10.0 (*mean ± stddev*) for answering (rows) and evaluating (columns) LLM pairs.

Answ./Eval.	gpt-4o-20240513	Llama3 70B Instr.	Mixtral 8x22B	Mixtral 8x7B	Qwen2 72B Instr.
Llama3 70B Instr.	7.4 ± 1.5	**8.8 ± 0.5**	8.6 ± 1.4	8.7 ± 1.3	7.7 ± 2.4
WizardLM-2-8x22B	7.5 ± 1.7	7.2 ± 3.0	7.2 ± 2.7	8.3 ± 1.3	7.1 ± 2.9
Mixtral 8x22B	7.5 ± 1.6	7.8 ± 2.3	7.5 ± 3.1	8.5 ± 1.3	7.6 ± 2.4
Mixtral 8x7B	6.9 ± 1.7	7.7 ± 2.3	7.4 ± 2.9	8.1 ± 1.7	7.1 ± 2.8
Qwen2 72B Instr.	7.6 ± 1.4	7.9 ± 2.3	8.6 ± 1.3	8.3 ± 1.9	**8.0 ± 2.5**

Table 5. Scores between 1.0 and 10.0 (*mean ± stddev*) for different model categories and single prompts (using *gpt-4o-20240513* as a judge).

Prompt	Comm.	Big OS	Small	Tiny
cat01_01_variants_bpic2020_rca	8.6 ± 0.4	6.9 ± 1.4	5.7 ± 2.9	3.2 ± 1.7
cat01_02_variants_roadtraffic_anomalies	6.5 ± 1.6	6.1 ± 1.8	4.3 ± 2.4	2.2 ± 0.9
cat01_03_bpic2020_var_descr	7.8 ± 1.6	7.5 ± 0.9	7.0 ± 1.3	3.4 ± 1.4
cat01_04_roadtraffic_var_descr	8.3 ± 0.6	7.4 ± 0.9	6.8 ± 1.4	3.2 ± 1.6
cat01_05_bpic2020_dfg_descr	8.2 ± 0.6	8.2 ± 0.7	7.4 ± 1.8	3.8 ± 2.1
cat01_06_roadtraffic_dfg_descr	7.8 ± 0.6	6.4 ± 1.8	5.1 ± 2.1	3.9 ± 1.9
cat01_07_ocel_container_description	7.2 ± 0.9	6.6 ± 1.5	4.9 ± 1.2	4.0 ± 1.3
cat01_08_ocel_order_description	7.7 ± 0.7	6.8 ± 1.4	4.8 ± 2.3	3.5 ± 1.6
cat01_09_ocel_container_rca	7.2 ± 1.2	7.5 ± 0.8	5.4 ± 2.1	2.6 ± 0.9
cat01_10_ocel_order_rca	7.2 ± 0.7	6.7 ± 1.8	3.5 ± 1.3	2.5 ± 1.0
cat02_01_open_event_abstraction	8.7 ± 0.4	8.4 ± 0.6	8.7 ± 0.4	6.6 ± 1.8
cat02_02_open_process_cubes	8.9 ± 0.2	8.4 ± 0.5	8.5 ± 0.5	5.8 ± 1.8
cat02_03_open_decomposition_strategies	8.7 ± 0.9	8.5 ± 0.3	8.6 ± 0.3	7.2 ± 1.2
cat02_04_open_trace_clustering	8.5 ± 0.7	8.4 ± 0.5	8.7 ± 0.7	7.7 ± 0.9
cat02_05_open_rpa	9.1 ± 0.2	8.8 ± 0.4	9.0 ± 0.5	8.2 ± 1.2
cat02_06_open_anomaly_detection	8.6 ± 0.5	8.7 ± 0.4	8.1 ± 1.0	8.0 ± 1.4
cat02_07_open_process_enhancement	8.9 ± 0.3	8.7 ± 0.4	8.7 ± 0.7	6.4 ± 1.0
cat02_08_closed_process_mining	8.8 ± 0.6	8.0 ± 1.1	8.8 ± 0.7	6.0 ± 2.7
cat02_09_closed_petri_nets	8.1 ± 0.6	7.2 ± 1.8	6.9 ± 1.3	2.9 ± 1.2
cat03_01_temp_profile_generation	9.0 ± 0.1	7.8 ± 0.9	7.8 ± 1.2	3.4 ± 1.6
cat03_02_declare_generation	6.8 ± 1.5	5.8 ± 1.2	4.8 ± 1.4	2.7 ± 0.9
cat03_03_log_skeleton_generation	8.2 ± 1.2	7.3 ± 1.2	5.8 ± 1.7	3.2 ± 1.6
cat03_04_process_tree_generation	7.4 ± 1.2	5.6 ± 2.0	5.6 ± 1.6	3.4 ± 1.4
cat03_05_powl_generation	6.6 ± 1.2	6.5 ± 1.5	6.9 ± 2.0	2.5 ± 1.4
cat03_06_temp_profile_discovery	5.5 ± 1.8	4.2 ± 1.7	2.4 ± 0.7	1.7 ± 0.7
cat03_07_declare_discovery	7.4 ± 1.3	4.3 ± 1.4	1.9 ± 1.0	1.0 ± 0.0
cat03_08_log_skeleton_discovery	5.8 ± 1.2	4.1 ± 1.4	2.2 ± 1.1	1.2 ± 0.6
cat04_01_bpmn_xml_tasks	9.2 ± 0.6	7.8 ± 3.1	1.3 ± 0.5	1.7 ± 0.7
cat04_02_bpmn_json_description	7.9 ± 1.0	6.3 ± 2.0	2.9 ± 1.5	2.8 ± 2.1
cat04_03_bpmn_simp_xml_description	8.2 ± 0.6	6.7 ± 1.2	3.6 ± 1.9	2.6 ± 1.4
cat04_04_declare_description	7.3 ± 1.1	7.1 ± 1.1	5.7 ± 1.6	3.6 ± 1.4
cat04_05_declare_anomalies	6.8 ± 2.0	5.9 ± 1.6	3.4 ± 0.9	3.2 ± 1.3
cat04_06_log_skeleton_description	7.9 ± 1.3	6.6 ± 1.4	5.2 ± 1.9	3.3 ± 1.7
cat04_07_log_skeleton_anomalies	6.5 ± 1.3	6.5 ± 1.6	4.0 ± 1.9	2.9 ± 0.7
cat05_01_hypothesis_bpic2020	8.2 ± 0.4	7.4 ± 1.4	7.6 ± 0.7	4.6 ± 1.7
cat05_02_hypothesis_roadtraffic	8.1 ± 1.0	6.6 ± 1.7	6.8 ± 2.2	4.7 ± 2.3
cat05_03_hypothesis_bpmn_json	7.5 ± 1.6	7.7 ± 1.2	5.2 ± 2.2	4.5 ± 2.3
cat05_04_hypothesis_bpmn_simpl_xml	7.2 ± 2.9	7.4 ± 1.9	4.6 ± 2.9	4.5 ± 2.4
cat06_01_renting_attributes	8.8 ± 0.6	8.2 ± 1.4	4.1 ± 2.0	2.5 ± 1.1
cat06_02_hiring_attributes	8.9 ± 0.7	8.6 ± 0.8	6.1 ± 2.4	5.0 ± 2.2
cat06_03_lending_attributes	8.3 ± 0.5	8.3 ± 1.1	7.1 ± 2.3	2.8 ± 1.2
cat06_04_hospital_attributes	8.8 ± 0.5	8.4 ± 0.7	6.3 ± 1.8	4.4 ± 2.1
cat06_05_renting_prot_comp	7.5 ± 1.2	5.8 ± 1.8	3.9 ± 1.1	2.0 ± 0.0
cat06_06_hiring_prot_comp	7.2 ± 1.4	6.1 ± 2.5	4.4 ± 1.7	2.9 ± 0.9
cat06_07_lending_prot_comp	8.3 ± 0.6	6.5 ± 1.8	3.6 ± 1.6	2.3 ± 0.5
cat06_08_hospital_prot_comp	7.0 ± 1.6	5.8 ± 1.8	4.4 ± 1.6	2.7 ± 0.9
cat07_01_dotted_chart	8.3 ± 0.7	–	–	–
cat07_02_perf_spectrum	8.5 ± 0.8	–	–	–
cat07_03_running-example	8.9 ± 0.5	–	–	–
cat07_04_credit-score	8.6 ± 0.6	–	–	–
cat07_05_dfg_ru	7.4 ± 2.3	–	–	–
cat07_06_process_tree_ru	7.8 ± 1.0	–	–	–

In Table 2, we collect the evaluation results (using *gpt-4o-20240513* as a judge) for different LLMs of different sizes. In particular, we divide between *commercial models* (usually ranging hundreds of billions of parameters), *big open-source LLMs*, *small LLMs* (≤ 8 GB of RAM), and *tiny LLMs* (≤ 4 GB of RAM).

We tested some LLMs with different levels of quantization. Quantization refers to the process of reducing the precision of the model's weights and activations from higher bit-widths (such as 16-bit floating point) to lower bit-widths (such as 8-bit or even lower). This technique aims to decrease the model's memory footprint and computational requirements, making it more efficient to run on hardware with limited resources. While quantization can lead to a slight loss in model accuracy, it often significantly improves the model's speed and reduces power consumption, enabling more practical and scalable deployment of LLMs.

In general, we see that commercial and big open-source models can perform process mining tasks adequately well. The winners among commercial models seem to be *gpt-4o-20240513* and *claude-3.5-sonnet*. The best of the open-source models seem to be *Qwen2 72B Instruct* (occupying 145 GB of memory at full quantization). Some small LLMs also report an overall sufficient score. For instance, *Qwen2 7B Instruct* at *Q6K* quantization is process-mining-capable while occupying just 6.3 GB of memory. However, tiny LLMs are still inadequate for process mining tasks.

Overall, we found that aggressive quantization has a severe impact on LLMs' abilities in the proposed benchmark. While we do not have precise explanations for this phenomenon, the benchmarks' prompt requires significant attention to some elements of the input prompt (e.g., the semantic anomalies), and quantization impacts such ability.

In Table 3, we report the scores for every model category and question category. In Table 5, the scores for every prompt of the benchmark are averaged over a model category.

We notice that question category **C2** (open/closed process mining domain knowledge questions) is answered adequately by all the model categories. Also, currently, only commercial models could answer to **C7** (visual prompts). Surprisingly, most of the considered LLMs could automatically generate hypotheses over the provided process models and event data (**C5**). Categories **C3** (process model generation) and **C4** (process model understanding) have high variance between the different model categories. While commercial and big open-source LLMs can perform the tasks adequately, small and tiny models fail to generate/understand the information provided in the prompt. Categories **C1** (general-purpose qualitative tasks) and **C6** (fairness assessment) have similar outcomes. Commercial and big open-source LLMs successfully execute such tasks, while small/tiny LLMs usually fail.

To further assess the validity of LLMs-as-Judges, we report in Table 4 a cross-validation based on five open-source answering models and five evaluation models (including *gpt-4o-20240513*). We see that only *Llama 3 70B Instruct* display the egocentric bias. The models tend to agree on the scores. The smallest considered model (*Mixtral 8x7B*) reports lower scores than its bigger counterpart (*Mixtral*

8x22B) and other state-of-the-art models (*Llama 3 70B Instruct* and *Qwen2 72B Instruct*). Notably, *WizardLM2 8x22B* achieves lower overall scores than *Mixtral 8x7B*. This could be explained by the model being a fine-tuned version of *Mixtral 8x22B* favoring more verbose responses. Overall, only *Qwen2 72B Instruct* and *gpt-4o-20240513* favor Qwen2 over Llama3, while Qwen2 is an overall better-performing model in general-purpose benchmarks[8]. As the models and responses become more advanced, it becomes complicated for lower-performing models to judge the differences between them. Using the less advanced *Mixtral 8x7B*, the "plateauing" of the scores becomes evident, highlighting the importance of using advanced LLMs as judges. Therefore, Table 4 justifies LLMs-as-Judges, but points to the importance of choosing advanced LLMs for the task.

5   Future Benchmarking Strategies

Benchmarking Retrieval-Augmented Generation (RAG): while LLMs have been trained on generic process-specific knowledge, the implementation of business processes in real-life organizations could be different. Therefore, Retrieval-Augmented Generation (RAG) techniques have been used to dynamically inject process-specific knowledge to the prompts provided by process mining analysts [5]. As the correct retrieval of the information is crucial for the quality of the answers, benchmarks should also assess the capabilities of the RAG pipeline.

Benchmarking LLM-Based Agent Crews: Our benchmark focuses on executing a prompt, recording the answer, and evaluating it. The *agents crew* paradigm [12] involves workflows with specialized or role-specific LLMs performing analytical tasks. For instance, estimating the level of discrimination in an event log involves identifying the protected group and comparing differences between groups. An agents crew could consist of one agent creating the SQL statement to filter the protected group and another specializing in process comparison. Each agent's performance is crucial for accurate benchmarking, as evaluating only the final output may be misleading.

Benchmarking Hypotheses Refinement: Hypotheses generation involves creating and verifying hypotheses against event data. If a hypothesis is invalid, the LLM refines it based on feedback. This process may lead to specific hypotheses that perform poorly on imseem data. Thus, it is important to test the entire hypothesis feedback and verification cycle, not just hypotheses generation.

Data Generation with Relevant Semantic Anomalies or Root Causes: Our benchmark uses publicly available event data and process models. Including these datasets in LLM training data, even without ground truth answers, can lead to higher benchmark scores. Therefore, it is important to dynamically generate novel event data for LLM benchmarking. Current simulation solutions lack the semantic understanding needed to generate data suitable for process

---

[8] https://qwenlm.github.io/blog/qwen2/.

mining assessment. LLMs should be considered for the goal of generating data with various semantic anomalies and root causes.

6   Conclusion

We proposed *PM-LLM-Benchmark*, a benchmark for process mining on LLMs, utilizing LLMs-as-Judges for scalable evaluation. This benchmark does not provide ground truth answers, relying instead on the "judge" LLM's capabilities, addressing the open-ended nature of the inquiries. The benchmark includes various task categories to assess LLMs' abilities in process mining, modeling, and comprehension. Applied to several commercial and open-source LLMs, we found most models perform well in process mining tasks, with bigger models achieving higher scores. Smaller models (≤ 8 GB or ≤ 4 GB of RAM) struggle with complex tasks. We also suggest improvements in benchmarking strategies, including enhanced hypotheses generation, agent-crew-based benchmarks, and dynamic dataset generation with semantic anomalies. To our knowledge, this is the first general-purpose process mining benchmark focusing on different implementation strategies. While it has limitations in evaluating well-performing LLMs, it is a useful tool for assessing smaller LLMs and evaluating the current state of PM-on-LLMs.

References

1. Barbieri, L., Madeira, E.R.M., Stroeh, K., van der Aalst, W.M.P.: A natural language querying interface for process mining. J. Intell. Inf. Syst. **61**(1), 113–142 (2023)
2. Berti, A., Kourani, H., Hafke, H., Yun-Li, C., Schuster, D.: Evaluating large language models in process mining: capabilities, benchmarks, evaluation strategies, and future challenges. In: BPM-DS 2024 Working Conference. Springer (2024)
3. Berti, A., Qafari, M.S.: Leveraging large language models (LLMs) for process mining (technical report) (2023)
4. Berti, A., Schuster, D., van der Aalst, W.M.P.: Abstractions, scenarios, and prompt definitions for process mining with LLMs: a case study. In: BPM 2023, vol. 492, pp. 427–439. Springer (2023)
5. Chen, B., Zhang, Z., Langrené, N., Zhu, S.: Unleashing the potential of prompt engineering in large language models: a comprehensive review (2023)
6. Dhurandhar, A., Nair, R., Singh, M., Daly, E., Ramamurthy, K.N.: Ranking large language models without ground truth (2024)
7. Dixit, P.M., Buijs, J.C.A.M., van der Aalst, W.M.P., Hompes, B.F.A., Buurman, J.: Using domain knowledge to enhance process mining results. In: SIMPDA 2015, vol. 244, pp. 76–104. Springer (2015)
8. Dong, Y.R., Hu, T., Collier, N.: Can LLM be a personalized judge? arXiv preprint arXiv:2406.11657 (2024)
9. Fahland, D., Fournier, F., Limonad, L., Skarbovsky, I., Swevels, A.J.E.: How well can large language models explain business processes? (2024)
10. Fournier, F., Limonad, L., Skarbovsky, I.: Towards a benchmark for causal business process reasoning with LLMs (2024)

11. Grohs, M., Abb, L., Elsayed, N., Rehse, J.: Large language models can accomplish business process management tasks. In: BPM 2023 Workshops, vol. 492, pp. 453–465. Springer (2023)
12. Guo, T., Chen, X., Wang, Y., et al., R.C.: Large language model based multi-agents: a survey of progress and challenges (2024)
13. Jessen, U., Sroka, M., Fahland, D.: Chit-chat or deep talk: prompt engineering for process mining (2023)
14. Koo, R., Lee, M., Raheja, V., Park, J.I., Kim, Z.M., Kang, D.: Benchmarking cognitive biases in large language models as evaluators (2023)
15. Kourani, H., Berti, A., Schuster, D., van der Aalst, W.M.P.: Process modeling with large language models. In: EMMSAD 2024. Springer (2024)
16. Kourani, H., Berti, A., Schuster, D., van der Aalst, W.M.P.: ProMoAI: Process modeling with generative AI. In: IJCAI 2024 Demo Track (2024)
17. Kourani, H., van Zelst, S.J.: POWL: partially ordered workflow language. In: BPM 2023 Proceedings, vol. 14159, pp. 92–108. Springer (2023)
18. Maggi, F.M.: Declarative process mining with the declare component of ProM. In: BPM Demos sessions 2013, vol. 1021. CEUR-WS.org (2013)
19. Pohl, T., Berti, A., Qafari, M.S., van der Aalst, W.M.P.: A collection of simulated event logs for fairness assessment in process mining. In: BPM 2023 Resources. vol. 3469, pp. 87–91. CEUR-WS.org (2023)
20. Raina, V., Liusie, A., Gales, M.J.F.: Is LLM-as-a-Judge Robust? Investigating universal adversarial attacks on zero-shot LLM assessment (2024)
21. Rebmann, A., Schmidt, F.D., Glavaš, G., van der Aa, H.: Evaluating the ability of LLMs to solve semantics-aware process mining tasks. arXiv preprint arXiv:2407.02310 (2024)
22. Singh, A.K., Devkota, S., Lamichhane, B., Dhakal, U., Dhakal, C.: The confidence-competence gap in large language models: a cognitive study (2023)
23. Thakur, A.S., Choudhary, K., Ramayapally, V.S., Vaidyanathan, S., Hupkes, D.: Judging the judges: evaluating alignment and vulnerabilities in LLMs-as-judges. arXiv preprint arXiv:2406.12624 (2024)
24. Vidgof, M., Bachhofner, S., Mendling, J.: Large language models for business process management: opportunities and challenges. In: BPM 2023 Forum, vol. 490, pp. 107–123. Springer (2023)
25. Wang, P., Li, L., Chen, L., et al., D.Z.: Large language models are not fair evaluators (2023)
26. Wornow, M., Narayan, A., et al., B.V.: Do multimodal foundation models understand enterprise workflows? A benchmark for business process management tasks (2024)
27. Zerbato, F., Soffer, P., Weber, B.: Initial insights into exploratory process mining practices. In: BPM Forum 2021, vol. 427, pp. 145–161. Springer (2021)
28. Zheng, L., Chiang, W., Sheng, Y., et al., S.Z.: Judging LLM-as-a-Judge with MT-Bench and Chatbot Arena. In: NeurIPS 2023 (2023)

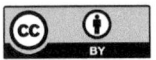

Terpsichora: A Tool to Generate Synthetic MP-Declare Process Models

Wesley da Silva Santos[1]([✉]), Juliana Rezende Coutinho[2], Fernanda Baião[2], Georges Miranda Spyrides[1], and Hélio Côrtes Vieira Lopes[1]

[1] Department of Informatics, PUC-Rio, Rio de Janeiro, Brazil
{wsantos,gspyrides,lopes}@inf.puc-rio.br
[2] Department of Industrial Engineering, PUC-Rio, Rio de Janeiro, Brazil
julianarezendecoutinho@aluno.puc-rio.br, fbaiao@puc-rio.br

Abstract. Process models play a fundamental role in the Business Process Management lifecycle and are crucial for assessing the robustness of proposed algorithms and conducting benchmarks among different tools. However, public models are limited as they expose strategic knowledge. While some researchers developed public repositories of imperative models, there remains a lack of diverse, publicly available multi-perspective declarative models. Our work aims to bridge this gap by providing a tool for generating synthetic MP-Declare process models. We leverage Large Language Models to generate these models, ensuring coverage of diverse aspects and enhancing the resource pool for the BPM community.

Keywords: declarative process management · process models · mp-declare · synthetically generated data · large language models

1 Introduction

Business Process Management (BPM) is a systematic approach to improve an organization's business processes [1]. It involves modeling, automation, execution, control, measurement, and optimization of business processes. A key component of BPM is the use of process models, which serve as blueprints for how processes should be executed. These models are essential for understanding, analyzing, and enhancing the efficiency of a company's operations.

Process models are generally categorized into imperative or declarative models [2]. Imperative models specify the exact sequence of tasks to be performed, whereas declarative models define constraints that specify what should and should not happen during the process execution. Declarative models, such as

W. da Silva Santos—Partially funded by National Council for Scientific and Technological Development (CNPq) grant 131447/2022-0.
F. Baião—Partially funded by Rio de Janeiro State Funding Agency (FAPERJ) grants 200.514/2023 and 211.308/2019) and CNPq grants 312059/2022-1 and 422810/2021-5.
H. C. V. Lopes—Partially funded by CNPq and Coordination for the Improvement of Higher Education Personnel (CAPES).

A. Delgado and T. Slaats (Eds.): ICPM 2024 Workshops, LNBIP 533, pp. 624–636, 2025.
https://doi.org/10.1007/978-3-031-82225-4_46

those using the Declare language, are particularly suited for environments where flexibility and adaptability are crucial. They allow for more dynamic and flexible process execution by focusing on the rules and constraints governing the process rather than the exact flow of activities.

Declare comprises constraints and templates to define the permissible behavior within a process, allowing for greater adaptability and exception handling [3]. Multi-perspective process modeling incorporates various dimensions of process execution, including control-flow, data, and resources. This holistic approach provides a more comprehensive understanding of business processes, which is essential for accurate analysis and optimization [4]. MP-Declare is the multi-perspective version of Declare [5] which allows the specification of relationships between many entities that are involved in business processes, such as actors, control-flow, rules, and attributes.

Despite their advantages, the availability of public multi-perspective declarative process models is limited. This scarcity is primarily because process models can reveal strategic knowledge about how organizations operate, making companies reluctant to share them publicly [6]. While some repositories of imperative models have been developed [7,8] and [9], there is still a significant gap in the availability of diverse multi-perspective declarative models, as most of the available models were extracted from mining techniques and are in repositories of declarative process mining tools, such as RuM Toolkit and Declare4Py [10].

On the other hand, recent advancements in AI, particularly in generative AI (GAI), have shown promise in generating complex data structures, including process models [6]. These models can learn from vast amounts of data and generate new instances that are both diverse and representative of real-world scenarios, unlike traditional approaches [11]. The use of synthetic data and models is gaining traction in BPM research, with an emphasis on many artifacts, such as log generations [12,13] and [14]. Synthetic data generation enhanced with GAI allows the creation of diverse and representative datasets without compromising proprietary business information [15] and [16], thereby enabling robust testing, development, and benchmarking.

Our work addresses this gap by providing `Terpsichora`[1], a tool capable of generating synthetic MP-Declare models. By leveraging GAI, specifically large language models (LLM), we systematically generated a wide range of MP-Declare models that cover diverse aspects of business processes and domains. This approach not only enriches the resources available to the BPM community but also demonstrates the potential of using advanced AI techniques in process model generation [17]. Our work builds on these foundations by integrating large language models to generate MP-Declare models, thus addressing the need for diverse, public multi-perspective declarative process models.

---

[1] Available at: https://github.com/santos-wesley/Terpsichora.

2   Related Work

In the field of BPM, synthetic data generation has become increasingly important for research and algorithm evaluation. This trend spans various aspects of BPM life-cycle, from event logs and process models to improvements and redesign suggestions. Loreti et al. [18] introduced an innovative method for generating synthetic logs with both positive and negative business process traces using abductive reasoning, addressing limitations in existing log generation techniques. Li et al. proposed a new paradigm for automating business process model discovery from natural language documents, creating the MaD dataset [19] to support this approach. Their work highlights the potential of large-scale datasets in training NLP models for BPM applications. Similarly, Yan et al. developed a technique for generating synthetic collections of business process models that mimic real-world properties, providing researchers with realistic datasets for evaluating process management techniques [20].

Leveraging advanced machine learning techniques, Van Dun et al. introduced ProcessGAN [21], a novel approach using generative adversarial networks (GANs) to support business process improvement. Their work demonstrates the potential of AI in enhancing creative aspects of BPM, such as generating improvement ideas. These studies collectively showcase the growing integration of AI and machine learning techniques in BPM, from automating model discovery and improvement suggestions to generating synthetic data for research and evaluation purposes. They highlight the potential for more efficient, accurate, and innovative approaches to process modeling, analysis, and improvement in the field of Business Process Management.

Over the years, research in synthetic data generation for BPM has advanced significantly, evolving from log generation to tackling specific challenges such as process improvement and redesign. However, despite these advancements, many approaches still rely on classical synthetic data generation techniques, which carry inherent limitations rooted in the characteristics of the trained data and the paradigms of the generation methods [22]. These limitations include difficulties in accurately modeling and reproducing complex, multidimensional relationships between variables, challenges in ensuring evaluation and consistency for complex pipelines, and the risk of overfitting, where models trained on synthetic data may become too tailored to the specifics of the generation process and thus fail to generalize effectively to real-world data. Additionally, accurately representing rare but important events or outliers in synthetic data is particularly challenging. Furthermore, adapting these models to new domains often necessitates extensive retraining, requiring handcrafted linguistic features and rules that are labor-intensive to create and maintain.

3   Data Model, LLM Configuration and Prompt Engineering Techniques

To interplay with large language models, we created a metamodel (Fig. 1) representing the structural definition of an MP-Declare model [4] and [5]. This metamodel specifies the constructs involved in MP-Declare in the form of classes and their relationships and was converted to a data model using Pydantic[2], a data validation library for Python which we used to validate if the data complies with our metamodel. Following, we explain the implementation of each construct in the metamodel, detailing the goal of each class, its rules, and attributes.

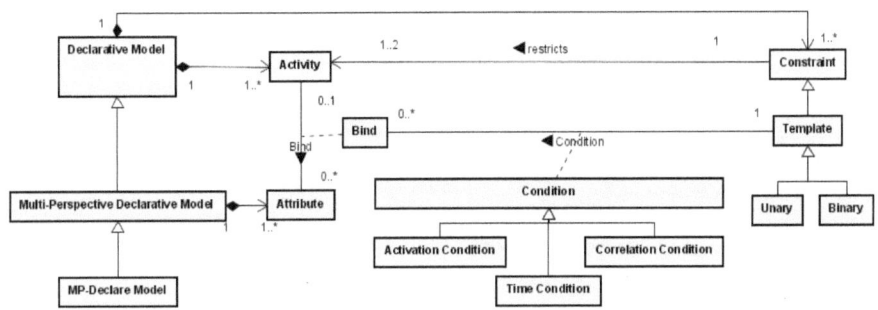

Fig. 1. The UML metamodel for the generation of MP-Declare process models.

The `Activity` class represents an activity within a process model. It is characterized by its `name` (a string that follows the format "<Action Verb> <Object>", suggested by [23] as a good pattern for naming an activity), and `description` (which provides a detailed explanation of the activity's purpose). The `Attribute` class defines attributes of a process, characterized by its `type` (which indicates whether the attribute is an integer, float, or enumeration), `name` (specifying the attribute's name) and `description` (providing a detailed explanation of the attribute); optionally, `min_value` and `max_value` fields define the range for integer or float attributes, while `enumeration_values` is a list of possible values for enumeration attributes.

The `Bind` class represents the linkage between activities and their attributes in a model. Hence, each bind is defined by an `Activity` (which represents the `Activity` involved in the binding), `attributes` (a list of `Attribute` objects bound to the activity), and a `description` (providing a description of the bind's purpose). The `Constraint` class models the constraints governing process execution, characterized by its `type` (specifying if the constraint is unary or binary), `description` (a detailed explanation of the constraint), `template` (which specifies the constraint's template), `activation` (representing the activation activity, required for both unary and binary constraints), its `target`

---

[2] Available at: https://docs.pydantic.dev/latest/.

(representing the target activity, required for binary constraints); in particular, the `activation_condition`, `correlation_condition`, and `time_condition` are optional fields for specifying specific conditions that govern the constraint's execution. Finally, `cardinality` defines the cardinality for certain unary templates. The `MPDeclareModel` is the main class and encapsulates the entire MP-Declare process model.

In addition to the structural metamodel illustrated in Fig. 1, our implementation of the proposed repository comprises validators to ensure appropriate types for each type of construct of the model, using logical and pattern methods. The `convert_to_string` method provides a string representation of the process model, formatting activities, binds, attributes, and constraints into a coherent textual format suitable for parsing to `Declare4Py`.

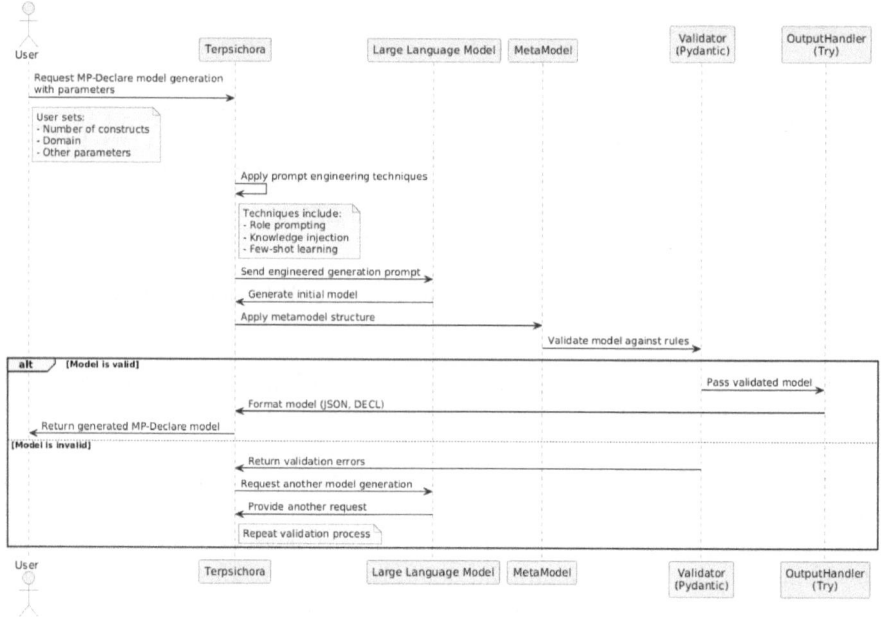

Fig. 2. The generation sequence diagram.

We used **gpt-4o-2024-05-13**, the flagship model of OpenAI, and ChatGPT[3] to generate 500 random domains to feed the generation prompt with a diverse set of domains to generate the models. Alongside with that, we modified the temperature parameter, which is used in the sampling process when generating text to control the randomness or entropy of the text [24]. A higher temperature value increases the randomness, while a lower value makes the model's output

---

[3] Available at: https://chatgpt.com/.

more deterministic. We used lower values of temperature (0.2) to make our outputs more reproducible and replicable [25].

We leveraged some prompt engineering (PE) techniques to understand the MP-Declare nuances and generate process models, without the extensive computational and data resources requirements of fine-tuning [24] and [26]. We used role-prompting [27], which goal is to assign a specific role to the LLM. In our case, we guided the LLM to generate data as an expert in process modeling and analysis and domain expertise using natural language instruction. Knowledge injection [28] involves providing the LLM with specific information that may not have been explored during its training.

In our case, we injected knowledge from MP-Declare's constraints templates in the pipeline, explaining them in natural language through an assistant prompt and converted the model from Pydantic to infuse the model with adequate expected generation, through the function call feature of OpenAI [29]. Function calling enables the integration of LLMs with external tools and systems. This capability has wide-ranging applications, including enhancing AI assistants with expanded functionalities and facilitating seamless interactions between applications and these models.

A set of few-shot learning was prepared to instruct the LLM of expected input and outputs. Few-shot learning in LLMs refers to the ability of these models to perform new tasks with only a small number of examples or demonstrations [30]. In our case, we used few-shots to enhance model's capability of generating data with quality to our proposed metamodel implementation.

4   Synthetic Model Generation and Quality Assessment

A pipeline was developed in a Jupyter Notebook[4], comprising all the steps for generating MP-Declare models guided by our proposed metamodel, the required packages, PE configurations, and post-processing techniques that were created. Figure 2 depicts a sequence diagram of the generation process, showing the interactions between the user, tool, and metamodel, pydantic and Output Handler.

We generated 500 process models in two batches[5], varying quantity of activities, constraint types, conditions, business domains, and complexity through prompts[6]. The models were used to assess the tool and were exported and saved to `decl` and `JSON` formats. The `JSON` file contains descriptions of the process constructs. We used the guidelines of Sandve et al. [31] to make our experiment reproducible, using version control system, log of generation of process models, error handling in tool and open access scripts.

With regard to quality assessment, the discussion about quality of declarative process models is almost absent in the literature. de Oca et al. [32] systematically reviewed the literature on business process modeling quality, investigating

---

[4] Available at: https://github.com/santos-wesley/Terpsichora/blob/main/Terpsichora_The_Pipeline.ipynb.

[5] Available at: https://github.com/santos-wesley/Terpsichora/tree/main/Models.

[6] Generation prompts can be found in the batch subfolders in each model directory.

Table 1. Overall Statistics (Batch 1 vs Batch 2)

Metric	Min		Mean		Median		Max		Std	
	Batch 1	Batch 2	Batch 1	Batch 2	Batch 1	Batch 2	Batch 1	Batch 2	Batch 1	Batch 2
Activities	8	10	9.904	14.888	10	15	10	19	0.356	0.807
Attributes	5	5	9.296	9.768	10	10	11	11	1.329	0.821
Binds	3	3	8.38	10.18	9	9.5	10	16	1.858	3.220
Attributes per Bind	1	1	1.863	1.711	2	2	5	4	0.659	0.661
Constraints	7	11	9.948	14.96	10	15	11	19	0.324	0.611
Unary Constraints	1	2	2.964	4.060	3	4	5	7	0.755	1.058
Binary Constraints	4	8	6.984	10.90	7	11	9	17	0.794	1.167
Integer Attributes	1	1	3.084	3.204	3	3	6	7	0.961	0.886
Float Attributes	0	0	1.512	1.616	1	2	3	4	0.633	0.718
Enumeration Attributes	2	2	4.7	4.948	5	5	8	8	1.220	1.036
Cardinality	1	1	1.817	4.042	1	1	50	1000	3.347	44.07
Activation Conditions	0	0	0.196	0.204	0	0	3	4	0.511	0.553
Correlation Conditions	0	0	0.016	0.016	0	0	1	1	0.125	0.125
Time Conditions	0	0	2.524	3.104	2	3	6	6	0.964	0.945
Templates per Model	3	3	7.492	9.516	8	9	10	15	1.473	2.248

Table 2. Template Usage Statistics (Batch 1 vs Batch 2)

Template	Count		Percentage of Total Constraints		Models Using Template	
	Batch 1	Batch 2	Batch 1	Batch 2	Batch 1	Batch 2
Precedence	498	773	20.02412545	20.6684492	238	242
Response	378	591	15.19903498	15.80213904	219	234
Chain Response	314	426	12.6256534	11.39037433	194	216
Init	251	252	10.0924809	6.737967914	250	247
End	231	232	9.288299156	6.203208556	230	231
Chain Succession	212	305	8.524326498	8.155080214	162	188
Existence	148	254	5.950944914	6.79144385	141	196
Alternate Response	101	159	4.061117813	4.251336898	94	127
Absence	62	172	2.49296341	4.598930481	62	163
Exactly	49	105	1.970245275	2.807486631	47	97
Succession	45	88	1.809408926	2.352941176	41	78
Chain Precedence	37	63	1.487736228	1.684491979	37	57
Responded Existence	29	54	1.16606353	1.443850267	28	49
Not Co-Existence	28	53	1.125854443	1.417112299	28	53
Co-Existence	24	46	0.965018094	1.229946524	23	42
Alternate Succession	22	46	0.88459992	1.229946524	22	42
Alternate Precedence	17	20	0.683554483	0.534759358	16	19
Choice	10	20	0.402090873	0.534759358	10	20
Not Precedence	9	8	0.361881785	0.213903743	9	8
Not Succession	8	26	0.321672698	0.695187166	8	23
Not Responded Existence	6	1	0.241254524	0.026737968	6	1
Exclusive Choice	4	19	0.160836349	0.50802139	4	19
Not Chain Succession	2	13	0.080418175	0.347593583	2	13
Not Response	1	4	0.040209087	0.106951872	1	4
Not Chain Response	1	7	0.040209087	0.187165775	1	7
Not Chain Precedence	0	3	0	0.080213904	0	3

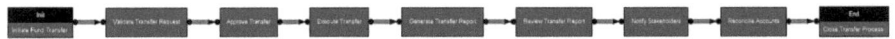

Fig. 3. A model discovered from log of synthetically generated process by Terpsichora.

Table 3. Complexity Metrics (Batch 1 vs Batch 2)

Metric	Min		Mean		Median		Max		Std	
	Batch 1	Batch 2	Batch 1	Batch 2	Batch 1	Batch 2	Batch 1	Batch 2	Batch 1	Batch 2
Size	17	22	19.852	29.848	20	30	21	34	0.513	1.072
Density	0.5	0.667	0.822	0.888	0.833	0.875	1	1.333	0.081	0.081
Separability	0.05	0.029	0.160	0.156	0.150	0.167	0.353	0.308	0.048	0.047
Constraint Variability	0	0	0.768	0.789	0.802	0.826	1	1	0.211	0.172

quality issues, relevant frameworks, and gaps. They showed there is no generally accepted framework for process model quality assessment and this is still a broader issue in the BPM field, even in the imperative paradigm. Some aspects of the Seven Process Modeling Guidelines (7PMG), proposed by Mendling et al. [33], were used to evaluate the generated models. The 7PMG proposes guidelines to assess quality of process constructs, such as elements usage, routing paths, model structuring, and so on. Although 7PMG are tailored to imperative languages and typically assume control-flow, we used two guidelines to assess our models quality: **G3: Use one start and one end event** and **G6: Use verb-object activity labels.**

We enforced the activities' names to have more than one word and use the verb-object pattern through PE and assessed a sample of the models. Every activity name has between 2 and 5 words, complying with our instruction and guideline G6. Most of the models comply with G3, but some generated models (batch 1: 72 and 77; batch 2: 100, 165, 211, 82, 86 and 87) have not more than two init or end constraints, and their usage relates to real-world possibilities. Table 1 and Table 2 present statistics about the model generation process of the two batches. For the two batches, we observed that the tool were capable of following our instructions regarding the quantity of elements of the model and the variety of constraints. The data of the two batches reveals that the tool progressively enhanced its model generation capabilities, as evidenced by the increase in complexity and diversity of the generated models. This progression demonstrates the tool's robustness in handling a wider range of process scenarios. The adherence to guidelines instructed with PE, coupled with the generation of models that closely resemble real-world processes.

Additionaly to these statistics, we used metrics of declarative models already employed and validated in literature proposed by Abbad-Andaloussi et al. [34]. Table 3 show these metrics, which explore the models in therms of size, density, separability and constraint variability. A comparative analysis of Batch 1 and Batch 2 reveals significant differences in model complexity and structure. Batch 2 models are notably larger, with a mean size of 29.848 compared to 19.852 in Batch 1, and exhibit greater size variability (std dev 1.072 vs 0.513). This substantial size increase suggests that Batch 2 represents more complex processes, and thus reflect that the strategy we employed in PE worked.

Interestingly, despite this size difference, both batches maintain similar density characteristics (means of 0.822 and 0.888), indicating a consistent ratio of constraints to activities. However, Batch 2's higher maximum density (1.333) points to some instances of highly constrained models, potentially reflecting more intricate rule structures in certain cases. The separability metric shows a slight decrease in Batch 2 (mean 0.156 vs 0.160), suggesting that the additional elements in these larger models are integrated into existing components rather than forming discrete sub-processes. This integration trend implies more interconnected and complex process representations in Batch 2. Both batches demonstrate high constraint variability (means of 0.768 and 0.789), indicating the use of diverse constraint types across models. Notably, Batch 2 shows slightly more consistency in this diversity (std dev 0.172 vs 0.211), suggesting a more uniform application of varied constraints across its models.

Collectively, these metrics reflect increased complexity in Batch 2, characterized by larger, more integrated models with consistently diverse constraint usage. The similarities in density and separability metrics between batches, despite the significant size difference, suggest that the modeling approach scales effectively to larger, more complex processes without fundamentally altering the model structure. This scalability, combined with the trend towards integration rather than fragmentation as processes grow more complex, indicates that the modeling technique is well-suited for representing increasingly sophisticated business processes while maintaining structural integrity and coherence.

We used several models (batch 1: 135, 250; batch 2: 39, 240) to generate logs and rediscover them[7]. We visually assessed them, and they were similar in terms of discovered constraints and control flow. Figure 3 shows a discovered model that appears very imperative. When compared with the synthetically generated model (model 250 from batch 1), it has the same constructs.

We inspected the generated JSON of these models to assess the descriptions and determine if they fit the knowledge we injected into the model. An example of a constraint description generated by Terpsichora for model 250 is: `Chain Succession[Approve Transfer, Execute Transfer] | | |0,2h`, described as "**Execute Transfer must directly follow Approve Transfer within 2 h.**" This description is compliant with our instructions and aligns with the semantics of the constraint.

5   Conclusions

In this work we presented Terpsichora, a tool for generating MP-Declare models leveraging LLM capabilities of PE and function calling. To evaluate the proposal, we generated 500 models and assessed them using statistics of output, metrics established in literature and visually assessed a sample of these models qualitatively to attest that they are real-world related.

---

[7] Available at: https://github.com/santos-wesley/Terpsichora/tree/main/Logs.

Our proposal enables a novel generation of a diverse set of MP-Declare models, representing a resource for assessing the robustness of new algorithms, benchmarking tools, and generating logs for simulation purposes, among others. Our pipeline is both reproducible and customizable, allowing users to generate models while overcoming the classic limitations of synthetic data generation, which often requires data acquisition and model training.

Terpsichora's utilization of Large Language Models (LLMs) offers significant advantages in addressing key challenges in synthetic process model generation. By leveraging the complex pattern recognition capabilities of LLMs, Terpsichora can capture and reproduce intricate multidimensional relationships between process elements, as evidenced by the diverse constraint types and their distributions shown in Table 2. This approach not only generates models with sophisticated control-flow patterns and multi-perspective aspects but also enhances adaptability to new domains. Unlike traditional methods that require extensive retraining and domain-specific adjustments, Terpsichora's prompt-based generation allows for quick adaptation to different business contexts simply by modifying the input prompts. This flexibility is particularly valuable for researchers and practitioners working across various industries.

Furthermore, the use of LLMs significantly reduces the need for handcrafted linguistic features and rules, which are often labor-intensive to create and maintain in traditional synthetic data generation methods. By automating the interpretation and application of process semantics with a metamodel and coding it into a datamodel in Pydantic, Terpsichora offers a more efficient and scalable approach to generating diverse, realistic MP-Declare models, potentially accelerating research and development in the context of model generation.

Along with the traditional constructs of MP-Declare, we add a new attribute to generate descriptions for each construct. This resource enables semantic anomaly detection not only for activities, as proposed by [35], but also for constraints. Another potential application is in generating multi-perspective process logs, incorporating additional perspectives inexistent in traditional log generation from structured models.

However, there are limitations. First, the current output context window of the model is limited to 4096 tokens, which restricts the ability to generate larger models and to test the LLM capacity to produce and maintain coherence in extensive, real-world models. Second, to ensure reproducibility, we kept a low temperature. Higher temperatures generally lead to more creative outputs, which could be beneficial for evaluating different generations of the same process.

Future work include testing with other models, including the newest OpenAi gpt-4o-2024-08-06, which implemented structured outputs techniques to enhance model inference in a given structured schema with complex rules [36] and increased the output tokens to 16384. Also, the usage of other prompt techniques to evaluate model quality at a semantic level, such as LLM-as-a-Judge [37], which enables open-ended questions evaluation using LLMs. Finally, addressing the understandability and cognitive impact of models generated by Terpsichora.

References

1. Dumas, M., Rosa, L.M., Mendling, J., Reijers, H.A.: Fundamentals of Business Process Management. Springer (2018)
2. van der Aalst, W.M.P., Pesic, M., Schonenberg, H.: Declarative workflows: balancing between flexibility and support. Comput. Sci.-Res. Dev. **23**, 99–113 (2009)
3. Di Ciccio, C., Montali, M.: Declarative process specifications: reasoning, discovery, monitoring. In: van der Aalst, W.M.P., Carmona, J. (eds.) Process Mining Handbook. LNBIP, vol. 448, pp. 108–152. Springer, Cham (2022). https://doi.org/10.1007/978-3-031-08848-3_4
4. Schönig, S., Di Ciccio, C., Maggi, F.M., Mendling, J.: Discovery of multi-perspective declarative process models. In: Service-Oriented Computing, pp. 87–103. Springer, Cham (2016)
5. Burattin, A., Maggi, F.M., Sperduti, A.: Conformance checking based on multi-perspective declarative process models. Expert Syst. Appl. **65**, 194–211 (2016)
6. Feuerriegel, S., Hartmann, J., Janiesch, C., Zschech, P.: Generative AI. Bus. Inf. Syst. Eng. **66**(1), 111–126 (2024)
7. Corradini, F., Fornari, F., Polini, A., Re, B., Tiezzi, F., et al.: RePROSitory: a repository platform for sharing business PROcess modelS. In: BPM (PhD/Demos), vol. 2420, pp. 149–153 (2019)
8. Weske, M., Decker, G., Dumas, M., Rosa, L., Mendling, J., Reijers, H.A.: Model collection of the business process management academic initiative. Zenodo (2020). https://doi.org/10.5281/zenodo.3758705
9. Sola, D., Warmuth, C., Schäfer, B., Badakhshan, P., Rehse, J.R., Kampik, T.: SAP signavio academic models: a large process model dataset. In: International Conference on Process Mining, pp. 453–465. Springer (2022)
10. Alman, A., Donadello, I., Maggi, F.M., Montali, M.: Declarative process mining for software processes: the RuM toolkit and the Declare4Py python library. In: International Conference on Product-Focused Software Process Improvement, pp. 13–19. Springer (2023)
11. Sutton, R., Barto, A.: Reinforcement Learning: An Introduction. MIT Press (2018)
12. Skydanienko, V., Di Francescomarino, C., Ghidini, C., Maggi, F.M.: A tool for generating event logs from multi-perspective declare models. In: BPM (Dissertation/Demos/Industry), vol. 2196, pp. 111–115 (2018)
13. Donadello, I., Maggi, F.M., Riva, F., Singh, M.: ASP-based log generation with purposes in Declare4Py. In: ICPM Doctoral Consortium/Demo (2023)
14. Di Ciccio, C., Bernardi, M.L., Cimitile, M., Maggi, F.M.: Generating event logs through the simulation of declare models. In: Enterprise and Organizational Modeling and Simulation: 11th International Workshop, EOMAS: Held at CAiSE 2015, Stockholm, 2015, Selected Papers 11, pp. 20–36. Springer (2015)
15. Recker, J., Indulska, M., Rosemann, M., Green, P.: How good is BPMN really? Insights from theory and practice. In: Ljungberg, J., Andersson, M. (eds.) Proceedings 14th European Conference on Information Systems, Goeteborg (2006)
16. Burattin, A.: Artificial datasets for multi-perspective declare analysis. Zenodo (2015). https://doi.org/10.5281/zenodo.20030
17. van der Aa, H., Di Ciccio, C., Leopold, H., Reijers, H.A.: Extracting declarative process models from natural language. In: Advanced Information Systems Engineering: 31st International Conference, CAiSE: Rome, Italy, 3–7 June 2019, Proceedings 31, pp. 365–382. Springer (2019)
18. Loreti, D., Chesani, F., Ciampolini, A., Mello, P.: Generating synthetic positive and negative business process traces through abduction. Knowl. Inf. Syst. **62**, 813–839 (2020)

19. Li, X., Ni, L., Li, R., Liu, J., Zhang, M.: MaD: a dataset for interview-based bpm in business process management. In: 2023 International Joint Conference on Neural Networks (IJCNN), pp. 1–8. IEEE (2023)

20. Yan, Z., Dijkman, R., Grefen, P.: Generating synthetic process model collections with properties of labeled real-life models. In: Asia Pacific Business Process Management: Second Asia Pacific Conference, AP-BPM, Brisbane, QLD, Australia, 3–4 July 2014. Proceedings 2, pp. 74–88. Springer (2014)

21. van Dun, C., Moder, L., Kratsch, W., Röglinger, M.: ProcessGAN: supporting the creation of business process improvement ideas through generative machine learning. Decis. Support Syst. **165**, 113880 (2023)

22. Nikolenko, S.I.: Synthetic Data for Deep Learning, vol. 174, Springer (2021)

23. Leopold, H., Eid-Sabbagh, R.H., Mendling, J., Azevedo, L.G., Baiao, F.A.: Detection of naming convention violations in process models for different languages. Decis. Support Syst. **56**, 310–325 (2013)

24. Li, C., et al.: Parameter-efficient sparsity for large language models fine-tuning. In: De Raedt, L. (ed.) Proceedings of the Thirty-First International Joint Conference on Artificial Intelligence, IJCAI 2022, Vienna, Austria, 23–29 July 2022, pp. 4223–4229. ijcai.org (2022)

25. Ivie, P., Thain, D.: Reproducibility in scientific computing. ACM Comput. Surv. (CSUR) **51**(3), 1–36 (2018)

26. Thangarasa, I., et al.: SPDF: sparse pre-training and dense fine-tuning for large language models. In: Evans, R.J., Shpitser, I. (eds.) Uncertainty in Artificial Intelligence, UAI 2023, 31 July–4 August 2023, Pittsburgh, PA, USA, vol. 216, pp. 2134–2146. Proceedings of Machine Learning Research. PMLR (2023)

27. Xu, B., et al.: ExpertPrompting: instructing large language models to be distinguished experts. CoRR, abs/2305.14688 (2023)

28. Martino, A., Iannelli, M., Truong, C.: Knowledge injection to counter large language model (LLM) hallucination. In: European Semantic Web Conference, pp. 182–185. Springer (2023)

29. OpenAI. Function Calling Guide (2024). https://platform.openai.com/docs/guides/function-calling. Accessed 03 July 2024

30. Brown, T., et al.: Language models are few-shot learners. Adv. Neural. Inf. Process. Syst. **33**, 1877–1901 (2020)

31. Sandve, G.K., Nekrutenko, A., Taylor, J., Hovig, E.: Ten simple rules for reproducible computational research. PLoS Comput. Biol. **9**(10), e1003285 (2013)

32. Moreno-Montes de Oca, I., Snoeck, M., Reijers, H.A., Rodríguez-Morffi, A.: A systematic literature review of studies on business process modeling quality. Inf. Softw. Technol. **58**, 187–205 (2015)

33. Mendling, J., Reijers, H., van der Aalst, W.: Seven process modeling guidelines (7PMG). Inf. Softw. Technol. **52**(2), 127–136 (2010)

34. Abbad-Andaloussi, A., Burattin, A., Slaats, T., Kindler, E., Weber, B.: Complexity in declarative process models: metrics and multi-modal assessment of cognitive load. Expert Syst. Appl. **233**, 120924 (2023)

35. van der Aa, H., Rebmann, A., Leopold, H.: Natural language-based detection of semantic execution anomalies in event logs. Inf. Syst. **102**, 101824 (2021). https://doi.org/10.1016/j.is.2021.101824

36. OpenAI. Introducing structured outputs in the API (2024). https://openai.com/index/introducing-structured-outputs-in-the-api/. Accessed 11 Aug 2024

37. Zheng, L., et al.: Judging LLM-as-a-judge with MT-bench and chatbot arena. Adv. Neural Inf. Process. Syst. **36** (2024)

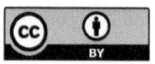

Process Modeler vs. Chatbot: Is Generative AI Taking over Process Modeling?

Nataliia Klievtsova[1]([✉])(iD), Janik-Vasily Benzin[1](iD), Juergen Mangler[1](iD), Timotheus Kampik[2](iD), and Stefanie Rinderle-Ma[1](iD)

[1] TUM School of Computation, Information and Technology, Technical University of Munich, Garching, Germany
{nataliia.klievtsova,janik-vasily.benzin,juergen.mangler, stefanie.rinderle-ma}@tum.de
[2] SAP Signavio, Berlin, Germany
timotheus.kampik@sap.com

Abstract. Large language models (LLMs) have become a promising tool for automating complex tasks such as process model generation from text. In order to evaluate the capabilities of LLMs in generating process models, it is crucial to provide means to assess the output quality. A few studies have already provided key performance indicators for assessing aspects such as completeness of the models in a quantitative way. In this paper, we focus on the qualitative assessment of generated process models generated by LLMs based on a user survey. By analyzing user preferences, we aim to determine whether LLM-generated process models meet the needs and expectations of experts. Our analysis reveals that 60% of users, regardless of their modeling experience, prefer LLM-generated models over human-created ground truth models.

Keywords: Business Process Engineering and Management · Process Modeling · Generative AI · Large Language Models · User study

1 Introduction

Process descriptions are textual descriptions of organizational routines that can serve as, e.g., manuals and learning materials for participants, as well as foundations for process optimization, redesign, automation, and execution. Process descriptions have to be comprehensible to multiple stakeholders from diverse backgrounds and knowledge cultures [10]. However, due to their flexible nature they often leave space for interpretation, resulting in arguably subjective representations and a lack of objectivity [3] leading to ambiguity.

Thus, process descriptions are transformed into *process models* [26] in order to improve the clarity of the described processes and to enable their analysis, facilitate decision-making about the processes, and aid the development of process software and documentation, as well as workflow management [19]. However, transforming process descriptions into models can be challenging, as domain

© The Author(s) 2025
A. Delgado and T. Slaats (Eds.): ICPM 2024 Workshops, LNBIP 533, pp. 637–649, 2025.
https://doi.org/10.1007/978-3-031-82225-4_47

experts and process modelers have to continuously communicate using different languages (i.e., domain-specific natural language vs. modeling languages) to exchange their knowledge and vision [25].

The inherent ambiguity in process descriptions complicates this transformation, as the modeler must decide which aspects to include, the level of abstraction, and the perspectives to consider [3]. These decisions can negatively impact the comprehension and application of the models [18]. For instance, if the modeler omits important details or includes unnecessary information, the resulting model can either be too simplistic or overly complex. A model that is too abstract may lack sufficient detail for practical application.

Therefore, it is crucial to ensure that domain knowledge is accessible during modeling [18]. One proposed solution is to equip domain experts with a modeling tool that allows them to create process models using natural language instructions through a conversational user interface, such as a chatbot [8,11]. LLMs such as ChatGPT have emerged as potential candidates for this task due to their capability to understand unstructured natural language text.

In order to evaluate whether domain experts can independently design high-quality process models using generative AI, it is paramount to assess the quality of these process models compared to those produced by humans. In previous work [20,21], we have suggested quantitative metrics such as model completeness and structural similarity. In this work, we conduct a survey with process modelers of different skills, focusing on qualitative aspects of the model and user satisfaction. One finding is that 60% of the participants—regardless of their modeling experience—prefer LLM-generated models over human-created ground truth models.

The paper is structured as follows: Sect. 2 describes the survey design and Sect. 3 the survey results. The latter are discussed in Sect. 4, followed by related work in Sect. 5, and a conclusion in Sect. 6.

2   Survey Design

Following [12], this section presents details of the survey design in Sect. 2.1 and the questionnaire design in Sect. 2.2.

2.1   Goal, Participants, and Data Collection

The main purpose of the survey is to perform a qualitative evaluation of process models generated by LLMs. The study participants are a group of students and professionals with different programming and modeling background. Their task is to select the one process model out of a list of given process models, which corresponds best to the provided process description (see Fig. 1). All data were collected electronically. The survey was performed anonymously and online by means of a questionnaire designed in Microsoft Forms[1].

---

[1] https://forms.office.com/e/Y55jyNuPi2.

The collected data are then analyzed to identify preferences among respondents regarding selected process models. Statistical methods (i.e., tests of independence and goodness-of-fit tests) are applied to determine which models are most frequently selected as the best match to the provided descriptions.

2.2 Questionnaire Design

The survey questionnaire is divided into three parts. First, we collect demographic information about participants regarding their modeling and programming experience. Second, we provide a brief description of the standardized BPMN (Business Process Model and Notation) notation and a simple process model to rate the general level of understanding of this description. We also ask which additional information is potentially required by the modeler to create a good process model. Finally, we provide several process descriptions and multiple process models associated with them. Figure 1 illustrates an example from the survey, where one model is always generated by a human modeler (see Data Set), while the others are generated by an LLM given the process description and a prompt (see Prompts and generated models).

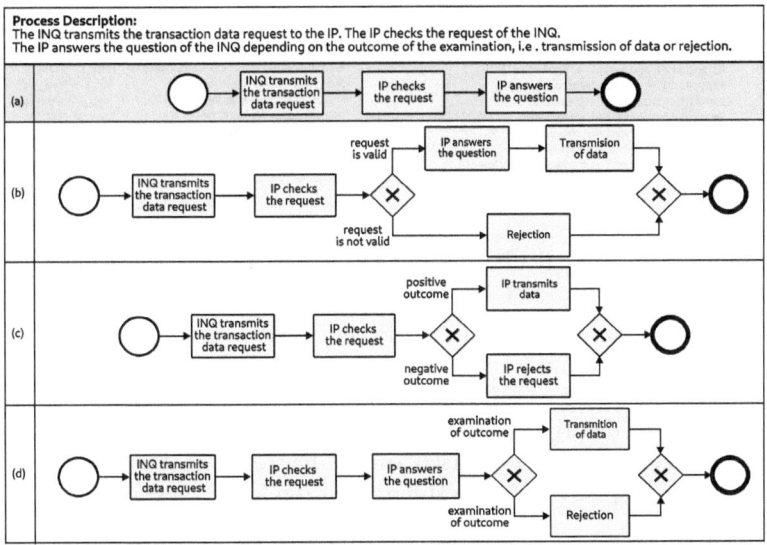

Fig. 1. Process Description and Associated Process Models, where (a) is a ground truth model; (b-d) are LLM-generated models

Participants are then asked to select the model from the set of proposed models that best matches the process description. In the following, we describe the data set with process descriptions and human-modeled process models as well as the approach to LLM-generated process models.

Data Set: We use the PET data set[2] [4] for process model generation. The PET data set only contains textual process descriptions. As ground truth models, we thus utilize BPMN process models created manually based on the existing human annotation of activities, gateways, and control flow provided in the PET dataset. Seven examples from the PET dataset are taken over from [5], as they are of different lengths and complexity.

Model Representation: The context window of an LLM (i.e., the total amount of text, including both the user's prompt and the model's generated output), typically ranging from 1,000 to 8,000 tokens, limits processing due to fixed sequence lengths used during training. As LLMs scale up, they can generate more extensive and longer responses. However it can impact the output quality, potentially introducing issues such as hallucinations and incurring significant costs. Therefore, it is necessary to use a simplified representation of traditional XML-based BPMN 2.0 models to facilitate efficient process model generation and visualization. In this survey, as introduced in [21], we utilize two intermediate process model representations for model generation: Mermaid.js[3] (MER) and Graphviz[4] (GV).

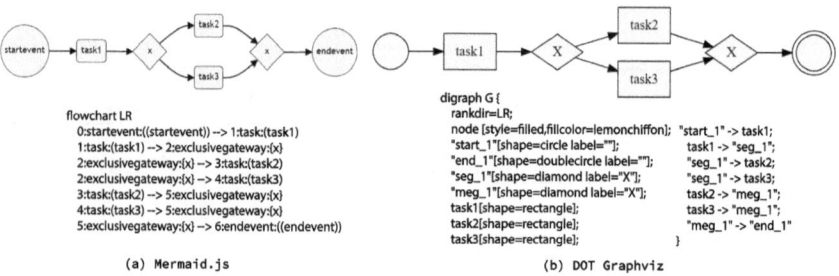

(a) Mermaid.js   (b) DOT Graphviz

Fig. 2. Selected Model Representations of Text Fragment given in TF1

Selected representations contain the orientation of the graph and custom structure for all nodes and edges in it. For every node, the specific features (e.g., type, color) are assigned to represent a particular BPMN element. For example, the simple process description

"After task1, either task2 or task3 are conducted." (Text Fragment TF1)

can be converted by an LLM into the process model as shown in Fig. 2.

Prompts and Generated Models: All models generated in the scope of this survey are based on the zero-shot principle, utilizing GPT-4 and three types of prompts developed in [21].

Figure 3 shows which prompts were used to generate models for the survey and their structure. Each prompt consists of three parts: [1] a process description, [2] some additional information, and [3] the actual task that should be solved by

---

[2] https://huggingface.co/datasets/patriziobellan/PET.

[3] https://mermaid.js.org/.

[4] https://graphviz.org/doc/info/lang.html.

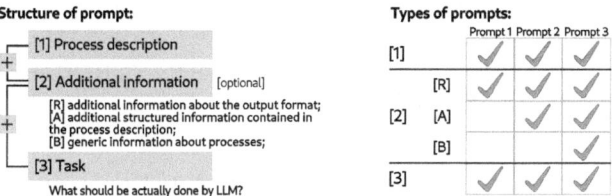

Fig. 3. Prompt Structure and Utilized Prompt Types

the LLM, i.e. "generate a graph" (cmp.[5]). The processes description [1] and the actual task to be performed [3] by the LLM are included in each prompt type. Multiple, optional pieces of information (see Fig. 3 [R, A, B]) can also be passed to the LLMs to influence the quality of the generated model.

All generated models contain two categories of BPMN elements: (a) flow objects (start and end events, tasks, exclusive and parallel gateways) and (b) connecting objects (sequence flows). Only models that were evaluated as correct and complete in [21] are taken into account[6]. Based on seven selected process descriptions from the PET data set, the two model representations (MER and GV), and the three prompts (cf. Fig. 3), 42 models were generated. Models identical to the ground truth and those that were incorrect or incomplete (only 26% of all generated models) were excluded from the survey, as they would provide no basis for distinction or could lead to biased results. Identical models do not provide any basis for distinction. Incorrect or incomplete models do not provide accurate representations of relevant process descriptions, which could lead to confusion among participants or biased results. Hence, including these models would not yield meaningful insights into preferences, as the choices would be arbitrary or redundant. In the end, 5 examples and 19 models were used for the survey.

3   Survey Results

Participant Background: A total of 40 respondents took part in the survey. Around 60% of respondents are familiar with various graphical modeling languages (e.g., UML, ER, or BPMN). 80% of them have more than 3 years of modeling experience or were applying modeling languages in class and industry projects and could be considered as confident modelers. Other participants either have no modeling experience or have few modeling skills. 29 out of 40 participants have more than 3 years of programming experience. 17.5% of all participants are not familiar with markup languages. Out of those familiar with markup languages, 15% have used MER and 42% have used GV.

Prompt Engineering: The assessments of completeness and correctness performed in [21] showed that GPT4 yields the best results using Prompt 1 (P1).

---

[5] https://github.com/com-pot-93/convermod/tree/main/prompt_engineering.
[6] https://github.com/com-pot-93/convermod/tree/main/survey/models.

Table 1. Percentage Distribution of Frequencies For Additional Information

Type–	R	A	B	R+A	R+B	A+B	R+A+B	Other
%	12.5	7.5	22.5	2.5	22.5	7.5	5	7.5	12.5

The second best results were achieved by Prompt 2 (P2). In order to gauge these results with human intuition, participants are asked to select one of the proposed types of additional information or their combination in the prompt template described in Fig. 3. The options were: [R] a set of rules of how to represent a particular text as a graph; [A] an explicit list of process activities; [B] a summary of the BPMN standard in addition to a textual process description.

Most of the respondents selected [A] or [R]+[A] (22.5% each). Notably, [R]+[A] corresponds to the achieved results, as Prompt 2 uses [R]+[A] and provides the second-best results. In contrast, only 7.5% of all respondents consider using [R] independently, despite the fact best results are achieved by using P1, which utilizes [R] (see Table 1).

Furthermore, 12.5% of all respondents suggest using other combinations of proposed information types like [A]+[B] or [R]+[B]. About 12.5% of all participants suggest including additional information or methods as process model examples or a workshop with a domain expert (again, see Tab. 1).

Model Representation: Respondents are also asked to rate their level of understanding when utilizing [R] (i.e., MER and GV) and [B] with respect to the 5-point scale in the survey. Only 2 participants rated [B] as poor. Out of 26 respondents, that were rating [R], 23% (MER) and 38% (GV) consider them as unclear (i.e., rated as poor or very poor). Nevertheless, 70% of respondents rate MER [R] as good or very good. At the same time, only 30% of participants acknowledge GV [R] as good or very good.

Interestingly, a majority of participants (17) find MER representation to be easier to read and understand and express a preference for using it over GV. In contrast, only 20% (5 participants) prefer GV representation, and 15% (4 participants) did not have any preference. However, it is essential to highlight that the representation preference distribution might be linked to the prior experience and comprehension of the provided information (i.e., [R]), observed during its evaluation.

Let us note that in a highly integrated prototype for using LLMs to create graphical models out of text, neither GV nor MER [R] would be visible to the user. Even so, another thing to highlight is that LLMs demonstrate a reduced occurrence of syntax errors using GV's representation, but generate semantically better models using MER representation.

Hypothesis Testing: To assess whether LLM-generated models could be deemed to be of similar quality as models designed by a human modeler, we ask participants to read a process description and to select the one of several proposed models that, in their opinion, corresponds best to it. For every process description, participants could select one model out of 2–5 associated models, where one model is always the ground truth model and the others are generated by LLMs (cf. Fig. 1).

To determine whether the actual data conforms to an expected pattern or distribution, the Pearson's chi-squared goodness-of-fit test is used. This test is chosen because we are examining just one categorical variable and comparing its observed frequencies to expected frequencies. Mostly, sources suggest to apply the chi-squared test for larger sample sizes, but there is no agreement on a "large" and "small" sample size definition or its boundaries [7]. According to [29] no expected frequency should fall below 5.

For every case, all collected responses ($N = 40$) fall into three groups: ground truth model (**ground**), LLM-generated model (**llm**), or other (**other**, i.e., a model suggested by a user and not included in the proposed options). The "I don't know" option was removed from the observations since, participants tend to select it for all the cases (or its majority) due to limited experience, lack of motivation, or time constraints. Only a small number of all responses (10%) correspond to the "I don't know" option.

Our null hypothesis is based on the assumption that the majority of people prefer the ground truth models over the LLM-generated ones and states the probabilities for each group as follows:

$$H_0 : P = (P_1, P_2, P_3) = (0.8, 0.15, 0.05) \tag{1}$$

where P_1 is the probability that the ground truth model is selected, P_2 stands for the LLM-generated model, and P_3 for "other".

Our alternative hypothesis suggest that the distribution of responses differs from our null hypothesis. In other words, we suspect that people do not predominantly select the ground truth models, and there is a change in the distribution among the three groups:

$$H_1 : P \neq (0.8, 0.15, 0.05) \tag{2}$$

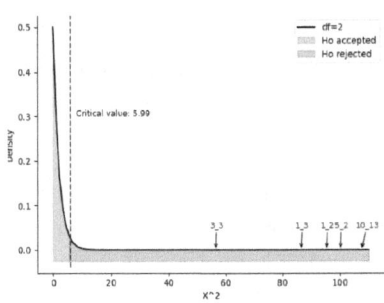

To determine the validity of the null hypothesis and whether it should be rejected, we compute the critical value for the goodness-of-fit test and compare it to the value obtained for each case.

For every model, the goodness-of-fit is significantly larger than its critical value, and the p-value is well below the selected level of significance (p = 0.0001). Hence, we reject the null hypothesis in all cases.

Fig. 4. Pearson's Chi-Squared Test Results: Model Preference

(see Fig. 4) It appears that only 19% of the responses recognize the ground truth models as the most suitable for the provided process descriptions. In contrast, 69% of the responses identify the models generated by LLMs as the most suitable (Fig.5).

Modeling Experience: Since only half of the participants possess modeling experience and are familiar with BPMN, we aim to investigate whether an association exists between the choice of model type (**ground, llm, or other**) and the level of modeling experience (i.e., (ne) no experience, (crb) learned in class or from book, (cp) used on a class project, (pi) used on one project in industry, (mp) used on multiple projects in industry). Our inference is that individuals with more modeling experience are more likely to choose other or ground choices, while those with less experience tend to prefer llm models.

To investigate whether there is a true relation between modeling experience and selected model type, we employ two tests of independence: the Pearson's chi-squared test and the Fisher's exact test. In both cases, our null hypothesis states that these variables are independent from each other:

$$H_0 : A \perp B, \tag{3}$$

where A is type of the chosen model and B is the level of modeling experience. Conversely, the alternative hypothesis claims that there is a connection between A and B.

Considering the individual results for both Fisher and Pearson tests (see Tab. 2), there is not enough evidence to reject the null hypothesis in 9 out of 10 cases. This indicates that we do not have sufficient confirmation to claim a significant connection between the chosen model type and a level of modeling skills. In simpler terms, these two variables are not considered to be dependent.

Table 2. Relationship Between Modeling Experience and Selected Model Type: p-values (LS = level of significance)

Case	LS	1.2	1.3	3.3	5.2	10.13	Total
Fisher	0.05	0.387	0.129	0.03	0.336	0.06	0.044
Pearson	0.05	0.306	0.179	0.053	0.292	0.111	0.054

However, when we consider all cases collectively as a single sample, the overall picture undergoes a substantial shift. According to the Fisher test, the null hypothesis is expected to be rejected, suggesting a potential dependency between modeling experience and choice of a model type. Based on the Pearson test, the null hypothesis remains valid, but the p-value is only slightly higher than the initially set level of significance. However, these results require careful interpretation. Combining all process models into a single sample for the independence test may compromise the assumption of independent observations, as multiple process models were evaluated by the same individuals.

Intriguingly, the current relationship between model type and modeling experience differs from our initial expectations. Participants with no modeling experience (ne) and those with a more academic background (crb and cp) tend to choose ground models more frequently compared to individuals with real-life experience (pi and mp). Conversely, more experienced respondents show a preference for the other option over the ground models. However, all groups consistently vote for llm models. The distribution of llm model selections remains consistent (~60%) across all groups (see Fig. 5).

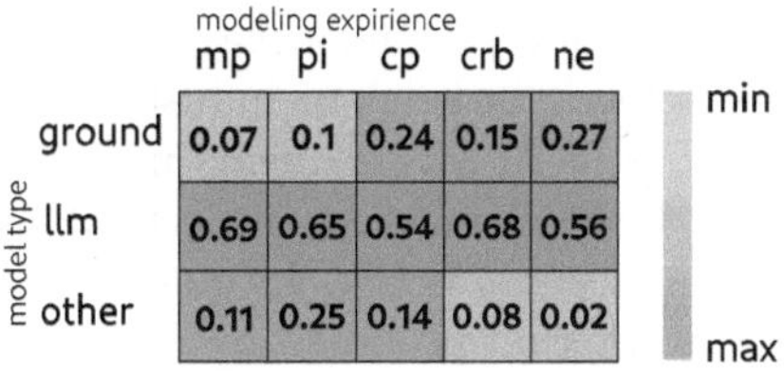

Fig. 5. Percentage Distribution of Frequencies For Modeling Experience and Selected Model Type

Concerns: It is essential to mention that these results should be considered with caution, due to relatively small sample size. With half of the respondents being limited familiar with the subject matter, it is important to acknowledge the potential influence of various response biases.

Manually filtering out incorrect or incomplete LLM-generated models can bias the results in favor of LLM-generated models by showcasing only the most accurate and complete outputs, which does not reflect the full range of the LLM's performance.

In addition, the variability caused by the probabilistic nature of the LLM and the lack of control over its evolution (i.e., release of new versions that impact significant changes in its output) can lead to reproducibility issues [28]. Furthermore, survey respondents' engagement and data quality can be compromised by survey length and complexity, potentially resulting in rushed or incomplete responses. Misinterpretation of questions and the influence of social desirability bias may introduce inaccuracies.

4   Discussion

Around 60% of the participants prefer models generated by LLMs over the models created based on human annotations or suggesting their solutions (see Sect. 3). This preference remains consistent regardless of modeling experience. These results highlight the capabilities of LLMs in generating models with a quality comparable to human-generated models. Still, our results should be interpreted with caution: the examples from the PET dataset may be overly simplistic compared to real-world use cases, and LLMs may perform exceptionally well on these simplified examples such that the same performance might not be achieved in more complex cases. Additionally, while LLMs demonstrate high performance in model generation for simple process descriptions, their efficiency is questionable when higher levels of abstraction or multiple perspectives are involved.

However, while the overall preference leans towards LLM-generated models, it is crucial to examine the cases in which human-generated models were chosen. Understanding these scenarios can provide insights into the limitations of LLMs and areas where human intuition and expertise still play a crucial role. Models created by humans might be preferred in scenarios involving high complexity where human intuition and judgment play a significant role and scenarios requiring deep domain-specific knowledge or industry expertise.

Furthermore, the number of BPMN elements utilized during model generation was restricted to the basic elements (see Sect. 2.2). Introducing a greater variety of model elements may compromise the quality of the results. During the survey, respondents were aware that proposed models were generated by humans or LLMs. This could significantly influence the survey results, potentially introducing bias into the evaluation process. Participants' perceptions and expectations can affect their judgments. For instance, they might assume that LLM-generated models are more simple or sophisticated or that human-generated models are more detailed and better structured, influencing their choice respectively.

5   Related Work

According to [16] business process models can be generated from different sources, such as business rules, standard operating procedures, spreadsheets and unstructured text. In the scope of this paper we focus on unstructured text (i.e., T2M transformation), as not everyone understands specific formats and notations, but essentially everyone understands at least one natural language [9].

The idea of transforming unstructured text into a structured, diagram-based representation such as UML (Unified Modeling Language), ER diagrams (Entity–relationship), BPMN, and DECLARE (Declarative Process Modeling), is not novel. Most existing methods rely on text pattern search, rule-based approaches, or semantic analysis (e.g., [13,14,30]). [1,27] propose techniques for automatic annotation of textual process descriptions utilising classical supervised machine learning-based approaches. Nonetheless, due to the absence of suitable publicly available datasets containing real-life complex data, applying these machine learning techniques becomes challenging [6].

Hence, the rise and evolution of natural language processing (NLP) holds additional promise for research, particularly when applied in the context of utilizing LLMs. In [6,20], language models are utilized to extract entities and relationships from textual process descriptions and in [15,21] a method for generating a process model in a pre-specified intermediary notation as an output format of LLMs (particularly GPT4) is proposed and show-cased. Additionally, several online tools for conversational process modeling were introduced in [22,23].

However, not only the generation of models is a challenge, but also their evaluation presents significant difficulties and demands considerable effort. Mostly, the evaluation tends to be more quantitative, focusing on measurable aspects like model complexity, execution time, and compliance with syntactical rules, rather than qualitative semantic evaluation [2,17,24]. In [22], the effectiveness of the tool and its technological acceptance are also taken into consideration. Yet, during evaluation it must be ensured that the models accurately reflect the intended processes and are useful to stakeholders (i.e., model correctness regarding provided process description and stakeholder's satisfaction with it).

6   Conclusions and Future Research Directions

The results of the evaluation indicate that chatbots for conversational process modeling are ready to be applied in practice. The LLMs demonstrate a strong capability to handle model generation tasks, confirmed by the high accuracy of the generated models—74% were both complete and correct in representing the provided process descriptions. The survey results show that distinguishing a ground truth model from a set of LLM-generated models is not straightforward, and interestingly, the ability to select the correct model does not depend on modeling experience.

The probabilistic nature of LLMs necessitates that domain experts check the results. However, since acquiring as-is models consumes up to 60% of the time spent on process management projects [13], chatbot-based partial automation can be sufficiently impactful, even if substantial human refinement is required.

Future research will focus on integrating the strong language capabilities of chatbots into the iterative process of model generation, where users create process models with the help of chatbots and then refine them. Additionally, the set of utilized business process elements should be extended to include at least pools and lanes. There is also a necessity to enhance the ability of LLM-generated models to handle more complex use cases and integrate diverse viewpoints based on stakeholder perspectives and modeling purposes.

References

1. Ackermann, L., Neuberger, J., Jablonski, S.: Data-driven annotation of textual process descriptions based on formal meaning representations. In: Advanced Information Systems Engineering, pp. 75–90 (2021)
2. Avila, D.T., dos Santos, R.I., Mendling, J., Thom, L.H.: A systematic literature review of process modeling guidelines and their empirical support. Bus. Process. Manag. J. **27**(1), 1–23 (2021). https://doi.org/10.1108/BPMJ-10-2019-0407
3. Beerepoot, I., Ciccio, C.D., Reijers, H.A., et al.: The biggest business process management problems to solve before we die. Comput. Ind. **146**, 103837 (2023)
4. Bellan, P., van der Aa, H., Dragoni, M., Ghidini, C., Ponzetto, S.P.: PET: an annotated dataset for process extraction from natural language text tasks. In: Business Process Management Workshops, pp. 315–321 (2022)
5. Bellan, P., Dragoni, M., Ghidini, C.: A qualitative analysis of the state of the art in process extraction from text. In: Italian Association for Artificial Intelligence, pp. 19–30. CEUR Workshop Proceedings (2020)
6. Bellan, P., Dragoni, M., Ghidini, C.: Extracting business process entities and relations from text using pre-trained language models and in-context learning. In: Enterprise Design, Operations, and Computing, pp. 182–199 (2022)
7. Campbell, I.: Chi-squared and Fisher-Irwin tests of two-by-two tables with small sample recommendations. Stat. Med. **26**(19), 3661–3675 (2007)
8. Casciani, A., Bernardi, M.L., Cimitile, M., Marrella, A.: Conversational systems for AI-augmented business process management. In: Research Challenges in Information Science, pp. 183–200 (2024)

9. Dalianis, H.: A method for validating a conceptual model by natural language discourse generation. In: Advanced Information Systems Engineering, pp. 425–444 (1992)

10. Dehnert, J., van der Aalst, W.M.P.: Bridging the gap between business models and workflow specifications. Int. J. Coop. Inf. Syst. **13**(3), 289–332 (2004)

11. Dumas, M., et al.: AI-augmented business process management systems: a research manifesto. ACM Trans. Manage. Inf. Syst. **14**, 1–19 (2022)

12. Fowler Jr, F.J.: Survey Research Methods. Sage Publications (2013)

13. Friedrich, F.: Automated generation of business process models from natural language input. Master's thesis, Humbold-University zu Berlin (2010)

14. Ghose, A., Koliadis, G., Chueng, A.: Process discovery from model and text artefacts. In: Services Computing Workshops, pp. 167–174 (2007)

15. Grohs, M., Abb, L., Elsayed, N., Rehse, J.: Large language models can accomplish business process management tasks. CoRR abs/2307.09923 (2023)

16. Honkisz, K., Kluza, K., Wisniewski, P.: A concept for generating business process models from natural language description. In: Knowledge Science, Engineering and Management, pp. 91–103 (2018)

17. Kahloun, F., Ghannouchi, S.A.: Improvement of quality for business process modeling driven by guidelines. Procedia Comput. Sci. **126**, 39–48 (2018)

18. Kannengiesser, U., Oppl, S.: Business processes to touch: Engaging domain experts in process modelling, vol. 1418 (2015)

19. Kesari, M., Chang, S., Seddon, P.B.: A content-analytic study of the advantages and disadvantages of process modelling. In: Australasian Conference on Information Systems, ACIS 2003, Perth, Australia, 26–28 November 2003 (2003)

20. Klievtsova, N., Benzin, J., Kampik, T., Mangler, J., Rinderle-Ma, S.: Conversational process modelling: state of the art, applications, and implications in practice. In: Business Process Management Forum, pp. 319–336 (2023)

21. Klievtsova, N., Mangler, J., Kampik, T., Benzin, J.V., Rinderle-Ma, S.: How can generative AI empower domain experts in creating process models? In: Wirtschaftsinformatik (2024)

22. Koepke, J., Safan, A.: Efficient LLM-based conversational process modeling. In: Business Process Management Workshops (2024)

23. Kourani, H., Berti, A., Schuster, D., van der Aalst, W.M.P.: ProMoAI: process modeling with generative AI. CoRR abs/2403.04327 (2024)

24. de Oca, I.M.M., Snoeck, M., Reijers, H.A., Rodríguez-Morffi, A.: A systematic literature review of studies on business process modeling quality. Inf. Softw. Technol. **58**, 187–205 (2015)

25. Odeh, Y.: BPMN in engineering software requirements: an introductory brief guide. In: International Conference on Information Management and Engineering (2017)

26. Polyvyanyy, A., Smirnov, S., Weske, M.: Business process model abstraction. In: Handbook on Business Process Management. Introduction, Methods, and Information Systems. International Handbooks on Information Systems, pp. 147–165. Springer (2015)

27. Qian, C., et al.: An approach for process model extraction by multi-grained text classification. In: Advanced Information Systems Engineering, pp. 268–282 (2020)

28. Sallou, J., Durieux, T., Panichella, A.: Breaking the silence: the threats of using LLMs in software engineering. In: Proceedings of the 2024 ACM/IEEE 44th International Conference on Software Engineering, NIER@ICSE 2024, Lisbon, Portugal, 14–20 April 2024, pp. 102–106. ACM (2024). https://doi.org/10.1145/3639476.3639764

29. VanVoorhis, C.W., Morgan, B.L., et al.: Understanding power and rules of thumb for determining sample sizes. Tutor. Quant. Methods Psychol. **3**(2), 43–50 (2007)
30. Yue, T., Briand, L.C., Labiche, Y.: An automated approach to transform use cases into activity diagrams. In: Modelling Foundations and Applications, pp. 337–353 (2010)

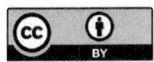

Skill Learning Using Process Mining for Large Language Model Plan Generation

Andrei Cosmin Redis[1]([✉]), Mohammadreza Fani Sani[2]([✉]), Bahram Zarrin[2]([✉]), and Andrea Burattin[1]([✉])

[1] Technical University of Denmark, Lyngby, Denmark
andreiredis@gmail.com, andbur@dtu.dk
[2] Microsoft Development Center Copenhagen, Lyngby, Denmark
{mfanisani,bahram.zarrin}@microsoft.com

Abstract. Large language models (LLMs) hold promise for generating plans for complex tasks, but their effectiveness is limited by sequential execution, lack of control flow models, and difficulties in skill retrieval. Addressing these issues is crucial for improving the efficiency and interpretability of plan generation as LLMs become more central to automation and decision-making. We introduce a novel approach to skill learning in LLMs by integrating process mining techniques, leveraging process discovery for skill acquisition, process models for skill storage, and conformance checking for skill retrieval. Our methods enhance text-based plan generation by enabling flexible skill discovery, parallel execution, and improved interpretability. Experimental results suggest the effectiveness of our approach, with our skill retrieval method surpassing state-of-the-art accuracy baselines under specific conditions.

Keywords: Large Language Model · Plan Generation · Process Mining · Agentic Context Retrieval · Skill Learning

1 Introduction

Large language models (LLMs) have demonstrated remarkable capabilities in natural language processing tasks and have shown some capacity for logical reasoning [12,22]. However, their performance tends to decline as the complexity of problems increases, particularly in tasks requiring intricate reasoning or multi-step planning [8,20]. To enhance LLM performance on reasoning tasks, researchers have incorporated tools and plan generation capabilities, enabling LLMs to function as agents that generate sequences of tool invocations to solve given problems [2,5,24].

Despite these advancements, existing plan generation methods, especially text-based planners, face significant challenges when dealing with complex tasks [20]. Text-based planners typically produce flat sequences of actions without an underlying structured control flow model [24]. This lack of control flow

© The Author(s) 2025
A. Delgado and T. Slaats (Eds.): ICPM 2024 Workshops, LNBIP 533, pp. 650–662, 2025.
https://doi.org/10.1007/978-3-031-82225-4_48

limits their ability to generalize plans to other problems, making them less adaptable to varying parameters and conditions. Although these plans may include parameters, they are still less generalizable and often require adjustments or replanning when faced with new tasks. Additionally, the linear sequences are less interpretable, as the absence of logical structure makes it challenging for humans to understand the rationale behind the plans. Furthermore, the inability to identify parallelizable actions leads to less efficient execution, as tasks are processed sequentially without exploiting opportunities for concurrent execution.

In contrast, code-based planners [24] inherently incorporate structured control flow models, such as functions, loops, and conditionals, allowing for flexible and adaptable plan generation. This flexibility likely enables effective skill learning, as observed in works like Voyager by Wang et al. [21], where previously generated plans (skills) can be reused and adapted to new problems. The structured control flow in code-based planners facilitates the grouping of related plans and the dynamic adjustment of actions based on different parameters and conditions.

The problem we address in this paper is the lack of structured control flow models in text-based LLM planners, which hinders their ability to perform efficient skill learning and limits their effectiveness in generating plans for complex tasks. Without a control flow model, text-based planners cannot effectively group related plans or identify parallelizable actions, resulting in sequential execution and increased latency.

To overcome this limitation, we propose a novel skill learning framework for text-based LLM planners that integrates process mining techniques [1] to extract structured control flow models from flat action sequences. Process mining allows us to discover process models from execution traces, providing a structured representation of the control flow underlying the sequences generated by text-based planners. By incorporating these process models, we enable text-based planners to benefit from structured control flow, similar to code-based planners, thereby enhancing skill learning and plan generation capabilities.

Our approach addresses the limitations of text-based planners by:

1. **Enabling flexible skill discovery and storage:** By discovering process models from action sequences, we can capture general behaviors and reuse skills across similar problems, reducing the reliance on generating plans from scratch.
2. **Supporting parallel execution of actions:** The structured control flow models identify ordering constraints and parallelizable tasks, allowing for parallel execution where appropriate, thus reducing execution time and service latency.[1]
3. **Improving interpretability and reliability:** Structured process models could enhance the interpretability of the LLM's decision-making process, facilitating debugging and optimization by developers and users.

---

[1] For example, in the TaskBench dataset [18], enabling parallel execution could potentially answer queries 1.43 times faster, assuming equal execution time for all actions. The time to execute a process model where groups of actions without ordering constraints can be executed in parallel is equal to the longest path of the plan in process model format (e.g., BPMN).

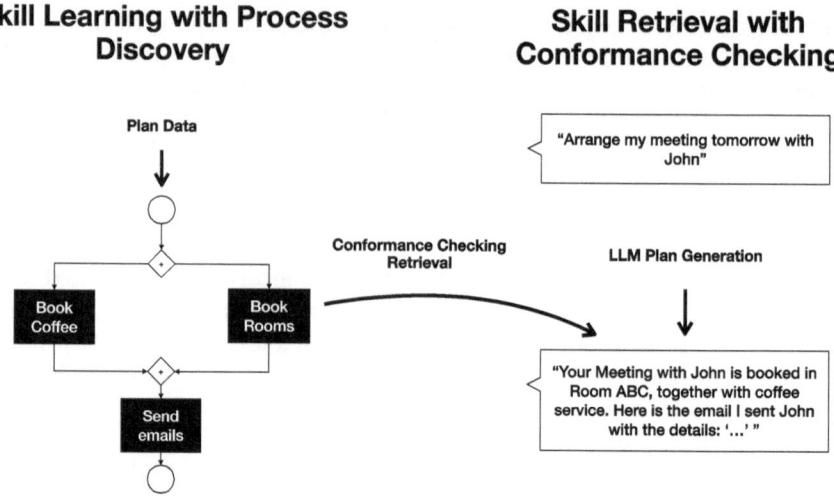

Fig. 1. In the skill learning approach, when given a prompt such as 'Arrange my meeting tomorrow with John', the LLM plan generator retrieves the 'meeting' skill to enhance its response. This paper introduces process mining techniques to discover this skill in a process model format, facilitating its retrieval and offering additional advantages, such as enabling parallelism in plan execution.

As illustrated in Fig. 1, when given a prompt such as "Arrange my meeting tomorrow with John", the LLM plan generator can retrieve the "meeting" skill represented as a process model. This additional context enhances its response by leveraging the structured control flow and enabling parallel execution where appropriate.

Throughout this paper, we will use the terms *plans*, *traces*, and *cases* interchangeably. Similarly, the terms *process*, *problem*, *query*, and *task*. That is also the case for *action*, *activity*, and *step*, as well as in equal measure *planner*, *agent*, and *LLM plan generator*. This is to reflect on the close relationship between the fields of planning and process mining and the overlap in the concepts they deal with.

2   Related Work

In addition to the related work discussed in the introduction, several other studies intersect with the field of process mining. Fettke et al. corroborate our findings from developing our approach, asserting that despite the compartmentalized research, AI planning, machine learning, and process mining share common objectives, making collaboration advantageous [7]. Moreover, [6] explores the potential of utilizing LLMs for event log abstraction and process automation.

Regarding process mining and LLMs, research has primarily concentrated on employing LLMs to perform process mining tasks. Despite the existing research into prompt engineering for process mining [11], process question answering [3], and event log data pre-processing [9], the application of process mining methods to assist with LLM tasks remains largely uncharted.

3   Skill Learning Using Process Discovery

Text-based LLM planners typically generate flat sequences of actions to solve tasks. While effective for simple scenarios, these linear plans lack the structured control flow needed for complex tasks involving parallelism and reusability. To address this limitation, we propose a process mining method to discover structured control flow models - *skills* - from these flat action sequences.

Our approach takes the action sequences generated by the LLM planner as input and applies process discovery techniques, such as the Inductive Miner algorithm [13], to infer general process models. These models capture the underlying control flow, including sequential and parallel relations between actions, providing a more expressive and flexible representation than flat plans.

Storing these skills as process models in a skill library enable the LLM planner to reuse previous solutions when faced with similar problems, reducing the need to generate new plans from scratch. This approach is analogous to the skill learning observed in code-based planners like Voyager [21] but applied to text-based planners without requiring them to generate code.

The skill learning framework overview is shown in Fig. 2. The inputs are problems, and their corresponding flat plans are generated by the LLM. We transform these plans into structured process models (skills) through process mining, which are then stored in the skill library for future retrieval.

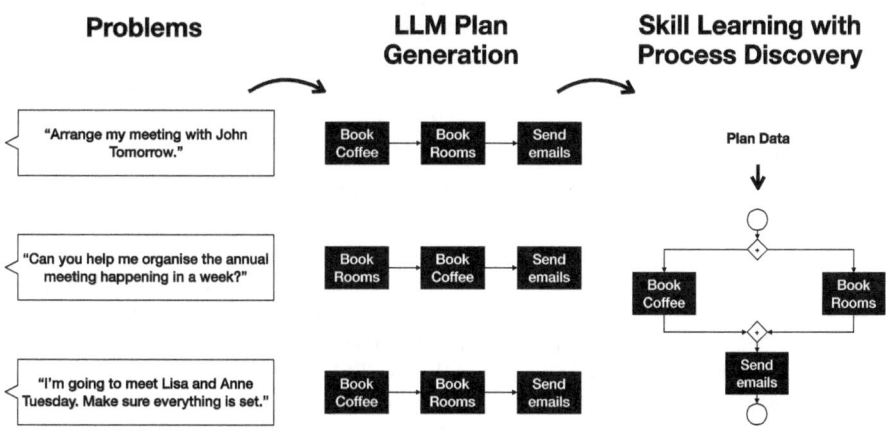

Fig. 2. Schematic view of the skill learning process using process discovery.

By integrating process mining into the skill learning process, our method enhances text-based LLM planners by providing them with reusable, interpretable, and parallelizable skills derived from their own generated plans. This bridges the gap between text-based and code-based planners, enabling text-based planners to handle more complex tasks effectively while maintaining their simplicity.

4   Skill Retrieval Using Conformance Checking

To enhance both the accuracy and interpretability of skill retrieval in LLMs, we propose two methods based on conformance checking: (1) retrieval solely using conformance checking and (2) a two-stage retrieval method that combines text semantic similarity with conformance checking. The overall pipeline is shown in Fig. 1.

1. Conformance Checking Only: This method exclusively relies on conformance checking. This process mining technique assesses how well the control flow of a candidate skill's process model aligns with a bare-bones LLM-generated plan, referred to as a *thought*. We define *thought* as a partial plan embodying a full planning trace but not needing to be fully grounded in the state space. I.e., a plan that does not consider information received from the execution of tools, such as would be the case with [23]. The key metric is alignment fitness, which measures the degree of structural match between the generated plan and the stored process models. Focusing on structural alignment rather than textual similarity offers superior interpretability, making it easier to understand why a particular skill was retrieved. The direct comparison of control flows ensures that the retrieved skills are relevant and logically compatible with the problem at hand.
2. Two-Stage Retrieval: This hybrid method begins with a rapid filtering stage using text semantic similarity. Embedding models like the Universal Sentence Encoder (USE) or OpenAI's ada-002 generate vector representations of the problem description, and cosine similarity is used to identify the top-k candidates. These shortlisted candidates are then reranked using conformance checking based on alignment fitness. This two-stage approach balances computational efficiency with high retrieval accuracy and enhanced interpretability, as the final ranking is based on the logical structure of the process models rather than solely on textual descriptions.

Both methods aim to outperform existing baselines that rely primarily on semantic similarity between text descriptions. By integrating process model alignment, these methods improve the precision of skill retrieval and significantly enhance the retrieval process's interpretability. This ensures that the logic behind the skill selection is transparent, which is crucial for debugging and optimizing LLM-driven plan executions. Additionally, the alignment values obtained from conformance checking can help assess the quality of the generated plan.

5   Evaluation and Discussion

In this section, we aim to answer the following questions: Given the current state of LLM plan generation, how feasible is it to learn skills using our proposed skill learning method? And, enabled by the skills learned, how does the accuracy of the proposed skill retrieval methods compare with previous approaches?

5.1   Experiments

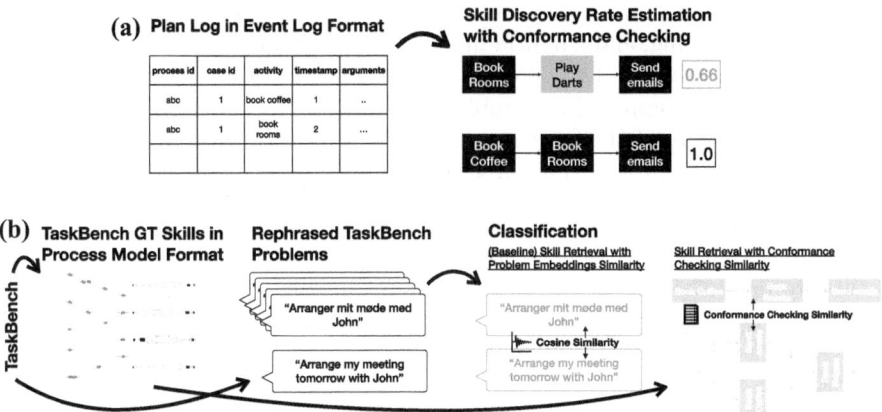

Fig. 3. (a) Schematic view of the experimental pipeline for skill learning with process discovery. (b) Schematic view of the experimental skill retrieval pipeline with conformance checking.

Skill Learning with Process Discovery. To evaluate the feasibility and effectiveness of our proposed skill learning method, we conducted experiments using the ProcessTBench synthetic dataset [16]. This experiment aimed to determine whether our method could reliably generate accurate process models (skills). We used conformance checking of the generated action sequences (traces) compared to ground-truth process models provided in the dataset.

The ProcessTBench synthetic dataset includes queries requiring LLM-generated plans, with corresponding solutions provided as action sequences using predefined tools. Each of the 532 problems represents a distinct process instance, with 5–6 LLM-generated action sequences serving as individual cases within these instances. The dataset simulates multiple process executions, where different paraphrasings of a query and various plans are treated as execution instances of the same process.

To evaluate the feasibility of our skill learning method, we used conformance checking to compare the LLM-generated plans (traces) from ProcessTBench with the ground truth process models provided by TaskBench. This part is illustrated in Fig. 3a. We employed two widely-used conformance checking metrics, *Replay Fitness* and *Alignment Fitness* [10], to assess how well the generated plans align with the known process models. High conformance values indicate that accurate process models could be derived from these traces using process discovery, supporting our method's viability. For this task, ProcessTBench uses the GPT-4-0613 model.

Skill Retrieval with Conformance Checking. We conducted experiments using the TaskBench dataset, rephrasing 533 problems (queries) 5–6 times each to simulate scenarios where a similar problem requires a relevant solution from the skill library. We then tested different skill retrieval methods. We compared the baseline method that uses problem embeddings, our proposed model using conformance checking, and a hybrid model combining both approaches (i.e., two-stage retrieval). We aimed to determine if conformance checking could enhance retrieval accuracy compared to established similarity methods.

The architecture of the Skill Retrieval With Conformance Checking experiment is depicted in Fig. 3b. This architecture has the following components.

1. **LLM Rephraser:** Generates paraphrased descriptions of problems in English, Danish, and French. To improve its accuracy, the model was asked first to reason about the problem, as shown in [14].

     Input: Problem description from the TaskBench dataset [18]

     Output: Rephrased problem descriptions

2. **DAG to Petri net Converter:** Converts reference DAG process models to Petri nets.

     Input: A reference process model presented in the DAG format

     Output: A process model presented in the Petri net format

3. **LLM plan (*thought*) generator:** Generates partial plans (*thoughts*) using the given problem description and tools available in the TaskBench domain. We call these plans *thoughts* and partial to distinguish them from the output of more thorough and widely used planners such as ReAct [23]. I.e., due to experimental constraints, the thought generator is asked to return a full trace solution in one inference session, while ReAct builds the plan more thoroughly in inference iterations.

     Input: Problem description and all available tools in the TaskBench domain

     Output: Plan that solves the problem as a sequence of actions.

4. **Classifier:** Calculates a distance distribution between rephrased and original TaskBench problems. For conformance checking retrieval, we first generate a thought-a partial plan representing the solution before calculating the distance. This thought is then used to compare the rephrased problem to other problems.

     Input: Rephrased problem

     Output: Distance distribution over original problems.

For the classifier, the following two baseline and proposed models were used:

1. **Universal Sentence Encoder (USE):** Measures semantic similarity using cosine distance between problem and skill embeddings [4].
2. **ada-002:** A more recent embedding model by OpenAI[2].
3. **Conformance checking:** Measures the alignment between the LLM-generated plan (*thought*) and the stored process models, using alignment fitness as a similarity measure [10].

---

[2] https://openai.com/blog/new-and-improved-embedding-model.

Table 1. Descriptive statistics of the dataset used to evaluate the feasibility of skill acquisition through process discovery.

	Mean	Std.	Min.	Median	Max.
Cases (Plans)/Process	4.08	1.27	2	4	11
Activities (Actions)/Process	3.79	0.89	2	4	8
Case Variants/Process	2.68	0.97	1	3	5
Replay Fitness/Case	0.96	0.09	0.25	1.00	1.00
Alignments Fitness/Case	0.94	0.12	0.40	1.00	1.00

4. **Hybrid (ada-002 + Conformance checking):** Candidates are pre-filtered using ada-002 and re-ranked using conformance checking.

The retrieval models' performance was evaluated using two state-of-the-art metrics for multi-class classification and next-item recommender systems: F1-score and Mean Reciprocal Rank (MRR) [19].

Each of these evaluation metrics serves different purposes. For a given rephrased query, the models output a ranked list of process models based on their similarity scores. The F1-score measures the accuracy when considering only the top-ranked prediction, counting it as correct if it matches the actual class. The Mean Reciprocal Rank (MRR) provides a more nuanced assessment by evaluating the average inverse rank position of the correct class in the ranked list, thus accounting for how high the correct class appears in the recommendations.

5.2 Skill Learning with Process Discovery

In this study, we evaluated the feasibility of our proposed skill learning method using the TaskBench [18] and the ProcessTBench [16] synthetic datasets. TaskBench contains various queries and their corresponding process models. Each query represents a separate process, and each specific instance of solving that query is considered a case. ProcessTBench extends TaskBench by providing repeated sequential planning traces for the problems.

Table 1 summarizes the dataset characteristics, including the average number of cases per process, the number of activities (actions) per process, and the fitness metrics for conformance checking. The mean number of cases per process was 4.08, indicating a relatively small dataset, especially compared to popular real-world process mining datasets like the BPI Challenges, where the number of cases is significantly larger [17]. Despite the dataset's small size, the high average replay fitness (0.96) and alignment fitness (0.94) suggest that our skill learning method is feasible. These metrics indicate that the discovered skills closely matched the ground truth in many cases, with 75% processes achieving a perfect fitness score for all associated cases.

Figure 4 illustrates the accuracy distribution of the generated traces. Replay fitness tends to be higher than alignments, suggesting the planner's difficulty

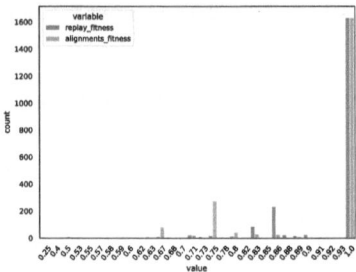

Fig. 4. Summary of the overall accuracy of the traces generated by the planner for n = 2173 cases.

Table 2. F1 score and MRR for the four retrieval methods. The best result across each metric is highlighted in bold. The ada-002 X Conformance Checking @ 3 is the hybrid model described in Sect. 5.1, with 3 nearest neighbors retrieved during the first stage.

	F1	MRR
USE	0.66	0.71
ada-002	**0.91**	**0.94**
Conformance Checking	0.75	0.84
ada-002 X Conformance Checking @ 3	0.90	0.93

assembling individual components into a coherent sequence. E.g., for a specific query in ProcessTBench, the ground truth process model was $\wedge(\to (A,B), \to (C,D,E,F))$, but the planner produced the sequence E, F, A, B, C, D, resulting in a replay fitness of 0.9 and an alignment fitness of 0.66. Although the planner accurately captured most relationships between actions, it struggled with correctly ordering them. This suggests that sequence alignment, and consequently the creation of complete control flow models, could be particularly challenging for LLMs - a challenge that is somewhat expected given that reasoning is a known weakness.

The experiment aimed to demonstrate that a real-life dataset of 'similar problems' would exhibit sufficient variance to allow the capture of accurate process models. However, in this study, the variance was artificially generated using the synthetic ProcessTBench dataset, where an LLM was prompted to 'generate more plan variants', which may not fully replicate real-world conditions. Finally, although ProcessTBench contains a relatively low number of traces, process discovery algorithms are not the sole real-life contributors to skill learning. Human experts can also play a crucial role in defining the correct skills. Overall, the evidence suggests that when automated process discovery tools are combined with additional data and expert input, it is likely feasible to construct a robust skill library using our proposed skill learning method.

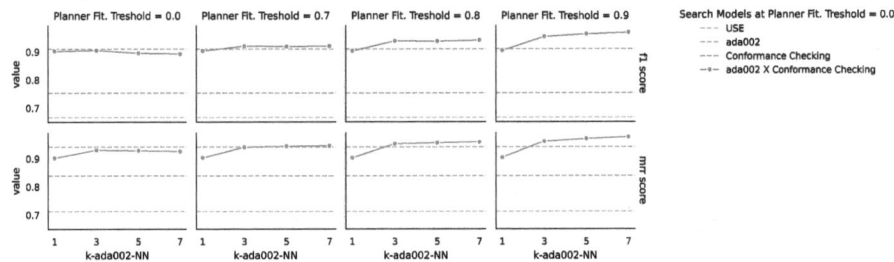

Fig. 5. performance of the proposed ada-002 and conformance hybrid model, given different planner accuracies. The columns represent different planner accuracies, while the rows represent the metric, f1, or MRR. The x-axis represents the nearest neighbors retrieved by the first stage retrieval model, ada-002. The y-axis represents the final result of the respective metric after reranking with Conformance Checking. The reference lines show the results at the baseline planner accuracy (fitness) threshold = 0.0. The figure reveals that with a counterfactual conformance checking threshold of 0.7 alignment fitness, the combined ada-002 and Conformance Checking would outperform all other methods.

5.3 Skill Retrieval with Conformance Checking

The results in Table 2 show that the ada-002 model outperforms the other models in terms of F1 score and MRR. The combination of ada-002 and Conformance Checking also delivers strong performance, nearly matching the accuracy of the ada-002 model. This suggests at first glance that the baseline method, using ada-002, is better for Skill Retrieval than our proposed methods using conformance checking.

It is worth observing that ada-002 performs 11% better than in the documentation provided by OpenAI, the model's creators. This suggests that our rephrased queries were less complex than what was used in their benchmark (sentence similarity); see Footnote 2. We couldn't find previous work on a comparable experiment for conformance checking.

Finally, we show that the results above might change when relaxing one experimental constraint: the accuracy of the planner. To understand the impact of the plan (*thought*) generator accuracy on the relative performance of our models, we did a sensitivity analysis, shown in Fig. 5. It turns out that the combined ada-002 and conformance-checking model would outperform ada-002, given a generator accuracy of 0.7 or more. In our opinion, a threshold of 0.7 is not too low. It could be realistically achieved with better planner design (cp. with the planner accuracy 1 with an average of 0.94 and std of 0.12, and with TaskBench achieving 0.9 node and 0.71 edge prediction [18]).

These findings lead us to believe that, with better "thought" generator design, integrating conformance checking with other retrieval models could be a promising direction for future research. As discussed in Sect. 4, the proposed Skill Retrieval approach is also more interpretable and accurate.

While generating 'thoughts' initially introduces additional LLM inference overhead, this investment can lead to overall inference savings compared to methods like ReAct. Since the generated plans can be stored and reused for similar problems in the future, the need for repeated inference is reduced. Additionally, the ability to identify and execute parallelizable actions within these plans allows for concurrency savings, further enhancing efficiency.

Finally, it's important to note that ada-002 has been outperformed by newer embedding models since conducting these experiments, with improvements of up to 25% [15]. Similarly, more recent LLMs have surpassed the one used for skill retrieval in this study. These advancements could significantly impact the results, suggesting that future research should evaluate the effects of these newer models on skill learning and retrieval.

6 Conclusion

Our experiments suggest the feasibility of using process mining techniques for skill learning in text-based LLM planners. By integrating conformance checking into skill retrieval, we may improve the accuracy and interpretability of plan generation. These advancements could pave the way for more efficient and reliable LLM-driven automation solutions. More interpretable LLM plan generation can give businesses greater control and transparency over automated processes. As LLMs' role in decision-making expands, effectively managing and understanding these systems will be increasingly important.

In the future, we aim to develop our experimental framework further. Generating more data and creating more sophisticated LLM plan generators will enable more general conclusions. Furthermore, controlling for more confounding variables, such as LLM and embedding models, would increase the robustness of the observed effects. We have developed a skill learning framework and presented its theoretical properties. Still, we have not created a skill "usage" framework to gather evidence for our approach's end-to-end effectiveness. Lastly, we have tested skill retrieval in a closed-set classification setting, but the open-set classification is also a realistic use case worth exploring.

References

1. van der Aalst, W.: Process Mining. Springer, Heidelberg (2016). https://doi.org/10.1007/978-3-662-49851-4
2. Ahn, M., et al.: Do as i can, not as i say: grounding language in robotic affordances (2022). http://arxiv.org/abs/2204.01691
3. Berti, A., Schuster, D., van der Aalst, W.M.P.: Abstractions, scenarios, and prompt definitions for process mining with LLMs: a case study. In: De Weerdt, J., Pufahl, L. (eds.) BPM 2023. LNBIP, vol. 492, pp. 427–439. Springer, Cham (2024). https://doi.org/10.1007/978-3-031-50974-2_32
4. Cer, D., et al.: Universal sentence encoder (2018). https://arxiv.org/abs/1803.11175v2

5. Chang, Y., et al.: A survey on evaluation of large language models (2023). http://arxiv.org/abs/2307.03109

6. Fani Sani, M., Sroka, M., Burattin, A.: LLMs and process mining: challenges in RPA: task grouping, labelling and connector recommendation. In: ICPM Workshop Proceedings, pp. 379–391. Springer (2023)

7. Fettke, P., Rombach, A.: Towards automated process planning and mining (2022). http://arxiv.org/abs/2208.08943

8. Gendron, G., Bao, Q., Witbrock, M., Dobbie, G.: Large language models are not abstract reasoners (2023). http://arxiv.org/abs/2305.19555

9. Grohs, M., Abb, L., Elsayed, N., Rehse, J.R.: Large language models can accomplish business process management tasks. In: De Weerdt, J., Pufahl, L. (eds.) BPM 2023. LNBIP, vol. 492, pp. 453–465. Springer, Cham (2024). https://doi.org/10.1007/978-3-031-50974-2_34

10. Jagadeesh Chandra Bose, R., van der Aalst, W.: Trace alignment in process mining: opportunities for process diagnostics. In: International Conference on Business Process Management, pp. 227–242. Springer (2010)

11. Jessen, U., Sroka, M., Fahland, D.: Chit-chat or deep talk: prompt engineering for process mining (2023). https://arxiv.org/abs/2307.09909

12. Kojima, T., Gu, S.S., Reid, M., Matsuo, Y., Iwasawa, Y.: Large language models are zero-shot reasoners. In: NeurIPS 2022 (2022)

13. Leemans, S.J.J., van Zelst, S.J., Lu, X.: Partial-order-based process mining: a survey and outlook. Knowl. Inf. Syst. **65**(1), 1–29 (2023). https://doi.org/10.1007/s10115-022-01777-3

14. Mizrahi, M., Kaplan, G., Malkin, D., Dror, R., Shahaf, D., Stanovsky, G.: State of what art? A call for multi-prompt LLM evaluation (2023). http://arxiv.org/abs/2401.00595

15. Muennighoff, N., Tazi, N., Magne, L., Reimers, N.: MTEB: massive text embedding benchmark (2022). https://arxiv.org/abs/2210.07316

16. Redis, A.C., Sani, M.F., Zarrin, B., Burattin, A.: ProcessTBench: an LLM plan generation dataset for process mining (2024). https://doi.org/10.48550/arXiv.2409.09191

17. Sani, M.F., Boltenhagen, M., van der Aalst, W.: Prototype selection based on clustering and conformance metrics for model discovery (2019). http://arxiv.org/abs/1912.00736

18. Shen, Y., et al.: TaskBench: benchmarking large language models for task automation (2023). http://arxiv.org/abs/2311.18760

19. Taha, A.A., Hanbury, A.: Metrics for evaluating 3D medical image segmentation: analysis, selection, and tool. BMC Med. Imaging **15**, 29 (2015). https://doi.org/10.1186/s12880-015-0068-x

20. Valmeekam, K., Olmo, A., Sreedharan, S., Kambhampati, S.: Large language models still can't plan (a benchmark for LLMs on planning and reasoning about change) (2023). http://arxiv.org/abs/2206.10498

21. Wang, G., et al.: Voyager: an open-ended embodied agent with large language models. arXiv:2305.16291 [cs] (2023)

22. Wei, J., et al.: Chain-of-thought prompting elicits reasoning in large language models. In: Proceedings of NIPS, pp. 24824–24837. Curran Associates Inc. (2024)

23. Yao, S., et al.: ReAct: synergizing reasoning and acting in language models (2023). http://arxiv.org/abs/2210.03629

24. Zhao, et al.: A survey of large language models (2023). http://arxiv.org/abs/2303.18223

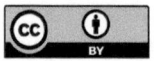

Providing Domain Knowledge for Process Mining with ReWOO-Based Agents

Max W. Vogt[1], Peter van der Putten[1(✉)] ⓘ, and Hajo A. Reijers[2] ⓘ

[1] LIACS, Leiden University, Leiden, The Netherlands
m.w.vogt@umail.leidenuniv.nl, p.w.h.van.der.putten@liacs.leidenuniv.nl
[2] Department of Information and Computing Sciences, Utrecht University,
Utrecht, The Netherlands
h.a.reijers@uu.nl

Abstract. Process mining practitioners often face the challenge of interpreting complex process data and driving process improvements with limited expertise in process optimization, tools, and the application domain of the process. This study explores the integration of LLM-based agentic frameworks in process mining to bridge this gap and democratize access to process optimization. We developed a Proof-of-Concept that leverages a Reasoning WithOut Observation (ReWOO)-based agent to perform process discovery, problem identification, generate ecosystem domain knowledge, and propose potential process improvements. Our experiments on a range of business processes suggest that LLM-based agent systems can insert meaningful domain knowledge into process mining tool interactions.

Keywords: Process mining · LLM · ReWOO · Domain knowledge · Agents

1 Introduction

Process mining offers several benefits for organizations, such as fact-based insights into processes, alignment with process models, and process improvement. It can improve productivity and business outcomes, and reduce risks. However, organizations often encounter obstacles when trying to derive value from process mining. One issue Zerbato et al. found is the lack of domain knowledge[17]. Similarly, Andrews et al. found that process improvements are largely proposed by domain experts and that process mining tools themselves do not provide direction for these improvements [1].

We propose to explore the potential of using LLMs to provide domain knowledge in process mining tools. We validated the lack of domain knowledge in process mining and the potential of using LLMs to fill this gap through in-depth interviews with a small set of process mining practitioners.

Several studies have been done about using LLMs in combination with process mining, such as connecting the open-source process mining tool PM4PY to

A. Delgado and T. Slaats (Eds.): ICPM 2024 Workshops, LNBIP 533, pp. 663–676, 2025.
https://doi.org/10.1007/978-3-031-82225-4_49

an LLM [2]. Not only academics are looking into using LLMs in process mining, but we also see interest from commercial companies. For instance, process mining vendors Celonis[1] and Pegasystems[2] are currently developing LLM capabilities in their process mining solutions. However, these efforts are mainly focusing on using LLMs for descriptive tasks in process mining tools, e.g. 'How long does my process take?' or answering questions regarding process mining expertise, e.g. 'What is conformance checking?'.

We propose a different approach. We use LLMs-based agents to fill the observed gap in domain knowledge in process mining tools, the type of knowledge that would traditionally come from a human domain expert, e.g. knowledge about the sector of the organization. Hence our research question is, 'How can LLMs provide domain knowledge to help users of process mining tools understand and improve processes?'. To study this, we follow the principles of a research by design study as proposed by Peffers et al. [11]. We developed a Proof-of-Concept (PoC) and evaluated this with a limited set of experiments. The results indicate that LLM-based systems can generate domain knowledge and give directions for future work.

The remainder of this paper is as follows: Sect. 2 discusses background and Sect. 3 related work. Next we present our conceptual vision (Sect. 4), the PoC (Sect. 5) and evaluation (Section (6), followed by a discussion of limitations and future work (Sect. 7) and a conclusion (Sect. 8).

2   Background

In this section, we discuss LLM-based agents, and the ReWOO agentic framework as a special case.

2.1   LLM-Based Agents

AI agents are systems that can make decisions and take actions, based on their perception of their environment [16]. The development of LLMs led to an increasing interest in LLM-based agents, as these models allow for the creation of more powerful agents. LLM-based agents can interact via natural language with a human user, making the agent easier to use and more explainable [13], and can leverage generative capabilities to create plans, understand tool capabilities, build up context and memory, and interpret feedback.

2.2   Reasoning WithOut Observation

Reasoning WithOut Observation (ReWOO) is an LLM-based agent framework proposed by Xu et al. as an improved version of Reasoning and Acting (ReAct)

---

[1] https://accelerationeconomy.com/ai/process-mining-meets-generative-ai-celonis-rides-industry-wave-to-democratize-core-tech/.

[2] https://docs.pega.com/bundle/process-mining/page/process-mining/content/process-mining-assistant-basics.html.

[15]. ReAct proposes that the agent has reasoning steps in between the execution of tools and then observes the generated output [16]. While this approach allows an agent to solve more complex tasks there are some drawbacks. For instance, ReAct calls the LLM at each step of the process, creating more computational complexity and increasing token usage.

ReWOO decouples the reasoning and acting parts of the agent. A ReWOO agent consists of three main instances: a (1) planner, (2) worker, and (3) solver. The planner creates a plan for the execution of the task provided by the user, the worker iteratively executes the tools of the agent based on the generated plan, and the solver generates the final output and returns that to the user. According to experiments by Xu et al. ReWOO achieved a 5x token efficiency and 4% accuracy improvement compared to ReAct.

3   Related Work

Both business and academia have been exploring the use of LLMs in process mining, such as using LLMs to interpret process models via textual abstractions of these models [2,3]. This approach allows the model to interpret the process model and answer user queries about it, but it does not utilize more advanced prompt engineering techniques and uses a 'zero-shot' prompting approach. Busch et al. provided an overview of the potentials and challenges for using prompt engineering techniques in BPM [4], and Jessen et al. developed an approach for using LLMs in process mining, aiming to make process mining tools more accessible [7]. Their approach focuses on using LLMs to create a conversational agent that can answer questions about the process model or event log.

Eichele et al. studied the potential of adding domain knowledge to event logs, using Web Ontology Language (OWL) ontologies [5]. With this approach, they can map the domain knowledge to specific cases and activities. This angle differs from our approach as it focuses on the manner of supplementing domain knowledge and not on the automatic generation of domain knowledge. Therefore, these two different angles can potentially benefit from each other.

Current studies are focused on using LLMs in process mining tools for generating process models, providing process mining and process domain knowledge. Our approach proposes to use LLMs to provide another type of domain knowledge into process mining tools: delivering specific domain knowledge, for instance, based on characteristics of the sector or the specific organization, that is relevant to the generated process model. The provided domain knowledge allows a user to interpret the process model or make process improvements, making process mining tools more user-friendly, time-efficient, and accessible.

4   Conceptual Vision

In this section, we first present the different types of domain knowledge that we distinguish. Then we present our conceptual framework that shows where and how domain knowledge, generated by an LLM, can be incorporated into a process mining tool to solve the observed scarcity of domain knowledge.

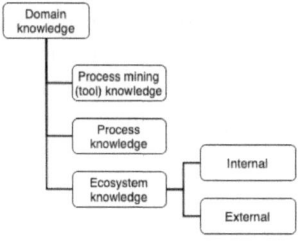

Fig. 1. Types of domain knowledge

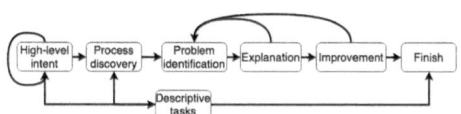

Fig. 2. Proposed conceptual framework

4.1 Domain Knowledge

Domain knowledge in process mining is knowledge about the context of the process and knowledge that is necessary to analyze and fully understand the generated processes [5]. We make the distinction between three types of domain knowledge (Fig. 1). Firstly, process mining knowledge: Knowledge about the domain of process mining itself, which can be an inaccessible field for non-experts [8]. So this can include knowledge about the use of a specific process mining tool.

Secondly, process optimization knowledge: Knowledge about process optimization, regardless of the process mining tool used, and mostly independent of the specific problem domain or industry. E.g., knowledge of Lean Six Sigma, a set of techniques for process improvements and waste elimination [18].

Thirdly, ecosystem knowledge: Knowledge about the domain and business of the organization and the ecosystem surrounding the process (e.g. regulation). This knowledge is important when interpreting the process model and when trying to make changes to the process. The lack of this knowledge has been identified in practice as an issue in current implementations of process mining [9]. Within this type of domain knowledge, we make the distinction between external and internal. Internal ecosystem domain knowledge consists of knowledge only available within an organization, e.g. internal documentation of an organization. External ecosystem domain knowledge is publicly available knowledge, e.g. regulatory documents or sector reports published online.

4.2 Framework

The framework (Fig. 2) consists of seven main components.

The first one is the 'high-level intent', the user specifies what the goal of the analysis is and potentially what tools should be used. This can be done by using a single prompt or by having a conversation with the system. In this conversation, the user can express the desired output and usage of tools, ask clarifying questions, and the system can inform the user about the available options. Furthermore, the system can ask questions to the user to obtain the most complete picture of the high-level intent, e.g. asking the name of the organization or the type of process.

In the 'process discovery' component, the system will generate the process model from the event log that was provided by the user. If the user specifies a preference for a specific approach, that approach will be used. Otherwise, the system will pick an approach, based on process mining domain knowledge.

The third component of the framework is 'problem identification', the system will analyze the generated process from the previous step and identify the relevant information. What this relevant information is and how it is identified depends on the preferences of the user from the high-level intent. If the user does not specify a preference, the system will determine what type of analysis should be used, based on ecosystem domain knowledge. For instance, for spotting process inefficiencies, an analysis based on the frequency and duration of the process and its activities could be the best option.

In the fourth component, the 'explanation', the system generates relevant ecosystem domain knowledge for the user based on the results of the problem identification phase. For instance, if the problem identification phase has identified inefficient process components, the explanation phase can provide explanations about why these inefficiencies might be happening in the process. Based on the explanations that the system provides, the user can refine the problem identification, e.g., by applying a filter.

The fifth component is 'improvements', an extension of the explanation phase where the system will generate potential solutions addressing the identified problems in the process, e.g. improvements for removing bottlenecks, addressing risks or improving business outcomes. The user can refine the problem identification during this phase, e.g., by letting the system update the process with the proposed process improvements and execute problem identification on the updated process. If the user does not want to refine the problem identification and is content with the output from the system, the final result will be generated and returned to the user (sixth component, 'Finish').

Besides the mentioned components, there is another one that can be used, the 'descriptive tasks' component. This represents the option for the user to ask descriptive questions about the event log (before process discovery) or generated process model (after process discovery), for instance, 'How many activities are between A and B in the process model?'. These are the types of questions that can be answered with process mining domain knowledge and process domain knowledge. The capacity to answer these types of questions with LLMs is already being studied and developed by others (e.g., [2,7]).

With this framework, we allow the execution process mining techniques and incorporate the different types of domain knowledge. During the execution of the system, the user can still interact with the system, for instance, to change the type of analysis or ask clarifying questions. This design should help to address the mentioned shortage of domain knowledge in current process mining tools.

5   Proof of Concept

Based on the conceptual vision and framework, we developed a PoC to explore the value of a system that provides domain knowledge in a process mining tool.[3] The framework is a vision of a system that can execute all process mining techniques integrating all types of domain knowledge (Fig. 1), but for our PoC we focused on a process mining system integrating ecosystem domain knowledge, as the generation of this type of knowledge has not been studied yet. To keep the approach generic, we zoomed in on external ecosystem domain knowledge (through GPT Researcher, see below). This approach could easily be extended by adding documentation internal to an organization. Our PoC contains all components of the framework (Fig. 2) except 'descriptive tasks' and all the code is ours (except the mentioned libraries). Requirements for the PoC were gathered through a small set of in-depth interviews with process mining practitioners.

We use a ReWOO-based agent to let the system execute external functions (e.g. process mining techniques) and solve more complex tasks. We use ReWOO to lower the computational complexity and costs of running the agent, while maintaining the quality of performance (compared to ReAct). When the agent receives the high-level intent from the user, it will generate a plan. The generated plan consists of Plan and #E steps. Plan steps contain the goal of the step and the #E step contains the tool with the input the agent shall use to reach this goal. The outcome is captured in the #E variable and can be used in later steps. E.g. the first step of such a plan: 'Plan: Create a process model using the DFG approach and identify the top 3 IT and cyber risks. #E1 = ProcessDiscovery_DFG[file_path]'.

With the available tools, the agent can fulfill the steps in our framework (Fig. 2). From the user (in the 'high-level intent'), the system requires the file path to the event log, the name of the organization, the type of the process, and the type of analysis that should be conducted. The user can also express a preference for the approach that should be used for problem identification (DFG, temporal profile, or variants), otherwise, the system will pick one (Technique Selector tool). Our agent has the following tools at its disposal.

In Fig. 3, the tools of the agent are shown under the 'Worker' instance, we will now discuss the purpose of each of these tools. For each tool, we will also discuss which part of our framework it represents.Our ReWOO-based agent has the following tools at its disposal.

The **Process Discovery** tool generates a process model from an event log ('process discovery' and 'problem identification' in Fig. 2). It uses the textual abstraction functionalities of PM4PY [3], visualizes the process model in multiple formats (DFG, Petri net, BPMN, heuristic net, and decision tree) and provides statistics about the event log, like the distribution of events over time.

The **Technique Selector** selects the appropriate basis for the problem identification technique (DFG, temporal profile, or variants) for the analysis that the

---

[3] For links to architecture, code, input event logs, experimental set up and outputs of experiments see https://github.com/maxvogt12/ReWOO_agent_for_PM.

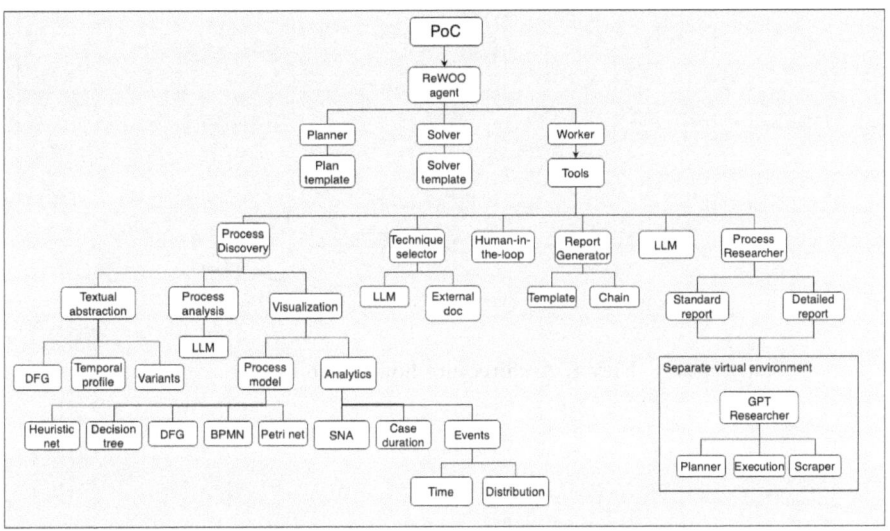

Fig. 3. Architecture of the PoC

user has requested, e.g. focusing on process inefficiencies. The user can request a specific technique that should be used by the agent. If the user does not specify a preference, the tool uses internal ecosystem domain knowledge in the form of a document ('Prototype/Tools/Process_Mining/PM_approach_mapping.txt' on GitHub) that the tool analyses to base its decision on, simulating the use of internal documents of an organization. If the document does not contain any useful information to base the decision on and the user does not provide a preference the agent will pick the default technique (DFG).

The **Process Researcher** tool generates research reports about the identified process components, supplying explanations and potential improvements for the identified process issues ('explanations' and 'improvements', Fig. 2). For each provided process component one report is generated, based on external ecosystem domain knowledge from the internet. Reports are generated by the GPT Researcher module, an open-source project of an LLM-based research assistant [6], the information within the reports is referenced to reduce hallucination. The reports can have two levels of detail: standard (one GPT Researcher run, inspired by the Plan-and-Solve approach [14]) or detailed (multiple GPT Researcher runs, inspired by the STORM approach [12]).

The **LLM** allows the agent to ask simple questions to an LLM, e.g. to find the sector of an organization.

The **Human-in-the-loop** allows the agent to interact with the human user for input if it requires that, the response of the user is then used in the execution of the agent.

The **Report Generator** generates the final report, which aligns with the 'explanations' and 'improvements' steps of the framework (Fig. 2) as this report

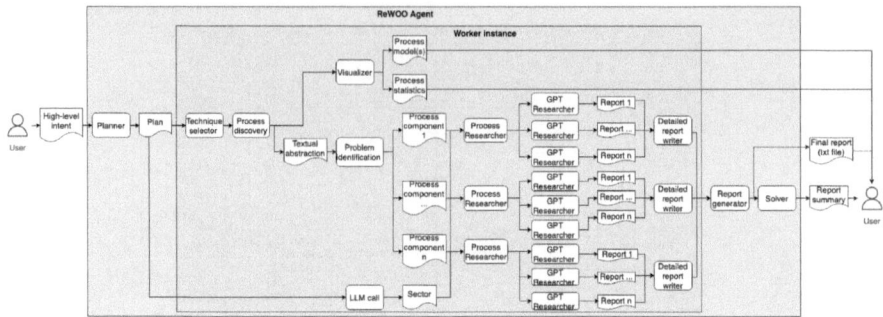

Fig. 4. Architecture flow of the PoC

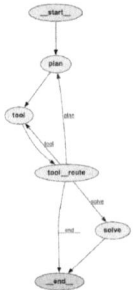

Fig. 5. Graph representation of the ReWOO agent

includes potential explanations and improvements. The final report is returned as a separate text file because these files are too large to be returned to the user as the output of the agent.

Figure 4 shows an overview of the sequential steps of an execution of the agent using the mentioned tools (see the GitHub for a more detailed description of these steps), although this is not a static order of steps as the agent constructs a plan of action each time it is run. If the constructed plan is insufficient for solving the task, the agent can go back to the planner instance and change it. This type of looping within the agent is controlled through a graph structure [19]. Figure 5 shows an overview of the graph structure of the agent, where it can be seen that the agent can go back to the 'plan' node after the tool execution has begun.

The PoC is based on the LangChain[4] framework, because this framework is open-source, regularly updated, and offers a versatile set of functionalities. We use OpenAI's, GPT-3.5 for simple tasks that do not require a lot of input and output tokens and GPT-4 for the more complex tasks that require a lot of input and output tokens [10]. We chose these models, as they are well-integrated into the LangChain framework and GPT Researcher module.

---

[4] https://www.langchain.com.

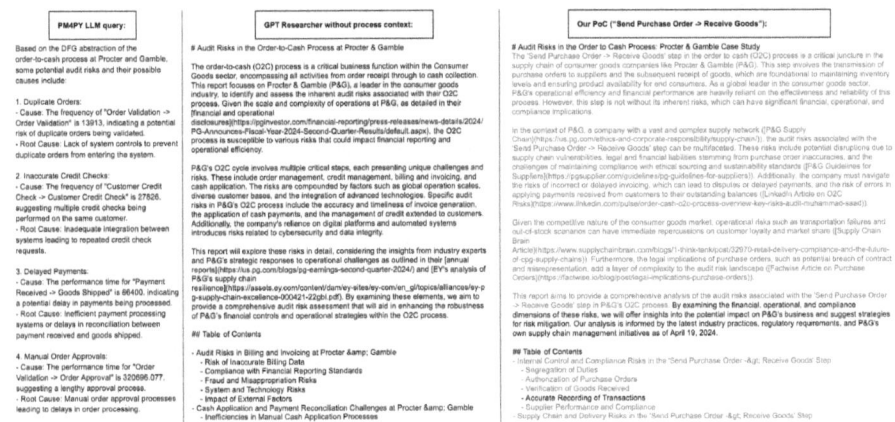

Fig. 6. Sample from the generated reports from the experiments

6   Evaluation

In this section, we discuss the methods we used to evaluate the PoC. We conducted two experiments: an ablation experiment and a qualitative analysis of the output of our PoC across different executions (see Github for full details).

6.1   Ablation Experiment

We tested three different ablations to compare their outputs. The outputs that were generated are too large to fully display in this paper, therefore, we present the first part of the outputs. The three ablations that we tested are: (1) the PM4PY LLM query functionality [2], (2) GPT Researcher [6], and (3) our PoC. We selected these three systems because PM4PY represents the process mining capabilities and GPT Researcher the domain knowledge generation capabilities of our PoC. We compared these two to our PoC to see if the construction of our PoC offers additional value compared to these separate components of our PoC.

We used the same prompt for all three systems, asking what the audit risks are in an order-to-cash (O2C) process at Procter and Gamble (P&G), and what could be causing them. The dataset that we used can be found on our GitHub page ('/Event_Logs/O2C.csv'). The data is about an O2C process but not specifically at P&G, we added this for testing purposes. The beginning of the output is shown in Fig. 6 and our analysis of the output is shown in Table 1.

The PM4PY LLM query system was able to execute process discovery and problem identification but could not generate in-depth domain knowledge. GPT Researcher was able to generate more in-depth domain knowledge about O2C processes. However, because it cannot execute process discovery and problem identification, the domain knowledge is superficial in the sense that it is not focused on specific activities or parts of the O2C process. Our PoC combines the strengths of these two systems, leading to in-depth domain knowledge that

Table 1. Analysis of the output of the ablation experiment

Ablation	Analysis of output (see Fig. 6 **for output**)
PM4PY LLM Query	The textual abstraction (DFG) allows the LLM to analyze the process model and reason which activities in the process could form an audit risk based on the DFG (process domain knowledge). However, the explanations about the causes of these audit risks (ecosystem domain knowledge) are superficial compared to the other systems
GPT Researcher	Generates more in-depth knowledge for the provided question. However, it is unaware of the components of the system and that makes the answers more superficial, the information is just about an O2C process but not about specific components within this process. GPT Researcher provides references for the information that it generates
PoC	Executes process discovery and problem identification and can then provide relevant process components to the GPT Researcher. This allows for the generation of in-depth knowledge that is focused on the relevant parts of the process, in this case, the 'Send Purchase Order ->Receive Goods' step. Our PoC provides references for the information that it generates

is focused on a specific part of the O2C process that was identified using process discovery and problem identification. The beginning of this report is shown on the right in Fig. 6; we marked all information green that was specific for the process component that was passed along, compared to the 'generic' report of the GPT Researcher ablation (middle part of Fig. 6).

In the output of our PoC, we see more detailed information, e.g. focusing on a specific risk for receiving goods: "Given P&G's global operations, purchase orders often involve transactions in foreign currencies. Fluctuations in exchange rates can significantly impact the cost of goods received, leading to financial statement volatility.".

The system can combine information about the organization with current trends to identify risks for P&G. The report mentioned that P&G is active in over 70 countries and therefore faces geopolitical risks like the war in the Middle East and the Houthi attacks on cargo ships. The used source is an example of RAG, the article[5] is from February 2024 and the pre-trained knowledge of the GPT-4 model used is cut off in December 2023 [10]. The reports also include potential improvements for the observed audit risks in the process, e.g. that P&G can use the Third-Party Risk Management (TPRM) process and internal control frameworks that it has in place to mitigate some of the mentioned risks (including a reference to the website mentioning this framework).

Another ablation experiment was carried out asking what the risks are in context of an automotive IT incidents handling process, with similar results, for instance pointing out that an observed delay in assessing a recorded incident leads to increased cyber security risks (see Github for full results).

6.2 Qualitative Analysis

With the qualitative analysis, we evaluate if the PoC performs differently across various problem identification types or use cases compared to others. This is

---

[5] https://sphera.com/spark/top-10-operational-risks-for-2024/.

Table 2. Compared results of our PoC

Problem identification	Sector/use case	Process type	Technique	Average
Environmental risk	Retail	Purchase-to-Pay (P2P)	DFG	92.58%
Audit risk	Consumer goods	Order-to-Cash (O2C)	DFG	90.07%
IT & cyber risk	Automotive	IT incident handling	Temporal profile	82.10%
Process inefficiencies	Manufacturing	Accounts Payable (AP)	Variants	74.37%
Operational risk	Technology	Travel expenses	Variants	68.64%
Regulatory risk	Financial services	Loan application	Temporal profile	66.96%

important for determining whether or not the PoC offers additional value in all areas or specific ones. Furthermore, we use different process types (event logs can be found on GitHub at 'Experiments/Prototype_exp') and different techniques and execute multiple runs to see if this influences the results.

We let our PoC generate a report and then we analyzed how much of the content of the report contains information that is specific to the process component that the system analyzed. We used this approach since LLMs and LLM-based systems tend to generate generic knowledge and therefore a challenge is to let such a system generate specific information. Generic information could be removing manual processing (can be applied to many processes and activities). Process (component) specific information could be the impact of return policies on the carbon footprint of an organization ('Return Goods' step in a P2P process). For this experiment, process component-specific information is information where the report names the process component or argues about it. We used this same approach in Fig. 6, the green marked text on the right indicates process (component) specific. As an extension, it would be useful to study the portion of the report that contains useful domain knowledge (see Sect. 7).

Table 2 shows the average results of the qualitative analysis for all the reports we generated (multiple reports per row, see GitHub). We observe that the average scores for Audit risk and Environmental risk are higher than those for Process inefficiencies and Regulatory risk. This could be because there are more online sources available about these problem identification types, the organization, or the process type. Another interesting thing is that the higher-scoring ones both used the DFG technique, while the other two did not. We see that all averages are above 65%, so 65% of the report contained specific information. For the full reports, see the 'Experiments/Prototype_exp' folder on GitHub.

Overall, the ablation experiment showed that our PoC offers additional value over some of its components, PM4PY LLM query, and GPT Researcher. The qualitative analysis indicated that within all reports across different problem identification types, over 65% of the content represented information (external ecosystem domain knowledge) specific to the process component(s).

7   Discussion, Limitations and Future Work

Although our research presents a novel way to generate domain knowledge within process mining tools, it has its limitations. First, as the goal was to design and deliver initial proof for the concept, we haven't run a full end-user test with domain experts. Iterative development and validation with an end-user group would be an interesting next step.

Our PoC works best for organizations with sufficient online resources, although the industrial sector is used if the organization is not known. A real-life system could rely on documentation of the organization (internal ecosystem domain knowledge) to fill this gap. We demonstrated this by using a document as the information source for the Technique Selector tool.

The PoC bases the generated domain knowledge on the outcomes of the process discovery and problem identification phases but does not allow refinement of the problem identification phase based on the generated domain knowledge. We did include this option in our conceptual vision (Fig. 2) but it would be interesting to develop this functionality, where the user could demand a new analysis (e.g. filtering) based on the generated domain knowledge.

For the experiments, we assessed three ablations of the system and conducted a qualitative analysis on multiple reports. To get a more complete picture of the added value of our approach, it could prove useful to conduct user tests with people who do and who do not have a lot of process mining experience.

The output of the PoC is rather large (often 10+ pages) as we tried to generate as much relevant domain knowledge as possible to study the potential of LLMs for this task. However, for a business user, it might prove useful to investigate a filter for this large output and to just return the most useful output for a specific user. This can be realized by changing the prompts of the 'Solver' instance (Fig. 4), to let it write a summary.

8   Conclusion

In this paper, we have explored if and how LLMs can improve the current state of process mining by generating domain knowledge for process mining tools. We have presented a conceptual vision that shows the design of such a system and its components. Our PoC is a tangible system that demonstrates that our vision can already be developed and offer additional value compared to current LLM implementations in process mining. Through our experiments, we observed that our PoC provided more in-depth external ecosystem domain knowledge about specific process components compared to the other systems in the experiment. We believe that if the mentioned challenges are overcome, our proposition can offer even more value to process mining practitioners.

References

1. Andrews, R., Wynn, M.T., Vallmuur, K., ter Hofstede, A.H.M., Bosley, E.: A comparative process mining analysis of road trauma patient pathways. Int. J. Environ. Res. Public Health **17**(10) (2020)
2. Berti, A., Qafari, M.S.: Leveraging large language models (LLMs) for process mining (technical report) (2023). https://arxiv.org/abs/2307.12701
3. Berti, A., Schuster, D., van der Aalst, W.M.P.: Abstractions, scenarios, and prompt definitions for process mining with LLMs: a case study. In: De Weerdt, J., Pufahl, L. (eds.) Business Process Management Workshops, pp. 427–439. Cham (2024)
4. Busch, K., Rochlitzer, A., Sola, D., Leopold, H.: Just tell me: prompt engineering in business process management. In: International Conference on Business Process Modeling, Development and Support, pp. 3–11. Springer (2023)
5. Eichele, S., Hinkelmann, K., Spahic-Bogdanovic, M.: Ontology-driven enhancement of process mining with domain knowledge. In: AAAI 2023 Spring Symposium on Challenges Requiring the Combination of Machine Learning and Knowledge Engineering (2023)
6. Elovic, A.: GPT Researcher (2024). https://github.com/assafelovic/gpt-researcher?ref=blog.langchain.dev. Accessed 26 Apr 2024
7. Jessen, U., Sroka, M., Fahland, D.: Chit-chat or deep talk: prompt engineering for process mining (2023). https://arxiv.org/abs/2307.09909
8. Kampik, T., et al.: Large process models: Business process management in the age of generative AI (2023). https://arxiv.org/abs/2309.00900
9. Martin, N., et al.: Opportunities and challenges for process mining in organizations: results of a Delphi study. Bus. Inf. Syst. Eng. **63**, 511–527 (2021)
10. OpenAI: Models (2024). https://platform.openai.com/docs/models/overview. Accessed 28 Apr 2024
11. Peffers, K., Tuunanen, T., Rothenberger, M.A., Chatterjee, S.: A design science research methodology for information systems research. J. Manag. Inf. Syst. **24**(3), 45–77 (2007)
12. Shao, Y., Jiang, Y., Kanell, T., Xu, P., Khattab, O., Lam, M.: Assisting in writing Wikipedia-like articles from scratch with large language models. In: Duh, K., Gomez, H., Bethard, S. (eds.) Proceedings of the NAACL (Vol 1: Long Papers), pp. 6252–6278. Mexico City, Mexico (2024)
13. Wang, L., et al.: A survey on large language model based autonomous agents. Front. Comp. Sci. **18**(6), 186345 (2024)
14. Wang, L., et al.: Plan-and-Solve prompting: Improving zero-shot chain-of-thought reasoning by large language models. In: Annual Meeting of the Association for Computational Linguistics (2023)
15. Xu, B., Peng, Z., Lei, B., Mukherjee, S., Liu, Y., Xu, D.: ReWOO: decoupling reasoning from observations for efficient augmented language models (2023). https://arxiv.org/abs/2305.18323
16. Yao, S., et al.: ReAct: synergizing reasoning and acting in language models. In: International Conference on Learning Representations (ICLR) (2023)
17. Zerbato, F., Soffer, P., Weber, B.: Process mining practices: evidence from interviews. In: International Conference on Business Process Management, pp. 268–285. Springer (2022)

18. Zhang, Q., Irfan, M., Khattak, M.A.O., Zhu, X., Hassan, M.: Lean six sigma: a literature review. Interdisc. J. Contemp. Res. Bus. **3**(10), 599–605 (2012)
19. Zhuge, M., Wang, W., Kirsch, L., Faccio, F., Khizbullin, D., Schmidhuber, J.: Language agents as optimizable graphs. arXiv preprint arXiv:2402.16823 (2024)

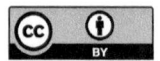

International Workshop on Stream Management and Analytics for Process Mining (SMA4PM 2024)

Preface

4th International Workshop on Streaming Management and Analytics for Process Mining (SMA4PM 2024)

Streaming Process Mining is an emerging area in process mining that spans data mining (e.g. stream data mining; mining time series; evolving graph mining), process mining (e.g., process discovery; conformance checking; predictive analytics; efficient mining of big log data; online feature selection; online outlier detection; concept drift detection; online recommender systems for processes), scalable big data solutions for process mining and the general scope of online event mining, in addition to many other techniques that are all gaining interest and importance in industry and academia. Recently, event streams are gaining attention in the process management and mining community not only for analytics but also for the management and orchestration of business processes. Examples are online event correlation as a preprocessing step for online process mining, using flexible rule-based event consumption and generation for enacting process instances, and decentralized process execution.

The SMA4PM workshop aims to promote the use and the development of new techniques to support the management and analysis of streaming-based processes. We aim to bring together practitioners and researchers from different communities, e.g., Process Mining, Stream Data Mining, Case Management, Business Process Management, Complex Event Processing, Database Systems, and Information Systems, who share an interest in online analysis and optimization of business processes and process-aware information systems with time, storage, or complexity restrictions. Additionally, SMA4PM aims to attract research results on scalable algorithmic process mining solutions in general, given that the work addresses how such efficient solution would function under streaming settings. The workshop aims to discuss the current state of ongoing research and to share practical experiences, exchange ideas, and set up future research directions.

This 4th edition of the workshop attracted 3 international submissions. Each paper was reviewed by 2–3 members of the Program Committee. From these submissions, the top 2 were accepted as full papers for presentation at the workshop. The papers presented at SMA4PM 2024 provided a mix of novel research ideas and focused on two main aspects of the workshop. One paper represented the streaming analytics aspect of the workshop, while the other represented the stream management aspect. Both presenters got the chance to interact with the audience through extensive discussions. At the end of the workshop, the audience reflected on the field's recent and near-future challenges in the light of the two talks.

Christian Imenkamp et al. address the online stream management aspect of the workshop. The paper observes the challenges streaming analytics algorithms face due to the requirements in terms of scalability and accuracy imposed by processes in Internet-of-Things environments. Against this observation, this paper presents an approach for online process analysis that is based on standard models and systems for complex event processing (CEP). The authors present the "Detect and Conquer" approach that includes generic process templates to accurately capture behavioral regularities or deviations, which are then mapped to CEP queries to achieve their efficient evaluation. The authors evaluated their approach against synthetic and real-world datasets. The results demonstrate the feasibility and efficiency of the introduced approach.

Next, *Tamara Verbeek et al.* focus on applying a continual learning model for next activity prediction. Continual learning, known also as lifelong learning, aims to design learning models that can continuously and autonomously adapt to varying data concepts without forgetting previously collected knowledge. The authors observe the problems in many existing frameworks that assume a static setting, ignoring dynamic nature and concept drifts in processes, leading to catastrophic forgetting where training over new data adversely affects the performance on previously learned data distributions. This paper presents TFCLPM, a framework for online next activity prediction that operates without relying on predefined tasks and employs continual learning techniques to reduce catastrophic forgetting. The methodology combines a Single Dense Layer neural network with a continual learning algorithm designed to retain challenging historical samples and include a regularizer to stabilize model parameters. Extensive experimental evaluations with synthetic and real-world event logs highlight the superiority of the introduced method wrt the literature in particular with recurrent drifts.

We hope that the reader will find this selection of papers useful to keep track of the latest advances in the stream process mining & management area. We are looking forward to seeing new advances in future editions of the SMA4PM workshop.

November 2024

Marwan Hassani
Thomas Seidl
Ahmed Awad

Organization

Workshop Chairs

Marwan Hassani	Eindhoven University of Technology, The Netherlands
Thomas Seidl	Ludwig-Maximilians-Univ. München, Germany
Ahmed Awad	British University in Dubai, UAE

Program Committee

Toon Calders	University of Antwerp, Belgium
Marco Comuzzi	Ulsan National Institute of Science and Technology, South Korea
Massimiliano de Leoni	University of Padua, Italy
Jochen De Weerdt	Katholieke Universiteit Leuven, Belgium
Francesco Folino	ICAR -CNR, Italy
Agnes Koschmider	University of Bayreuth, Germany
Xixi Lu	Utrecht University, The Netherlands
Boudewijn Van Dongen	Eindhoven University of Technology, The Netherlands
Eric Verbeek	Eindhoven University of Technology, The Netherlands
Matthias Weidlich	Humboldt-Universität zu Berlin, Germany

Detect and Conquer: Template-Based Analysis of Processes Using Complex Event Processing

Christian Imenkamp[1] , Samira Akili[2]([envelope]) , Matthias Weidlich[2]([envelope]) ,
and Agnes Koschmider[1]([envelope])

[1] Business Informatics and Process Analytics, University of Bayreuth,
Bayreuth, Germany
{christian.imenkamp,agnes.koschmider}@uni-bayreuth.de
[2] Department of Computer Science, Humboldt-Universität zu Berlin,
Berlin, Germany
{akilsami,matthias.weidlich}@hu-berlin.de
https://www.pa.uni-bayreuth.de/en/

Abstract. Online process analysis aims at identifying behavioral regularities or abnormalities in processes in near-real-time from continuous event streams. Yet, its realization is challenging, due to the requirements in terms of scalability and accuracy imposed by processes in Internet-of-Things environments. Against this background, this paper presents an approach for online process analysis that is based on standard models and systems for complex event processing (CEP). We present the "Detect and Conquer" approach that includes generic process templates to accurately capture behavioral regularities or deviations, which are then mapped to CEP queries to achieve their efficient evaluation. We evaluated our approach against synthetic and real-world datasets. The results demonstrate the feasibility and efficiency of our approach.

Keywords: Process Querying · Complex Event Processing · Control-Flow Patterns · Event Stream Processing

1 Introduction

With the rise of the Internet-of-Things (IoT), the volume of data that can be exploited for process analysis has increased significantly. Specifically, IoT environments include sensor-based systems that produce continuous streams of data [11]. While such a setting provides unique opportunities for online process analysis [9], it also imposes challenges in terms of accuracy, i.e., how to identify behavioral regularities or abnormalities, and in terms of scalability, i.e., how to scale the analysis to high-velocity data streams.

Most existing techniques for online process analysis are based on approaches that have originally been developed for static data and subsequently been lifted to online settings [16,17]. However, these techniques are tailored for

© The Author(s) 2025
A. Delgado and T. Slaats (Eds.): ICPM 2024 Workshops, LNBIP 533, pp. 681–692, 2025.
https://doi.org/10.1007/978-3-031-82225-4_50

a specific analysis task, and do not provide a generic mechanism that may be instantiated for a wide range of analysis needs. In addition, their execution over streams of data requires dedicated optimizations to achieve scalability, instead of employing technical infrastructures for efficient stream processing.

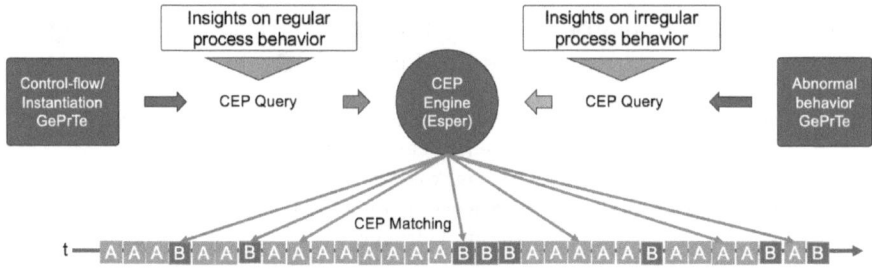

Fig. 1. Conceptual visualization of the "Detect and Conquer" approach.

In this paper, we outline the "Detect and Conquer" approach as a generic mechanism for accurate and scalable online process analysis. In essence, our idea is to facilitate accurate online process analysis through a collection of *generic process templates* that capture behavioral dependencies that signal both, the regular progress of process execution as well as abnormal behavior. Once these templates have been instantiated for a specific process, they are translated into queries for complex event processing (CEP). This way, standard models and systems for CEP, which have been designed for high-throughput, low-latency processing of event streams, can be leveraged for online process analysis.

Figure 1 provides a conceptual overview of our approach. It operates over a stream of events that are emitted continuously (bottom). Then, user-defined patterns that capture behavioral dependencies between activities as well as abnormal behavior are mapped onto a set of generic process templates (GePrTe). The instantiated templates are then translated into CEP queries, which are processed by a CEP engine.

To realize this vision, this paper introduces 17 generic process templates and their mapping to CEP queries. The templates correspond to common behavioral dependencies of process activities, e.g., related to process instantiation, basic control-flow patterns, and behavioral anomalies. To map these templates onto CEP queries, we introduce a conceptual model that aligns the most important concepts of either area. Based thereon, we operationalize the mapping and formulate the CEP queries in the Esper Query Language (EPL), i.e., the query language of Esper, a generic, open-source CEP engine.

We evaluated our approach using synthetic data and the Sepsis event log. The results highlight the general feasibility of our approach and illustrate its runtime efficiency in terms of latency.

The remainder is structured as follows. Section 2 introduces our template-based approach for online process analysis. The evaluation results are given in Sect. 3. Section 4 reviews related work, before Sect. 5 concludes the paper.

2   The Detect and Conquer Approach

This section presents our "Detect and Conquer" approach to online process analysis. We first introduce our model for generic process templates, before turning to their translation into CEP queries.

2.1   The Notion of a Generic Process Template (GePrTe)

A generic process template (GePrTe) captures the essence of common behavioral dependencies between process activities. It is wrapped in a query that is formulated using the Esper Query Language (EPL), as follows. The **SELECT** clause captures the input, while the **FROM** clause contains the actual template definition. In addition, a template must be assigned a name.

```
<independent_templates>

@Name(<template_name>)
SELECT *
FROM PATTERN [
    EVERY ( <event_definition> )
]
.WIN:TIME(<time_window>)
```

The `<template_name>` corresponds to one of the 17 generic process templates (e.g., SingleEventTrigger), as extracted from the literature and summarized in Table 1. The `<time_window>` defines the temporal context, e.g., in terms of the duration of a sliding window (e.g., '60 sec', '2 h', or '2 days 3 h').

A query might require the output of another query as input. Therefore, it must be possible to define an order of execution. Unless mentioned explicitly, by a `<independent_templates>` statement, multiple queries may be defined and their execution order follows from the order of their definition.

The actual template definition, captured as `<event_definition>` is given in terms of the following scheme:

```
(
<event_id> = <event_class_ref>(<event_attributes>)
<operator> <negation> <predicate>

<operator> <event_definition>
)
```

Here, the `<event_id>` is a unique identifier for the respective event. Moreover, `<event_class_ref>` is a reference to the class that defines a single event in the stream, thereby linking the template to a particular schema of the stream. `<event_attributes>`, in turn, defines the specific event that should be matched in the query. `<operator>` captures the behavioral relation between the events/predicates, with examples being conjunction ('AND'), disjunction ('OR'), and sequencing ('-¿'), while `<negation>` potentially negates a statement (i.e., using 'NOT'). In addition, a `<predicate>` is defined through the following scheme:

```
(
    <event_id>.<event_attributes>
        <comparison_operator>
    <event_id>.<event_attributes>
) <operator>
<predicate>
```

Here, the `<comparison_operator>` is used to compare the attribute values of two events, e.g., using '<', '>', '=', or '!='.

Table 1 shows the set of generic process templates that we implemented as part of our approach. They cover various behavioral dependencies that capture regular process execution in terms of its basic control-flow and instantiation, as well as abnormal process execution.

Next, exemplify **occurred event**, one of the generic process templates. It is shown in Fig. 2 and, once instantiated, can be used to discover specific events that trigger the instantiation of a process.

```
@Name('OccurredEventsActivation')                                    A
select *
from pattern [
    every (
    #foreach($i in [0..$eventCount])
        $eventKeys[$i] = ${EPPMEventType}(activity = '$eventValues[$i]')   B
        #if($i < $eventCount) or #end
    #end
    )
].win:time($time_window)                                              C
```

Fig. 2. Example template that triggers when a specific event is observed

The template consists of three parts: (A) the pattern name and core EPL logic; (B) the template engine syntax, which converts the GePrTe into a CEP query; and (C) the time window, which allows the user to define the duration for the sliding window. In (B), the template engine uses a *#foreach* loop to create assignments for the events, based on user input. Additionally, the *#if* condition appends an 'or' operator between event assignments, except for the last one.

Next, we define how to map the generic process templates onto CEP queries.

2.2   Mapping GePrTe Onto CEP Queries

The mapping relies on the Esper Query Language (EPL). The CEP queries are written in EPL syntax accordingly. The following query illustrates the EPL syntax definition for the pattern that an event of type "A" is followed by event of type "B" within 5 min:

```
SELECT * FROM PATTERN [every a=A -> b=B(a.end + 5 min >= b.start)]
```

Table 1. List of generic process templates

Template Name	Description
Basic Control-Flow	
Exclusive Choice [1]	One of several possible paths is selected
Parallel Split [1]	A single path branches into multiple parallel paths
Simple Merge [1]	Merges multiple branches into a single branch
Synchronization [1]	Synchronize multiple parallel branches into one
Process Instantiation	
Occurred Events (conditional) [6]	Triggers a process when specific events happen
Single Event Trigger [6]	Starts a process upon a single event
Multi Event Trigger [6]	Requires multiple events to start a process, using all events at once
All Subscriptions [6]	Creates event subscriptions for all non-triggered start events
No Subscriptions [6]	No event subscriptions are created for the process instance
Reachable Subscription [6]	Activates event subscriptions only for necessary process completion
Until Consumption [6]	Subscriptions remain active until the relevant event is consumed
Event-based Unsubscription [6]	Cancels remaining subscriptions after one of several events occurs
Abnormal Behavior	
Deadlock [8]	An exclusive choice followed by a parallel merge
Infinite Loop [8]	A loop begins with an and join and ends with a XOR split
Missing Events [12]	Triggering an event that requires follow-up actions but no subsequent event occurs
Unexpected Sequence [12]	A sequence of events that should occur
Unattended Decision Points [12]	Only positive outcomes are logged, and failures are unaddressed

We defined EPL queries that correspond to the discovery of process tasks like finding behavior dependencies. Table 2 illustrates this. For example, the first row defines the EPL syntax to find events that follow each other. This corresponds to the control-flow pattern sequence. The second row defines the EPL syntax to detect parallel events corresponding to control-flow patterns Parallel Split or Synchronization.

Table 2. Mapping of Esper EPL Syntax to Process Discovery Tasks

(Esper) EPL Syntax	Task
`PATTERN [every a=EventA -> b=EventB]`	Discovery of sequence activities [5]
`PATTERN [every (a=EventA AND b=EventB)]`	Discovery of parallel activities [5]
`PATTERN [every (EventA and not EventB or EventB and not EventA)]`	Discovery of alternative activities [5]
`SELECT COUNT(*) FROM EventA`	Discovery of frequent activities [5]
`WHERE EventA.timestamp < EventB.timestamp`	Discovery of temporal dependencies [5]
`WHERE EventA.activity ='Approval'`	Filtering of relevant cases [5]
`PATTERN [every a=EventA -> (b=EventB AND c=EventC)]`	Discovery of complex control-flow patterns [5]

To clarify the correspondence of concepts from the domain of CEP and process mining, we defined a conceptual model. Each entity in the model is either attributed to the CEP, PM or has a meaning in both contexts. While the notion of an *event* is central to our model, its meaning is defined on a different level of abstraction in the context of CEP and PM. That is, for CEP an event stands for the change of a state or the occurrence of a situation of interest within some system. For PM, an event denotes a recorded activity of a business process. As such, it comes with an *activity* and *case* identifiers, as well as a *timestamp*. The former attributes define a certain event class from the perspective of CEP based on which arbitrary *patterns* can be constructed, based on CEP *operators*. Those patterns again, can be used to encode temporal behavior among certain activities. Matches of such patterns over some *event stream* are referred to as *complex events* and consequently, correspond to the instantiation of control flows within process models (Fig. 3).

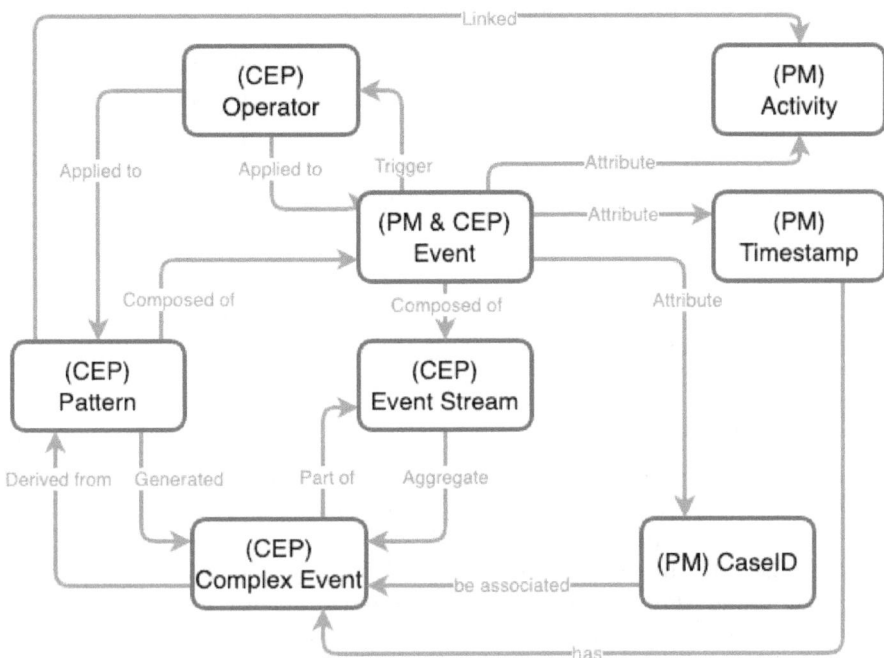

Fig. 3. Conceptual model of CEP query constructs and the inclusion of event log attributes.

3   Evaluation

This section summarizes the evaluation results. We implemented a prototype in Java[1]. The implementation integrates Esper for event processing and analysis[2]. We applied our approach on publicly accessible event logs and synthetically generated event logs of different variety in terms of variability, length of traces. Table 3 summarizes the properties of the event logs that we used for evaluation. The implementation can be found in a publicly available repository[3].

The evaluation results and queries for the synthetic event logs are summarized in (Sect. 3.1). Next, we applied our approach on the Sepsis event log and used the online heuristics miner to evaluate the discovery result, see (Sect. 3.2). Due to page limitations, we only present an excerpt of results. However, all results (e.g., queries) can be found in the repository along the prototype implementation. Finally, we evaluated the runtime efficiency (Sect. 3.3)

---

[1] https://www.java.com/en/.
[2] https://github.com/espertechinc/esper.
[3] https://github.com/chimenkamp/detect-and-conquer---Esper.

Table 3. Synthetic and real-world event logs

Log Name	Mean Trace Length	Number of Activities	Number of Events
Deadlock, Loop, and Conditions (Synthetic)	7.12	19	71212
Subscriptions and Choices (Synthetic)	24.55	29	1227635
Sepsis Cases [15]	14.48	16	15214

3.1 Generation of Different Queries and the Application to an Event Stream

This section summarizes the results of the generated queries and shows how we matched them on the event stream. The following query aims to identify a deadlock (i.e., and AND join is used for synchronization although a XOR has been used for branching). The query consists of three sub-queries for control-flow detection (i.e., "ExclusiveChoiceAsStreamactivity_2", "ExclusiveChoiceAsStreamactivity_1" and "ParallelMergeAsStream") and one query to detect the deadlock (i.e., see subquery "DeadlockDetection"). "DeadlockDetection" provides the output stream:

Listing 1.1. Generated Query to detect deadlocks

```
@Name('ExclusiveChoiceAsStreamactivity_2')
SELECT * FROM PATTERN 2
INSERT INTO ExclusiveChoiceStream
SELECT *
FROM EventRef.win:time(50 sec) as event
WHERE event.activity = 'Electronic␣invoice␣received'
HAVING NOT EXISTS (
    SELECT *
    FROM EventRef.win:time(50 sec) as subEvent
    WHERE subEvent.caseID = event.caseID
        AND subEvent.activity = 'Paper␣invoice␣received'
);

@Name('ExclusiveChoiceAsStreamactivity_1')
...

@Name('ParallelMergeAsStream')
INSERT INTO ParallelMergeStream
SELECT *
FROM EventRef.win:time(50 sec) as event
WHERE event.activity IN (
    'Order␣Amendment␣Confirmation'
,    'Clarification␣Sent␣to␣Supplier'
    )
```

```
GROUP BY event.caseID
HAVING COUNT(DISTINCT event.activity) = 2;

@Name('DeadlockDetection')
INSERT INTO DeadlockStream
SELECT ex.caseID, 'DeadlockDetected' AS DeadlockType
FROM ExclusiveChoiceStream.win:time(50 sec) AS ex
INNER JOIN ParallelMergeStream.win:time(50 sec) AS pm
ON ex.caseID = pm.caseID
    OUTPUT LAST EVERY 5 SECONDS;
```

We applied, i.e., matched, our generated queries against the considered event streams using Esper. The exemplary event stream, over which the above query was matched, can be found in our repository.

3.2   Application of the Online Heuristics Miner for Query Generation

Our CEP pattern generation relies on a predefined set of control-flow patterns. To construct such patterns from a given event stream, we implement the online heuristic miner, a state-of-the-art approach for online control flow discovery. As the online heuristic miner has limited performance on high-rate event streams, we ran it on a 20 second's long snippet from the Sepsis event log. Given that, the heuristic's miner identifies *84* control flow patterns (i.e., sequential: *28*, or: *28*, and: *28*). 1.2 shows one of the simplified queries generated from control-flow fragments discovered by the heuristic miner with ($\varepsilon = 0.01$). ¡consistency check¿ is a placeholder to turn the inclusive OR into an exclusive OR. The query is derived by the following control-flow fragment: *"OR(ER Triage, IV Liquid)"*

Listing 1.2. Exemplary query generated from the sepsis dataset

```
SELECT * FROM PATTERN [
EVERY(
    (a1 = EPPMEventType('IV␣Liquid') -> <consistency check>)
    OR
    (a2 = EPPMEventType('IV␣Liquid') -> <consistency check>)
    OR
    (a1 = EPPMEventType('ER␣Triage') -> <consistency check>))
)].win:time(50 sec)
```

3.3   Performance Evaluation

This section presents the evaluation results in terms of runtime efficiency. Following [10], we evaluated information latency, which refers to the time between where an event occurred and its processing by the system. The experiments were run on a MacBook Pro (Apple M2 and 16 GB of RAM). The system processed a stream of over two million events. Figure 4 illustrates the latency during the experiment. The plots were smoothed with (1) a rolling mean and (2) a rolling maximum approach (with window size of 5000 events). Please note that the 14 selected queries have (on average) lower latencies than two queries, which might be counterintuitive, but can be explained due optimization efficiency and parallelism across the queries. However, the 14 queries configurations demonstrate more frequently and higher latency spikes. This can be attributed to occasional resource contention or synchronization overhead. Additionally, the triggering of complex events may temporarily increase processing time.

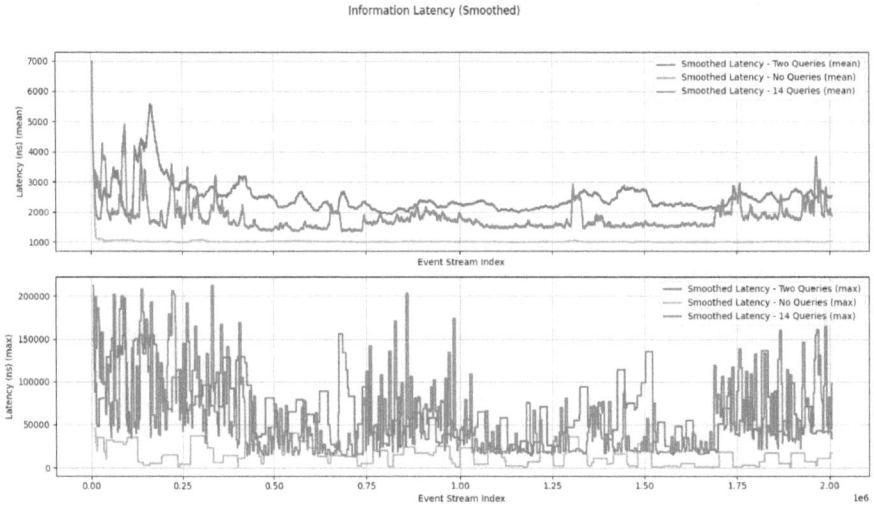

Fig. 4. Latency plots for the average and maximal latency inside a window size of 5000 events

4   Related Work

Several approaches exist that aim to identifying behavioral regularities or abnormalities in an offline setting. For instance, [13] introduced an approach to discovering behavioral models from software execution data.

[7] propose a method to repair outlier behaviors in event logs by removing infrequent events. Furthermore, [16] addressed the detection of structural behavioral flaws (e.g., deadlocks and lack of synchronization) from business process event logs. Additionally, approaches have been proposed, which address certain properties unique to the online setting. For instance, [4] discuss techniques for discovering processes that change over time. [2] introduced an online framework for process mining over unordered event streams. In the same vein, [14] introduces a framework for online concept drift detection in processes based on event

streams. Moreover, [3] adapts the heuristic miner that incrementally mines processes from event streams. However, as also observed in our experiments, the respective approach does not meet the scalability requirements of online data processing in the long term.

Despite these advances, there is a notable gap between classical process mining algorithms adapted for online settings and native online approaches. Classical algorithms, even when adapted, often struggle with efficiency and flexibility when confronted with the highly dynamic nature of real-time processing. Native online approaches, while designed to handle real-time data, sometimes lack the robustness and explainable pattern recognition capabilities of traditional methods.

5 Conclusion

Online process analysis seeks to identify behavioral regularities or abnormalities in processes in near-real-time from continuous event streams, a task that remains challenging. This paper introduced an approach for an online behavioral analysis. Through the "Detect and Conquer" approach, generic process templates are defined that capture most behavioral dependencies of process activities and are subsequently translated into CEP queries. These queries are then applied to streams of events. The approach has been evaluated using both synthetic and real-world datasets, and the results demonstrate its feasibility and efficiency.

Acknowledgements. This work received funding by the Deutsche Forschungsgemeinschaft (DFG), grant 496119880. The responsibility for the content of this publication remains with the authors.

References

1. van der Aalst, W.M.P., ter Hofstede, A.H.M., Kiepuszewski, B., Barros, A.P.: Workflow patterns. Distrib. Parall. Databases **14**(1), 5-51 (2003). https://doi.org/10.1023/A:1022883727209

2. Awad, A., Weidlich, M., Sakr, S.: Process mining over unordered event streams. In: 2020 2nd International Conference on Process Mining (ICPM), pp. 81–88, October 2020. https://ieeexplore.ieee.org/document/9230157/?arnumber=9230157, 13 Aug 2024

3. Burattin, A., Sperduti, A., van der Aalst, W.M.: Heuristics miners for streaming event data. *CoRR* abs/1212.6383 (2012). arXiv: 1212.6383

4. Carmona, J., Gavaldà, R.: Online techniques for dealing with concept drift in process mining. In: Hollmén, J., Klawonn, F., Tucker, A. (ed.) Advances in Intelligent Data Analysis XI, pp. 90–102. Springer, Berlin, Heidelberg (2012)

5. Chapela-Campa, D., Mucientes, M., Lama, M.: Mining frequent patterns in process models. Inf. Sci. **472**, 235–257 (2019). https://www.sciencedirect.com/science/article/pii/S0020025517304875

6. Decker, G., Mendling, J.: Instantiation semantics for process models. In: Dumas, M., Reichert, M., Shan, M.-C. (eds.) BPM 2008. LNCS, vol. 5240, pp. 164–179. Springer, Heidelberg (2008). https://doi.org/10.1007/978-3-540-85758-7_14

7. Fani Sani, M., van Zelst, S.J., van der Aalst, W.M.P.: Repairing outlier behaviour in event logs. In: Abramowicz, W., Paschke, A. (eds.) BIS 2018. LNBIP, vol. 320, pp. 115–131. Springer, Cham (2018). https://doi.org/10.1007/978-3-319-93931-5_9

8. Han, Z., et al.: Definition and detection of control-flow antipatterns in process models. In: 2013 IEEE 37th Annual Computer Software and Applications Conference Workshops. pp. 433–438 (2013)

9. Janiesch, C., Koschmider et al.: The internet of things meets business process management: a manifesto. In: IEEE Syst. Man Cybern. Mag. **6**(4), 34–44 (2020). http://dx.doi.org/10.1109/MSMC.2020.3003135

10. Karimov, J., et al.: Benchmarking distributed stream data processing systems. In: 2018 IEEE 34th International Conference on Data Engineering (ICDE), pp. 1507–1518 (2018)

11. Koschmider, A., et al.: Process mining for unstructured data: challenges and research directions. In: Michael, J., Weske, M. (ed.) Modellierung 2024, Potsdam, Germany, 12–15 March 2024, vol. p.-348, LNI. Gesellschaft für Informatik e.V., pp. 119–136 (2024). https://doi.org/10.18420/modellierung2024

12. Laue, R., Koop, W., Gruhn, V.: Indicators for open issues in business process models. In: Daneva, M., Pastor, O. (eds.) REFSQ 2016. LNCS, vol. 9619, pp. 102–116. Springer, Cham (2016). https://doi.org/10.1007/978-3-319-30282-9_7

13. Liu, C.: Automatic discovery of behavioral models from software execution data. In: IEEE Trans. Autom. Sci. Eng. **15**(4), 1897–1908 (2018)

14. Liu, N., Huang, J., Cui, L.: A framework for online process concept drift detection from event streams. In: pp. 105–112, July 2018

15. Felix Mannhardt. Sepsis Cases - Event Log (2016). https://data.4tu.nl/articles/dataset/Sepsis_Cases_-_Event_Log/12707639/1

16. Song, W., Chang, Z., Jacobsen, H.-A., Zhang, P.: Discovering structural errors from business process event logs. IEEE Trans. Knowl. Data Eng. **34**(11), 5293–5306 (2022)

17. Tavares, G.M., et al.: Overlapping analytic stages in online process mining. In: 2019 IEEE International Conference on Services Computing (SCC), pp. 167–175, July 2019, ISSN: 2474–2473. https://ieeexplore.ieee.org/document/8813959/footnotes#footnotes, Accessed 02 Aug 2024

Task-Free Continual Learning with Dynamic Loss for Online Next Activity Prediction

Tamara Verbeek, Ruozhu Yao, and Marwan Hassani[✉]

Eindhoven University of Technology, Eindhoven, The Netherlands
{t.a.m.verbeek,r.yao}@student.tue.nl, m.hassani@tue.nl

Abstract. Continual learning, known also as lifelong learning, aims at designing learning models that can continuously and autonomously adapt to varying data concepts without forgetting previously collected knowledge. Such concepts are referred to as tasks. Predictive business process monitoring, which predicts future process steps, is crucial in dynamic environments where tasks are not previously specified and processes frequently change or face unpredictability. However, many existing frameworks assume a static setting, ignoring dynamic nature and concept drifts in processes, leading to catastrophic forgetting—where training over new data adversely affects the performance on previously learned tasks. This paper presents TFCLPM, a framework for online next activity prediction that operates without relying on predefined tasks and employs continual learning techniques to reduce catastrophic forgetting. The methodology combines a Single Dense Layer neural network with a continual learning algorithm designed to retain challenging historical samples and include a regularizer to stabilize model parameters. Extensive experimental evaluations with synthetic and real-world event logs highlight our optimal configurations. The proposed framework's performance is compared against three existing online next activity prediction methodologies. Results show significant improvements in prediction accuracy, especially in scenarios with gradual or recurrent drifts, highlighting the framework's robustness and efficiency, even with large datasets.

Keywords: Next-Activity Prediction · Concept Drift · Catastrophic Forgetting · Continual Learning · Task-free Learning · Dynamic Loss Function

1 Introduction

Process mining involves analyzing event logs from business processes to discover, monitor, and improve real processes by extracting valuable insights and patterns. It bridges the gap between data and process management, enabling organizations to visualize, understand, and optimize their operational workflows [18]. A recent focus on predictive process monitoring underscores its vital significance, as it

© The Author(s) 2025
A. Delgado and T. Slaats (Eds.): ICPM 2024 Workshops, LNBIP 533, pp. 693–705, 2025.
https://doi.org/10.1007/978-3-031-82225-4_51

allows organizations to dynamically predict the future paths of individual process instances [5]. The ability to predict the next activity in predictive process monitoring is crucial for foreseeing and preparing for future actions in business processes. By leveraging this predictive power, organizations can manage resources such as manpower, materials, and time proactively, ensuring they are utilized effectively to address upcoming needs.

Traditionally, machine learning models are trained with separate training and test sets, assuming all data is available upfront. However, in real-world business scenarios (e.g. [6]), next activity prediction is more effective in an online setting, where the model continuously learns from incoming data. This allows the model to stay current with the latest information and adapt to changes in the data, known as concept drifts [21], which occur when the statistical properties of the target variable change over time. By continually integrating new data, the model maintains accuracy and relevance, effectively responding to dynamic business environments.

Continual learning, or lifelong learning, is essential for improving online prediction. It allows models to retain past knowledge while adapting to new data, maintaining a deep understanding of evolving data. In dynamic real-world environments, predicting next activities accurately is crucial, as it ensures that models remain effective and relevant amid changing patterns. This adaptability is vital for maintaining efficiency, enhancing decision-making, and enabling proactive responses in areas like business workflows, manufacturing, and customer service, where timely predictions directly affect performance. Various strategies for predicting future activities in an online context are discussed in [7,9,22].

In the context of this paper, a *task* is not conceptualized as a step in a process, but as a learning task where a model must execute actions like next activity prediction on a given data distribution. In dynamic environments with continuously evolving data, traditional next activity prediction methods often rely on predefined tasks or concept drift detection to trigger model updates. However, these approaches have limitations, as defining tasks in advance or detecting drifts can be impractical in real-world scenarios where changes are subtle and unpredictable. A task-free approach to continual next activity prediction offers significant advantages. It eliminates the need for explicit task definitions, allowing the model to adapt seamlessly to shifting data distributions without manual intervention. This flexibility is essential in environments where activities are not clearly split into specific tasks or where drifts occur gradually.

Rather than waiting for concept drift detection, it is more effective to update the model based on loss function behavior [3]. By monitoring for *plateaus* followed by *peaks*, we can pinpoint when the model's performance stabilizes and then declines, indicating that an update is needed. This method ensures timely updates, maintaining model accuracy while avoiding unnecessary updates that could lead to overfitting or resource waste. Additionally, it is advantageous to use a dynamic loss function that adapts based on the significance of the model's parameters [1] because it helps the model to selectively retain critical knowledge while adapting to new information. By weighting the loss according to parameter importance, the model can prioritize preserving crucial parameters that have a significant impact on performance, thereby minimizing catastrophic forgetting.

The contributions of this paper include: i) introducing the first use of continual learning through a dynamic loss function for task-free online next activity prediction; ii) conducting a comprehensive experimental evaluation using both synthetic and real-world datasets with various types of concept drifts; and, iii) demonstrating that our approach outperforms existing methods.

The remainder of the paper is organized as follows: Sect. 2 reviews a required background and most related work, followed by preliminaries and problem formulation in Sect. 3. Section 4 details our main approach, TFCLPM (Task-Free Continual Learning for predictive Process Mining). A extensive experimental evaluation is presented in Sect. 5 while a conclusion of this paper is presented in Sect. 6.

2 Background and Memory Aware Synapses

Studies explore incremental techniques to update predictive models with new process execution data. Pauwels et al. [14] compare various update strategies, including re-training with and without hyperoptimization and incremental updates, demonstrating the effectiveness of incremental updates in maintaining model quality while offering real-time adaptability.

Continual learning aims to enable machine learning models to learn and adapt continuously over time, much like how humans assimilate knowledge throughout their lives. Within this framework, researchers have explored various methods, each offering unique perspectives and strategies. These methods include memory-based, architecture-based, regularization-based, and prompt-based approaches.

Memory-based approaches involve storing and retrieving past experiences or knowledge. These approaches can be divided into two categories: the first retains actual past experiences, as seen in methods like Experience Replay [16], iCaRL [15], DynaTrainCDD [9], Maximally Interfered Retrieval [2], and Gradient Episodic Memory [12]. The second category generates past experiences during training, exemplified by Generative Replay [10].

Regularization-based methods aim to prevent catastrophic forgetting by constraining weight updates during training. This constraint can be achieved by determining the significance of each parameter for past tasks, like in Elastic Weight Consolidation [8] or determining how crucial each weight in the network is, such as Memory Aware Synapses [1]. Alternatively, the importance of parameters can be assessed based on their impact on output sensitivity, with selective penalties applied to key parameters to mitigate forgetting, which is done in Learning without Forgetting [11].

Architecture-based approaches, in contrast, prioritize adjusting the neural network's structure to integrate new data while preserving existing knowledge. One approach involves dynamic architectures, which expand the network by adding more neurons or layers for each task. This allows the model to continuously grow and adapt without forgetting previous knowledge, as exemplified by methods such as Progressive Neural Networks [17].

Prompt-based approaches (e.g. DualPrompt [20]), a more recent addition to the continuum, introduce a novel perspective on continual learning challenges. These methods entail attaching static or adaptable "instructions", also referred to as prompts, to direct the model's behavior. These prompts can take various forms, such as specific input patterns, embeddings, or task-specific tokens which help the model to recall and apply knowledge from earlier tasks.

We further elaborate on Memory Aware Synapses (MAS) [1] as a memory-based technique that our method, TFCLPM, builds on. First, it evaluates the significance of each weight, also called parameter, in the network. Once the network has been trained on a task, the importance of a parameter is assessed by determining how changes to it could impact the network's overall performance. The importance Ω_{ij} of a particular parameter θ_{ij} is calculated using Eq. 1:

$$\Omega_{ij} = \frac{1}{N} \sum_{k=1}^{N} ||g_{ij}(x_k)|| \tag{1}$$

where N represents the total number of data samples and $g_{ij}(x_k)$ indicates how the network's output changes for a given input x_k when θ_{ij} is adjusted (see Eq. 2). For networks with multiple outputs, a simplified approach is recommended. Instead of evaluating changes for each output separately, the overall magnitude of the output change is measured with:

$$g_{ij}(x_k) = \frac{\partial[\ell_2^2(F(x_k; \theta))]}{\partial \theta_{ij}} \tag{2}$$

where ℓ_2^2 is the squared l_2 norm of the function output.

This approach reduces complexity by concentrating on the total change rather than individual output variations. When the network is trained on a new task, MAS prevents the forgetting of previously learned tasks by penalizing significant changes to important parameters. The model's objective is thus a balance between performing well on the new task and preserving crucial parameters: Objective = $Ln(\theta) + \lambda \times$ Penalty, where λ is a regularization parameter that controls the penalty for altering important parameters.

A modified version of MAS eliminates the need for explicit task definitions by continuously learning from a data stream and adapting to evolving data distributions [3]. The system identifies plateaus—moments when the network's performance stabilizes—by tracking the mean and variance of losses in a sliding window (cf. Figure 1). During these plateaus, the system saves snapshots of the network's weights to compare current and past data streams, updating the importance weights of neurons to preserve knowledge while adapting to new data.

Additionally a "hard buffer" with a small set of challenging samples retained based on their high loss is introduced. This buffer helps evaluate neuron importance and contributes to creating a retraining dataset. Importance weights are calculated using a cumulative moving average, preventing rapid fluctuations and supporting stable learning. A regularization term is added to the loss function

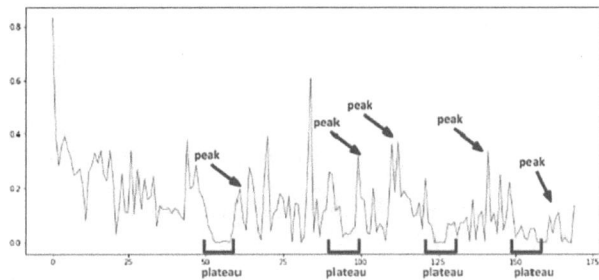

Fig. 1. Distinct plateaus and peaks are shown in loss values, which signal when to update the importance weights. X-axis represents update steps while y-axis shows the loss values [3].

to retain critical parameters, avoiding overfitting. Overall, the system enables continual learning without predefined tasks, adapting to gradual data shifts and supporting continuous model retraining and performance improvement.

3 Preliminaries and Problem Formulation

In this section we delve into the problem of utilising continual learning in process prediction. Assume we aim to develop an algorithm that continuously processes an event stream $S = \{e_1, e_2, ...\}$ as events are generated, where $e = (c, a, t, v_1, ..., v_A)$. An event e is a tuple of case identifier c, activity label a, timestamp t, and the values of the event attributes $v_1, ..., v_A$. A case refers to a single instance of the process being analyzed or executed, encompassing all events, attributes, and contextual information associated with that instance. A case can include multiple traces, each representing different sequences of activities within the same instance. The stream S contains multiple traces. A trace $\sigma^{(i)} = \langle e_{1i}, ..., e_{ni} \rangle$ denotes any finite sequence over the set of all events, related to a case. Given $\sigma^{(i)}$, the prefix represents the sequence of activities executed up to a certain point in a trace's lifecycle. The prefix of length k is defined by $\sigma_{\leq k}^{(i)} = \langle e_{1i}, ..., e_{ki} \rangle$. On the other hand, a suffix refers to the part of a process trace that occurs after a particular event or activity in that trace. Given $\sigma^{(i)}$, the suffix of events of length k is defined by $\sigma_{>n-k}^{(i)} = \langle e_{(n-k)i}, ..., e_{ni} \rangle$. For each event e_i that occurs in stream S, the general problem is that we want to predict the next activity happening in the suffix $\sigma_{>n-k}^{(i)}$ based on the prefix $\sigma_{\leq k}^{(i)}$.

Definition 1 (Next activity prediction). *Let there be a sample of prefixes of sequences* $\mathcal{P} = \{\sigma_{\leq k}^{(i)}\}_{i=1}^{i=m}$ *where* $2 \leq k < |\sigma^{(i)}|$ *is the prefix length and m is the sample size. Given a prefix of an events sequence* $\sigma_{\leq k}^{(i)}$, *the next activity prediction is* $\hat{a}_{(k+1)i}$ *of the activity* $a_{(k+1)i}$ *happening in the beginning of the suffix* $\sigma_{>n-k}^{(i)}$.

Definition 2 (Online Next Activity Prediction). *We aim to perform ongoing predictions of the next activity on a stream of events. Upon the arrival* *of each new event e_{ki}, we utilize the prefix $\sigma_{\leq k}^{(i)}$ to forecast the subsequent activity $\hat{a}_{(k+1)i}$. The stream S may encompass multiple learning tasks $\mathcal{T}_j$ that the prediction model has to learn. We say that $\mathcal{T}_p$ and $\mathcal{T}_r$, where $p \neq r$ represent two different learning tasks if they belong to two different processes separated by a concept drift, implying there is no relationship between these learning tasks.*

In the context of a stream of events involving multiple learning tasks, the distribution evolves over time, necessitating continuous updates to the model. In many scenarios, the model has to handle entirely new tasks that are distinct from previously encountered ones. This necessitates task incremental learning.

Definition 3 (Task Incremental Learning). *In task incremental learning, two tasks $n, m \in [1, ..., \mathcal{N}]$ have no correspondence to each other if $n \neq m$. Each task possesses unique objectives and is associated with a separate process, potentially necessitating the model to acquire new patterns, features, or behaviors.*

If we want to update the model after a concept drift, we aim to use as much data as possible. If a task reappears in a recurrent concept drift setup, it is advantageous to have stored data about this task to ensure that it is not forgotten. However, this poses challenges such as storage limitations or privacy concerns. Those often prevent the model from keeping all past data, letting it rely instead merely on recent data. This causes catastrophic forgetting [4].

Definition 4 (Catastrophic Forgetting). *Let there be a prediction model at any point in time that has learned a sequence of $\mathcal{T}_1 \cdots \mathcal{T}_n$ learning tasks. When faced with the $\mathcal{T}_{n+1}$th task, a typical model tends to forget how to predict the next activities of the previously learned tasks.*

This phenomenon poses a significant challenge in dynamic environments. To address the issue of catastrophic forgetting, continual learning enables models to retain and incorporate knowledge from previous tasks while learning new ones.

Definition 5 (Continual Learning). *In continual learning, the model is designed to mainly mitigate catastrophic forgetting while quickly adapting to emerging tasks. This is done by leveraging the past knowledge in the knowledge base to help learn recurrent tasks. The objective is to optimize the performance of new tasks while minimizing performance degradation of previously learned tasks.*

Definition 6 (Continual Learning for Next Activity Prediction). *Consider a model that has learned to predict the next activities for an event stream S. Throughout S, concept drifts may occur. These concept drifts refer to the alteration in the learning task. The event stream contains a sequence of $\mathcal{T}_1 \cdots \mathcal{T}_n$ learning tasks, where each learning task represents an individual process. A learning task for next activity prediction is defined by pairs of prefixes and suffixes of sequences $\mathcal{P}$. Given a prefix of an event sequence $\sigma_{\leq k}^{(i)}$, the learning task is to deliver a prediction $\hat{a}_{k+1}$ of the activity a_{k+1} occurring in the suffix $\sigma_{>n-k}^{(i)}$ such that when presented with the $\mathcal{T}_{n+1}$th task, the model must accurately predict next activities for this task without suffering from catastrophic forgetting if it was a* *recurrent one. This necessitates maintaining the ability to predict the next activities for past prefixes while adapting to new patterns and variations in the event sequences as new events e arrive from S.*

Task-Free Continual Learning: In this work, we are designing the model in such a way that tasks are neither previously specified, nor their starting and ending timestamps are given. We refer to this by task-free continual learning. This imposes further challenges to the designed model to detect the drift and to also recognize the task while facing other continual learning challenges.

4   Task-Free Continual Learning for Predictive Process Mining (TFCLPM)

We provide a comprehensive overview of the TFCLPM architecture, highlighting its critical components. The implementation is available on GitHub[1]. Figure 2 shows the framework architecture for training the model.

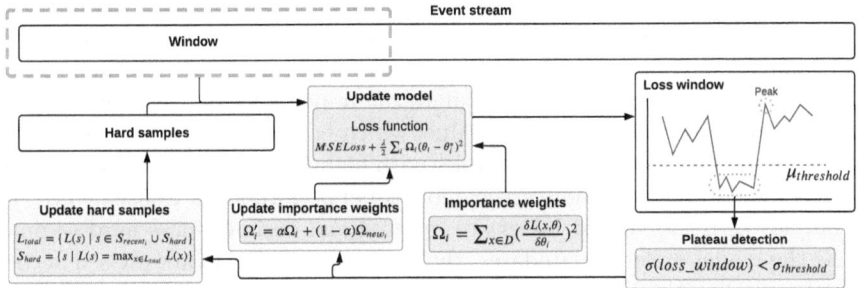

Fig. 2. Framework of the Task-Free Continual Learning for predictive Process Mining (TFCLPM).

Events from the event stream are stored in a window, which is a temporary storage for the most recent events. When 500 events accumulate, chosen following the experiments in [9], a model update is initiated. The events from the window are combined with hard samples to form the retraining dataset. At initialization, the hard samples dataset is empty. This retraining dataset is then fed into the Single Dense Layer (SDL) model, which undergoes several epochs to assimilate the new information. During model updates, a dynamic loss function is employed, combining the Mean Squared Error (MSE) loss with the Memory Aware Synapses (MAS) regularizer term defined as in Eq. 3:

$$MAS_{regularizer} = \frac{\lambda}{2} \sum_{i} \Omega_i (\theta_i - \theta_i^*)^2 \tag{3}$$

---

[1] https://github.com/TamaraVerbeek/TFCLPM.

where θ_i represents the current value of a model parameter and θ_i^* is the value of that parameter prior to the update. This regularizer applies the calculated importance weights Ω_i to penalize significant changes in critical weights.

After each model update, the loss values for all samples in the retraining dataset are computed. For each sample, we determine the loss by evaluating $L_n(F(x;\theta), y)$, and then plotting the resulting values. Once the plot is generated, we need to analyze it to identify whether it contains a peak or a plateau. This involves examining the plot to detect regions where the loss value either reaches a maximum (peak) or stabilizes (plateau). To detect if a peak occurred, the condition $\mu(loss\_window) > \mu' + \sigma'$ is checked, where μ' and σ' represent the mean and standard deviation of the previous window. Next, we calculate the variance of the losses from the retraining dataset. We then verify if the conditions $\mu(l\_window) < \mu_{th}$ and $\sigma(l\_window) < \sigma_{th}$ are met, where μ_{th} and σ_{th} represent the predefined thresholds. This step is crucial for assessing whether the variance and the mean of the loss values are within acceptable limits, which helps in determining if the model requires an update based on stability criteria. If both metrics fall below a predetermined threshold, the importance weights and hard samples are updated accordingly.

Importance Weights and Hard Samples Update. At initialization, the number of hard samples, denoted as H, is configured as a hyperparameter. To manage the hard samples effectively, we first calculate the importance of each sample in the retraining dataset based on its loss value, which has been previously assessed to determine the need for updates. Samples with higher loss values are deemed more challenging and therefore more critical for model performance. Consequently, the H samples with the highest losses are selected and designated as hard samples.

As the model undergoes updates, the importance weights are revised accordingly. In parallel, the Memory Aware Synapses (MAS) regularizer is adjusted to reflect these changes. The importance values used in the MAS regularizer are updated using Eq. 4:

$$\Omega_i' = \alpha\Omega_i + (1-\alpha)\Omega_{new_i} \tag{4}$$

where α is set to 0.5, indicating that the updated importance values are influenced equally by both the previous and current values. This balanced approach ensures that the regularizer effectively accounts for both historical and recent data, facilitating more stable and accurate model updates. The new importance values Ω_{new_i} are determined by the Eq. 1.

5   Experimental Evaluation

Evaluation Metrics. To effectively measure the performance of our proposed approach, it is essential to have evaluation metrics that offer a nuanced understanding of our model's performance dynamics.

Accuracy at a given event index is a performance metric used to assess the effectiveness of a predictive model at a specific position within the sequence of events. In mathematical terms, if we denote γ as the size of the average accuracy window, and $\hat{y}_j$ as the predicted event at index j based on preceding events, with y_j representing the actual event at index j, the accuracy at index i can be expressed as: $accuracy_i = \frac{1}{\gamma} \sum_{j=i-\gamma}^{i} \mathbb{1}\{\hat{y}_j = y_j\}$ (5). The formula computes the ratio of correct predictions from j up to event index i, averaging the predictions in the window. **Average accuracy** is calculated by averaging across all events to determine whether each one is predicted correctly. **Running Time** encapsulates the total duration the approach requires to process the entire event stream.

The Datasets. We provide an overview of the datasets utilized in our study comprising a diverse selection of both real-world and synthetic datasets.

Synthetic Datasets: Business Process Drift. The *Business Process Drift* dataset is a synthetic compilation designed to serve as a benchmark for the study of business process changes. To simulate drift in a log, the authors of [13] systematically altered a base model by applying one of twelve simple change patterns, resulting in a total of 5.000 events per simulated log containing 17 unique events. For more details on these simple change patterns, we refer interested readers to [13].

Real-World Datasets. The *BPI Challenge 2020* dataset captures two years of travel expense claims at a university, with 6.000 to 10.000 cases showing gradual drift. It includes five subsets where only three are used in this research: Domestic Declarations and Request for Payment average 5 events per case while International Declarations has 11 on average. The *BPI Challenge 2015* dataset merges building permit applications from five municipalities into one event stream, with four sudden concept drifts, 5.600 cases, 181 unique events, and an average of 37 events per case. The *BPI Challenge 2017* dataset includes 5.168 loan application cases with 45 unique events and avg of 18 events/case.

The Competitors. The performance of the model is compared with three competitors. Among these competitors are two baseline methods. The **Incremental Update (w = 1)** approach [14] involves updating the model every month to incorporate the most recent data. In the **Incremental Update (w = Last Drift)** approach [14], the model is updated after each window of data based on the historical data up to the last observed concept drift. Next to this, a state-of-the-art method is used as a competitor. The method **DynaTrainCDD** [9] distinguishes itself through its advanced concept drift detection algorithm called PrefixCDD [7]. It continually monitors process data for deviations and utilizes Prefix Trees to represent and analyze process sequences efficiently. These detected drifts dynamically dictate the frequency of updates and the selection of datasets for retraining.

Parameter Selection. The selection of parameters for our framework was driven by a combination of empirical experimentation and theoretical considerations. The primary goal was to optimize accuracy. After experimentation and analysis, the number of hard samples is set to 100, the MAS weight is set to 0.5, and the mean and variance thresholds for detecting a plateau are 0.2 and 0.1, respectively.

5.1   The Results

Tab. 1 displays the average accuracy across all methods and datasets. Notably, TFCLPM achieves the highest average accuracy for the synthetic datasets. Dyna-TrainCDD also shows strong performance, closely trailing TFCLPM. In contrast, both Incremental Update (w = 1) and Incremental Update (w = Last Drift) lag significantly behind TFCLPM and DynaTrainCDD. Since these datasets include recurring concept drifts, this metric demonstrates that our approach is highly effective in reducing catastrophic forgetting. For the real-world datasets, TFCLPM achieves the highest accuracy on the BPIC2020 datasets (DomesticDeclarations, InternationalDeclarations, and RequestForPayment), but not on BPIC2017 or BPIC2015. This indicates that TFCLPM maintains consistent performance in datasets with gradual drift. Similar to the synthetic datasets, DynaTrainCDD closely follows TFCLPM, while Incremental Update (w = 1) and Incremental Update (w = Last Drift) lag significantly behind the other two methods. Arguably, BPIC2017 lacks concept drifts, allowing us to evaluate if our approach remains effective in their absence. In this case, our approach ranks second-best, while DynaTrainCDD achieves the highest average accuracy. However, both of these leading methods significantly outperform the other two approaches, highlighting their advantages. BPIC2015 is a challenging dataset due to its inclusion of four distinct processes and many unique events, which poses difficulties for our approach in handling these variations which shows in the lower average accuracy.

Table 1. Average accuracy for all methods and datasets. **Bold** denotes the highest accuracy, *italic* the second highest, and underlined the third highest.

	[14] (w = Last Drift)	[14] (w = 1)	DynaTrainCDD [9]	TFCLPM
IRO5000	75.35	75.33	*79.61*	**80.43**
ORI5000	75.73	74.21	*80.84*	**81.88**
RIO5000	75.02	75.08	*80.15*	**81.06**
ROI5000	75.66	73.87	*81.27*	**82.85**
OIR5000	68.23	68.88	*75.73*	**77.36**
InternationalDeclarations	82.00	80.79	*82.30*	**82.83**
DomesticDeclarations	83.72	84.00	*87.93*	**88.69**
RequestForPayment	83.73	83.74	*85.33*	**87.65**
BPI Challenge 2017	75.47	69.59	**84.82**	*83.49*
BPI Challenge 2015	*74.75*	**75.25**	69.16	74.01

Figure 3a and Fig. 3c illustrate the advantages of avoiding reliance on concept drift detection systems. It is evident that our approach restores accuracy much more quickly compared to Incremental Update (w = 1), Incremental Update (w = Last Drift), and DynaTrainCDD. The competitors take longer to detect concept drift, resulting in a slower return to an acceptable accuracy.

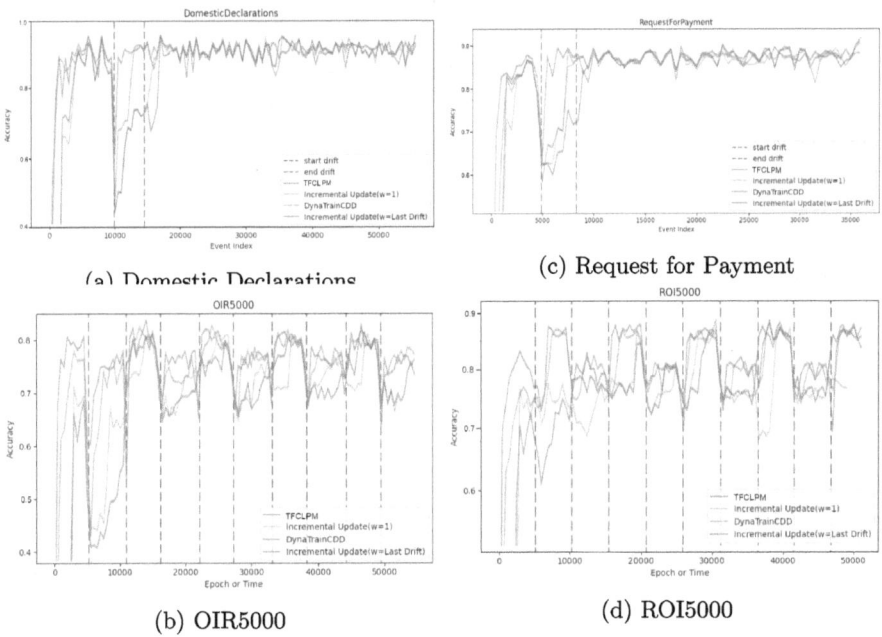

Fig. 3. Accuracy at a given event index for four different datasets. Vertical dashed lines represent a start (or an end) of a drift.

Figure 3b and Fig. 3d demonstrate the effectiveness of our approach on datasets with recurrent concept drifts, highlighting the significance of the hard buffer and importance weights. Our method consistently achieves high accuracy faster than the others. In the OIR5000 dataset, when the drift occurs from the first to the second concept, DynaTrainCDD, Incremental Update (w = 1), and Incremental Update (w = Last Drift) encounter difficulties, whereas our approach swiftly recovers to around 75%. Although DynaTrainCDD gradually improves and eventually matches TFCLPM's accuracy, our approach remains quicker to recover after each drift. A similar trend is observed in the ROI5000 dataset, where DynaTrainCDD lags slightly in regaining accuracy compared to our method's rapid recovery. Table 2 demonstrates the running time for all approaches. Incremental Update (w = 1) consistently performs efficiently across all scenarios while Incremental Update (w = Last Drift) often has longer running times, particularly with sudden drifts, due to its reliance on the last drift for updates. Our method offers stable and faster running times compared to DynaTrainCDD and Incremental Update (w = Last Drift). This is because our method maintains a constant retraining dataset size, ensuring a robust efficiency. On the other hand, Incremental Update (w = Last Drift) uses a varying dataset size based on drift detection, leading to longer running times in stable environments. Additionally, DynaTrainCDD runs a concept drift detection algorithm in parallel that further increases its running time. Our approach does not require an explicit drift detection component, resulting in its consistently higher efficiency.

Table 2. Running times in Seconds for all methods and datasets.

	[14] (w = Last Drift)	[14] (w = 1)	DynaTrainCDD [9]	TFCLPM
IOR5000	305.03	**48.35**	400.33	*112.67*
ORI5000	257.98	**39.06**	311.72	*131.76*
OIR5000	297.69	**29.54**	402.03	*104.33*
RIO5000	241.52	**26.31**	451.87	*97.33*
ROI5000	215.18	**45.87**	351.22	*120.11*
DomesticDeclarations	988.50	**69.44**	775.95	*267.69*
InternationalDeclarations	1801.68	**87.95**	953.96	*377.53*
RequestForPayment	517.30	**50.76**	530.05	*118.11*
BPI Challenge 2017	1605.53	**361.68**	3198.75	*1226.71*
BPI Challenge 2015	5893.64	**2774.51**	7194.67	*3518.07*

6 Conclusion

In this work, we proposed TFCLPM, a novel approach for continual next-activity prediction aimed at mitigating catastrophic forgetting. This approach operates without predefined tasks, allowing it to adapt flexibly to evolving data. It addresses catastrophic forgetting by maintaining a buffer of hard samples and employing a dynamic loss function. We evaluated its performance using various metrics, including average accuracy and accuracy at a given event index. Through experiments on multiple synthetic and real-life datasets, we observed that TFCLPM achieves the highest average accuracy on eight out of ten datasets. It quickly recovers high accuracies after experiencing a concept drift and demonstrates minimal forgetting in cases of recurrent drifts compared to other methods. Our method also shows stable running times compared to competitors. We plan to explore further continual learning methods for possibly other downstream prediction tasks, in a similar setup to [19] but for other prediction tasks.

References

1. Aljundi, R., Babiloni, F., Elhoseiny, M., Rohrbach, M., Tuytelaars, T.: Memory aware synapses: learning what (not) to forget. In: ECCV, pp. 139–154 (2018)
2. Aljundi, R., Caccia, L.: Online continual learning with maximally interfered retrieval. In: NeurIPS, pp. 11872–11883 (2019)
3. Aljundi, R., Kelchtermans, K., Tuytelaars, T.: Task-free continual learning. In: CVPR, pp. 11254–11263 (2019)
4. Chrysakis, A., Moens, M.F.: Online continual learning from imbalanced data. In: ICML, pp. 1952–1961. PMLR (2020)
5. Ferilli, S., Angelastro, S.: Activity prediction in process mining using the WoMan framework. J. Intell. Inf. Syst. **53**(1), 93–112 (2019). https://doi.org/10.1007/s10844-019-00543-2
6. Hassani, M., Habets, S.: Predicting next touch point in a customer journey: a use case in telecommunication. In: ECMS, pp. 48–54 (2021)

7. Huete, J., Qahtan, A.A., Hassani, M.: PrefixCDD: effective online concept drift detection over event streams using prefix trees. In: COMPSAC, pp. 328–333 (2023)
8. Kirkpatrick, J., Pascanu, R., Rabinowitz, N., et al.: Overcoming catastrophic forgetting in neural networks. CoRR **abs/1612.00796** (2016)
9. Kosciuszek, T., Hassani, M.: Online next activity prediction under concept drifts. In: CAiSE Workshops, pp. 335–346 (2024)
10. Lesort, T., Caselles-Dupré, H., Garcia-Ortiz, M., Stoian, A., Filliat, D.: Generative models from the perspective of continual learning. In: IJCNN, pp. 1–8. IEEE (2019)
11. Li, Z., Hoiem, D.: Learning without forgetting. IEEE Trans. Pattern Anal. Mach. Intell. **40**(12), 2935–2947 (2017)
12. Lopez-Paz, D., Ranzato, M.: Gradient episodic memory for continual learning. Adv. Neural. Inf. Process. Syst. **30**, 6470–6479 (2017)
13. Maaradji, A., Dumas, M., La Rosa, M., Ostovar, A.: Fast and accurate business process drift detection. In: BPM, pp. 406–422 (2015)
14. Pauwels, S., Calders, T.: Incremental predictive process monitoring: the next activity case. In: BPM, pp. 123–140 (2021)
15. Rebuffi, S., Kolesnikov, A., Sperl, G., Lampert, C.H.: iCaRL: incremental classifier and representation learning. In: CVPR, pp. 5533–5542 (2017)
16. Rolnick, D., Ahuja, A., Schwarz, J., Lillicrap, T., Wayne, G.: Experience replay for continual learning. In: Advances in Neural Information Processing Systems, vol. 32 (2019)
17. Rusu, A.A., et al.: Progressive neural networks. CoRR **abs/1606.04671** (2016), http://arxiv.org/abs/1606.04671
18. Van Der Aalst, W.: Process mining: overview and opportunities. ACM Trans. Manage. Inf. Syst. (TMIS) **3**(2), 1–17 (2012)
19. Verbeek, T., Hassani, M.: Handling catastrophic forgetting: online continual learning for next activity prediction. In: CoopIS, p. to appear (2024)
20. Wang, Z., et al.: DualPrompt: complementary prompting for rehearsal-free continual learning. In: ECCV, pp. 631–648 (2022)
21. Widmer, G., Kubat, M.: Learning in the presence of concept drift and hidden contexts. Mach. Learn. **23**(1), 69–101 (1996)
22. Wolters, L., Hassani, M.: Predicting activities of interest in the remainder of customer journeys under online settings. In: ICPM Workshops, pp. 145–157 (2022)

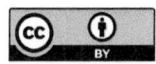

1st International Workshop on Process Mining for Sustainability (PM4S 2024)

Preface

1st International Workshop on Process Mining for Sustainability (PM4S 2024)

With increasing environmental and societal challenges, the urgency for sustainable development becomes paramount. Industries, responsible for a significant portion of global emissions and waste, play a crucial role in this transition. The First International Workshop on Process Mining for Sustainability (PM4S), organized at the Sixth International Conference on Process Mining, offered a platform to bridge the gap between technological advancement and sustainable practices, focusing on the transformative potential of process mining in fostering sustainable business processes. Besides the paper presentations, the workshop featured an interactive session in which the advancement of PM4S was discussed.

In the interactive session, the participants shared their vision for PM4S and discussed the communalities and differences among their understandings of PM4S. Based on these insights, different groups discussed methods and advancements, tools and applications, and community building. The workshop concluded with the intent of building and expanding a community of PM4S enthusiasts sharing news on this important topic and working on its advancement. To continue the momentum from the workshop, a LinkedIn group has been established as a community platform for further knowledge sharing and collaboration.

This volume presents the five accepted papers from the workshop, showing a broad perspective on issues of sustainability beyond mere process optimization for (economic) prosperity.

Dominik Schäfer et al. examine the feasibility of using data from ERP systems to calculate Key Ecological Indicators (KEIs) for assessing business process sustainability. Through a case study, the authors analyze real-world process data, finding current data availability insufficient for accurate sustainability assessments. They propose a conceptual model using proxy metrics to approximate KEIs and suggest refining data collection methods and leveraging expert knowledge to improve sustainability analysis.

Muskan et al. address unfairness in business processes, proposing an extension to a genetic process discovery algorithm that incorporates fairness-aware quality measures. The authors argue that traditional process discovery techniques might overlook unfair or discriminatory practices, particularly when they are infrequent. They test their approach on synthetic datasets containing instances of unfairness, showing that it reveals hidden biases that would remain undetected using traditional methods.

Fritsch introduces a set of process sustainability patterns that can be used to evaluate and improve the sustainability impact of processes. These patterns, inspired by "workflow patterns", integrate BPM concepts with existing sustainability analysis methods, particularly Life Cycle Assessment (LCA). The author applies the patterns to existing process modeling and mining approaches, showing how they can be used to assess and improve sustainability.

The paper by Costache et al. proposes guidelines for Greenhouse Gas Emission Management (PMG3), a structured approach for organizations to report and improve their sustainability performance through process mining. The authors validate PMG3 using real-world data from a business case in the consumer goods industry, finding high approval for its usefulness and ease of use.

González Moyano et al. propose the integration of nudging, a concept from psychology and behavioral economics, into the BPM lifecycle. The authors outline how nudging can be used to guide an organization, stakeholders, and process participants toward more sustainable business processes. They discuss specific examples, such as nudging employees to choose more environmentally friendly travel options.

These five contributions strongly support the advancement and awareness of the application of process mining to support the transformation towards more sustainable business processes. The interactive session fostered a shared understanding of PM4S and the development of a dedicated community. Hence, we consider this first edition of the PM4S Workshop a great success and thank the authors for their high-quality submissions. We also express our gratitude to the members of the Program Committee for using their time and expertise to review the submissions.

October 2024

István Koren
Janina Bauer
Nina Graves
Birgit Penzenstadler

Organization

Workshop Chairs

István Koren   RWTH Aachen University, Germany
Janina Bauer   Celonis, Germany
Nina Graves   RWTH Aachen University, Germany
Birgit Penzenstadler   Chalmers University, Sweden

Program Committee

Andrea Burattin   TU Denmark, Denmark
Adam Burke   Queensland University of Technology,
                                    Australia
Chiara Di Francescomarino   University of Trento, Italy
Andreas Fritsch   Karlsruhe Institute of Technology,
                                    Germany
Sander Leemans   RWTH Aachen University, Germany
Felix Mannhardt   Eindhoven University of Technology,
                                    Netherlands
Jari Peeperkorn   KU Leuven, Belgium
Luise Pufahl   TU Munich, Germany
Majid Rafiei   SAP, Germany
Stefanie Rinderle-Ma   TU Munich, Germany
Niek Tax   Meta, London

Process Mining Guidelines for Greenhouse Gas Emission Management in Production Processes

Ioana Costache$^{(\boxtimes)}$, Oktay Turetken , Banu Aysolmaz , and Karolin Winter

Eindhoven University of Technology, Eindhoven, The Netherlands
{i.costache,o.turetken,b.e.aysolmaz,k.m.winter}@tue.nl

Abstract. Despite the urgent need for becoming more sustainable and enhancing sustainability reporting induced by, e.g., the Corporate Sustainability Reporting Directive effective from January 2024, there exists a lack in research and industry efforts for integrating sustainability metrics into business processes. One particular reporting requirement entails that large EU companies must disclose their sustainability metrics for greenhouse gas (GHG) emissions across their supply chains. To address this challenging task, this paper presents the Process Mining Guidelines for Greenhouse Gas Emission Management (PMG3), helping companies implement process mining to meet GHG emissions targets in production processes. Thereby, the PMG3 provides detailed steps for defining business and data requirements, analyzing inefficiencies, and formulating recommendations to enhance sustainability reporting. To validate PMG3, a detailed demonstration was conducted using real-world data from a business case in the production process within the consumer goods industry. The utility evaluation revealed high approval for the PMG3's usefulness, ease of use, and practitioners' intention to use it in industry settings. Overall, this paper contributes a structured and applied approach for organizations to report GHG emissions and improve sustainability performance through process mining.

Keywords: green business process management · process mining · sustainability · production processes · design science research

1 Introduction

With the United Nations' 2030 Agenda for Sustainable Development and the European Green Deal aiming for climate neutrality by 2050, businesses are increasingly responsible for minimizing environmental impact [1]. Goal 12 encourages large companies to include sustainability indicators in their reports [2]. The Corporate Sustainability Reporting Directive (CSRD) takes effect in 2024, requiring large or publicly listed EU-based companies to apply new rules for environmental and social sustainability reporting [3]. Reporting must cover the entire value chain, including partners and suppliers, making tracking sustainability metrics, including CO_2e emissions, a high priority. As such, organizations face increasing reporting requirements, adopting IT-based business process management solutions to enhance sustainability performance. Double materiality, a concept in sustainability reporting, recognizes the broader impact of an organization's actions on the economy, society, and environment [4].

© The Author(s) 2025
A. Delgado and T. Slaats (Eds.): ICPM 2024 Workshops, LNBIP 533, pp. 711–724, 2025.
https://doi.org/10.1007/978-3-031-82225-4_52

In the EU, the manufacturing sector accounts for roughly 35% of total GHG emissions [5]. GHG emission scopes include Scope 1 (direct emissions from company-owned sources), Scope 2 (indirect emissions from purchased energy), and Scope 3 (all other indirect emissions in the value chain). The three-scope classification is the official classification defined by the GHG Protocol [6]. In light of the CSRD, companies must report on emissions originating from their entire value chain, including production processes that generate emissions of various scopes (Scope 1 and Scope 3). Due to Scope 3 emissions being indirect emissions, their calculation is less straightforward. Recent emission reduction efforts in the manufacturing sector led to a decrease in value-added due to high start-up costs of emission reduction initiatives, lack of innovation, and low digital maturity [5]. This indicates challenges in developing and adopting economically efficient environmental sustainability practices in this sector. In the first stages of adopting sustainability practices, such an effect is not unexpected. In line with the devil's pentagon [7], an extension of the devil's quadrangle [8], improvements to the sustainability of processes can come at the cost of the other dimensions – time, flexibility, cost, and quality. In the long run, due to lower operating costs, emission reduction initiatives should turn out to be cost-effective [9].

Sustainability metrics are rarely tracked along business processes [10], posing a problem as the CSRD requires large companies to report on sustainability metrics starting January 1, 2024. The lack of consistent guidelines and industry-specific reporting standards complicates tracking and quantifying sustainability KPIs. Process mining techniques can provide solutions for measuring sustainability KPIs of business processes by achieving full process transparency [11]. Traditional process mining offers transparency into process flow rather than material flow, making it difficult to determine materials' contribution to the carbon footprint of products [12].

Accordingly, the research objective of this study is to *provide guidelines for organizations to implement process mining for GHG emissions goals reporting and improvement in production processes*. To achieve the research objective, a set of Process Mining Guidelines for GHG management (PMG3) is developed following design science research. PMG3 is applied in a business case to demonstrate its applicability in real-life business settings and evaluated for its validity and utility through interviews and focus groups. The result is a set of guidelines for implementing process mining projects for sustainability, particularly GHG reporting in production processes, with a focus on addressing data quality and availability issues.

2   Related Work on Process Mining and Sustainability

Applying process mining techniques for sustainability is part of the broader research area of Green Business Process Management (Green BPM). Green BPM is a multidisciplinary field that integrates BPM principles with environmental sustainability considerations. Its focus is optimizing business processes in an environmentally responsible manner. The priority is the design, analysis, and improvement of business processes while minimizing their environmental impact, such as reducing resource consumption, waste generation, and carbon emissions [13]. Green BPM strives to strike a harmonious equilibrium between operational efficiency and sustainability goals, ensuring that businesses conduct their operations in an environmentally conscious manner. Recent studies show that a process-oriented strategy allows organizations to enhance their sustainability performance throughout all their operations rather than a narrow focus on the sustainability of end products and services [14].

One existing framework, PM4S, utilizes an object-centric approach to process mining, focusing on individual objects throughout the production cycle. Object-centric event logs enrich data on both the event and object levels, enabling use cases such as waste reduction and emission control. However, PM4S has not been tested in real-world scenarios, leaving its practical applicability unproven. Additionally, it highlights gaps in integrating sustainability with process mining, particularly in data enrichment and compliance checking [12]. The framework by Ortmeier et al. [15] integrates Process Mining Project Methodology (PM2) with Life Cycle Assessment (LCA), as defined by ISO 14044:2006, which evaluates the environmental impact of a product throughout its life cycle [16]. The framework proposes an iterative process for continuous hotspot analysis, while data availability challenges limit its real-life application [15].

To summarize, we observe two studies in the literature that provide methods and techniques for using process mining for sustainability purposes. Both frameworks recognize data availability and quality issues but lack comprehensive guidelines for addressing these issues. This study aims to provide guidelines for implementing process mining for sustainability in production and address related data availability and quality issues by demonstrating the applicability of the guidelines in real-life business settings.

3   Research Design

In developing PMG3, we followed the Design Science Research (DSR) methodology [17], adopting the DSR process by Peffers et al. [18]. The process depicted in Fig. 1 presents the research design that we followed. Accordingly, we identified the problem and defined our motivation, as we presented in Sect. 1. In the following sections, we describe the remaining research steps we followed.

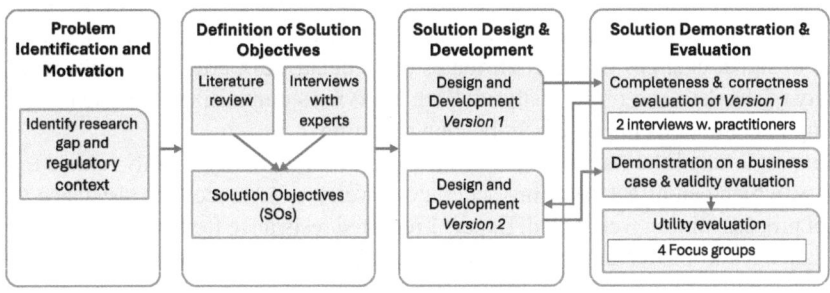

Fig. 1. Research design process.

3.1 Definition of Solution Objectives

The goal of this research step is to identify the objectives for an admissible solution (i.e., PMG3), which acts as the reference for the solution's validity [17]. To this end, we first reviewed the relevant literature on process mining methodologies and guidelines (e.g., [10–12, 15, 19]) as well as the regulatory aspects in the sustainability context. Due to limited existing research (as discussed in Sect. 2), we also performed interviews with two practitioners to gain insights into the success factors and challenges in the industry and the requirements for practical guidance to address them.

We interviewed two experts from different companies operating in the process mining industry. Both experts had over 4 years of experience in process mining consultancy and services, one acting as the 'sustainability lead' in the last 3 years, in charge of managing process mining implementation teams. The semi-structured interviews (recorded and transcribed) involved topics related to opportunity identification, methodologies, challenges, data availability and quality, continuous improvement, risk management, and process mining success factors. The first interview aimed at addressing the aforementioned topics in relation to the manufacturing and production processes, while the second interview focused on the same topics applied to sustainability goals.

Both experts confirmed the relevance of using process mining for sustainability reporting of production processes, particularly the ability of process mining techniques to improve process transparency and uncover hidden inefficiencies. Key challenges in process mining implementation were reported as data availability and quality. Business information systems like ERP and SCM are not designed for tracking sustainability metrics, resulting in fragmented or missing data, especially when combined with machine and sensor data. When available, machine and sensor data is relevant for tracking sustainability metrics, including GHG emissions, as the machines used in manufacturing can monitor not only parameters directly relevant for tracking emissions (e.g., chemical reactions) but also other parameters that can be used as contextual data to enhance the quality of the analysis (e.g., operating temperatures, fuel consumption). Manual input errors and system failures further compromise data quality. Both experts suggested using APIs to integrate external sustainability data, linking various data sources, and enabling change logs to address data challenges. Change logs are event logs that track changes made to the data. When not explicitly logged as activities in the IT systems, change logs serve to signal changes in object attributes (e.g., quantities), crucial for enhancing the quality of the data and of the analysis. Both interviews emphasized the role of process mining in continuous improvement beyond reporting.

Expert 2 noted the risks in process mining for sustainability, mainly related to data quality, which can affect reporting accuracy. Diverse experiences for resistance to the use of process mining were noted. Expert 1 reported resistance from IT departments due to challenges to the status quo and security concerns. Expert 2 noted some resistance and acknowledged that financial goals often precede sustainability goals due to stricter financial reporting guidelines. Based on our literature review and expert interviews, we defined the following solution objectives (SOs) for PMG3:

- SO1	PMG3 should give guidelines to address data availability, quality, and awareness challenges.
- SO2	... align with existing technology and security infrastructure of the organization.
- SO3	... support the integration of various systems and data sources.
- SO4	... be understandable and transparent for the user in terms of design and logic.
- SO5	...support sustainability domain experts in sustainability improvement decision-making processes.
- SO6	...support managerial involvement through feedback, decision-making, and project management
- SO7	...serve to identify carbon emissions throughout the target processes.

3.2 Solution Design and Development

Based on the solution objectives (Sect. 3.1), the first version (Version 1) of the guidelines was designed taking the existing research frameworks (e.g., the process mining project implementation process of [20]) as a basis. Following the evaluation of the first version for its completeness and correctness regarding its content and structure, the final version of the artifact (Version 2) was developed. The final version consists of a number of subprocesses for each step (represented using BPMN) and detailed guidelines for inputs and outputs. Various frameworks, concepts, and classifications (e.g., PPTI framework [21] and GHG emission scopes) have been incorporated to enhance the applicability and utility of the guidelines.

3.3 Solution Demonstration and Evaluation

The objective of this research step was to showcase the application of the artifact and evaluate it for its validity and utility [17], focusing on ex-post (post-design) evaluation [22]. The initial version (ver.1) was evaluated through unstructured interviews with process mining practitioners to refine its structure. Further evaluations of the final version, aligned with DSR guidelines, assessed the artifact's validity and utility through a business case demonstrating its applicability in reporting and tracking GHG emissions. Validity was measured by benchmarking outcomes against predefined objectives, while utility, emphasizing practical benefits, was assessed using the core constructs of the Technology Acceptance Model (TAM) [23], i.e., usefulness, ease-of-use, and target user's intention to use the guidelines. Participants' feedback on additional resources or adjustments needed for ease of use and integration was also collected through a 7-point Likert scale survey questions. The results are presented in Sect. 5.

4   PMG3: Description and Demonstration

The PMG3 includes a set of steps, each consisting of a subprocess and detailed guidelines for inputs and outputs. The final artifact's description shows how its steps address the solution objectives (SOs). Table 1 presents an overview of the main steps. While these steps are presented in sequence, the process is iterative. A detailed description of the artifact and a demonstration of its applicability can be found in the online Appendix (https://drive.google.com/drive/folders/1YsxzyavURN5IwoT4EIqE5-c6jTRae2Zu).

We demonstrate the application of the PMG3 using a business case in the consumer products industry using synthetic data. The datasets were created based on an anonymized data model used for Bill of Materials (BoM) explosions, preserving the structure of the data model (datasets, columns, and logical relationships) while using the U.S. Lifecycle Inventory database [24] to construct BoM alternatives. The business case aims to compare emissions for different BoM alternatives (ALT1 and ALT2 of product X) to inform future product composition decisions. Since the source database lacks product alternatives, some components and quantities were constructed to complete the comparison. While this approach involves some artificial data creation, it effectively demonstrates the artifact's applicability in guiding emission-related decision-making and showcasing how issues regarding data availability can be dealt with.

Table 1. Overview of PMG3 core process steps.

Step	Output	Involved Org. Roles	Tools/Resources
Step 1. Define business requirements	Business requirements	Process expert, project manager	
Step 2. Define data prerequisites/ requirements	Data requirements	Implementation expert, project manager, sustainability expert	
Step 3. Perform data pooling	Carbon-enriched event logs	Implementation expert, sustainability expert	Data sources, data pool
Step 4. Visualize target relationship	Process model/visualization	Implementation expert	Visualization tool/dashboard
Step 5. Analyze results & formulate recommendations	Result analysis, Recommendations	Implementation expert, project manager, sustainability expert	Visualization tool/dashboard

In Step 1, the business requirements are defined using the Pearson framework, focusing on key dimensions, such as people, processes, technology, and information. The project goal, target process, and sustainability metrics are established, followed by decisions on tracking levels, emission scopes, KPIs, and reporting frequency. Table 2 presents the sub-steps for this step. This step also aims to address SO1–3 (Sect. 3.1).

For the business case on which we applied our model, the goal was to compare CO_2e emissions of two product alternatives (ALT1 and ALT2) within the production process. CO_2e emissions were selected as the sustainability metric, with tracking at the *object level*. Emission scopes included *Scope 1* and *Scope 3*. Scope 2 emissions are also relevant, but are omitted in the absence of data... Resources included a project manager, an implementation, and a sustainability expert.

Table 2. Sub-steps of Step 1. Define business requirements.

Sub-steps of Step 1	Ouput	Involved Org. Roles
Set project goal	Project goal	Project mng., sustainability expert
Determine target process	Target process	Project manager
Determine sustainability metric	Sustainability metric	Sustainability expert
Determine tracking level	Tracking level	Sustainability expert, project mng
Determine GHG emission scope	Emission scope	Sustainability expert
Determine KPIs & exp. Outcomes	KPIs, Expected outcomes	Project mng., sustainability expert
Determine reporting frequency	Reporting frequency	Sustainability expert
Determine required resources	Resources	Project manager
Determine tasks	Tasks	Project manager
Determine involved business units	Business units, data sources	Project manager
Determine infrastr. Requirements	Infrastructure requirements	Project manager

Step 2 involves determining the data fields required for analysis, including process, contextual, and sustainability metrics. Data availability is checked internally, with external sources used if necessary. Quality standards are set, and data is enhanced and validated to meet these standards. Figure 2 presents a process model (in BPMN) for the sub-steps of Step 2 (more details are available in the online Appendix.)

In the business case, process and contextual data were available internally, while GHG emissions data was sourced externally from databases such as CBAM (https://publications.jrc.ec.europa.eu/repository/handle/JRC134682), GHG (https://ghg protocol.org/calculation-tools-and-guidance), and Climate Trace (https://climatetrace. org/data). The data was then prepared for pooling.

During Step 3, the retrieved data is integrated to form carbon-enriched event logs. These logs are the fundamental data structure for PMG3 and are achieved by mapping the sustainability metric to the process data. They are event logs with an additional event attribute (carbon emissions quantified per event or object). The data flow diagram representing the creation of the carbon-enriched event logs of the data pooling step is

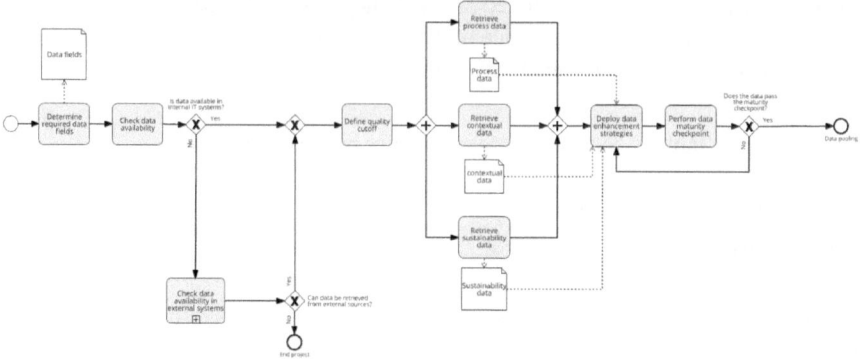

Fig. 2. Process model for the sub-steps of Step 2.

represented in Fig. 3. The data is mapped to the appropriate tracking level and adjusted for contextual factors like material weight. This forms the foundation for the analysis. In the business case, the emission factors were mapped to product subcomponents at the object level, ensuring accurate CO_2e calculations. Despite the absence of activity-level emissions data, the approach provided a comprehensive view of the emissions for each product alternative.

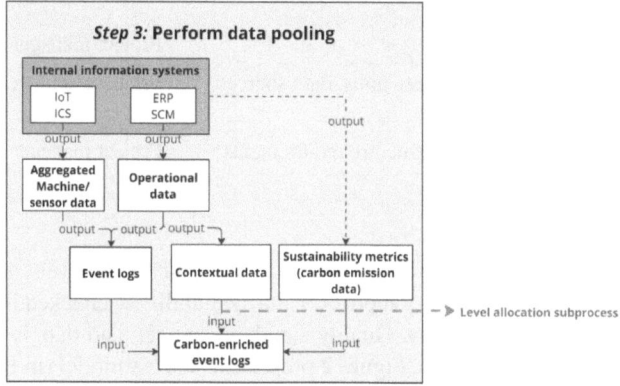

Fig. 3. Data flow of retrieved and pooled data.

In Step 4, relationships between events, objects, and activities related to GHG emissions are visually represented. This helps in understanding material flows, identifying emissions hotspots, and comparing process variants. In the business case, the visualizations were created using Celonis EMS to represent the object-to-object relationships for the two product alternatives, providing insights into which materials contributed most to overall emissions. Figure 4 presents the final output for both alternatives.

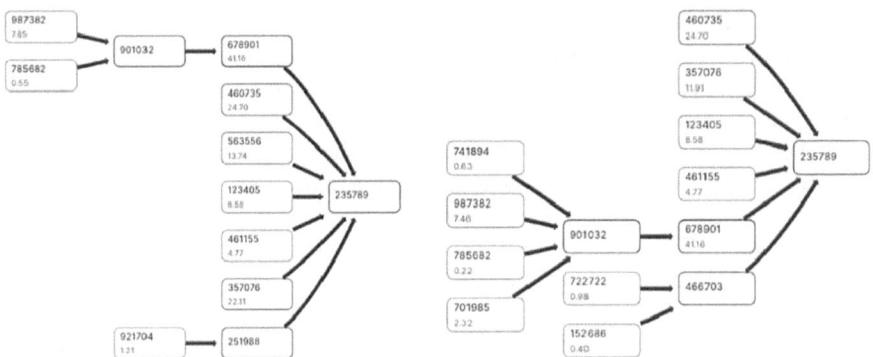

Fig. 4. Network representation of the BoM explosion of the product alternatives (up: material number, down: emissions (CO_2e kg/ kg of material)): ALT1 (left), ALT2 (right).

Aiming to address SO5–6 (Sect. 3.1), Step 5 involves analyzing the pooled data to identify inefficiencies and improvement areas. Process discrepancies and KPI inefficiencies are examined, and recommendations are formulated to improve the process. In the business case, CO_2e emissions for the two product alternatives were calculated, revealing opportunities for improvement, such as reducing component weights and improving waste management. These recommendations were prioritized based on their potential impact on emissions reduction to help address SO7.

5   Evaluation

5.1   Evaluation of Version 1

The evaluation of the first version of PMG3 was conducted through two unstructured interviews with practitioners who were target users of the guidelines, aiming to assess completeness. The first interviewee had 9 years of experience as aaa process improvement manager, and the second interviewee had 3 years of experience as a process intelligence consultant. Subprocesses as a part of the guidelines (detailed in the online Appendix were not yet included and were added following this initial evaluation. Interviewees advised differentiating business and data requirements by type, such as infrastructure and resources, in Steps 1 and 2, and suggested using a sequential representation for defining data maturity requirements. They also recommended providing detailed guidelines for sustainability-specific concepts throughout these steps. Additionally, for Steps 2 and 3, they emphasized the importance of focusing on specific requirements and guidelines for retrieving sustainability data. For Step 3, they advised adopting a sequential approach for selecting and retrieving sustainability data sources.

5.2   Evaluation of the Final Version

The final version was evaluated for its utility through four focus groups (FGs), which included process mining and improvement experts of varying expertise. (FG 1 involved three experts with 1 to 5 years of experience in process mining, FG 2–4 involved three experts with 1 to 3 years of experience in process mining, and one project manager with 4 years of experience. The expertise was assessed through tenure, field experience, and job title, while interest in sustainability was gauged via a pre-focus group survey. Each session began with a walk-through of the main process of the guidelines and specific subprocesses based on participants' interests and qualifications. Questions were asked regarding the method's completeness, ease of understanding, and necessary modifications for adoption. Two focus groups (FG1 and FG3) focused on Steps 1, 2, and 3 of the guidelines, with FG1 also evaluating guidelines for GHG data requirements in detail. FG2 reviewed Steps 1, 2, and 5, and FG4 focused on Steps 3, 4, and 5.

After the focus groups, we asked practitioners to provide a more structured view of the utility of the guidelines through a questionnaire involving the core constructs of the Technology Acceptance Model (TAM) [23]. Accordingly, the questionnaire assessed practitioners' perceived usefulness, ease of use, and intention to use the guidelines. Statements in the questionnaire were crafted based on the extended TAM questionnaire [25] (Table 3). Respondents rated the statements on a 7-point Likert scale, with 1 being 'Completely disagree' and 7 being 'Completely agree'. Table 4 presents the survey results, including the distribution of ratings, average scores, and standard deviations.

Table 3. Statements in the Questionnaire.

Perceived usefulness	1. I think this method supports a more efficient and effective implementation of Process Mining techniques for sustainability/ GHG emission (reporting) goals? 2. The way this method shows how to conduct a Process Mining for sustainability/ GHG emission (reporting) goals would be difficult for users to understand. (*) 3. Using this approach would make it more difficult to communicate how Process Mining implementation techniques can help organizations achieve sustainability/ GHG emission (reporting) goals. (*) 4. Overall, I find this process useful
Perceived ease of use	5. Learning to use this method would be easy for me 6. I found the method unclear and difficult to understand. (*) 7. It would be easy for me to become skillful at using this method 8. Overall, I find this method difficult to use. (*)
Intention to use	9. I would use this approach to implement a PM project for sustainability/ GHG emission goals 10. I would intend to use this approach in preference to another approach

Reversed questions, marked with an asterisk had their scores adjusted to mitigate response bias

With average scores above 5 for all *Perceived Usefulness* questions, respondents generally find the guidelines beneficial, though two noted some difficulty in understanding them. The method's structured, step-by-step guidance is particularly appreciated by those new to sustainability data, while even experienced experts found it helpful for decision-making on data sources and validation. However, additional sustainability training was suggested despite the guidelines being perceived as flexible.

Perceived Ease of Use received lower scores, though still positive. Two respondents found the artifact challenging, primarily due to difficulties in understanding sustainability concepts, which one attributed to a lack of process or industry-specific knowledge. Respondents recommended more detailed documentation and sustainability training to improve ease of use. Despite these issues, the level of detail in the subprocess steps, as illustrated by BPMN, was considered appropriate.

Table 4. Questionnaire results: # of respondents per rating and rating statistics per question (r).

	Ques	Completely disagree ←→ Completely agree							Avg	Std.Dev
Perceived usefulness	1	0	0	0	0	3	9	5	6.1	0.70
	2 (*)	1	8	4	2	1	1	0	5.2	1.29
	3 (*)	3	11	1	2	0	0	0	5.9	0.86
	4	0	0	0	0	4	5	8	6.2	0.83
Perceived ease of use	5	0	0	1	3	6	6	1	4.2	1.00
	6 (*)	4	8	2	2	1	0	0	4.7	1.20
	7	0	0	1	1	7	4	4	4.7	1.10
	8 (*)	2	8	5	0	0	1	1	4.3	1.60
Intention to use	9	0	0	0	0	6	6	5	5.9	0.83
	10	0	0	0	3	6	7	1	5.4	0.86

The *Intention to Use* the guidelines is relatively high, but adoption challenges include costs and the framework's complexity. While the detailed guidelines enhance usefulness, they can increase implementation costs, particularly for IT systems for sustainability metrics and API licenses. Despite these barriers, the guidelines align with sustainability strategies and are expected to integrate well with current methods.

The evaluation shows that PMG3 is generally considered useful, with interest in adopting the guidelines. However, ease of use (EoU) received lower and varied scores, likely due to differences in seniority, technical skills, and sustainability knowledge. The need for clearer instructions on selecting emission factor databases and additional sustainability training was noted. Data validation challenges, especially when mapping internal data to third-party emission factors, highlight the importance of basic sustainability knowledge. Challenges in adopting the guidelines align with findings from the literature review, particularly regarding data availability and ERP systems' capacity to store sustainability data. Respondents also stressed the need for strategic alignment, as financial goals often overshadow sustainability objectives.

6 Conclusion

Despite growing interest in Green BPM, the use of process mining for sustainability and carbon accounting is underexplored. Process mining typically focuses on financial goals and lacks real-life applicability for sustainability. Frameworks like PM4S introduce OCPM for tracking GHG emissions, energy consumption, and waste but struggle with data availability and quality issues [12]. To address these gaps, we developed guidelines following design science research, focusing on GHG emissions in response to evolving sustainability regulations like the CSRD. Our literature review and exploratory interviews identified key challenges—such as data availability and process complexity—and success factors like system integration and management support. These insights shaped the development of the objectives of the solution and its design.

The guidelines consist of five steps essential for successful implementation. A business case comparing CO_2e emissions of two product alternatives demonstrated the need for contextual data, such as waste and inventory data, for effective decision-making. Evaluation through focus groups and surveys confirmed the guidelines' utility and ease of use, though challenges remain, particularly in data maturity and strategic alignment. This research contributes by developing and demonstrating the applicability of guidelines for process mining projects focused on GHG emissions. These guidelines provide detailed instructions for data requirements definition, process data retrieval, contextual data enrichment, and analysis. The artifact supports process mining practitioners in implementing sustainability projects, addressing data challenges, and ensuring accurate reporting. The demonstrated application in a business case adds to previous research by proving the guidelines' practical utility. Moreover, the research offers concrete examples of measuring and calculating sustainability KPIs, expanding process mining techniques to sustainability use cases, and aiding practitioners in meeting emerging legal requirements for sustainability reporting. Further research is needed to refine team roles, skills, and organizational attributes necessary for successful sustainable development projects using process mining. Our research extends prior frameworks like [12] and [15], which lacked real-life testing, by providing evaluated guidelines demonstrated in GHG emission projects. The artifact addresses data quality challenges through comprehensive data pooling guidelines and is structured around a five-step process: defining business and data requirements, data pooling, process model mapping, and result analysis to formulate recommendations.

This research has limitations related to both the artifact and the research design. While the artifact generally applies to various processes, it does not fully develop the object-centric perspective, which is important for accurate sustainability reporting. Future research could enhance the guidelines by integrating OCPM techniques for a more comprehensive implementation. The business case's narrow geographical and industry focus limits the generalizability of the findings. Although the geographical scope aligns with European CSRD coverage, further research is needed to test the guidelines in other industries, particularly highly regulated ones like pharmaceuticals. Additionally, the artifact has not addressed the complexities of emissions tracking in service industries. The empirical nature of the study, with focus groups, interviews, and surveys involving only 17 respondents from the same organization, also presents limitations. The small sample size and the homogeneity in tenure of the respondents restrict the diversity of insights. Future studies should expand to multiple organizations and include more senior practitioners to provide a broader validation of the findings.

References

1. UN General Assembly: Transforming our world: the 2030 Agenda for Sustainable Development A/RES/70/1
2. The United Nations: Goal 12: Ensure sustainable consumption and production patterns
3. The European Parliament, The Council of The European Union: Corporate Sustainability Reporting Directive (EU) 2022/2464. The European Comission (2022)
4. UNEP: Guidelines for social life cycle assessment of products and organisations 2020, (2020)
5. Central Bureau of Statistics: Greenhouse gas emissions 5 percent lower in Q2 2023
6. GHG Protocol: Greenhouse Gas Protocol: FAQ (2011)
7. Seidel, S., Recker, J., vom Brocke, J.: Green business process management. In: Green Business Process Management, pp. 3–13. Springer, Berlin Heidelberg (2012). https://doi.org/10.1007/978-3-642-27488-6_1
8. Reijers, H.A., Liman Mansar, S.: Best practices in business process redesign: an overview and qualitative evaluation of successful redesign heuristics. Omega (Westport). **33**, 283–306 (2005). https://doi.org/10.1016/j.omega.2004.04.012
9. Hechelmann, R.-H., Paris, A., Buchenau, N., Ebersold, F.: Decarbonisation strategies for manufacturing: a technical and economic compariso. Renew. Sustain. Energy Rev. **188** (2023)
10. Brehm, L., Slamka, J., Nickmann, A.: Process mining for carbon accounting: an analysis of requirements and potentials (2022). https://doi.org/10.1007/978-3-031-06543-9_9
11. Steinhöfel, E., Galeitzke, M., Kohl, H., Orth, R.: Sustainability reporting in german manufacturing SMEs. Procedia Manuf. **33**, 610–617 (2019). https://doi.org/10.1016/j.promfg.2019.04.076
12. Graves, N., Koren, I., van der Aalst, W.M.P.: ReThink your processes! A review of process mining for sustainability. In: 2023 International Conference on ICT for Sustainability (ICT4S). pp. 164–175. IEEE (2023). https://doi.org/10.1109/ICT4S58814.2023.00025
13. Couckuyt, D., Looy, A. Van: Green BPM as a business-oriented discipline: a systematic mapping study and research agenda. Sustainability (Switzerland). **11** (2019). https://doi.org/10.3390/su11154200
14. Sohns, T.M., Aysolmaz, B., Figge, L., Joshi, A.: Green business process management for business sustainability: a case study of manufacturing small and medium-sized enterprises (SMEs) from Germany. J. Clean. Prod. **401**, 136667 (2023). https://doi.org/10.1016/j.jclepro.2023.136667
15. Ortmeier, C., Henningsen, N., Langer, A., Reiswich, A., Karl, A., Herrmann, C.: Framework for the integration of process mining into life cycle assessment. Procedia CIRP. **98**, 163–168 (2021). https://doi.org/10.1016/j.procir.2021.01.024
16. ISO 14044:2006: Environmental management — Life cycle assessment — Requirements and guidelines (2006)
17. Hevner, M., Park, R.: Design science in information systems research. MIS Quarterly. **28**, 75 (2004)
18. Peffers, K., Tuunanen, T., Rothenberger, M.A., Chatterjee, S.: A design science research methodology for information systems research. J. Manag. Inf. Syst. **24**, 45–77 (2007). https://doi.org/10.2753/MIS0742-1222240302
19. Graafmans, T., Turetken, O., Poppelaars, H., Fahland, D.: Process mining for six sigma: a guideline and tool support. Bus. Inf. Syst. Eng. **63**, 277–300 (2021). https://doi.org/10.1007/s12599-020-00649-w

20. van der Aalst, W.: Process mining: a 360 degree overview. In: Process Mining Handbook, pp. 3–34 (2022)

21. Pearson, J.: People – Process – Technology – The eternal triangle

22. Sonnenberg, C., vom Brocke, J.: Evaluations in the science of the artificial – reconsidering the build-evaluate pattern in design science research. Presented at the (2012)

23. Davis, F.D.: Perceived usefulness, perceived ease of use, and user acceptance of information technology. MIS Q. **13**, 319 (1989). https://doi.org/10.2307/249008

24. NREL: U.S. Unit & system life cycle inventory (USLCI)

25. Venkatesh, V., Davis, F.D.: A theoretical extension of the technology acceptance model: four longitudinal field studies. Manage. Sci. **46**, 186–204 (2000). https://doi.org/10.1287/mnsc.46.2.186.11926

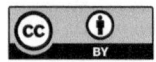

Sustainability Analysis Patterns for Process Mining and Process Modelling Approaches

Andreas Fritsch$^{(\boxtimes)}$ (iD)

Karlsruhe Institute of Technology, Institute AIFB, Karlsruhe, Germany
`andreas.fritsch@kit.edu`

Abstract. Business Process Management (BPM) has the potential to help companies manage and reduce their activities' negative social and environmental impacts. However, so far, only limited capabilities for analysing the sustainability impacts of processes have been integrated into established BPM methods and tools. One of the main challenges of existing Sustainable BPM approaches is the lack of a sound conception of sustainability impacts. This paper describes a set of sustainability analysis patterns that integrate BPM concepts with concepts from existing sustainability analysis methods to address this challenge. The patterns provide a framework to evaluate and develop process modelling and process mining approaches for discovering, analysing and improving the sustainability impacts of processes. It is shown how the patterns can be used to evaluate existing process modelling and process mining approaches.

Keywords: Process Patterns · Business Process Management · Process Mining · Sustainable Development · Life Cycle Assessment

1 Introduction

The demand for more sustainability is being put forward to companies from various sides, be it from politics, non-governmental organisations, customers or the company's workforce [12]. The term sustainability or Sustainable Development stands for a long-term perspective to satisfy human needs today and in the future in light of escalating global challenges such as the climate crisis [33]. From a company's point of view, contributing to sustainable development means considering the (negative) effects of its activities on humans (social justice) and the environment (environmental protection) [33]. A consequence of this perspective is that the area of responsibility for a company expands [13]. It is not enough to consider only the direct impacts within the company's boundaries, such as wages to the company's workforce or pollutant emissions on its premises. Rather, the effects triggered by the company's activities along its value chain must also be considered [16,30]. For example, a company that manufactures batteries bears responsibility for lithium mining and the associated contamination

© The Author(s) 2025
A. Delgado and T. Slaats (Eds.): ICPM 2024 Workshops, LNBIP 533, pp. 725–737, 2025.
https://doi.org/10.1007/978-3-031-82225-4_53

of water resources [22]. This idea is central to existing sustainability analysis methods, such as Life Cycle Assessment (LCA) [16,30,35].

Business Process Management (BPM) concepts, methods, and tools have the potential to help companies become more sustainable. BPM aims to analyse and improve the activities of companies [36]. While traditionally improvements in terms of costs, lead times, and error rates are being sought [7], researchers have begun to include sustainability aspects in their approaches [5,10]. These Sustainable BPM approaches include concepts, methods and tools to support the modelling, analysis, improvement, implementation and management of business processes [7,36], taking into account their environmental and social impacts. One of the challenges of existing Sustainable BPM approaches is the lack of a sound conception of how to measure the impacts of a business process [5,10].

This paper provides a set of sustainability analysis patterns to address this challenge. The definition of the patterns is inspired by "workflow patterns" that have been used to evaluate process modelling and process mining approaches regarding their capabilities to represent control flow and data flow aspects of business processes [27,28]. Similarly, the sustainability analysis patterns describe different aspects of a process' environmental and social impacts. Note that the patterns are not intended as *design* patterns, meaning they do not describe how an organisation can operate sustainably. Rather, they describe what aspects a business process *model* should represent to provide a foundation for a sound, comparable and transparent sustainability analysis. This way, they guide (1) process analysts who aim to analyse the sustainability of business processes and (2) developers and researchers who integrate sustainability analysis capabilities in process modelling and process mining approaches. The patterns are derived by mapping a meta-model of BPM concepts with a meta-model of concepts from existing sustainability analysis methods (i.e. LCA). They are evaluated by applying them to compare the capabilities of existing process modelling and mining approaches and derive improvement possibilities for future developments.

In Sect. 2, we provide background on BPM and LCA as well as an overview of related pattern proposals. Section 3 provides a synopsis of BPM and LCA meta-models. Section 4 presents the developed sustainability analysis patterns, and in Sect. 5, the patterns are applied to a review of existing process modelling and mining approaches. Finally, we conclude in Sect. 6 and provide an overview of future work.

2   Background and Related Work

2.1   Business Process Management (BPM) and Process Mining

BPM is concerned with improving business processes and thus the performance of a company [7,36]. A distinction can be made between management and technical BPM approaches [5]. Management approaches address issues such as organisational structure, values, roles, and responsibilities within a company [34]. Technical approaches are concerned with the modelling, analysis, improvement and implementation of business processes [7,36]. Process mining is a branch of BPM

[1]. The basic idea of process mining is to automatically create business process models from event log data (e.g. events logged by IT systems) [1].

2.2 Sustainability Analysis and Life Cycle Assessment (LCA)

In the so-called Brundtland report, the term Sustainable Development was coined as a guiding principle for global change [33]. The goal is to satisfy the needs of current generations without endangering the ability of future generations to satisfy their needs [33]. The joint consideration of social, environmental, and economic factors is an essential aspect of the sustainability concept described in the Brundtland report [25].

It is important to consider that an activity's sustainability impacts may occur outside the company's boundaries. An important concept in this context is life cycle thinking [13]. It means that a systemic perspective is adopted when analysing the sustainability of a product or a company. This includes the interactions between the product or company under consideration, the environment, and other stakeholders along its value chain (also called life cycle) [16]. The goal is to improve the entire system [16]. Life Cycle Assessment (LCA) is a method for conducting such an investigation [16].

The LCA method was initially developed to analyse the environmental impacts of products, e.g., contribution to climate change, acidification, ecotoxicity and waste [16,18]. The method was adapted and extended for analysing the environmental impacts of an entire company [17], as well as social impacts [30]. The corresponding standards and guidelines define that an LCA study consists of four phases [16,17,30]. The first phase is the *definition of goal and scope*. Here, the system boundaries, as well as basic requirements and assumptions, are defined. Second, *inventory analysis* is carried out, in which data about the system is collected, and calculations are made to quantify relevant inputs and outputs. The third phase is the *impact assessment*, where the significance of sustainability impacts is evaluated. And finally, as the last step, the *interpretation* of the results, where improvement potential is identified. The GHG Protocol [35] guidelines can be considered as a restricted variant of LCA since it only considers one impact category (climate change) [32]. It largely follows the structure outlined by the LCA standards and provides definitions for different assessment scopes regarding GHG emissions [35]: *Scope 1* refers to direct GHG emissions within the premises of a company, *Scope 2* refers to indirect GHG emissions that stem from the generation of energy consumed by a company, and *Scope 3* addresses further indirect GHG emissions in the value chain.

2.3 Related Work

In Sustainable BPM literature, several proposals for sustainable or green business process patterns can be found [19–21]. These proposals for patterns describe, in a structured way, how the sustainability of a business process can be improved (e.g. using resources with reduced environmental impact [21]). In each case, it is implicitly assumed that the impacts of a business process *have already been measured.* The patterns described in this paper focus on the more fundamental question, *how* the sustainability impacts of a business process should be measured.

3   Mapping of BPM and LCA Meta-models

3.1   Meta-models for BPM and LCA

This section maps basic concepts from the BPM and LCA disciplines using meta-models. This way, a synopsis of concepts from both disciplines is constructed that allows for adapting insights from LCA for Sustainable BPM. From this synopsis, patterns that describe how the sustainability impacts of a process can be modelled are derived in the next section.

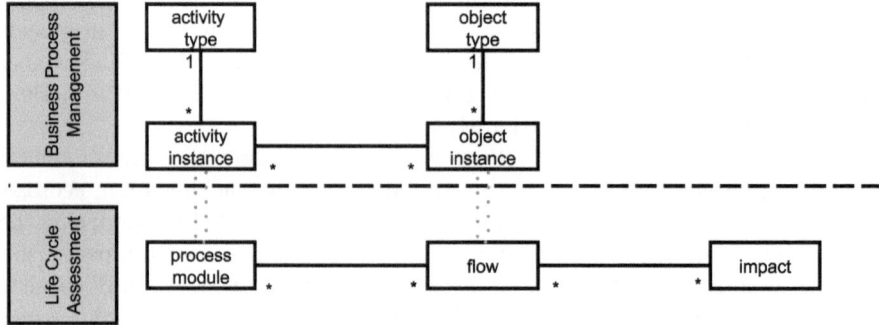

Fig. 1. Mapping of BPM and LCA meta-models.

Figure 1 shows a mapping between the meta-models of BPM and LCA. From left to right, it shows similar concepts in the respective disciplines. As a basis for describing BPM concepts, we refer to the OCEL 2.0 standard [3]. The choice is motivated by the concise form of the given meta-model and its interoperability between BPM technologies. Similarly, as a basis for describing LCA concepts, we refer to a description of the ILCD standard [38], which is used to exchange data between LCA tools. Note that in both cases, some of the terminology has been adapted for consistency and clarity within this paper. For example, the OCEL standard defines a concept *event* as an execution of an activity. In Fig. 1, this concept is called an *activity instance*. In the following description of Fig. 1, we additionally refer to basic sources of BPM [23,36] and LCA [16,18] to explain the concepts and conclusions.

In BPM, the notion of a process refers to a business process, i.e. a set of *activities* that are performed by a company to realise a business goal [36]. Processes are modelled and analysed to improve a company's performance or to support the development of information systems [36]. Activities may be associated with *objects*: objects can be inputs or outputs of an activity, they may be altered by an activity, or they may be resources (machines, humans) that are needed to execute an activity [3,36]. It is common to differentiate between *activity and object types and instances* [3,36]. Typically, a business process is modelled at the type level, where the model describes a general frame for executing the process [23]. Activity instances refer to executions of an activity at a specific time [3]. BPM traditionally focuses on causal and temporal relationships between activities (control flow) [7,36]. However, several approaches aim to integrate the data flow perspective more tightly [29]. Similarly, the early focus of process mining approaches was on the relationships between activities, with a recent uptake of interest in analysing the relationships between activities and objects [3].

In LCA, process models are created to analyse the sustainability impacts of a product, service or company [16,17,30]. Different to how processes are typically modelled in BPM, these process models represent the phases of a value chain (also called life cycle) and are built from *process modules* [18,38]. A process module may represent a phenomenon similar to an activity in BPM (e.g. manufacturing of a workpiece), but it may also represent a whole industry (e.g. energy generation in Germany) [18]. Process modules are associated with *flows* [38]. Similar to the object concept in BPM, flows may be products, information or data, but the focus is on material and energy flows [16,18]. When modelling processes, LCA doesn't distinguish between types and instances. Instead, a process model represents the quantified flows along a value chain relative to a "functional unit" (e.g. the flows required to provide a certain amount of mineral water) [16]. The identified flows are then associated with different *impacts* [16,38]. The resulting impact indicators quantify the extent of a certain flow's impact on an environmental or social problem area [16]. For example, emissions of $CO2$ and other GHG emissions ("flows") contribute to the problem area *climate change* (an "impact"). This impact is typically measured in CO2 equivalents (CO2e) [18]. Other environmental impacts include ozone depletion, land use, ecotoxicity and acidification. Examples of impacts addressed in social LCA are excessive working hours, work accidents or discrimination [31]. Note that any list of considered impacts depends on scientific progress and societal awareness [18]. For an overview of environmental impact lists, see [18]. For a list of impacts considered in social LCA, see [31].

3.2 Specific Characteristics of Process Modelling in LCA

Several notable aspects of process modelling in LCA are relevant when considering how to model sustainability aspects in BPM. In particular, the relevant flows depend on the assessed impacts. For example, the assessment of climate change requires the identification of GHG emissions, while the assessment of ozone depletion requires the identification of gas emissions that damage the ozone layer [18].

The scope definition is another important factor in the identification of relevant flows. For example, a "gate-to-gate" analysis only considers flows within a company [16]. A "cradle-to-gate" analysis extends the scope of considered flows to include the upstream value chain of the company (the company's suppliers and their suppliers etc.) [16]. Scopes 1 to 3, as defined in the GHG Protocol, are another example of a scope definition specific to climate change impacts [35].

A further important aspect is the allocation of impacts. When dealing with process modules that have multiple inputs or outputs (e.g. mining produces diamonds and rubble), it needs to be decided how the associated impacts are distributed [18]. This is a central problem in LCA and conventions exist how to handle these situations (e.g. allocation by weight or economic value) [16,18]. In any case, allocation decisions can have significant consequences in the resulting assessment, so they must be carefully considered and documented [16,18].

3.3   Conclusion: Sustainability Impacts of a Business Process

In both disciplines, BPM and LCA, processes are modelled and analysed. The observed similarities allow for using LCA as a reference to reason about how to measure sustainability impacts in BPM [5,10,11]. From the mapping conducted above, there are several lessons to be learned. First, Sustainable BPM requires some kind of object or data flow perspective to capture impacts (see also [11]).

Second, Sustainable BPM needs a conception of the scope of an analysis. Speaking in LCA terms, a gate-to-gate analysis may yield significantly different results than a cradle-to-gate analysis. Taking, for example, a business process supported by IT, it needs to be clarified if an analysis considers Scope 2 (electricity would be the main relevant input) or Scope 3 (the IT infrastructure and its impact along the value chain would have to be considered as well).

Third, allocation is an important challenge to be addressed by Sustainable BPM. In the BPM modelling perspective, multi-input and multi-output processes are commonplace (e.g., a resource is used by multiple activity instances, an activity may have multiple object outputs). Thus, mechanisms for transparently and consistently allocating impacts are required.

4   Sustainability Analysis Patterns

Based on the results of Sect. 3, the following sustainability analysis patterns for business processes are defined. They describe different sustainability-relevant aspects of business processes and adapt concepts of LCA for BPM. Their implementation in approaches for Sustainable BPM thus enables the analysis of process sustainability from a life cycle perspective. For the four patterns, a description, a motivation and variants (if applicable) are provided. In the following, the term *process component* refers to any of the BPM concepts shown in Fig. 1.

(AP 1) Sustainability-Relevant Inputs and Outputs: A process component can be assigned sustainability-relevant inputs and outputs (see Fig. 2a). For example, an activity instance requires a certain amount of energy as input or produces a certain amount of waste as output.

Motivation: The recording of inputs and outputs of a business process corresponds to the inventory analysis of LCA. It is a basic requirement to enable reasoning about the sustainability impacts of a process.

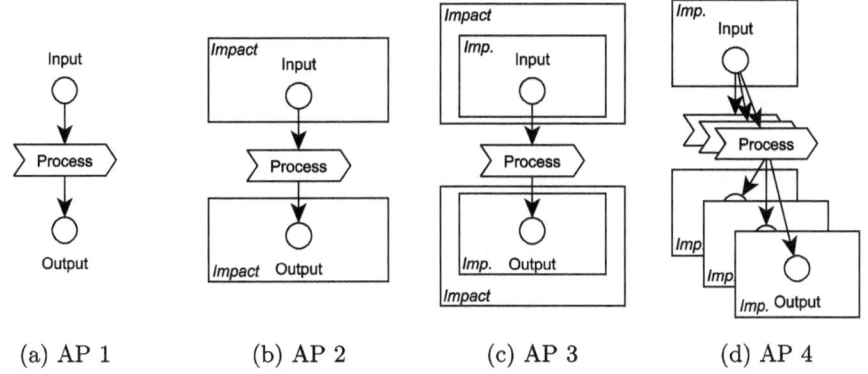

(a) AP 1   (b) AP 2   (c) AP 3   (d) AP 4

Fig. 2. Sustainability Anaylsis Patterns

(AP 2) Sustainability Impacts: A process component can be assigned sustainability impacts (see Fig. 2b). Different environmental and social impacts can be distinguished (see the following variants).

AP 2-Env: A process component can be assigned environmental impacts (e.g., an activity instance contributes to ozone depletion with 3 kg CFCe).

AP 2-Climate: A process component can be assigned a climate impact (e.g., an activity instance causes a climate impact of 5 kg CO2e).

AP 2-Social: A process component can be assigned social impacts (e.g., an activity instance causes work accidents).

Motivation: The assignment of impacts to a process component corresponds to the impact assessment in LCA. The assessment of impacts is to be differentiated from the mere recording of inputs and outputs. A comprehensive assessment of impacts allows for identifying shifts between them. AP 2-Climate is defined as a special case of AP 2-Env because climate impacts are particularly relevant in the context of sustainability analysis [35].

(AP 3) Scoping of Sustainability Impacts: A process component can be assigned impacts for different scopes (see Fig. 2c). This scope definition can be made for different sustainability impacts (see the following variants of AP 3).

AP 3-Env: A process component can be assigned environmental impacts for different scopes (e.g., an activity instance contributes to ozone depletion with 3 kg CFCe when including direct emissions, and 15 kg CFCe when including emissions in the value chain).

AP 3-Climate: A process component can be assigned climate impacts for different scopes (e.g., following the scoping concept of the GHG Protocol an activity instance causes a Scope 1 impact of 5 kg CO2e and a Scope 3 impact of 30 kg CO2e).

AP 3-Social: A process component can be assigned social impacts for different scopes (e.g. an activity instance causes an average of 0.00001 work accidents within the company and 0.00002 work accidents when considering the value chain of used resources).

Motivation: Following the idea of life cycle thinking, Sustainable BPM should enable the identification of impact shifts along value chains. However, fully considering the value chain may not always be feasible. Still, a transparent definition of the considered scopes should be supported for comparability.

(AP 4) Allocation of Sustainability Impacts: Sustainability impacts assigned to a process component can be (partially) allocated to other process components (see Fig. 2d). For example, the impact associated with the production of a resource can be allocated to individual activity instances.

Motivation: To identify improvement potential in a business process, an analysis should yield results on which process components are responsible (to what extent) for various impacts. For this, transparent mechanisms are needed to allocate impact assessment between process components.

5   Application of Sustainability Analysis Patterns

5.1   Criteria and Overview

To show the utility of the proposed sustainability analysis patterns, they are applied to evaluate existing Sustainable BPM approaches. The evaluation focuses on modelling approaches since this has been the focus of Sustainable BPM literature [10]. Corresponding publications were extracted from a literature review on Sustainable BPM [10]. In the extracted publications, it can be seen that various authors developed their approaches across several publications. Due to space restrictions, we only reference selected publications for each approach. For an overview of all publications on Sustainable BPM identified in [10], see [9]. The modelling approaches considered were examined based on the sustainability analysis patterns described in Sect. 4. The criteria and their evaluation are explained in the following.

Regarding *AP 1* an approach is evaluated ● if modelling of inputs/outputs is supported, and ○ if not. For *AP 2* an approach is evaluated ● if modelling of impacts is supported, and ○ if modelling of impacts is not supported. The evaluation for *AP 3* distinguishes between ● if scoping is supported, ◗ if scoping is considered but explicitly limited, and ○ if scoping is not supported. Finally, for *AP 4* an approach is evaluated ● if allocation is supported, and ○ if not.

5.2   Evaluation of Sustainable Process Modelling Approaches

Table 1 provides an overview of existing modelling approaches for Sustainable BPM, the respective modelling languages used, and the evaluation according to the described criteria.

Houy et al. [15] describe the idea of annotating activities in EPC models with indicators such as resource consumption or energy demand. The publications describe an initial concept. Various sustainability-relevant inputs and

Table 1. Review of existing sustainable process modelling approaches.

Approach	AP 1	AP 2			AP 3			AP 4
		Climate	Env	Social	Climate	Env	Social	
Houy et al.	●	○	○	○	○	○	○	○
Hoesch-Klohe et al.	●	●	○	○	◑	○	○	●
Recker et al.	●	●	○	○	●	○	○	●
Wesumperuma et al.	●	●	○	○	●	○	○	●
Zhu et al.	●	○	○	○	○	○	○	○
Betz	○	●	●	●	●	●	●	○

outputs, such as water consumption, energy demand, and CO2 emissions, are mentioned as possibilities for annotation (● for AP 1), but the measurement of sustainability impacts is not addressed (○ for AP 2). No modelling support is provided for scoping or allocating impacts (○ for AP 3 and AP 4).

In the publications of *Houy et al.* [14], activities are also annotated with sustainability indicators, in this case, in BPMN process models. For the considered indicators, a distinction is made between sustainability-relevant inputs and outputs (such as energy demands) and climate impacts (measured in CO2e) (● for AP 1 and AP 2-Climate). The consideration of climate impacts is explicitly limited to Scopes 1 and 2 of the GHG Protocol (◑ for AP 3-Climate). Other sustainability impacts are not addressed (○ for AP 2-Env, AP 2-Social, AP 3-Env and AP 3-Social). Regarding allocation, [14] proposes a resource modelling concept (● for AP 4). With these models, the total impacts for different process instances can then be calculated.

In the approach of *Recker et al.* [26], a BPMN extension for sustainability aspects is proposed. With these new notation elements, activities can be marked, as paper-consuming or fuel-consuming (● for AP 1). Furthermore, the resulting climate impact for different groups of activities is displayed in a special notation element (● for AP 2-Climate). The calculated climate impacts also consider the production of used resources, i.e. Scope 3 (● for AP 3-Climate). Concepts for considering additional impacts are not developed (○ for AP 2-Env, AP 2-Social, AP 3-Env and AP 3-Social). A procedure is proposed in which the climate impacts of resources are allocated (● for AP 4).

Closely related to *Recker et al.* is the approach of *Wesumperuma et al.* [37], which also proposes and elaborates an extension of BPMN with notation elements for capturing climate impacts (● for AP 2-Climate). A procedure is described in which the climate impact is summed up for individual activities, and processes. Furthermore, a calculation method is proposed that can be used to allocate the sustainability impacts caused by resources to individual activities (● for AP 1 and AP 4). As with *Recker et al.*, the approach considers different scopes of climate impacts, including Scope 3 (● for AP 3-Climate). Other environmental or social impacts are not considered (○ for AP 2-Env, AP 2-Social, AP 3-Env and AP 3-Social).

The approach of *Zhu et al.* [39] involves enriching BPMN process models with sustainability-relevant context data such as resources, countries, or people (● for AP 1). In terms of impacts, the approach remains unspecific. It is shown that integration of data from environmental information systems is possible, but the adequate integration of sustainability data in terms of allocation, different impacts, and scoping is not addressed (○ for AP 2, AP 3 and AP 4).

Betz [4] describes the idea of modelling sustainability aspects of business processes with a variant of high-level Petri Nets. It is mentioned that various environmental and social impact indicators can be integrated into a process model. A distinction is made between direct, indirect, and socio-economic impacts (● for AP 2 and AP 3). However, the identification of sustainability-relevant inputs/outputs and allocation are not considered (○ for AP 1 and AP 4).

The identified modelling approaches have only reached a limited degree of maturity. The majority of developed concepts focus on energy aspects and GHG emissions. Apart from measuring climate impacts based on the GHG Protocol, a systematic distinction between inputs/outputs and impacts, as well as concepts for impact scopes, are missing. The approach from *Betz* is an exception with its distinction of direct, indirect and socio-economic impacts. This scoping concept takes an even broader perspective than conventional LCA analyses since it does not only consider the value chain. Of the approaches that consider the allocation of sustainability impacts, *Hoesch-Klohe et al.* appears to be the most sophisticated with detailed resource modelling concepts.

5.3   Evaluation of Sustainable Process Mining Approaches

So far, sustainability aspects have only been addressed to a limited extent in process mining. A systematic literature review on Sustainable Process Mining approaches [11] finds that existing publications on the topic provide mainly high-level descriptions. Four case studies identified in the review directly address social or environmental sustainability aspects. Three of them, however, only address sustainability-related domains (health and safety [24], wind turbine maintenance [6] and sustainable agriculture [8]). The described approaches do not attempt to measure sustainability aspects in processes. Rather, conventional measures (e.g. time usage) are applied. Only [2] addresses measuring sustainability aspects in processes by relating energy needs to identified process models (AP 1). This shows that further work is required to provide more expressive sustainability analyses with process mining. One solution proposed by [11] is to enrich process models with object quantities. This, in turn, would enable future approaches that provide support for allocating impacts between process components (AP 4).

6   Conclusion and Outlook

Sustainable BPM approaches need a solid concept of sustainability impact measurement to provide meaningful and comparable analyses. The sustainability analysis patterns proposed in this paper provide an initial framework to critically assess Sustainable BPM approaches. The mapping provided in Sect. 3 shows that Sustainable BPM and LCA share common goals and concepts. Therefore, in the future, further insights from LCA can be adapted for Sustainable BPM to elaborate and extend the proposed patterns. The LCA standard [16] primarily defines certain principles but does not prescribe specific techniques. In this sense, Sustainable BPM approaches can be seen as a technical variant of other LCA approaches. However, the BPM (modelling) perspective provides specific advantages regarding the continuous support of process changes, as well as the implementation of tools and IT support [36]. Sustainable BPM thus brings a unique and promising contribution to effectively improving the sustainability performance of companies.

References

1. van der Aalst, W.: Process mining. Springer (2016)
2. Acerbi, F., Polenghi, A., Quadrini, W., Macchi, M., Taisch, M.: Fostering circular manufacturing through the integration of genetic algorithm and process mining. In: APMS. Gyeongju, South Korea (2022)
3. Berti, A., et al.: OCEL (Object-Centric Event Log) 2.0 Specification (2023)
4. Betz, S.: Sustainability aware process management using XML-Nets. In: EnviroInfo, Oldenburg, Germany (2014)
5. Couckuyt, D., Van Looy, A.: Green BPM as a business-oriented discipline: a systematic mapping study and research agenda. Sustainability 11(15) (2019)
6. Du, L., Cheng, L., Liu, C.: Process mining for wind turbine maintenance process analysis: a case study. In: EI2. Taiyuan, China (2021)
7. Dumas, M., La Rosa, M., Mendling, J., Reijers, H.A.: Fundamentals of business process management. Springer (2018)
8. Dupuis, A., Dadouchi, C., Agard, B.: Predicting crop rotations using process mining techniques and Markov principals. Comput. Electron. Agric. 194 (2022)
9. Fritsch, A., von Hammerstein, J., Schreiber, C., Betz, S., Oberweis, A.: Sustainable BPM primary papers. https://figshare.com/s/83840f7f29cb0f04240b (2021)
10. Fritsch, A., von Hammerstein, J., Schreiber, C., Betz, S., Oberweis, A.: Pathways to greener pastures: research opportunities to integrate life cycle assessment and sustainable business process management based on a systematic tertiary literature review. Sustainability 14(18) (2022)
11. Graves, N., Koren, I., van der Aalst, W.M.: ReThink your processes! A review of process mining for sustainability. In: ICT4S. Rennes, France (2023)
12. Haldar, S.: Towards a conceptual understanding of sustainability-driven entrepreneurship. Corp. Soc Resp. Env. Ma 26(6) (2019)
13. Heiskanen, E.: The institutional logic of life cycle thinking. J. Clean Prod. 10(5) (2002)
14. Hoesch-Klohe, K., Ghose, A., Lê, L.S.: Towards green business process management. In: ICSOC, Miami, FL, USA (2010)
15. Houy, C., Reiter, M., Fettke, P., Loos, P.: Towards green BPM - sustainability and resource efficiency through business process management. In: BPM Workshops. Hoboken, NJ, USA (2011)
16. ISO: ISO 14040:2006 Environmental management - Life cycle assessment - Principles and framework (2006)

17. ISO: ISO/TS 14072:2014 Environmental management - Life cycle assessment - requirements and guidelines for organizational life cycle assessment (2014)
18. Klöpffer, W., Grahl, B.: Life Cycle Assessment (LCA) a Guide to Best Practice. Wiley-VCH (2014)
19. Larsch, S., Betz, S., Duboc, L., Magdaleno, A.M., Bomfim, C.: Integrating sustainability aspects in business process management. In: BPM Workshops. Rio de Janeiro, Brazil (2016)
20. Lubbecke, P., Fettke, P., Loos, P.: Towards ecological workflow patterns as an instrument to optimize business processes with respect to ecological goals. In: HICSS. Koloa, HI, USA (2016)
21. Nowak, A., Leymann, F., Schleicher, D., Schumm, D., Wagner, S.: Green business process patterns. In: PLoP, Portland, OR, USA (2011)
22. NRDC: lithium mining is leaving chile's indigenous communities high and dry. https://www.nrdc.org/stories/lithium-mining-leaving-chiles-indigenous-communities-high-and-dry-literally, April 2022
23. Oberweis, A.: Modellierung und Ausführung von Workflows Mit Petri-Netzen. B. G. Teubner (1996)
24. Pika, A., Ter Hofstede, A.H., Perrons, R.K., Grossmann, G., Stumptner, M., Cooley, J.: Using big data to improve safety performance: an application of process mining to enhance data visualisation. Big Data Res. **25** (2021)
25. Purvis, B., Mao, Y., Robinson, D.: Three pillars of sustainability: in search of conceptual origins. Sustain Sci. **14**(3) (2019)
26. Recker, J., Rosemann, M., Gohar, E.R.: Measuring the carbon footprint of business processes. In: BPM Workshops. Hoboken, NJ, USA (2011)
27. Russell, N.: Workflow data patterns. In: ER. Shanghai, China (2004)
28. Russell, N., ter Hofstede, A.H.M., van der Aalst, W.M.P., Mulyar, N.: Workflow control-flow patterns: a revised view. BPM Center Rep. (2006)
29. Steinau, S., Marrella, A., Andrews, K., Leotta, F., Mecella, M., Reichert, M.: DALEC: a framework for the systematic evaluation of data-centric approaches to process management software. Softw. Syst. Model **18**(4) (2019)
30. UNEP: guidelines for social life cycle assessment of products and organizations (2020)
31. UNEP: methodological sheets for subcategories in social life cycle assessment (S-LCA) (2021)
32. UNEP, SETAC: guidance on organizational life cycle assessment (2015)
33. United nations general assembly: report of the world commission on environment and development: our common future (A/42/427) (1987)
34. Van Looy, A., De Backer, M., Poels, G.: A conceptual framework and classification of capability areas for business process maturity. Enterp. Inform. Syst. **8**(2) (2014)
35. WBCSD, WRI: the greenhouse gas protocol (2004)
36. Weske, M.: Business Process Management: Concepts, Languages. Architectures, Springer (2019)
37. Wesumperuma, A., Ginige, A., Ginige, J.A., Hol, A.: Green activity based management (ABM) for organisations. In: ACIS. Melbourne, Australia (2013)
38. Wolf, M.A., Düpmeier, C., Kusche, O.: The international reference life cycle data system (ILCD) format. In: EnviroInfo. Ispra, Italy (2011)
39. Zhu, X., Zhu, G., Broucke, S.V., Recker, J.: On merging business process management and geographic information systems: modeling and execution of ecological concerns in processes. In: GRMSE. Ypsilanti, MI, USA (2015)

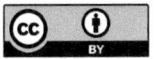

Towards Nudging in BPM: A Human-Centric Approach for Sustainable Business Processes

Cielo González Moyano[1], Finn Klessascheck[2,3(✉)], Saimir Bala[1], Stephan A. Fahrenkrog-Petersen[1,3], and Jan Mendling[1,3]

[1] Humboldt-Universität zu Berlin, Berlin, Germany
{c.gonzalez.moyano,saimir.bala,stephan.fahrenkrog-petersen,
jan.mendling}@hu-berlin.de
[2] Technical University of Munich, School of CIT, Heilbronn, Germany
finn.klessascheck@tum.de
[3] Weizenbaum Institute, Berlin, Germany

Abstract. Business Process Management (BPM) is mostly centered around finding technical solutions. Nudging is an approach from psychology and behavioral economics to guide people's behavior. In this paper, we show how nudging can be integrated into the different phases of the BPM lifecycle. Further, we outline how nudging can be an alternative strategy for more sustainable business processes. We show how the integration of nudging offers significant opportunities for process mining and business process management in general to be more human-centric. We also discuss challenges that come with the adoption of nudging.

Keywords: Nudging · BPM Lifecycle · Green BPM

1 Introduction

Business Process Management (BPM) aims at governing business processes throughout their lifecycle, with a continuous focus on their improvement. Business processes describe work undertaken for achieving specific goals for the organization, such as delivering a product to the customer. To this end, BPM develops novel techniques for the analysis and optimization of all aspects related to this work. An established category of process analysis techniques is process mining [1], which has the goal of providing data-driven insights about the process.

Research on process mining and other BPM techniques focuses on event data and the development of techniques to extract insights and recommendations from this data. As a result, a number of highly technical solutions to a various BPM problems have been developed. In many scenarios, considering human aspects can bring additional opportunities for process improvements. This is observed, among others, in the space of prescriptive process monitoring [2,3], where human actions shall be triggered based on process predictions. In other words, while the techniques developed in BPM may provide important actionable insights into the

© The Author(s) 2025
A. Delgado and T. Slaats (Eds.): ICPM 2024 Workshops, LNBIP 533, pp. 738–750, 2025.
https://doi.org/10.1007/978-3-031-82225-4_54

process, they become futile if not put into practice by stakeholders. Furthermore, by focusing on optimization, BPM endeavors often overlook their environmental impact [4,5].

To address this issue, we propose the integration of nudges [6,7] into BPM. Take for example the process of requesting, conducting, and reimbursing business trips, which is important for organizations so that they can correctly handle and recompense travel costs [8]. Notably, business travel, which has been linked with facilitating innovation and technology transfer [9], is predicted to account for 1 to 4% of global greenhouse gas emissions in 2050 [10]. Through nudging, employees requesting and reimbursing their business travels can be guided towards certain behavior that may contribute towards reducing the emission of business travel, and thus, the environmental impact. For example, they might be nudged to 1) conduct non-essential or domestic business trips via rail instead of plane (i.e., a mode of travel that causes fewer emissions), 2) voluntarily reimburse CO_2 emissions from their flights [11], 3) forego some business trips entirely in favor of e.g. video-conferencing, or 4) book flights that may be unfavorable for their travel experience, but cause fewer emissions, and 5) request reimbursement digitally instead of via a printed form.

In this work, we will show how nudging can be integrated into the BPM life-cycle to guide an organization, its stakeholders and process participants towards better and environmentally aware business processes [12]. Figure 1 illustrates the idea of nudging for sustainable business processes and the main concepts we draw upon: By influencing process participants and stakeholders to take sustainability issues into account, nudging influences an organization's business processes to be more environmentally aware. Further, by integrating sustainability concerns into business processes and their management, nudging ultimately influences the way an organization and its business processes impact sustainability.

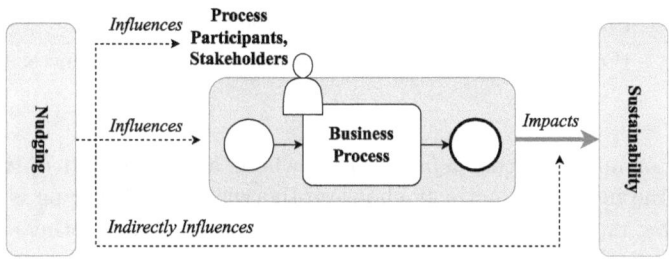

Fig. 1. Conceptual overview of Nudging for Sustainable Business Processes

The remainder of the paper is structured as follows. In Sect. 2, we provide a background on nudging and different types of nudges. In Sect. 3, we show how nudges can be integrated into different phases of the BPM lifecycle. Section 3 we highlight potential research directions for process mining researchers in the area of digital nudges. In Sect. 4, we discuss the implications of integrating nudging into BPM. In Sect. 5 we draw conclusions.

2   Background

Only a few works explore nudging in BPM [4,13]. In the following, Sect. 2.1 introduces nudging, Sect. 2.2 discusses its relevance on decision-making in BPM, and Sect. 2.3 highlights its potentials for Green BPM.

2.1   What Is Nudging?

Nudging is a term coined in behavioral economics and social psychology where people are subtly guided toward desired behaviors or decisions without restricting their choices or significantly changing the incentives [6,14]. A nudge increases the probability that an individual will make a specific choice or act in a particular way by modifying the environment to trigger an automatic cognitive response that favors a desired outcome [6]. To be considered as a nudge, the intervention must be simple and allow people to make their decisions [14]. Table 1 presents a categorization of the nudges based on some of the strategies that are employed to influence behavior. We briefly describe these the various types of nudge below.

Table 1. Types of nudges to guide user behavior

Category	Description
Default effect	Automatically select a particular option.
Social norms	Influence individual behavior according to the group behavior.
Framing effect	Alter the interpretation of information by changing its presentation.
Salience	Capture attention by making certain choices more visually prominent.
Priming	Trigger certain associations in the mind.
Simplification	Reduce the complexity of a choice.
Reminders	Produce timely notifications that encourage to act.
Feedback	Provide information about behavior and its consequences.

A type of nudge is the *default effect*, where a pre-selected option is chosen unless the individual actively chooses otherwise. Another type is the use of *social norms*, making people conform to what they perceive others are doing. For instance, informing individuals that a high percentage of their neighbors are donating to a fund-raiser program can significantly increase the donations [15]. Similarly, *framing effects*, where the way information is presented influences decision-making, is a commonly used type of nudge. For example, highlighting the benefits of taking a certain action (e.g., 90% success rate) in comparison to another option (e.g., 10% success rate) can influence the final decision [16].

Nudges commonly work because they inform people or make their decisions easier in an environment designed with that intent [6]. For instance, in *salience* nudges, placing healthier foods at eye-level in a store can increase their selection without removing less healthy options [17]. *Priming*, on the other hand, uses unconscious associations. Such associations have led participants in a diet study to change their eating behavior by being subtly exposed to diet-related words [18]. *Simplification* reduces the complexity of decisions, making it easier for individuals to make beneficial choices. An example is the simplification of health insurance plan options, where clear, concise information helps people choose plans that best meet their needs without feeling overwhelmed by complexity [19]. In a similar health context, an example for *reminders* is the notifications sent to patients to remind them to take medication, which has been shown to improve health outcomes [20]. As sending reminders brings advantages, providing *feedback* is also a nudging strategy that can positively influence behavior. For instance, providing households with feedback on their energy consumption compared to their neighbors has led to a significant reduction in consumption [21].

All the nudges depend on creating an environment that addresses the behavior simply and economically without limiting the choices [6,14]. To create this environment, nudging relies on an understanding of human behavior to design interventions that are both effective and ethical [22]. In this context, it cannot be considered a nudge if the intervention imposes significant restrictions on choices or introduces substantial economic incentives. For example, a mandatory policy that requires people to participate in a program is not a nudge given that it removes individual choice [14]. Similarly, offering large financial incentives to adopt a specific behavior, such as substantial subsidies for purchasing electric cars, does not qualify as a nudge. Although these alternatives are also effective, they align with traditional economic strategies rather than with nudging [23].

2.2   Why Is Nudging Relevant?

In their work, Thaler and Sunstein [6] argue that the necessity of nudging arises from fundamental aspects of human nature. Two systems characterize human thinking: the *reflective system* and the *automatic system* [24]. The first one, the *reflective system*, is deliberate and conscious. It requires individuals to process information carefully and consider the consequences of their actions. This system is typically associated with a slow and rigorous decision-making process.

On the other hand, the *automatic system* is quick and intuitive. It relies on heuristics to make decisions with minimal cognitive effort [24]. This system is typically used to make decisions that do not require exhaustive processing. However, humans do not always make complex decisions based on rationalization [25]. When situations are highly complex, uncertain, or overwhelming, and there is pressure to make a decision, humans tend to rely on the *automatic system* [6,24,26]. This results in faster decisions, but it can also lead to inadequate outcomes by relying on heuristics and biases or simply giving in to pressure.

Nudging strategies can effectively target these inadequate outcomes and support automatic decision-making by subtly guiding behavior through small changes in the environment or choice of architecture [6,24]. This makes nudging particularly powerful, aligning with how people naturally think and make decisions. Using nudging, it is possible to achieve various BPM goals [13], such as improving productivity with cost-effective approaches [6], promoting healthy and sustainable behaviors [20,21], and executing scale interventions with technology [27].

2.3   What Can Nudging Do for Green BPM?

Considering the environmental impact of businesses and their processes has become increasingly important, especially in light of climate change [28]. As a response, the field of *Green BPM* has emerged, which explicitly aims to incorporate the issue of environmental sustainability into the traditional notion of BPM [5] in order to increase the environmental performance of organizations [28].

Concretely, Green BPM is concerned with the modeling, deployment, optimization, and management of business processes in a way that particularly takes consequences on the environment into account. Further, organizational aspects beyond technical capabilities, such as culture (here, related to questions such as how "green" values can be communicated or individual stances of an organization's members can be influenced to favor less environmentally impactful behavior [5]), play an important role for a successful adoption of Green BPM [29]. However, existing research has mostly focused on technical aspects, such as modeling capabilities, with little focus on organizational culture [30,31].

As a consequence, we see significant potential in approaches such as nudging, in order to engage with BPM in general, and Green BPM in particular, in a way that goes beyond technical concerns and addresses cultural aspects. Notably, this would contribute to paving the way for further research on how attitudes and behaviors related to sustainable business processes can be shaped.

3   Nudging and the BPM Lifecycle

The BPM lifecycle consists of six phases: identification, discovery, analysis, redesign, implementation, and monitoring [32]. This section explores how nudging can be incorporated into each phase, providing a comprehensive framework for a human-centric and sustainable BPM approach.

3.1   Identification

As a first step, a process needs to be *identified*. The goal of this phase is to define what a specific process is. To this end, existing knowledge of what work is being carried out in the organization has to be rationalized. This requires managers to think about the status quo of how work is carried out in the organization. Before any BPM initiative occurs, knowledge about the processes may be fully unstructured and not explicit. Nudging can come into play to aid BPM initiatives' success by guiding an organization to learn and adopt BPM concepts and methods.

Helping Process Thinking. A starting point for process identification is *process thinking*. Typical process thinkers are able to identify the various ingredients of processes, such as actors, customers, value delivered to customers, and its possible outcomes. To change an organization's mindset toward process thinking, challenges must be faced. One big challenge is the *status quo* bias. This represents a cognitive challenge and can be addressed by designing specific learning nudges [33].

In more practical terms, processes are often pre-defined and identified within the functional silos of an organization. Nudging is used to break up this silos and promote the end-to-end vision of the process. To this end, different nudging strategies can be applied. For instance, *framing* the benefits of integrated processes in terms of improved efficiency and satisfaction of process participants can motivate stakeholders to adopt a broader view. *Priming* can be used to subtly influence stakeholders to think beyond their immediate functional areas. For instance, workshops and training sessions can start with examples and case studies that emphasize the importance and benefits of cross-functional processes. *Simplifying* the language and tools for describing and modeling processes can make it easier for users to create a shared understanding of the functions.

Once there is a holistic view of the process, nudging can help ensure that sustainability considerations are included. For instance, *framing* the business problem in terms of environmental impact can nudge stakeholders to consider sustainable practices when identifying relevant processes. Additionally, *default options* can prioritize the processes that have the potential for the highest environmental benefits. This can guide the selection of processes for the next phases of the BPM lifecycle.

Avoiding Scoping Mistakes. Scoping the process is key to the identification phase. Not any arbitrary chunk of work is considered a business process. To avoid mistakes in this phase, the BPM team takes a structured approach. Questions posed here are the following: Is it a process at all? Can the process be controlled? Is the process important enough to manage? Is the scope of the process not too big or not too small? Challenges are associated with all these questions.

One big problem in this phase is that the scope of the process is inappropriate, resulting in processes that are not in line with the organization's values. Nudges such as *framing*, *feedback*, and *social norms* are all useful in this phase. In the case of *framing*, presenting the criteria for process identification within the context of the goals of the organization, can help stakeholders to align their scope definitions. For example, framing the discussion around how the process contributes to sustainability goals can help ensure that the scoped processes are environmentally aligned. Implementing *feedback* loops where the initial scoping decisions are assessed can help in refining the scope over time. Providing feedback on the effectiveness and alignment of scoped processes with sustainability organizational values can nudge the BPM team to make necessary adjustments. With a similar approach, highlighting examples of well-scoped processes from within the organization or industry can serve as *social norms* that nudge the BPM team towards best practices. Sharing success stories and case studies where proper scoping led to significant improvements can create normative pressure to follow similar approaches.

3.2   Discovery

In the process discovery phase, the current state of relevant processes is documented, typically in the form of as-is process models. This can be done both through manual work, and automatically through process mining.

Mitigating Intrusiveness in Observation-Based Process Discovery. One method used for process discovery is the observation of the process workers. This method is often challenging since process workers find it intrusive and might behave differently when under observation. This issue can be mitigated by applying nudging techniques. First, an opt-out protocol can be used, where process workers by *default* participate in the observational study but can decide against their participation.

Furthermore, process workers might try to hide behavior that is considered unwanted. By explicitly encouraging them to show their workaround [34] a *social norm* could be introduced that ensures a feeling of safety necessary to understand how they act within the business process. Additionally, before the observation begins, *priming* workers with positive examples of how their input can lead to beneficial changes can help reducing anxiety and promoting honest behavior. This can be achieved via briefings or informational material.

Preventing Manipulation of the Event Logs. Automated techniques like process mining offer a less intrusive alternative to manual observation. However, process mining depends on event logs, which in turn depend on the interaction of the users with the system. Users might manipulate these logs or the interactions with the system to present a more favorable view of their actions [35,36]. In this context, providing users with regular *feedback* on how their accurate logging has contributed to process improvements can reinforce positive behavior and discourage manipulation.

3.3   Analysis

In the *analysis* phase, weaknesses of the processes are identified and reported, providing information about its alignment with the business goals.

Defining Goal-settings in Business Processes. The way goals are structured in a business can serve as a nudge. As an example, the aim could be that all processes produce zero waste, this would set a *primer* on what analytical questions might be asked in the analysis phase. Furthermore, certain goals can be the *default*, but it could be allowed to deviate from them, if they do not impact the goal of the business process, i.e., a zero-emissions goal might not be compatible to a process that requires employees to travel overseas within a set time frame.

Identifying Issues with the As-Is Process. Providing immediate *feedback* on the environmental performance of processes can motivate stakeholders to identify and prioritize issues related to sustainability. Comparative *feedback*, such as benchmarking against industry standards or best practices, can further drive improvement efforts.

Identifying Potential Use Cases for Nudges for Green BPM. Nudges can also be integrated into the business process, and the analysis phase can be used to identify the respective entry points. As an example, setting the *default* option in a process to sign a document electronically instead of requiring a signature on paper, or to book a means of transport with generally lower emissions for a business trip. The main task in the analysis point would be to identify areas where customers prefer non-sustainable options, and nudges could be used to encourage more sustainable behavior.

3.4 Redesign

The purpose of the redesign phase is to produce a newly designed process model, that overcomes the issues identified in the analysis phase. To this end, we identify two situations where nudging can help.

Tackling the Status Quo. Although there is a newly devised process model, resulting from the redesign, status quo bias within the organization can hinder its adoption by employees. Nudges can be designed to tackle this bias. For example, *default* settings can make the steps of the to-be process the first option. Additionally, *framing* can be used to highlight how the adoption of the to-be process improves certain issues or key performance indicators (KPIs). This can help shift the perception of the new process from a disruptive change to a beneficial enhancement.

Encouraging Sustainable Redesign Options. Nudging can promote the consideration of sustainable redesign options. Presenting *default* redesign templates that incorporate green practices can guide stakeholders toward more sustainable solutions.

Validating Redesign Choices. Leveraging *social norms*, redesign workshops can include examples of successful sustainable redesigns from other organizations. This can create a social expectation to adopt similar practices, thus nudging stakeholders toward environmentally friendly solutions.

Integrating Nudges into the Process. To ensure participants' conformance with the to-be process, nudges can be included in their personal workflows. For example, participants can be guided to perform tasks differently once the to-be process is adopted. Nudges such as *default* and *framing* are relevant here.

3.5 Implementation

In the process implementation phase, the changes required to move from the as-is process to the to-be process are prepared and performed, covering both organizational change management and automation. There are threats in the (mis-)use of information systems in which processes are implemented. We describe two main opportunities when an organization decides to implement its processes and what type of nudging can be used for that.

Addressing Potential Fears of Process Participants. Implementing new processes and executing them through information systems often encounters resistance from stakeholders who fear the unknown. This makes it hard to properly gather the correct requirements needed for the implementation of the process. Some of the nudges that may tackle this resistance are *default, framing,* and *simplification. Default* can be used to first describe the optimal process and then ask if the participants agree with this interpretation. *Framing* can be used to better gather information from participants. For example, framing questions in a way that emphasizes the positive outcomes of the new process can shift the focus from resistance to cooperation. Instead of asking, "What issues might arise from this new process?" a framing approach would be, "How will this new process help us achieve our goals and improve sustainability?". Complementing this, *simplification* may be used by providing participants with typical scenarios where they have to make a decision.

Avoiding Misuse of New Information System. The introduction of new information systems carries the risk that employees might misuse or underuse them due to a lack of understanding or intentional manipulation. Nudging strategies can help mitigate these risks. For instance, *salience* can guide the use of the system correctly. Visual cues such as color coding, bold text, or strategic placement can address the attention to critical features and usage guidelines. Additionally, *default options* to make the steps of the new process the primary option can reduce resistance to change and reduce mistakes. These default settings can also be used to support sustainable practices. For example, software systems can be pre-configured to optimize resource usage and reduce waste.

3.6   Monitoring

Process monitoring is the BPM phase in which data, typically stored in information systems, is used to analyze the status of the running business process.

Providing Transparent Feedback and Continuous Improvement. Providing transparent, real-time *feedback* on performance, including sustainability metrics, can nudge continuous improvement. Dashboards that visualize environmental performance can motivate ongoing adherence to sustainable practices.

Providing Timely Interventions Based on Monitoring Data. Using nudges such as timely *reminders* (i.e., alerts and notifications) when performance deviates from sustainability goals can prompt quick corrective actions. This ensures that the processes remain aligned with both operational and environmental objectives.

Supporting Data Collection and Reporting. Collecting data and reporting includes extracting and manipulating data from information systems event logs and presenting the analysis of the results to the user. Data collection may suffer from unsystematic and non-diligent behavior of the analyst in charge. Additionally, reporting may be of low-quality when results do not explain actual issues or fail to point to actionable items. The following nudges may be used. *Reminders* may help the analyst to act. This may be paired with defined data collection methodologies, such as [37]. For reporting, process mining results can be used to *frame* adherence to conformant behavior [38]. To aid this, a *feedback* nudge can be used, by providing direct information on the consequences of the the issues pointed out by process mining outputs.

4   Implications of Nudging for Green BPM

Next, we turn to discuss the opportunities (O) and challenges (C) of nudging for Green BPM:

O1 - Improved sustainability of processes. Nudging can be integrated into all phases of the BPM lifecycle. This allows us to incorporate ideas of sustainability within business processes. Therefore, nudging can be one tool towards sustainable business processes.

O2 - Designing interventions for more sustainability. Nudges can not only lead to more sustainable business processes at design time, but can also be integrated at runtime; leading to a more sustainable behavior of process workers and customers. Previous work showed how nudges can affect decisions for a desired outcome, and so far this type of intervention received limited attention in BPM.

O3 - Promote culture of sustainability. Nudges may help in raising consciousness in members of an organization that sustainability is an important aspect of business processes and their management. They may also influence individual stances and values towards sustainability-awareness, which is crucial for a successful adoption of Green BPM [29].

C1 - Nudges do not guarantee a desired outcome. The effectiveness of nudges can vary significantly depending on the context and individual differences [39]. Research has shown that not all nudges have the same impact across different cultures [40]. Therefore, what works in one company might not work in another. In this scenario, the design and testing of nudges are essential to ensure they achieve the intended result.

C2 - Evaluating effectiveness. Evaluating whether a nudge is achieving the desired outcomes, such as increased sustainability, presents another challenge. The methods used to measure the effectiveness of the nudge should take into consideration short and long-term sustainability results. Continuous monitoring and adjustment important to maintain the nudge's effectiveness.

C3 - Not a sole strategy Nudges should be seen as part of a broader strategy for promoting sustainable business processes. Relaying uniquely on nudging may jeopardize sustainability efforts. Other measures such as integrated sustainability management, eco-efficiency, sustainable innovation, and competitive advantage are crucial to have a holistic approach [41].

C4 - Ethical considerations One of the primary challenges in the application of nudging is the ethical implications of influencing behavior without explicit consent [14]. Thaler and Sunstein [6] argue that nudges should be transparent and not manipulative, but in practice, the boundary between acceptable influence and manipulation can be blurry. In the context of Green BPM, where the goal is to promote environmentally sustainable behavior, it is crucial to ensure that nudges do not infringe on individual autonomy or influence stakeholders to make unethical decisions. Therefore, transparency and preservation of freedom of choice must be an integral part of the implementation of the nudge. Additionally, nudges with illicit ends must be avoided even when there is general consent [14].

5 Conclusion

In this paper, we showed how nudging can be used alongside the BPM lifecycle. Especially, we argue how nudges can be used to as a tool to achieve more sustainable business processes and process mining. We discuss that, while providing opportunities for inducing stakeholders towards desired positive behavior, nudging comes along with challenges and ethical considerations. In future work, we plan to study specific instances of how nudges can be integrated into business process management tasks or specific business processes.

Acknowledgments. This research was supported by the Einstein Foundation Berlin under grant EPP-2019-524 and the BMBF under grant 16DII133.

References

1. van der Aalst, W.: Process mining: overview and opportunities. ACM TMIS **3**(2), 1–17 (2012)
2. Dees, M., de Leoni, M., van der Aalst, W.M.P., Reijers, H.A.: What if process predictions are not followed by good recommendations? In: BPM Industry Forum, CEUR-WS.org, pp. 61–72 (2019)
3. Fahrenkrog-Petersen, S.A., et al.: Fire now, fire later: alarm-based systems for prescriptive process monitoring. Knowl. Inf. Syst. **64**(2), 559–587 (2022)
4. Ghose, A., Hoesch-Klohe, K., Hinsche, L., Lê, L.: Green business process management: a research agenda. Australas. J. Inf. Syst. **16**(2) (2009)
5. vom Brocke, J., Seidel, S., Recker, J. (eds.): Green Business Process Management - Towards the Sustainable Enterprise. Springer (2012)
6. Thaler, R.H., Sunstein, C.R.: Nudge: The final edition. Yale University Press (2021)
7. Weinmann, M., Schneider, C., vom Brocke, J.: Digital nudging. BISE **58**(6), 433–436 (2016)
8. Pufahl, L., et al.: Performance variant and conformance analysis of an academic travel reimbursement process. In: BPI Challenge 2020 (2020)

9. Hovhannisyan, N., Keller, W.: International business travel: an engine of innovation? J. Econ. Growth **20**(1), 75–104 (2015)
10. McCain, M., Dowd, A., Salzer, D., Toothaker, E., Xu, S.: Business travel GHG emissions analysis: factors, tools, and cases for calculating GHG emissions and setting science-based targets for organizations. WRIPUB (2021)
11. Székely, N., Weinmann, M., vom Brocke, J.: Nudging people to pay CO_2 offsets - the effect of anchors in flight booking processes. In: ECIS (2016)
12. Klessascheck, F., Fahrenkrog-Petersen, S.A., Mendling, J., Pufahl, L.: Unlocking sustainability compliance: characterizing the EU taxonomy for business process management. In: Borbinha, J., Prince Sales, T., Da Silva, M.M., Proper, H.A., Schnellmann, M. (eds.) EDOC 2024. LNCS, vol. 15409, pp. 339–359. Springer, Cham (2025). https://doi.org/10.1007/978-3-031-78338-8_18
13. Bammert, S., König, U.M., Roeglinger, M., Wruck, T.: Exploring potentials of digital nudging for business processes. BPMJ **26**(6), 1329–1347 (2020)
14. Sunstein, C.R.: The ethics of nudging. Yale J. on Reg. **32**, 413 (2015)
15. Cialdini, R.B.: The science of persuasion. Sci. Am. **284**(2), 76–81 (2001)
16. Tversky, A., Kahneman, D.: Rational choice and the framing of decisions. In: Decision making: descriptive, normative, and prescriptive interactions, pp. 167–192 (1988)
17. Valenčič, E., Beckett, E., Collins, C.E., Seljak, B.K., Bucher, T.: Changing the default order of food items in an online grocery store may nudge healthier food choices. Appetite **192**, 107072 (2024)
18. Papies, E.K.: Goal priming in dieters: recent insights and applications. Curr. Obes. Rep. **1**(2), 99–105 (2012)
19. Handel, B.R.: Adverse selection and inertia in health insurance markets: when nudging hurts. Am. Econ. Rev. **103**(7), 2643–2682 (2013)
20. Pop-Eleches, C., et al.: Mobile phone technologies improve adherence to antiretroviral treatment in a resource-limited setting: a randomized controlled trial of text message reminders. AIDS **25**(6), 825–834 (2011)
21. Allcott, H.: Social norms and energy conservation. J. Public Econ. **95**(9–10), 1082–1095 (2011)
22. Bicchieri, C., Dimant, E.: Nudging with care: the risks and benefits of social information. Public Choice **191**(3), 443–464 (2022)
23. Thaler, R.H.: Misbehaving: the making of behavioral economics. WW Norton & Company (2015)
24. Kahneman, D.: Thinking, fast and slow. Macmillan (2011)
25. Gigerenzer, G., Gaissmaier, W.: Heuristic decision making. Annu. Rev. Psychol. **62**(1), 451–482 (2011)
26. Tversky, A., Kahneman, D.: Judgment under uncertainty: heuristics and biases: biases in judgments reveal some heuristics of thinking under uncertainty. Science **185**(4157), 1124–1131 (1974)
27. Weinmann, M., Schneider, C., vom Brocke, J.: Digital nudging. BISE **58**(6), 433–436 (2016)
28. Roohy Gohar, S., Indulska, M.: Environmental sustainability through green business process management. AJIS **24** (2020)
29. Couckuyt, D., Van Looy, A.: A systematic review of green business process management. BPMJ **26**(2), 421–446 (2019)
30. Couckuyt, D., Van Looy, A.: Green BPM as a business-oriented discipline: a systematic mapping study and research agenda. Sustainability (2019)

31. Fritsch, A., von Hammerstein, J., Schreiber, C., Betz, S., Oberweis, A.: Pathways to greener pastures: research opportunities to integrate life cycle assessment and sustainable business process management based on a systematic tertiary literature review. Sustainability **14**(18), 11164 (2022)
32. Dumas, M., Rosa, M.L., Mendling, J., Reijers, H.A.: Fundamentals of Business Process Management, 2nd Edn. Springer (2018)
33. Damgaard, M.T., Nielsen, H.S.: Nudging in education. Econ. Educ. Rev. **64**, 313–342 (2018)
34. Beerepoot, I., van de Weerd, I., Reijers, H.A.: The potential of workarounds for improving processes. In: BPM Workshops, pp. 338–350. Springer (2019)
35. Baier, T., Ciccio, C.D., Mendling, J., Weske, M.: Matching events and activities by integrating behavioral aspects and label analysis. SoSym **17**(2), 573–598 (2018)
36. Sinik, T., Beerepoot, I., Reijers, H.A.: A peek into the working day: comparing techniques for recording employee behaviour. In: RCIS, pp. 343–359. , Springer (2023)
37. van Eck, M.L., Lu, X., Leemans, S.J.J., van der Aalst, W.M.P.: PM^2 : A process mining project methodology. In: CAiSE, pp. 297–313. Springer (2015)
38. Hobeck, R., Pufahl, L., Weber, I.: Process mining on curriculum-based study data: a case study at a German university. In: ICPM Workshops, pp. 577–589. Springer (2022)
39. Hummel, D., Maedche, A.: How effective is nudging? a quantitative review on the effect sizes and limits of empirical nudging studies. J. Behav. Exp. Econ. **80**, 47–58 (2019)
40. Johnson, E.J., Goldstein, D.: Do defaults save lives? Science **302**(5649), 1338–1339 (2003)
41. Danciu, V., et al.: The sustainable company: new challenges and strategies for more sustainability. Theor. Appl. Econ. **20**(9), 7–26 (2013)

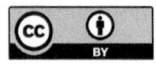

Extending Genetic Process Discovery to Reveal Unfairness in Processes

Muskan$^{(\boxtimes)}$ ⓘ, Felix Mannhardt ⓘ, and Boudewijn van Dongen ⓘ

Eindhoven University of Technology, Eindhoven, The Netherlands
m.muskan@tue.nl

Abstract. Fairness is an essential consideration for most processes in an organization since an equitable treatment of people involved in a process is often mandated by the rules or regulations. It is also desired from a social sustainability perspective. Many processes have a social impact on the actors performing the process activities and on the subjects affected by the process. We focus on the latter case in which a group of process subjects, such as citizens or patients, experiences unfair bias or discrimination during the execution of the process. Obvious instances of such discrimination in processes are negative decisions, but any change in process behavior for a certain group may be a symptom of unfairness. Process mining has been proposed as a method to analyze such unfairness. However, when considering the classical process discovery of a single overall process model, such hidden biases may get disregarded since they are relatively rare occurrences. To address unfairness in processes through process mining, we first need to reveal it in the process model. Towards this goal, we contribute a fairness-aware process discovery approach that extends a genetic algorithm with new quality measures for group fairness. We tested the approach on a set of synthetic but realistic benchmark datasets containing controlled cases of unfairness. The results indicate that in several cases our approach succeeds in revealing hidden biases against certain groups, which would remain hidden in state-of-the-art process discovery. We consider this as an initial step towards a comprehensive analysis of unfairness in processes.

Keywords: Evolutionary Tree Miner · Fairness · Genetic Algorithm

1 Introduction

Most business processes have a real-life impact on people. Consider a loan application process at a bank. The subject of each process case, the applicant, is an individual, and the decisions taken on the loan as well as the decision on which activities are performed bear direct consequences for them. Fairness [3] in such decision-making, both automated and non-automated, is an essential consideration for organizations from the viewpoint of the *social sustainability* of processes as well as often mandated by regulations.

Discrimination against process subjects is not only a matter in banking but is also present in other domains in which individuals are the main subject of a

ⓒ The Author(s) 2025
A. Delgado and T. Slaats (Eds.): ICPM 2024 Workshops, LNBIP 533, pp. 751–763, 2025.
https://doi.org/10.1007/978-3-031-82225-4_55

process, e.g., administration (citizens), healthcare (patients), or human resources (employees). Taking one of the group fairness notions, the decision to reject a loan based on the group membership of the applicant, e.g., their nationality, may be clearly unfair. However, in the enactment of processes, there are further decisions that possibly constitute unfair discrimination [11]. The repetition of certain activities, e.g., multiple background checks of the applicant, or the execution of certain activities, e.g., extensive documentation with wet-signed paperwork, may require the investment of additional resources (time and money) from the individual compared to other process cases. Conversely, skipping certain activities in a process case may also be considered unfair, e.g., skipping certain interviews that are part of a hiring process that leads to a rejection without due process.

Process mining can be used to scrutinize decision-making in the enactment of business processes and provide insight into the *social sustainability* of processes. An event log of the processes' control flow together with detailed information on process subjects may be sufficient information to reveal unfair discrimination. Indeed, process mining has been proposed to detect unfairness in processes [12]. Pohl et al. [12] show that it is possible to leverage traditional techniques and fairness definitions by building tabular representations of decisions or situations from event logs. However, such an approach is not positioned in the standard setting of process discovery in which the process is analyzed on the basis of a discovered process model. For process discovery to be useful in revealing unfairness it needs to clearly represent the discriminating behavior in the process model.

In this paper, we show that directly using process discovery for this purpose can be a challenge. Often, process discovery algorithms disregard the infrequently occurring discriminating process behavior as noise or fail to distinguish it from actual noise [8]. As a single process model is often the departure point of an analysis, this shortcoming of the process discovery may inhibit the detection and analysis of potential unfairness in processes. Therefore, we address the problem of revealing unfair discrimination experienced by subjects of a process through process discovery of a process model from an event log. We take on the setting of group fairness [3,12] in which the event log can be partitioned along the groups into sublogs. Then, the goal is to obtain a single process model that can be used to analyse unfair discrimination in process behavior towards one of the groups, which represents likely a minority of the cases in the event log.

Towards addressing this group fairness issue, we propose two novel quality measures that indicate how well the representation of process behavior in a process model is balanced among subsets of cases recorded in an event log. We integrate our proposed measures into the Evolutionary Tree Miner (ETM) [4], a genetic process discovery algorithm, and test if we can steer the process discovery to yield models that better represent the, possibly unfair, process behavior of the minority group. An experiment with a motivational example as well as four synthetic event logs recently proposed for fairness analysis [11] shows that process discovery algorithms, indeed, hide some kinds of unfair behavior. Our proposed measures can steer the ETM to discover a process model with a more balanced log fitness towards the groups and provides, in several cases, more useful models for analysing unfairness in processes.

The remainder of this paper is structured as follows. Section 2 further motivates our work with an example. Section 3 introduces two quality measures for fairness and Sect. 4 presents the results of the ETM.

2 Motivation

As indicated, we assume to be given a partition of an event log L into two sublogs L_a and L_b such that $L = L_a \cup L_b$. For our work, we take the standard definition of an event log as a finite multiset over finite sequences of activities. Given a set A of activities, $L \in \mathcal{B}(A^*)$ is an event log. Here, $\mathcal{B}(X)$ is the set of all multisets over set X. To motivate our approach, consider a process with activities $A = \{A, B, C, D, E, Y, N\}$ and a partition of event log L^1 into:

$$
\begin{aligned}
L_a^1 = [\langle A, B, D, E, N \rangle^{60}, & \qquad L_b^1 = [\langle A, B, D, E, B, N \rangle^5, & (1) \\
\langle A, B, D, E, Y \rangle^{40}, & \qquad \langle A, B, D, E, B, Y \rangle^1, & (2) \\
\langle A, C, D, E, N \rangle^{60}, & \qquad \langle A, C, D, E, B, N \rangle^5, & (3) \\
\langle A, C, D, E, Y \rangle^{40}, & \qquad \langle A, C, D, E, B, Y \rangle^1, & (4) \\
& \qquad \langle A, D, E, N \rangle^5, & (5) \\
& \qquad \langle A, D, E, Y \rangle^1, & (6) \\
\langle D, A, B \rangle^{10}] & \qquad \langle D, A, B \rangle^1] & (7)
\end{aligned}
$$

Note that the traces in L_b^1 are less frequent in the overall log $L^1 = L_a^1 \cup L_b^1$ and also show distinct process behavior that is not visible in L_a^1. In a real-world process, this log may be recorded by a hiring or loan application process and the partition may be the result of splitting the log into two groups based on *gender*, *race*, or *nationality* of the applicant. To illustrate it further, the applicant may not get invited for an interview, and/or a background check might be done twice for them. In our log, this is shown by the skipping of activities B and C, and another occurrence of B later in the process. Note that we also consider that some other, unrelated, infrequent behavior, which could be considered noise, namely $< D, A, B >$ may be contained as is often the case in real-world scenarios.

Applying process discovery to the overall event log L_1, for instance the Inductive Miner [9] and the ETM [4], returns the process models shown in Fig. 1. Both Inductive Miner and ETM do not yield a desired model for such event logs since the occurrence of the discriminatory behavior is usually a minority, which may be disregarded as noise by the algorithm. Moreover, when changing the noise filtering parameters to include all behavior other infrequent behavior that could be considered actual noise may obstruct the discovered model.

3 Equalised Log Fitness Using Genetic Process Discovery

We describe the proposed quality measures and how they can be used with the ETM approach to discover process models revealing unfairness. First, we briefly recall the ETM, then, we define the two measures.

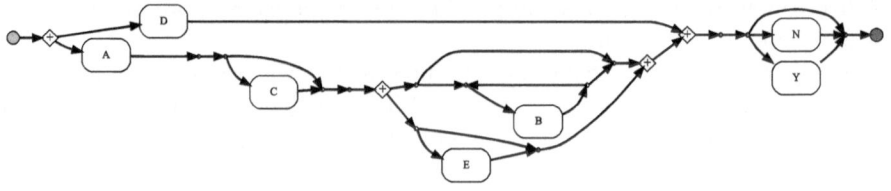

(a) Inductive Miner without filtering ($n = 0$).

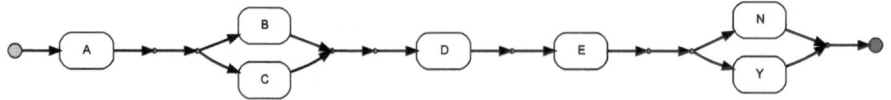

(b) Evolutionary Tree Miner and Inductive Miner with filtering ($n = 0.2$).

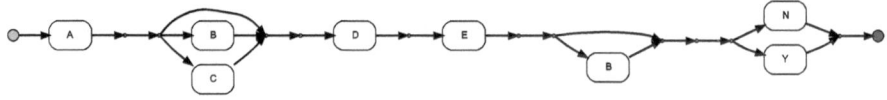

(c) Model discovered by our approach showing both kinds of unfair discrimination.

Fig. 1. Three process models discovered on L_1 by process discovery algorithms.

3.1   Evolutionary Tree Miner

The use of genetic or evolutionary algorithms for process discovery has been considered very early with the Genetic Miner [2,10] providing the first approach to discover Petri nets based on a genetic algorithm. The ETM [4] improved on this by providing a comprehensive framework for process discovery considering many different quality dimensions [5] such as *log fitness, precision, simplicity,* and *generalization.* The performance on these measures determines the survival of the candidates onto the next generation, hence, we refer to the combination of all dimensions as *survival fitness.* By using *process trees* as a block-structured representation, the search space of the ETM consists of only sound process models. This facilitates a more efficient exploration of the search space by guiding the *mutation* operations typical of a genetic algorithm [6]. Additionally, it allows more efficient computation of the proposed quality measures, for instance, computing the *log fitness* of a model via an *alignment* [1] between the event log and the model is faster for process trees and has seen recent improvements [13]. A recent development in genetic process discovery is X-Processes [7]. While it utilises a different survival fitness function and model representation, our quality measures can still applied to X-Processes. We leave a comparison of different genetic algorithms, including fairness considerations, for future work. As the primary goal of this paper is to demonstrate the feasibility of our approach and the relevance of our problem statement.

We briefly recall the approach followed by ETM as summarized by Fig. 2 taken from [4]. The ETM framework starts with *creating* an initial population of process tree models. Such population is typically random but could also be

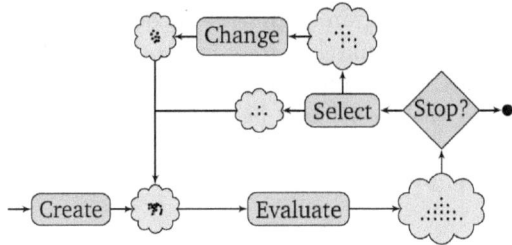

Fig. 2. The genetic algorithm in the ETM framework as illustrated in [4].

guided by the frequency of traces [6]. The main part of the generation loop is to evaluate the quality of all the models in the population according to a survival fitness function. Please note that here, *survival fitness* does not refer only to *log fitness* mentioned earlier but is determined as the weighted average of all selected quality measures, which should be normalized. Based on the evaluation of the population ETM checks a *stopping* criteria, e.g., a preset limit on the number of iterations of the loop also denoted as generations. Now, the main genetic part of the algorithm is concerned with selecting which candidate models to keep from the population and which of them to change through different operations. We are not further discussing the details of the change operations, which are explained in detail in [4], since they are not relevant to the presentation of our novel quality measure.

3.2   Proposed Measures for Equalising Log Fitness Between Groups

The quality of a process model is multi-faceted as shown in [4,5] which means that all of the quality measures are important and should be considered for process discovery. However, as a starting point for our research we selected *log fitness* as the most relevant measure to consider for uncovering unfair behavior. In fact, *log fitness* measures how much of the event log behavior is actually modelled and without unfair behavior being modelled it cannot be revealed. Of course, other quality dimensions are still relevant, e.g., *precision* is necessary such that we can better indicate in which part of the process unfair behavior was observed. Our quality measure can be used together with the regular *precision* measure and the investigation of additional measures for fairness is left for future work.

To ensure that the likely, infrequent unfair behavior is considered during the genetic search, we designed quality measures that aim to equalise the log fitness measured for both of the sublogs. We tested two formulas based on different considerations. The first formula for equalised log fitness is based on a normalised absolute difference EF_d and the second is based on a geometric argumentation EF_g. To define the measures, we briefly introduce *alignment costs* from which log fitness is typically determined and which we leverage directly. Given a process model M^1 and an event log L, an alignment [1] determines a model trace with the minimum number of mismatches to a log trace $\sigma \in L$. Each mismatch is typically assigned a cost, e.g., a unit cost of one, and the overall cost of aligning an individual trace to the model can be obtained. For our measure, we only require such cost function $cost(\sigma, M) \in \mathbb{Q}$ to be provided. Since the sublogs may be of different sizes, we are interested in the average alignment cost of a trace in a (sub) log.

Definition 1 (Average alignment cost). *Let L be an event log and let M be a process model. Let $cost(\sigma, M)$ be a function that returns the alignment cost, i.e., the cost of mismatches over some cost function, between any trace $\sigma \in L$ and the process model M. We denote with $avgCost(L, M) \in \mathbb{Q}$ the arithmetic mean of the cost of all traces in L:*

$$avgCost(L, M) = \frac{1}{|L|} \left(\sum_{\sigma \in L} cost(\sigma, M) \right)$$

We can now compute the average costs over all individual traces for each sublog and present our two quality measures in Definitions 2 and 3. Note that the two measures behave differently to small variations in average costs between the two group, as explained in more detail later.

Definition 2 (Equalised log fitness based on difference). *Let $L = L_a \cup L_b$ be an event log with a given partition into L_a and L_b. Let M be a process model. Let $\epsilon \in \mathbb{Q}_+$ be a small positive, non-zero constant. We define the equalised log fitness measure based on absolute difference $EF_d \in \mathbb{Q}$ in cost as:*

$$EF_d(L, M) = 1 - \left| \frac{avgCost(L_a, M) - avgCost(L_b, M)}{avgCost(L_a, M) + avgCost(L_b, M) + \epsilon} \right|$$

Definition 3 (Equalised log fitness based on geometry). *Let $L = L_a \cup L_b$ be an event log with a given partition into L_a and L_b. Let M be a process model. Let $\epsilon \in \mathbb{Q}_+$ be a small positive, non-zero constant. We define the equalised log fitness measure $EF_g \in \mathbb{Q}$ to be twice the angle in a right triangle spanned by both costs:*

$$EF_g(L, M) = \frac{2(avgCost(L_a, M) + \epsilon)(avgCost(L_b, M) + \epsilon)}{(avgCost(L_a, M) + \epsilon)^2 + (avgCost(L_b, M) + \epsilon)^2}$$

The addition of ϵ in Definitions 2 and 3, prevents undefined behaviour when both average costs are zero. In such cases, the equalised log fitness will be a perfect score of 1. The formula for EF_d may be more suitable than a normalized absolute difference if we want to penalize the differences while also considering

---

[1] In the ETM process trees are used as formalism but alignments make very few assumptions on the model only requiring every model trace to eventually properly finish. We do not further introduce process trees as our measure is independent of the modelling formalism used.

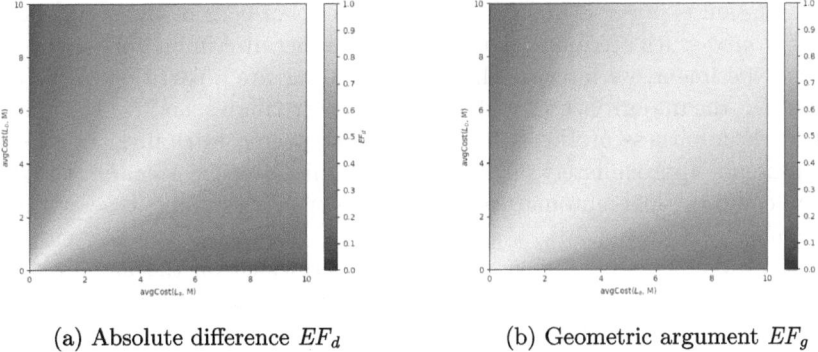

(a) Absolute difference EF_d (b) Geometric argument EF_g

Fig. 3. Values obtained for both EF_d and EF_g for cost varying from 0 to 10.

the overall magnitude of the two values, giving a more nuanced similarity metric than just the absolute difference alone. On the other hand, the formula for EF_g was obtained by following a geometric argumentation, i.e., it corresponds to $\sin(2\theta)$ where angle θ is in a right triangle spanned by both the average costs. This can be rewritten to the form in Definition 3 based on the identity $\sin(2\theta) = 2\sin\theta\cos\theta$.

Figures 3a and b visualise the proposed measures with $\epsilon = 1$ for the ranges of an average cost between 0 and 10 for each of the groups to facilitate their interpretation and show their unique characteristics. The graph for EF_d in Fig. 3a has a narrower yellow region, corresponding to an almost perfect score, whereas the graph for EF_g in Fig. 3b shows a broader area with a near-perfect score. EF_d hence punishes small differences more severely, which might be desirable in some scenarios. In contrast, EF_g has a relatively slow decrease of our measure for slightly different cost values. Consequently, we get a lower threshold for equalised log fitness measure, which might be desirable in certain real life applications where the notion of fairness is not so strict.

4   Evaluation

We implemented both proposed measures and added them to the ETM framework in ProM[2]. Then, we evaluated whether they, indeed, can help to reveal unfairness in processes based on event logs. The complete results are published as supplementary material[3].

4.1   Setup

Our evaluation builds on a recently published dataset [11] in which four exemplary processes, hiring, hospital, lending, and renting, are modeled, and unfair

---

[2] An updated ETM is available: https://github.com/promworkbench/Evolutionary TreeMiner/tree/etm-fairness and is added to ProM 6.14.

[3] Results are available at: https://dx.doi.org/10.5281/zenodo.13364712.

discrimination is injected in a controller manner. For each of the event logs, we have a ground truth attribute that indicates whether discrimination was applied. In this experiment, we leverage this attribute to create a partition of the event log into L_a, the majority cases with no protected attributes, and L_b, the minority cases with unfairness problems based on the protected attributes. In all cases, L_b represents approximately 30% of the data. In a real-life scenario, the partitioning could be done automatically using one or more suitable case attributes, e.g., gender or age.

The process discovery experiments were performed on the four event logs obtained from the benchmark dataset. Two process discovery algorithms were used: the ETM and the Inductive Miner infrequent (IMf). The regular ETM and the IMf were tested against the ETM having our equalised log fitness measures EF_d and EF_g. For evaluation, fitness and precision measures were computed on the overall logs and the two sublogs L_a and L_b.

The ETM results were computed over 3 repetitions with each 1000 generations for the benchmark log to mitigate the effect of randomness in the genetic algorithm. For the motivational example, we only used 300 generations once as it was sufficient to obtain stable results over this relatively small event log. The models for IMf were computed once for both of the event logs since it is deterministic. We use the default weight settings for the ETM, i.e., weight 10.0 for log fitness, weight 5.0 for precision and weight 1.0 for both generalisation and simplicity. The weight for the equalised log fitness measures was empirically chosen as 3.0 based only on the motivational example without any further optimisations.

4.2   Results

The performance of the discovered process models is evaluated by comparing the log fitness and precision values on our benchmark dataset. An overview of the results is presented in Table 1. Our primary goal is to minimize the difference in the log fitness between the two sublogs: L_a (the majority) and L_b (the minority or protected group), while still considering regular quality criteria such as log fitness and precision in the genetic search.

The hiring and lending logs show better performance with both our measures, especially with EF_d, as the fitness between the majority and minority sublogs is more equalised, with only a difference of 0.04 and 0.08. Surprisingly, for the hiring event log, our measures give an overall better fitting model on both L_a and L_b sublogs at the expense of precision. For the lending event log, our approach gives similar high fitness on L_b and slightly worse fitness on L_a. However, our measure, EF_g, gives slightly better precision. In case of the hospital log, we discovered that the simple process model is already perfectly fitting both sublogs. Only for the renting log, our approach resulted in a decrease in the log fitness with an increase in precision for both sublogs. Upon further investigated, we found out that it is likely due to difference in the way discrimination was introduced in this log, i.e., by the difference in the frequency of occurrence of some events. Furthermore, the renting log is different from the other logs, as it has two subprocesses. First, the process of getting the apartment after signing the contract.

Table 1. Result of four process discovery approaches: ETM with our proposed measures (EF_d, EF_g), without our measures (ETM) in the default configuration, and Inductive Miner infrequent (IMf) as a reference for a non-genetic approach. Average log fitness (fit_M) of the discovered models (M) is reported for both majority (L_a) and minority (L_b) sublogs, along with their difference $(\Delta_{fit_M}(L_a, L_b) = fit_M(L_a) - fit_M(L_b))$, and the precision (prc) is computed on the entire log.

Log	Metric	Model (M)			
		ETM	EF_d	EF_g	IMf
Hiring	$fit_M(L_a)$	0.89	**0.92**	0.91	0.93
	$fit_M(L_b)$	0.74	**0.88**	0.83	0.85
	$\Delta_{fit_M}(L_a, L_b)$	0.15	**0.04**	0.08	0.08
	$prc_M(L)$	**0.93**	0.55	0.71	0.71
Lending	$fit_M(L_a)$	**0.97**	0.91	0.91	1.00
	$fit_M(L_b)$	0.90	0.90	0.87	0.97
	$\Delta_{fit_M}(L_a, L_b)$	0.07	**0.01**	0.04	0.03
	$prc_M(L)$	0.82	0.76	**0.84**	0.90
Hospital	$fit_M(L_a)$	1.00	0.99	1.00	1.00
	$fit_M(L_b)$	1.00	0.99	1.00	0.97
	$\Delta_{fit_M}(L_a, L_b)$	0.00	0.00	0.00	0.03
	$prc_M(L)$	**1.00**	0.95	0.94	1.00
Renting	$fit_M(L_a)$	**0.95**	0.87	0.90	0.97
	$fit_M(L_b)$	**0.89**	0.77	0.83	0.86
	$\Delta_{fit_M}(L_a, L_b)$	**0.06**	0.10	0.07	0.11
	$prc_M(L)$	0.72	0.73	**0.79**	0.86

Second, the process of keeping the apartment by paying the rent on time, which is a repeating process. Additionally, the second sub-process is dependent on how often the late payment is accepted. Hence, the behavior in this log is more complex compared to other logs, which may necessitate additional generations for the ETM to converge. However, due to time restrictions, we limited ourselves to a thousand generations, as it gave a good model for all the other event logs.

Nonetheless, this is a side-affect of our approach that sometimes, it gives a reduced fitness on the sublog L_a compared to the model obtained with the regular ETM. Note that, this may be possible to mitigate by decreasing the weight of our measure EF from 3.0 or increasing the weight of log fitness from 10.0. However, the main aim of our approach is to have a discovered process model that can readily and clearly show the hidden discrimination.

To evaluate, whether the discovered process models are better suited to analyse unfair discrimination, we compared the process models discovered by regular ETM and our approach using the EF_d measure. We used EF_d instead of the EF_g since it achieved the best balance in fitness. The frequency annotated models are shown in Fig. 4. Clear differences can be seen in the discovered process models obtained with and without our measure. In contrast to the ETM, the

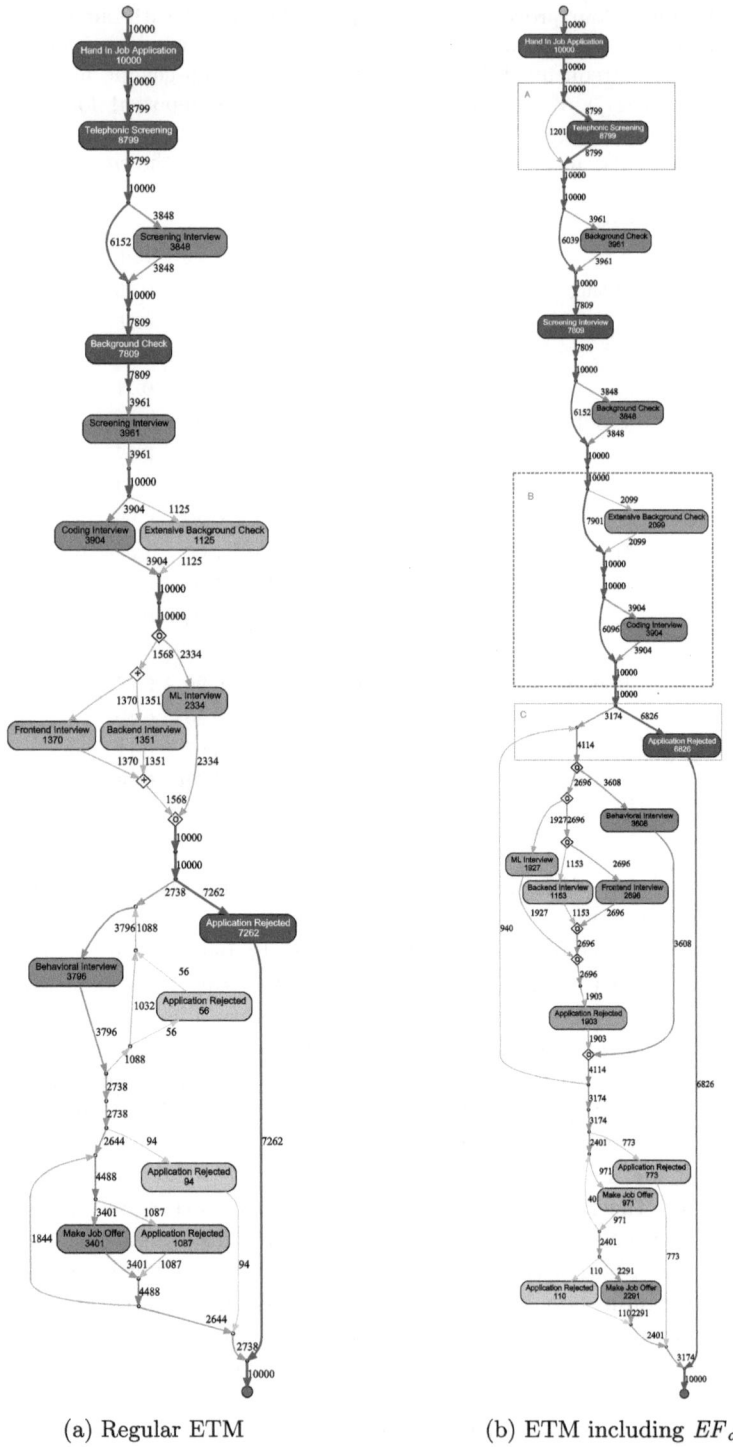

(a) Regular ETM   (b) ETM including EF_d

Fig. 4. Process models generated by ETM after 1000 generations with default configuration as well as including the quality measure EF_d on the hiring event log.

model returned by EF_d shows the possibility of skipping various activities such as, Telephonic interview (A, Fig. 4), Extensive background check, and Coding interview (B, Fig. 4). Additionally, it shows that the application can be rejected early on in the process i.e. without performing Frontend, Backend, or ML interviews (C, Fig. 4). Further, our approach depicted a second occurrence of Make job offer step. All these findings show the discriminatory behavior initially introduced in this unfair dataset. This includes higher rejection rates, fewer interview opportunities further leading to fewer job offers for the protected group [11].

5   Conclusion

This paper introduced two novel quality measures, denoted as *equalised log fitness*, that determine the balance in log fitness towards a process model for a partition of an event log into two sublogs. Our aim with this work was to more easily reveal any unfair discrimination in the process when using a single process model discovered from the overall log. By leveraging the measures, we guided a genetic process discovery approach towards returning a process model that strikes a better balance in representing the behavior of both groups. We evaluated our approach with a motivational example and a, recently published, benchmark event log. Our approach, indeed, improved the process model for some of the benchmark event logs and can re-discover all the unfair process behavior injected into the motivational example. The resulting process models showcased the hidden unfair behavior as well as improved the overall performance of the model for these logs.

Not all discrimination from the benchmark event logs was detected since our measures focus on *log fitness* which mainly detects missing or additional events. However, discrimination can also occur in terms of changes in the frequency of occurrence of some events, which would require a stochastic perspective on fairness in processes. This stochastic perspective is a possible avenue for extending this research by including a broader understanding of fairness and would help to reveal and explain the discrimination in some of our benchmark event logs such as the renting case. The dataset could also be varied by including more than two subsets of the event log, leading to a multi-class or multi-group problem with the aim of achieving a balanced log fitness among all of them. Additionally, the weight of the equalised fitness measures can be optimised or fine-tuned better with respect to the other quality measures. Finally, a more robust fairness metric can be investigated, and compared with the existing measures used in machine learning such as demographic parity, and equality of odds. Plus, the role of precision in such a fairness measure can further be discovered.

Acknowledgments. We thank Yi-Chiau Li for several discussions on fairness in the used benchmark dataset, which have greatly influenced this work. Part of this work is supported by the *Smart Journey Mining* project, funded by the Research Council of Norway (grant no. 312198).

References

1. van der Aalst, W.M.P., Adriansyah, A., van Dongen, B.F.: Replaying history on process models for conformance checking and performance analysis. WIREs Data Mining Knowl. Discov. **2**(2), 182–192 (2012)
2. van der Aalst, W.M.P., de Medeiros, A.K.A., Weijters, A.J.M.M.: Genetic process mining. In: Ciardo, G., Darondeau, P. (eds.) ICATPN 2005. LNCS, vol. 3536, pp. 48–69. Springer, Heidelberg (2005). https://doi.org/10.1007/11494744_5
3. Barocas, S., Hardt, M., Narayanan, A.: Fairness and Machine Learning: Limitations and Opportunities. MIT Press (2023)
4. Buijs, J.: Flexible evolutionary algorithms for mining structured process models. Ph.D. thesis, Mathematics and Computer Science (2014)
5. Buijs, J.C.A.M., van Dongen, B.F., van der Aalst, W.M.P.: Quality dimensions in process discovery: the importance of fitness, precision, generalization and simplicity. Int. J. Cooperative Inf. Syst. **23**(1) (2014)
6. van Eck, M.L., Buijs, J.C.A.M., van Dongen, B.F.: Genetic process mining: Alignment-based process model mutation. In: Business Process Management Workshops. Lecture Notes in Business Information Processing, vol. 202, pp. 291–303. Springer (2014)
7. Fantinato, M., Peres, S.M., Reijers, H.A.: X-processes: process model discovery with the best balance among fitness, precision, simplicity, and generalization through a genetic algorithm. Inf. Syst. **119**, 102247 (2023)
8. Koschmider, A., Kaczmarek, K., Krause, M., van Zelst, S.J.: Demystifying noise and outliers in event logs: review and future directions. In: Business Process Management Workshops. Lecture Notes in Business Information Processing, vol. 436, pp. 123–135. Springer (2021)
9. Leemans, S.J.J.: Robust process mining with guarantees - process discovery, conformance checking and enhancement, Lecture Notes in Business Information Processing, vol. 440. Springer (2022)
10. de Medeiros, A.K.A., Weijters, A.J.M.M., van der Aalst, W.M.P.: Genetic process mining: an experimental evaluation. Data Min. Knowl. Discov. **14**(2), 245–304 (2007)
11. Pohl, T., Berti, A., Qafari, M.S., van der Aalst, W.M.P.: A collection of simulated event logs for fairness assessment in process mining. In: BPM (Demos/Resources Forum), CEUR Workshop Proceedings, vol. 3469, pp. 87–91. CEUR-WS.org (2023)
12. Pohl, T., Qafari, M.S., van der Aalst, W.M.P.: Discrimination-aware process mining: a discussion. In: ICPM Workshops, LNBIP, vol. 468, pp. 101–113. Springer (2022)
13. Rocha, E.G., van der Aalst, W.M.P.: Polynomial-time conformance checking for process trees. In: BPM, LNCS, vol. 14159, pp. 109–125. Springer (2023)

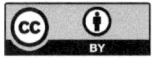

Can We Leverage Process Data from ERP Systems for Business Process Sustainability Analyses?

Dominik Schäfer[1,3]([envelope]), Finn Klessascheck[2,4]([envelope]), Timotheus Kampik[3,5], and Luise Pufahl[2,4]

[1] School of Management, Technical University of Munich, Munich, Germany
dominik.maximilian.schaefer@tum.de
[2] School of CIT, Technical University of Munich, Munich, Germany
luise.pufahl@tum.de
[3] SAP Signavio, Berlin, Germany
dominik.schaefer02@sap.com
[4] Weizenbaum Institute, Berlin, Germany
[5] Umeå University, Umeå, Sweden

Abstract. Sustainability is an increasingly important issue, which organizations need to take into account when assessing and improving their business processes. Doing so can contribute to enhancing an organisation's overall sustainability. *Green Business Process Management* is a line of research concerned with supporting organisations to integrate a sustainability perspective into their processes. However, existing approaches that assess sustainability on activity and process levels using, for instance, *Life-Cycle Assessment* (LCA) are often time-consuming and complex. Therefore, this work explores whether *Key Ecological Indicators* (KEIs) used to assess the sustainability of a business process can be calculated using data already available within an organisation. Following a case study methodology, we analyse nine real-world datasets extracted from a business process analysis system of a large enterprise software vendor. Results indicate that current data availability is insufficient for exact assessments. To address this issue, we introduce a high-level conceptual model and provide recommendations for action based on the observations of the case study.

Keywords: Sustainability · Green Business Process Management · Key Ecological Indicators · Process Data Analysis

1 Introduction

Five of the top ten global risks over a ten-year period can be assigned to environmental risks, highlighting the urgency of sustainability [1]. In addition, customers and society increase cultural pressures to drive sustainability [2]. Given the critical role of sustainability in today's world, organisations are increasingly

A. Delgado and T. Slaats (Eds.): ICPM 2024 Workshops, LNBIP 533, pp. 764–777, 2025.
https://doi.org/10.1007/978-3-031-82225-4_56

incentivised to identify their environmental impact [3]. Organisations can be viewed as collections of business processes designed to generate business value, and hence can improve their environmental footprint by enhancing these processes [4].

One promising approach for achieving this is *Green Business Process Management* [3]: it extends traditional Business Process Management (BPM), which focuses on concepts, methods, and techniques to design, execute and analyse business processes [5], by integrating a sustainability dimension and establishing sustainability as a business objective [6]. Central to this are Key Ecological Indicators (KEIs), e.g. Energy Consumption, which represent an extension of traditional Key Performance Indicators (KPIs) [7] and allow a quantitative assessment of business process sustainability [6]. KEIs are essential as, if reported and used correctly, they influence strategic decisions inside an organisation and thus can help to improve environmental performance [3].

Green BPM approaches include the introduction of *new notations*, such as emission annotations [8,9] to express sustainability aspects in process models, and the use of *Activity-based Costing (ABC)* approaches [8,9] or the integration with *Life Cycle Assessment (LCA)* [10], to quantify the environmental footprint of business processes. Notably, for many approaches which quantify the environmental footprint of business processes, the availability of data remains a critical issue: the Greenhouse Gas (GHG) protocol highlights that methodological rigour does not compensate for poor data quality [11]—indeed, related work such as [8,9] explicitly assume that key data such as carbon dioxide (CO_2) emissions of activity instances or power consumption data of machines involved in activity executions are known beforehand. However, it is unclear whether sufficient data of appropriate quality is actually available in practice.

To address this challenge, LCA databases have been developed, providing a wide range of data [12]. Notably, conducting an LCA study is usually complex and costly due to extensive data collection, stakeholder involvement, necessary reviews and updates [13]. These complexities underscore a significant research gap, particularly in situations where conducting a full LCA is not feasible, which is addressed in this work by answering the following Research Questions (RQs):

RQ1: To what extent is the data needed to calculate KEIs of Business Processes already present in large Business Process Analysis Systems?

RQ2: How could commonly found KEIs be approximated using real-world data?

To address these RQs, this work conducts a case study [14] in cooperation with one of the world's largest enterprise software vendors. The study performs a meta-data analysis of real-world process data to evaluate the feasibility of calculating common KEIs from this data. The process data is extracted from a Business Process Analysis tool, which sources its data from an Enterprise Resource Planning (ERP) system.

The paper is structured as follows: first, Sect. 2 introduces the theoretical background and related work, after which we identify common KEIs used in

Green BPM in Sect. 3. Subsequently, in Sect. 4, the methodology followed in the case study is presented and in Sect. 5, the results are described. Section 6 interprets these results and introduces a conceptual model for integrating KEIs in Green BPM while taking into account a lack of suitable data. Finally, we conclude the work and present future work in Sect. 7.

2   Background and Related Work

In the following, the research discipline *Green BPM* is introduced and common approaches to include a sustainability perspective into traditional BPM are presented.

2.1   Green BPM

Green Business Process Management is an emerging discipline that has increased in relevance over the years [4,7]. It extends traditional BPM by integrating a sustainability dimension [6] and putting this dimension into focus [3,6,13]. This work analyses business process data with respect to KEIs and evaluates whether commonly used KEIs are calculable with the given data. KEIs, also referred to as *Environmental Performance Indicators* [3,6], are indicators that organisations use to assess their environmental performance and to quantify their environmental impact [3].

2.2   Approaches for Incorporating Sustainability

Activity-based Costing. ABC aims at increasing the accuracy of product cost estimates by converting indirect costs in the traditional accounting system into direct costs [15]. This is achieved by allocating resource costs such as wages to cost objects based on their activity consumption [15]. It has found adoption in Green BPM, with multiple contributions leveraging ABC-based approaches to incorporate a sustainability perspective into business processes (e.g., [8–10]).

Life Cycle Assessment. LCA is a tool used to evaluate the environmental impact and resource utilisation across the entire life cycle of a product or service [12]. Fundamental to LCA is the *cradle-to-grave* perspective, meaning that it considers the entire life cycle of the process or product when assessing the environmental footprint [12]. In practice, LCA is widely used and specified by two international standards [12]. The cradle-to-grave perspective is also subject to some critique, as it is challenging to obtain all necessary data: LCA is extremely data-intensive and the reliability of its results highly depends on the data used [12]. To provide this data, several LCA databases have been developed, which provide environmental data on numerous products and essential services that are required in many LCAs [12].

Approaches for Green BPM. A tertiary literature review [13] clusters Green BPM approaches into the six capability areas of *modelling, deployment, optimisation, management, culture* and *structure*. For this work, especially the *modelling, deployment* and *management* areas are considered relevant. *Modelling* includes the three approaches [7] extending notations (e.g., [8,9]), adding notations (e.g., [16,17]), and adding patterns (e.g., [18]). *Deployment* and *management* both deal with KEIs, while the main difference is that the deployment area deals with the *application* of KEIs and the management area deals with the *definition* of them [13]. Relevant works in the *deployment* capability area include the measuring and controlling of emissions (e.g., [19]), whereas the *management* area includes the extension of the traditional business process lifecycle into the green business process lifecycle (e.g., [4]).

However, research so far does not explicitly address to which extent the data necessary for incorporating sustainability into business processes by calculating KEIs is available in average companies *without* relying on LCAs. Usually, the data needed to incorporate the sustainability dimensions is considered as given or is elicited manually (see, e.g., [8,9]). Even though using LCA databases to obtain the required data (see e.g., [10]) is feasible, a LCA study is still complex and costly, requiring extensive data collection, stakeholder involvement, and continuous reviews and updates [13]. To the best of our knowledge, there are no relevant studies focusing on whether KEIs, known from literature and useable for assessing the sustainability of a business process, can be calculated using data available within companies. Thus, this work addresses this research gap and focuses on KEIs. Focusing on KEIs has the advantages that they *i)* enable the assessment of whether a business process improves its sustainability over time [6]; *ii)* can serve as powerful tools that can influence the strategic decisions of organizations [3]; iii) align with the call made in [3] for research aimed at identifying the *right KEIs*.

3   Key Ecological Indicators in Green BPM

To analyse the availability of business process data needed for calculating KEIs, we first identify which KEIs are commonly used in Green BPM by drawing on existing Systematic Literature Reviews (SLRs).

KEI Identification. In a tertiary literature review, Fritsch et al. [13] observe that only three SLRs they analysed, namely [3,6,20], explicitly provide an overview of KEIs. However, as [3,20] display the same sustainability aspects only with a slightly different number of corresponding primary papers [13], only [3] is included here for further analysis. In addition, examining the references of the aforementioned SLRs led to the inclusion of [21]. Consequently, we identify KEIs commonly used in Green BPM based on the SLRs [3,6,21].

Table 1 presents the top three KEIs from each of these SLRs and their reported occurrences. To identify similarities across the SLRs, we assigned codes to unique KEIs. While the authors of [3] and [6] explicitly identify the top three KEIs and provide the percentage of their occurrence in the reviewed papers, Gräuler and Teuteberg [21] only display an absolute number of references per identified sustainability metric. Thus, in the latter case, the number of references per KEI was counted and divided by the total number of relevant papers identified by [21] and the top three KEIs with the most references are displayed. In total, [3] analysed 49 sources, [6] 56 sources, and [21] 31 sources.

Table 1. The top three KEIs identified in each SLR [3,6,21]

Roohy Gohar & Indulska [3]			Hernández González et al. [6]			Graeuler & Teuteberg [21]		
Code	Top KEIs	[%] ↓	Code	Top KEIs	[%] ↓	Code	Top KEIs	[%]↓
EC	Energy Consumption	31%	EM	Emissions	71%	EC	Energy Efficiency/ Consumption in e.g. kWh/unit	29%
C2	CO_2 footprint	22%	EC	Energy consumption	61%	GH	Emissions of greenhouse gases, ozone-depleting substances or other emissions in e.g. CO_2-equivalents	26%
GH	other GHG emissions	20%	UM	Use of materials	29%	WG	Waste Generation in e.g. kg/unit	13%

By examining how often each KEI occurred in Table 1, we aggregate the KEIs of the three Green BPM SLRs and arrive at a final set of common KEIs. *Energy Consumption* (*code: EC*) was found in all three SLRs and is a final KEI. GHG Emissions, Emissions and CO_2 (*codes: C2, GH & EM*) all refer to air quality and are summarised under the final KEI *Emission*. Material Use & Waste Generation (*codes: UM & WG*) both refer to physical goods and are related to each other as material use can also lead to waste, and thus are summarised under the final KEI *Material Use & Waste Generation*. The three *final KEIs* are only referred to as *KEIs* in the remainder of this paper.

KEI Calculation. For being able to assess whether the three KEIs identified above can be calculated using data from the case study, we first present approaches commonly used in the literature for calculating them.

Energy Consumption. To calculate the energy consumption of an activity, [9] examines energy-related parameters such as the wattage a machine utilises to perform a specific action expressed in kW, the total apparent power (KVA) or the ratio between both (power factor). Similarly, the GHG Protocol [11] suggests methods to gather energy consumption data, such as through meter readings or invoices. Once this data is obtained, energy data can further be used to calculate the resulting CO_2 emissions as demonstrated in [8]. They used data for energy consumption combined with a calculation tool provided by the GHG protocol [11] to calculate the resulting CO_2 emissions.

Emissions. When discussing emissions, this study understands *emissions* as GHGs as used in the GHG-Protocol [11]. It is a broad definition and includes both CO_2 *emissions* and *other emissions* as previously found in the literature (see Table 1). In general, to calculate the GHG emissions, the GHG Protocol [11] provides over 14 different calculation tools. For example, to calculate direct and indirect CO_2 emissions from the stationary equipment or to calculate the CO_2 emissions from the calcination process in cement production. More abstractly, [9] calculates GHG emissions of an activity as *activity data * emission factor*. Emission factors in this context are ratios that indicate how much, e.g. GHG emissions, per base unit or activity consumption, e.g. hour of use, are emitted [11].

Material Use and Waste Generation. To calculate material use & waste generation, again, it is essential to have access to data tracking the actual use or waste. In [8] the authors calculate the emission of paper consumption by using the formula *weight of paper * emission factors for manufacture of paper*. Thus, in order to calculate the environmental footprint, it is again necessary to determine an emission factor.

4   Methodology

To address the research questions we outline in Sect. 1, we conduct a *case study*, following the six-step methodology proposed by Recker [14].

For *planning* the study, we aimed to identify the extent to which data needed for calculating KEIs of business process is already present in real-world business process analysis systems and investigate how far common KEIs can be calculated using this data. With this, we justify the use of a case study methodology since case studies are well suited if the goal is to intensively study a contemporary case in its natural setting to understand its complexity [14], which applies to this work.

For the *design step*, we chose an *exploratory* research objective, a *positivist* epistemology, and a *holistic single case* design [14]. As a data source, we selected the pseudonymous *System Alpha*, which is a business process analysis system used worldwide by customers of the enterprise software vendor where the case study is conducted. It provides fast insights into the performance of over 100 defined business processes. The data required to display these business processes is exclusively collected from the underlying ERP system by using a data collector, which regularly gathers predefined process data from the different ERP tables.

As to the *preparation* stage, we first performed a preliminary inspection of the entire data inside System Alpha. Out of 104 available processes, nine were chosen with the support of internal experts. These nine processes focus on the domains of *transportation* and *logistics*, which significantly impact a company's environmental footprint [22], and are, according to internal experts of the case study's company, among the most commonly used transportation processes by customers.

The *collecting and analysing* stages were conducted iteratively, with each step informing the next. Initially, nine datasets in the form of CSV files were extracted from System Alpha for nine selected processes. To create the final meta-dataset, only the column names were retained from each process dataset, as these indicate which types of data are stored in each column, representing the data the customer has access to in their system. After data cleaning, all column headers were consolidated into a single meta-dataset, with each original column header transformed into an entry in the new meta-data analysis table. To enhance the interpretability of each original column, demo values were added by accessing an internal demo version of System Alpha containing example values for each column. Afterwards, the frequency of each column was counted and analysed.

After this first *collecting-analysing* iteration, a second iteration was done. First, a company-internal version of the Large Language Model (LLM) model of OpenAI, *GPT-4-Turbo*, was used to describe each column header in exactly one sentence and further enhance their interpretability. Subsequently, a categorisation of the data regarding the *Informative Value* was done. For this, a manual assessment was conducted identifying whether the information stored in an individual column contains useful information for calculating KEIs *by itself* (*e.g., the field 'delivery quantity (lfimg)' with the value '3.0'*) or whether the information must be *combined* with data from other systems—such as ERP systems—to become useful (*e.g., the field 'Company Code (BUKRS)' with the value 'F010'*). Additionally, a second categorisation, called *data-type* categorisation, was done by following a qualitative, inductive coding approach to identify the different data types existing in the meta-dataset, such as *Dates & Timestamps*. Using this categorisation, relevant units, such as *kWh* for *energy*, were searched in the analysis in Sect. 5.2. Finally, the meta-dataset was searched for relevant synonyms potentially containing information for calculating KEIs. These synonyms were generated using two online thesauruses,[1] and the meta-dataset was searched for these synonyms and their combinations. The detailed search protocol can be found online in a GitHub repository.[2]

After finishing the preceding steps, the meta-dataset was complete, with an excerpt provided in Table 2. It consists of six columns: *Column Name* stores the names of the original columns extracted from System Alpha, and is the primary key of this table. [#] counts the frequency with which each column occurs in the original nine datasets. *Demo Values* provides three, ideally non-null, demo values for each entry. *LLM-Description* contains one sentence describing each entry. *Informative Value* holds the assigned categorisation value for this entry. *Data Type* contains the assigned categorisation value for this entry.

Finally, the *sharing* stage, the sixth and final step proposed by Recker [14], is represented by the following sections displaying the case study's results and findings.

---

[1] See https://dictionary.com, https://www.collinsdictionary.com/dictionary/english-thesaurus [Accessed: 20/08/2024].

[2] https://github.com/dominik-maximilian-schaefer/icpm2024 [Accessed:22/08/2024].

Table 2. Excerpt of the final meta-dataset

Column Name	# ↓	Demo Values	LLM Description	Informative Value	Data Type
Currency (WAERS)	3	'EUR', 'RUB', 'USD'	Represents the currency used in the financial transactions, like USD or EUR.	direct	Amounts, Values & Units

5 Results

This section describes the result of our case study by first describing the dataset we created and subsequently analysing it regarding the question of which common KEIs can be calculated based on it.

5.1 Final Meta-Dataset

The final meta-dataset with 422 entries is provided in the GitHub repository linked above. When examining the *frequency* (#) of each column described, it is notable that approximately 32% of all column names appear in more than one of the original nine datasets. The majority of columns (68%) appear only once, while about 22% occur twice, 5% are found in three datasets, and the remaining 5% occur in four or more datasets.

The results of the *informative value categorisation* show that overall, 44% of all entries are considered to have direct value, while 56% are considered to have indirect value. This means that 56% of all 422 entries are considered to be not directly interpretable, and additional data sources, such as an ERP system or an LCA database, are required for deriving meaningful insights. Conversely, 44% of all entries are considered to have direct value, which means that the information is inherently interpretable.

The *data type categorisation* resulted in the following values: *Unique Identifiers (UIDs) (30%), Status & Indicators (28%), Dates & Timestamps (25%), Amounts, Values & Units (16%)* and *Ambiguous (1%)*. The significant proportion of information categorised under UIDs suggests that much of the data may not be directly useful for KEI calculation, as it cannot be further interpreted without additional context. This categorisation is mostly used to filter for relevant units in the next step.

5.2 Key Ecological Indicators

After describing the final meta-dataset, we now investigate it regarding data needed to calculate the KEIs of *Energy Consumption, Emissions* and *Material Use & Waste Generation*. The analysis is structured in two parts: First, based on the data type categorisation; second, based on the synonym analysis.

Analysis Based on Data Type. To identify energy-related parameters like *kWh* or other relevant units and quantities used for calculating the three KEIs (see Sect. 3), the meta-dataset was filtered according to the dimension *Amounts, Values & Units.* Of the 68 entries identified, 55 pertained to quantities or numerical data, while 13 related to units. However, none of these units were relevant to the KEIs, as they mainly referred to currencies or basic measurement units like *kilograms* or *liters.* The 55 entries on quantities were mainly pertinent to the KEI *Material Use & Waste Generation,* with fields like *withdrawal quantity (enmng), goods receipt quantity (gr_ amount),* and *delivery quantity (lfimg)* providing insights into material usage. Fields like *confirmed scrap (iasmg)* and *unplanned goods issue (unplanned_ gi)* were significant for understanding waste generation.

Analysis Based on Synonyms. The second approach for identifying relevant data for calculating the three KEIs involved using synonyms, as detailed in Sect. 4. In the GitHub repository linked above, the two tables depicting the results from the synonym search are provided. The first table depicts the synonyms (e.g. *power* and *electricity*) found for each single term (e.g. *Energy* and *Consumption*) of which the single KEIs (*e.g. Energy Consumption*) are composed of, while the second table depicts the synonyms that were found for each compound term of KEIs (e.g. *Energy Consumption*). Further, the final search protocol is provided there, outlining exactly which synonym sets were searched within the meta-dataset, with the search conducted using substring matching across the columns *Column Name, Demo Values,* and *LLM Description.* An excerpt of the search protocol is shown in Table 3. The first column is a continuous numbering, the second column indicates the corresponding KEI, the third column depicts which synonym set was used for the search (e.g. synonym set S1 contains all synonyms for energy; if two or more codes are combined with x, the cartesian product of the synonym sets was built, and subsequently, a search using all the resulting elements was done), the fourth column indicates an example word contained in the synonyms set, the last column contains the number of results found in the meta-dataset when searching for all synonyms under the respective code.

Table 3. Excerpt of the search protocol

Nr.	KEI	Code	Example	[#]
1	Energy Consumption	S1	"Energy"	29
7	Emissions	S5	"Emission"	30
21		S9	"Material"	142
23	Material Use &	S11	"Waste"	4
25	Waste Generation	S9 x S10	"Material" x "Use"	2
27		S20	"Material Use"	1

Analysing the results shows that for the KEI *Energy Consumption*, S1 found 29 unique column names. Examining all these matches shows that no column actually refers to energy consumption. Indeed, only matches for *potential* and *service* (as synonyms of Energy) were found. For the KEI *Emission*, only S5 has more than zero results. Examining these results, only matches for *issue, release, ejection and venting* were found, no match providing relevant information to calculate the KEI *emissions*. For the KEI *Material Use & Waste Generation*, *S9, S11, S9 x S10* and *S20* are relevant. The matches support the previous findings based on the *data type categorisation*, where a substantial number of columns were found by analysing *quantities*. All fields found there are also found examining the matches here. Thus, the preliminary conclusion can be drawn that data needed to calculate the KEI of *Material Use & Waste Generation* is available in the meta-dataset.

6   Discussion

This section discusses our results in the light of existing research, provides recommendations for action based on the findings of this case study and highlights limitations.

6.1   KEIs in Literature vs. Practice

Regardless of which KEI is considered, the literature typically calculates them by first gathering relevant *activity data* for each KEI, and then applying an *emission factor* to calculate the environmental footprint (see Sect. 3). The following discussion is structured according to these two steps:

Activity Data. Gathering *activity data* is the basis for the calculation of the KEIs and *must* be incorporated into the business process data so that it can effectively be used [23]. Primary activity data, particularly in the context of environmental footprints of products, is usually captured through equipment control sensors that measure i.a. flow rates and temperatures; however, this data is often *not* collected within the EPR system due to being perceived as having little value [24]. Examining the *activity data* available for *Energy Consumption* and *Emissions*, we find that the analysed meta-dataset does not provide useful data. Neither the analysis using the data type categorisation nor the analysis based on synonyms found any relevant fields that contain potential data that indicate one of these KEIs. For *Material Use & Waste Generation*, a substantial amount of data is found in the meta-dataset.

Emission Factors. Examining the *emission factors* which are used in literature when quantifying the environmental footprint of KEIs, the lack of data becomes even more salient: Data representing concrete emission factors is not found for any of the three KEIs. This possibly explains the success of LCA databases, as they provide the necessary emission factors [12], enabling such calculations to be performed (e.g., [10]).

From this case study, we can conclude that the availability of data required to calculate KEIs in large business process analysis systems is limited. Out of the three KEIs, *activity data* was only found for *Material Use & Waste management*, while data useful for *emission factors* was not found.

6.2 Recommendations for Action

Based on our findings, we propose three recommendations. First, use *indirect approximation* to quickly evaluate business process sustainability with *available* data, avoiding complex, time-consuming methods such as LCA. Second, *refine data collectors* to use more relevant data that is *available* in the ERP systems but not used in business process analysis systems. Third, *leverage expert knowledge* to improve the understanding of complex and partially ambiguous ERP data. These recommendations also address RQ2 and are explained in the following.

Indirect Approximation of KEIs. Our analysis indicates that data for exact sustainability analysis is not necessarily available in ERP systems. To mitigate this issue, it may be feasible to devise heuristics-based approaches that focus on inferring actions for sustainability improvements, given the data that is available. Therefore, we outline a conceptual model in Fig. 1 that might assist in improving the sustainability of business processes by using only available data.

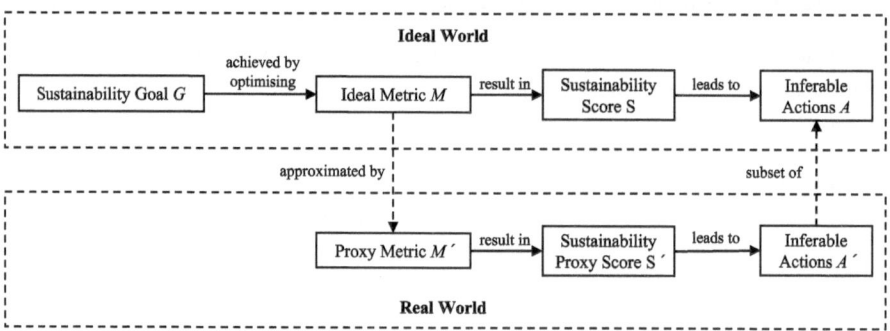

Fig. 1. Conceptual model for heuristics-based sustainability improvement in Green BPM.

The proposed solution involves setting a sustainability goal G, such as improving the environmental sustainability of a specific process. In an *ideal world*, this would be achieved by optimising *ideal metrics*, like the CO_2 emissions from transporting goods. These metrics form a *sustainability score S* which guides *inferable actions*. However, due to data limitations in the *real world*, *ideal metrics* often cannot be calculated. Instead, *proxy metrics* are used, such as the mode of transportation, to approximate the CO_2 footprint. By inferring the mode of transportation, such as inferring that a plane is used for transportation between Singapore and Munich based on a travel time of 20 h and the distance, we can make informed inferences about the environmental impact of the process, even without detailed CO_2 data or data specifying which transportation mode was used.

Refine Data Collectors. Enhancing the *data collectors*, which regularly collect data for systems such as System Alpha, is crucial: primary data central to sustainability assessments often does not penetrate the ERP system due to its historically low perceived value [24]. Additionally, about 50% of current entries offer only indirect informative value (see Sect. 5). By refining the data collector, we can increase the data's utility for sustainability assessments. For instance, extracting specific material details (e.g., type, weight) from the ERP system could enable rules that correlate larger or heavier items with a higher environmental footprint. Similarly, understanding delivery priorities could inform sustainability decisions, such as recognising that higher priority deliveries may have a greater environmental impact.

Leverage Expert Knowledge. Finally, evaluating the sustainability of business processes is complex and requires in-depth understanding of the data involved. For example, consultation with process experts revealed that depending on the process, 'scrap' can either be waste or be reintegrated into production, meaning it is no waste at all. This underscores the need for careful interpretation of process data by leveraging expert knowledge. When starting a new project, especially in specific sectors like transportation, it is essential to first understand the processes in detail, often through expert consultations.

6.3   Threats to Validity

This study is not without limitations: First, the data stored within each column is demo-data. However, as this case study analysed the column names and not the data within them, these demo-values are of secondary value and were only used to increase interpretability of each column. Second, the data analysis was done primarily by the first author. To mitigate this, the methodology is clearly documented, with additional materials provided in the GitHub repository linked above. Third, an LLM was used to enhance the data model with column descriptions. While LLMs can produce inaccurate information or hallucinate, this work mitigates that risk by using the LLM output as just one of five input sources, thoroughly reviewing it and cross-checking it against known attributes.

7   Conclusion

Our findings indicate that data for sound and complete sustainability analyses is not necessarily readily accessible in business process analysis systems, which extract their data from ERP systems. From a practice-oriented perspective, this limitation is crucial to acknowledge, as it highlights the importance of continued initiatives to increase sustainability data maturity and suggests that the data quality of existing sustainability reporting may be problematic. To still support

organisations in assessing the sustainability of their business processes, we introduce a high-level conceptual model using only available data, which may serve
as a starting point. Future work can: *i)* further expand research into data availability and quality for sustainability analysis, for example by analysing a variety
of source systems; *ii)* devise and evaluate frameworks and metamodels for the
extraction and analysis of sustainability data from ERP systems; *iii)* further
refine and evaluate heuristics-based approaches for sustainability analyses.

References

1. World economic forum: the global risks report 2024
2. Seidel, S., Recker, J., vom Brocke, J.: Sensemaking and sustainable practicing:
   functional affordances of information systems in green transformations. MIS Q.
   37, 1275–1299 (2013)
3. Roohy Gohar, S., Indulska, M.: Environmental sustainability through green business process management. Aust. J. Inf. Syst. **24** (2020)
4. Maciel, J.: The core capabilities of green business process management – a literature review (2017)
5. Weske, M.: Business Process Management: Concepts, Languages, Architectures,
   3rd edn. Springer, Berlin, Heidelberg (2019)
6. Hernández González, A., Calero, C., Pérez Parra, D., Mancebo, J.: Approaching
   green bpm characterisation. J. Softw. Evol. Process **31**(2), e2145 (2019)
7. Couckuyt, D., van Looy, A.: A systematic review of green business process management. Bus. Process. Manag. J. **26**(2), 421–446 (2020)
8. Recker, J., Rosemann, M., Hjalmarsson, A., Lind, M.: Modeling and analyzing the
   carbon footprint of business processes. In: vom Brocke, J., Seidel, S., Recker, J.
   (eds.) Green Business Process Management, pp. 93–109. Springer, Berlin, Heidelberg (2012)
9. Wesumperuma, A., Ginige, A., Ginige, J., Hol, A.: Green activity based management (ABM) for organisations. In: ACIS 2013 Proceedings (2013)
10. Klessascheck, F., Weber, I., Pufahl, L.: Sopa: a framework for sustainability-
    oriented process analysis and re-design in business process management. Inf. Syst.
    and e-Bus. Manag. (2025) https://link.springer.com/article/10.1007/s10257-024-
    00695-x
11. World resources institute and world business council for sustainable develop-
    ment: the greenhouse gas protocol: a corporate accounting and reporting standard.
    revised edition
12. Finnveden, G., et al.: Recent developments in life cycle assessment. J. Environ.
    Manage. **91**(1), 1–21 (2009)
13. Fritsch, A., von Hammerstein, J., Schreiber, C., Betz, S., Oberweis, A.: Pathways
    to greener pastures: research opportunities to integrate life cycle assessment and
    sustainable business process management based on a systematic tertiary literature
    review. Sustainability **14**(18) (2022)
14. Recker, J.: Scientific research in information systems: a beginner's guide, 2nd edn.
    Progress in IS. Springer, Cham (2021)
15. Tsai, W.H.: Activity-based costing model for joint products. Comput. Ind. Eng.
    31(3–4), 725–729 (1996)

16. Houy, C., Reiter, M., Fettke, P., Loos, P., Hoesch-Klohe, K., Ghose, A.: Advancing business process technology for humanity: opportunities and challenges of green bpm for sustainable business activities. In: vom Brocke, J., Seidel, S., Recker, J. (eds.) Green Business Process Management, pp. 75–92. Springer, Berlin Heidelberg (2012)
17. Hoesch-Klohe, K., Ghose, A., Le, L.-S.: Towards green business process management. In: 2010 IEEE International Conference on Services Computing, pp. 386–393 (2010)
18. Nowak, A., Leymann, F.: Green business process patterns – part ii (short paper). In: 2013 IEEE 6th International Conference on Service-Oriented Computing and Applications, pp. 168–173 (2013)
19. Ghose, A., Hoesch-Klohe, K., Hinsche, L., Le, L.S.: Green business process management: a research agenda. Aust. J. Inf. Syst. **16**(2) (2010)
20. Roohy Gohar, S., Indulska, M.: Business process management: saving the planet? (2015)
21. Gräuler, M., Teuteberg, F.: Experimental evaluation of a process benchmarking tool in a green business process management context. In: Wirtschaftsinformatik 2013 Proceedings, pp. 1083–1097 (2013)
22. Van Woensel, T., Creten, R., Vandaele, N.: Managing the environmental externalities of traffic logistics: the issue of emissions. Prod. Oper. Manag. **10**(2), 207–223 (2001)
23. Graves, N., Koren, I., van der Aalst, W.: Rethink your processes! a review of process mining for sustainability (postprint) (2023)
24. de Soete, W.: Towards a multidisciplinary approach on creating value: Sustainability through the supply chain and ERP systems. Systems **4**(1) (2016)

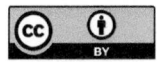

Author Index

A. Delgado and T. Slaats (Eds.): ICPM 2024 Workshops, LNBIP 533, pp. 779–781, 2025.
https://doi.org/10.1007/978-3-031-82225-4